Lord's
Health & Grace
Bill Kellas

SURVIVING THE TOXIC CRISIS

UNDERSTANDING, PREVENTING AND TREATING THE ROOT CAUSES OF CHRONIC ILLNESS

William Randall Kellas, Ph.D.
and
Andrea Sharon Dworkin, N.D.

Professional Preference
Olivenhain, CA

This book is not intended to replace the advice of your own doctor or to diagnose or prescribe, but rather to impart knowledge and understanding so you can make decisions that are right for you. You are ultimately responsible for your decisions and your own well-being. It is strongly suggested that you seek the advice of a practitioner or clinic that is in accord with these ideas.

Publisher's Cataloging in Publication
(Prepared by Quality Books Inc.)

Kellas, William Randall
    Surviving the toxic crisis : understanding, preventing and treating the root causes of chronic illness / William Randall Kellas and Andrea Sharon Dworkin.
    p. cm.
    Includes bibliographical references and index.
    ISBN 0-9636491-2-4

    1. Environmentally induced diseases. 2. Chemicals--Health aspects. 3. Toxicology. I. Dworkin, Andrea Sharon. II. Title

RB152.K455 1996   616.9'8
                           QB196-40537

Acknowledgments

This book and its companion volume *Thriving In A Toxic World* are a compilation of the knowledge, skills, clinical experience, and personal experience of the two authors. However, these books would not exist if it were not for the direct and indirect contributions of many others.

The chapters in both of these books cite about 1200 references. Each of these references is a book or article which itself is the product of the training and experience of one or more authors, and of the many reference sources they themselves used.

We would like to thank the doctors, dentists, and other practitioners at Comprehensive Health Centers for their input.

The artwork in this book is from several sources:

- Ed Silas Smith, who did many of the drawings.

- Nancy Henderson, who did many of the drawings in this book, especially in the Introduction chapter.

- The clipart files of CorelDraw 5, copyright Corel Corporation, 1994.

- Andrea S. Dworkin has done the design, book layout and computer graphics.

We are grateful to Oralee Archer, Ann Buller, and William Watt Lawrence, MS, for their editing and proofreading.

We can see so far because we stand on the shoulders of giants.

The pioneering work of many people has helped to make our work, and these books, what they are:

- Stephen Lawrence, DDS, who reviewed the Mercury and Nickel chapters.
- John Yiamouyiannis, PhD, who reviewed the Fluoride and AIDS chapters.
- Sherman Brees, MFC, who reviewed the Emotions Plus chapter.

• Dan Gole, DDS	• Devi Nambudripad, LAc
• Dave Kennedy, DDS	• John Davis, inventor
• David Olinger, DC	• Carl Mayer, PhD, JD
• Suzanne Fuselier, DC	• Hal Huggins, DDS
• Lowell Ward, DC	• Jim Kennedy, DDS
• Joe Smith, DDS	• Carol LaBate, DDS
• Joseph Lytle, DDS	• John Rothschild, DDS
• Jim Dobson, PhD	• Tim LeHay, PhD
• Alvin Dettloff, DC	• Jeffrey Bland, PhD
• Bill Timmins, ND	• Chris Katke
• Elias Illyia, PhD	

Last of all, we are grateful to those patients at Comprehensive Health Centers and elsewhere who have so much to teach those who will listen.

About the Authors

This book, several years in the making, is the melding of the skills, knowledge, and dedication of two gifted people. They both have scientific backgrounds consisting of five college degrees between them and considerable practical experience. This book and its companion volume *Thriving In A Toxic World* are their first books written together.

Both authors have personally triumphed over chronic illness using principles and methods described in these books.

William R. Kellas (Bill) has a Bachelor's degree in Business/Physics with a Premed minor and a Ph.D. in Nutritional Biochemistry. Over a decade ago he worked for IBM and became enormously successful in his field by looking for and working with the root causes of business problems as he now seeks out root causes of illness. However, his health was rapidly deteriorating. In the late 1970s he was diagnosed as having ankylosing spondylitis, a crippling autoimmune disease; his body was almost literally disintegrating. Although he appeared to be on a fast track to a wheelchair, he refused to accept the no-hope verdict offered by the medical establishment. He researched and tried progressive treatments, developed a deep understanding of how the body works, and over time has regained his health.

Bill's desire to use his knowledge to help others and his belief "To whom much is given, much is expected" led to his forming Comprehensive Health Center (CHC) in Encinitas, California. This clinic, which started in 1984 with two people, has grown to the point where it now employs about thirty people, including MDs, chiropractors, nutritionists, immunologists, naturopaths, and other progressive practitioners, and support staff. CHC also has proximity to a progressive dental center.

In addition to helping patients for the past ten years, he has written the *Toxic Immune Syndrome Cookbook*, has worked on this book and its companion volume for several years, hosts the syndicated radio program called *Health Talk: A Second Opinion* which originates in Southern California and is simulcast across the country, lectures throughout the country to both medical/dental and lay audiences, and is planning to coauthor other books on progressive health care with Andrea.

He lives in Olivenhain, California with his wife and three children.

Andrea Sharon Dworkin has a Doctorate in Naturopathic Medicine (N.D.). She also has Bachelor's and Master's degrees in Chemistry, which gives her a strong background in Toxicology and an understanding of how chemical toxins and nutrients affect the body. She is currently working on her Ph.D. in Nutrition, which she should complete in 1997.

Like Bill Kellas, Andrea has overcome personal health challenges. Years of working in chemistry laboratories in both school and work environments took their toll. The combination of chemical exposure and demanding schedule left her with debilitating chronic fatigue and life-threatening multiple chemical sensitivities. After about 18 months of treatment and healing with Dr. Bill Kellas and the CHC team, Andrea regained her health. She is strongly motivated to use her skills and knowledge to help others as she has been helped. She currently works as a practitioner and writer at Comprehensive Health Center.

This book and its companion volume are her first books. Other books in the progressive health care field and other fields are in the planning stages.

Andrea lives in Oceanside, California. In addition to consulting with patients, writing books, and studying nutrition and natural healing methods, she is an artist in various media.

Preface

Do they say you're not sick but you know you're not well?

Do you want to maintain your health to the greatest extent possible? The key is your body's environment.

Two controllable things must be considered in recovering and maintaining one's health:

- **Suppressors** - Those things that can interfere with health, such as toxins and structural misalignments, must be identified and removed from the environment and the body. These include the primary toxic suppressors such as chemicals and the secondary suppressors such as microorganisms which move in when the body is weakened by the primary suppressors.

- **Supporters** - Those things such as nutrients and necessities like air, water and sleep which support the body must be provided.

Surviving The Toxic Crisis focuses on the suppressors: how they can be identified, avoided, and removed from the body as the first necessary step to attaining or maintaining health.

Thriving In A Toxic World focuses on the supporters. The book also discusses how the body works, the mental/emotional/spiritual connection, and specific topics such as cancer, evaluating the validity of a scientific study, and complications from medical treatment.

The books *Surviving The Toxic Crisis* and *Thriving In A Toxic World* were originally written as one book, but the sheer volume of information necessitated the splitting into two books. These two books can each stand alone but work best together to provide the full picture. They are a compilation of what has proven successful in preventing and treating chronic illness and supporting the body's optimal function in a clinic that integrates medical, dental, chiropractic, nutrients, herbs, and other modalities.

These are possibly the only two books you'll need to survive the 21st century.

SURVIVING THE TOXIC CRISIS

Table of Contents

Secondary Toxic Suppressors - Microorganisms

Introduction
and
Overview

What Goes Around Comes Around

What kinds of illness are there?
Acute illness is defined as that which has lasted for less than 120 days, as the average cell lives that long. If it lasts for more than 120 days, then the illness is being passed from cell to cell. Other body systems start to get involved and the symptoms can be considered chronic. If untreated, a chronic illness may become long-term.

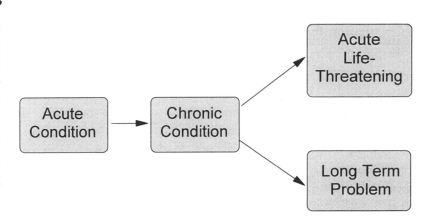

In some cases a chronic condition such as arteriosclerosis (hardening and blockage of the arteries) can lead to a condition which appears to be acute - a heart attack. Unfortunately, for some people the early warning sign of a heart attack is sudden death. But was it really the first sign?

Why are acute care specialists not appropriate for chronic illness?
Chronic illness affects the whole body, while acute care specialists focus on the heart, nervous system, joints, or another particular part of the body. These specialists are like racquetball players waiting for the ball to bounce off the ceiling and walls until it finally comes to their section of the court before they can or will act. In other words, they wait until the patient's symptoms match their area of expertise before they can treat, or refer you to another specialist. Specialists look at "what" without asking why, while the comprehensive practitioners look at "why".

If all you have is a hammer, everything looks like a nail. Restated, if you are, for example, a cardiologist, every chest pain looks suspiciously like a heart problem.

How is the whole body involved?
The circular chart that follows graphically shows how the different systems of the body are affected by what is going on elsewhere in the body. Many vicious cycles can be set up by untreated or improperly treated symptoms, leading to problems in other body systems which can then worsen what was going on originally.

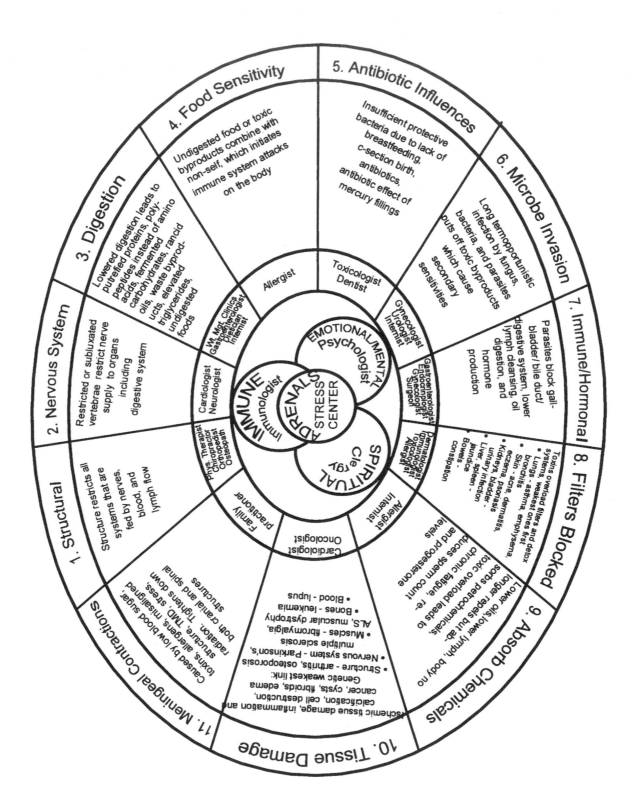

4. Food Sensitivity

Undigested food or toxic byproducts combine with non-self, which initiates immune system attacks on the body

5. Antibiotic Influences

Insufficient protective bacteria due to lack of breastfeeding, c-section birth, antibiotics, antibiotic effect of mercury fillings

3. Digestion

Lowered digestion leads to putrefied proteins, poly-peptides instead of amino acids, fermented carbohydrates, rancid oils, waste byproducts, elevated triglycerides, undigested foods

6. Microbe Invasion

Long termopportunistic infection by fungus, bacteria, and parasites puts off toxic byproducts which cause secondary sensitivities

2. Nervous System

Restricted or subluxated vertebrae restrict nerve supply to organs including digestive system

7. Immune/Hormonal

Parasites block gall-bladder/ bile duct/ digestive system, lower lymph cleansing, oil digestion, and hormone production

1. Structural

Structure restricts all systems that are fed by nerves, blood, and lymph flow

8. Filters Blocked

• Toxins overload filters and detox systems, weakest ones first
• Lungs - asthma, emphysema, bronchitis
• Skin - acne, dermatitis, eczema, psoriasis
• Kidneys, urinary infection
• Liver, bladder - jaundice
• Bowels, spleen - constipation

11. Meningeal Contractions

Caused by low blood sugar, toxins, allergens, TMD, stress, structure, radiation. Tightens down both cranial and spinal structures.

9. Absorb Chemicals

Lower oils lower lymph, body no longer repels but ab-sorbs petrochemicals, toxic overload leads to chronic fatigue, re-duces sperm count and progesterone levels

10. Tissue Damage

• Blood - lupus
• Bones - leukemia
• Muscles - fibromyalgia, ALS, muscular dystrophy
• Nervous system - Parkinson's, multiple sclerosis
• Structure - arthitis, osteoporosis
• Genetic weakest link: cancer, cysts, fibroids, edema calcification, cell destruction, Ischemic tissue damage, inflammation and

Allergist

Wt. Mgt. Clinics Gastroenterologist Dietician Internist

Cardiologist Neurologist

Phys. Therapist Chiropractor Orthopedist Osteopath

Family Practitioner

Cardiologist Oncologist

Toxicologist Dentist

Gynecologist Urologist Internist

Gastroenterologist Endocrinologist Gynecologist Surgeon

Dermatologist Immunologist Toxicologist Allergist

Allergist Internist

EMOTIONAL/MENTAL Psychologist

IMMUNE Immunologist

ADRENALS STRESS CENTER

SPIRITUAL Clergy

An acute illness affects a single part of the circle, and may involve most or all systems if it is un-treated and becomes chronic. For example, a whiplash injury which puts the neck out of alignment can, if untreated, become chronic, with headaches starting in about a month and the rest of the body being involved after about 120 days.

How is this circular chart read?
This chart can be read by starting anywhere and working around it clockwise. It may or may not be necessary to treat everything on this chart to achieve wellness. However, stopping treatment before all affected systems are brought back to health may result in the continuation of problems past that point in the chart as you cycle clockwise.

The body can correct itself at any point in the chart with or without treatment if the problem is acute, and even sometimes if it is chronic. But if a chronic problem is treated at only one point the patient can feel better for a while, and then go around the chart and start having symptoms again.

For example, if a spinal misalignment which has become a chronic problem is treated by itself, you will probably feel better for a few hours or days. But the other uncorrected problems originally caused by the misalignment can lead to toxic or allergic meningeal contractions, which can pull the spine out of alignment again. The pain or discomfort will then be felt. The best chiropractor in the world will probably not be able to bring about lasting healing if the related problems are not also treated.

The most common entry points to the chart are Structural and Antibiotic Influences (Low Beneficial Bacteria), although low beneficial bacteria is a condition which itself has a cause. The other points on the circle are usually not primary entry points, but rather are secondary to the initial problem.

> **Structural problems are one of the most common entry points to poor health.**

To show how problems can be interrelated, let's review the chart, starting at the top:

1. **Structure**: A problem with the structure or alignment of the spine can pinch the nerves leading to organs, including the digestive system, and other body structures. Such a structural disturbance can be the result of whiplash, concussion (primary), or can be secondary to other things that are going on in the body, discussed as we continue around the circle. If organs are affected, treatment in addition to structural adjustment may also be necessary. For this reason, any structural specialty including chiropractic and osteopathic care, although needed, may fail to give lasting relief.

2. **Nervous system**: Pinched nerves can affect organs. For example, cardiologists know that pain radiating down the left arm can be a warning of an impending heart attack. What is the connection? A subluxation, or misalignment, at the vertebrae T1 and C6 or C7 can pinch the nerve that feeds the heart and is also connected to the left arm. Nerve transmission or blood flow to the heart is impeded, leading to heart problems down the line.

3. **Digestion**: The subluxation lowers nerve and fluid flow to the digestive system, which can result in poor digestion, putrefied proteins and fermented carbohydrates in the gut, and higher triglycerides and low hormone levels from poor oil digestion. This sets up

conditions for food sensitivities to develop from poor digestion of food. A person thus affected may be too thin from malabsorption of nutrients or be puffy and overweight from accumulating water and/or fat to dilute toxins.

4. **Allergy**: Food which is not properly digested can lead to allergy-like reactions called food sensitivities by allergists. Improperly digested food is considered to be non-self, and is thus attacked by the immune system. This is sometimes called the leaky gut syndrome. The body is then in a constant state of readiness to fight the allergens, called sympathetic dominance, or the fight-or-flight reaction. The parasympathetic part of the nervous system, which works when the sympathetic part is not activated, is responsible for digesting food and repairing and restoring body tissues. If the sympathetic part is constantly "on", digestion, healing and restoration will not take place to the extent necessary for optimal functioning. In addition, the environment is not supportive for protective bacteria.

5. **Antibiotic influences / Low bacteria**: What you eat and chew your food with - specifically teeth filled with mercury fillings or nickel from stainless steel root canal posts or braces - can cause the leaching of these toxic metals into the body. These metals set up toxic allergies and act as an antibiotic which can kill healthy bacteria. Other causes of deficient beneficial bacteria are antibiotic use, Cesarean section birth and lack of breastfeeding. Poor digestion, which may be from deficient protective bacteria, can lead to milk allergy, which leads to ear infection, which is treated with antibiotics. This in turn then depletes the protective bacteria still more and worsens digestion in a vicious cycle. Taking acidophilus, which are protective bacteria, can help your body until the next time you eat and chew your food with mercury-filled teeth. This releases more mercury to be absorbed into the body.

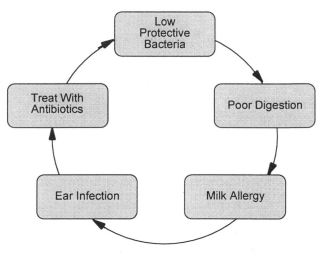

6. **Microbes**: Pathogenic (bad) bacteria and parasites gain a foothold in your body because of a deficiency of protective bacteria and because your body is in fight-or-flight mode from fighting allergens. These pathogenic bacteria live off undigested food and put out toxic waste byproducts. These byproducts can set up secondary allergies. Acetaldehyde, which can be poisonous and allergenic, is a byproduct of fungus growth and dieoff.

7. **Hormone balance**: Parasites such as helicobacter and fungus block the gallbladder and bile duct, and lower digestive enzymes because the bile duct carrying these enzymes is blocked. Carbohydrates and proteins may not be digested properly if the enzymes are deficient, leading to allergy as previously discussed. With a blocked gallbladder, good oils are not processed. Without enough good oils, hormone production is affected.

Lymph cleansing of the body is compromised and hormone levels are lowered because of poor oil digestion. Hormones called eicosanoids, or prostaglandins, regulate and balance many of the body's systems. An imbalance of eicosanoids in addition to sympathetic dominance (fight-or-flight) can weaken and burn out the adrenal glands. This leads to fatigue, as the adrenal glands put out adrenaline, the energy hormone.

8. **Filters blocked**: Oil deficiency sets up conditions for the body to absorb...

9. **Chemicals absorbed** ...toxic petrochemicals, which then overload the body's detoxification systems - skin, lungs, bowels, lymph, liver, kidneys. These are a few examples that can be seen:
    - *Skin* - *rashes, acne, psoriasis*
    - *Lymph* - *swollen lymph glands*
    - *Lungs* - *asthma, bronchitis*
    - *Digestive system* - *colitis, ileitis*
    - *Altered blood pressure*
    - *Constipation or diarrhea if the liver or kidneys are affected*

10. **Inflammatory tissue**: Inflammatory (ischemic or diseased) tissue develops because increased toxins from overloaded detox pathways and lowered nutrients from poor digestion lead to cell damage. Cysts and fibroids and ultimately cancer can result, as well as fibromyalgia (tissue pain) and edema (swelling) from water retention to dilute toxins. Inflammation can lead to calcification, which in turn becomes plaque on the arteries.

11. **Meningeal contraction**: Many stresses, including allergens, toxins, structural problems, and radiation cause tightening of the meningeal system surrounding the brain and spinal cord. This tightening can then cause or worsen structural problems by pulling vertebrae out of alignment, and so we have come full circle.

What systems will be affected?

The system or systems affected depend on the individual's genetically weakest link, although some toxins target certain organs or systems. Some people are most susceptible to heart and cardiovascular problems, some to joint and bone problems, and some to skin problems. Diseases which can result include:

- *Structure - arthritis, osteoporosis*
- *Bones - leukemia*
- *Blood - lupus*
- *Nervous system - multiple sclerosis (MS)*
- *Muscles - muscular dystrophy, ALS (amyotrophic lateral sclerosis, or Lou Gehrig's disease)*

How does the immune system fit in?

There are many components to the immune system, and these can be roughly correlated to the different body systems mentioned. The immune system is so all-pervasive in the cycles discussed in the chart that the name Toxic Immune Syndrome has been given to these processes.

If the nervous system is involved, immune system components called T-lymphocytes lose some of their ability to function. Digestive problems increase activity of IgA (mucosal lining defense), which leads to an overactive immune response, better known as an allergic reaction. When filters are blocked and chemicals get in, immune function as a whole is lowered.

Just as the problems listed on this chart can reduce effective immune system function, reduced immune function can lead to many of the problems and symptoms on the chart, such as cancer, allergies, arthritis, hormone imbalance, etc.

Mental or spiritual stress, in the center of the chart, can also suppress the immune system. The problems in the chart can result from this stress without attack from an outside source such as whiplash or antibiotics.

What if some of this doesn't make sense?
Many terms in this introduction may be unfamiliar to you. The information presented here is intended as an overview, and is discussed throughout the book in detail.

How this book is set up
This book is divided into six sections which explore the major suppressors and help you to further understand how chronic problems involve the entire body and the approaches and resolution necessary to help you survive in a toxic world.

Basic chemical concepts
Some basic chemical concepts are useful to understand material in the rest of the book. These concepts are presented in a way that assumes no prior chemical knowledge on the part of the reader, and in a way that is interesting and relevant.

Primary Toxic Suppressors
Nearly all of us have accumulated insults to our bodies over the years, as described in this introduction and throughout the book.

- *Antibiotics*
- *Electromagnetic radiation*
- *Pesticides*
- *Structural problems*
- *Emotional and spiritual stress*
- *Drugs*
- *Organs removed*
- *Chemicals and solvents*
- *Air and water pollution*
- *Metals*

All of these are considered to be primary toxic suppressors. They disturb immune function, which in turn sends us around the circle described earlier in this chapter until all of our organ systems may be affected.

Discussion of the primary toxic suppressors, their attendant symptoms, and solutions to the problems they cause form the major part of this book. They are presented in four sections: Chemicals, Metals, Electromagnetic Radiation, and Structural Problems.

Secondary Toxic Suppressors

Once the primary toxic suppressors take hold, conditions are set up for the colonization of your body by secondary toxic suppressors. These are considered to be secondary not because they are less important but because they move in after the primary damage has been done. They are like squatters who move into a rundown abandoned building, or looters who take over after the over-whelmed police (the immune system) leave the city to the rioters.

The secondary toxic suppressors are the parasites, including yeast and fungi, amoebas and proto-zoa, bacteria, viruses, and worms. Many of these exist together and feed off of each other. Once in your body they can invade and block organs such as the gallbladder, interfering with oil ab-sorption (in the case of the gallbladder) and paving the way for more chemical poisoning. They take nutrients intended for your body, so you can be in a state of nutrient deficiency in spite of an adequate dietary intake. They putrefy and ferment your food, and their life cycle processes and death put out toxic byproducts which keep you in a state of unwellness.

There are **References and Resources** listed at the end of most chapters for further information on the subject of the chapter (Numbered references within the chapter are found at the end of the book). A glossary, a list of abbreviations used in the book, and a list of sources for many of the supportive products named are also provided.

> **This book is not intended to replace the advice of your own doctor or to diagnose or prescribe, but rather to impart knowledge and understanding so you can make decisions that are right for you. You are ultimately responsible for your decisions and your own well-being.**

For a better understanding of much that has been covered in this introduction, it is suggested that you reread it after you have read the book and you will have a much greater understanding of how the pieces fall into place. The important point is the way in which the different systems of the body are interlinked. For lasting healing, chronic problems should be treated by involving the entire body, even if symptoms appear to be localized.

A paradigm shift

The comprehensive integrated approach is not just replacing drugs with herbs, but rather a re-thinking of the entire process and integrating the best of both as well as other therapies in a co-hesive plan based on setting priorities and beginning with the root cause.

You are probably being introduced to a new way of looking at things, a new way to approach your health which carries with it the possibility of a level of health and well-being that is within the realm of possibilities for your future. You may have felt so bad for so long, you've forgotten what it feels like to be healthy and filled with vitality. Let the possiblity sink into your mind for just a moment, and remember a time when you actually experienced that kind of existence. It's possible once again.

> **"The mind once expanded to the dimensions of a larger idea never returns to its original size."**
>
> - Oliver Wendell Holmes

Prepare to have your horizons expanded.

In finding solutions to chronic health problems it is important to get to the root causes. What are the primary and secondary suppressors that have set you up for chronic, long-term health problems that you have not been able to shake, and have caused you to almost give up hope that life can be good again? Well, take hope! As we take an in-depth look at these suppressors and how they have undermined your health, we will also find solutions that provide new ways of looking at what it means to achieve optimum health.

References and Resources

- The Burton Goldberg Group, *Alternative Medicine: The Definitive Guide*, Future Medicine Publishing Inc., Puyallup WA, 1994.

  *This excellent guide to alternative / progressive medicine is highly recommended for further understanding of the issues in this book. In addition, books, journals, and organizations pertinent to each chapter are found at the end of each chapter. Specific sections of **Alternative Medicine** will be referenced where applicable at the end of chapters in this book.*

- *Townsend Letter for Doctors is a monthly journal with many articles pertaining to issues raised in this book. Although the journal is geared towards progressive doctors and practitioners, much of the information would be understandable to the layperson.*

- Airola, Paavo, *How To Get Well*, Health Plus Publishers, Phoenix AZ, 1974.

- **American College of Advancement in Medicine**, P.O. Box 3427, Laguna Hills CA 92654. Phone 714-583-7666. *Provides worldwide listing of practitioners trained in nutritional and preventive medicine.*

- Austin, P., *Natural Remedies: A Manual*, Yuchi Pines Institute, Seale AL, 1983.

- Beasley, Joseph, *The Betrayal of Health*, Times Books, NY, 1991. *The effect of lifestyle and nutrition choices on health.*

- *Better Health Through Natural Healing: How To Get Well Without Drugs or Surgery*, McGraw-Hill, NY, 1985.

- Chopra, Deepak, *Quantum Healing: Exploring the Frontiers of Mind/Body Medicine*, Bantam Books, NY, 1989.

- Dirchfeld, Friedhelm and Wade Boyle, *Nature Doctors: Pioneers in Naturopathic Medicine*, Medicina Biologica, Portland OR, 1994.

- Goodheart, RS and MD Shils, *Health and Disease*, Lea and Febinger, Philadelphia PA, 1980.

- Heimlich, J., *What Your Doctors Won't Tell You*, Harper Perennial, NY, 1990.

- Hirschberg, Caryle and Marc Ian Barasch, *Remarkable Recovery*, G.P.Putman's Sons, NY, 1995. *Looks at survivors of cancer and other illnesses who were given a death sentence by their doctors. Discusses the many types of treatment, primarily "alternative", that the survivors credited with their recovery.*

- Moyers, Bill, *Healing and the Mind*, Doubleday, NY, 1993.

- Page, Melvin, *Degeneration and Regeneration*, St. Petersburg Beach, FL, 1949.

- Payer, Lynn, *Medicine and Culture: Varieties of Treatments in the United States, England, West Germany and France*, Henry Holt and Co., NY, 1988.

- Pizzorno, Joseph E. and Michael T. Murray, *A Textbook of Natural Medicine*, John Bastyr College Publications, Seattle WA, 1989.

- Pizzorno, Joseph E. and Michael T. Murray, *Encyclopedia of Natural Medicine*, Prima Publishing, Rocklin CA, 1991.

- Shannon, Sara, *Good Health In A Toxic World: The Complete Guide to Fighting Free Radicals*, Warner Books Inc., NY, 1994. *Fighting free radical damage. Has over 150 pages of resources and references.*

- Shreeve, Caroline M., *The Alternative Dictionary of Symptoms and Cures*, Century Hutchinson Publishing, London England, 1986.

- Simonton, O. Carl and S. Matthews, *Getting Well Again*, Jeremy P. Tarcher, Los Angeles CA, 1978.

- Sinclair, Brett Jason, *Alternative Health Care Resources*, Parker Publishing Co., West Nyack NY, 1992. *A directory of self-help groups, professional care providers, scientific journals, lay magazines and newsletters, and institutes / foundations. These are listed by subject heading.*

- Thomas, John, *Young Again!*, Plexus Press, Kelso WA, 1995. *Techniques and information to maintain youthfulness, including detoxification procedures, colon cleansing and nutrition.*

- Weil, Andrew, *Natural Health, Natural Medicine: A Comprehensive Manual for Wellness and Self-Care*, Houghton Mifflin, Boston MA, 1990.

- Wigmore, Ann, *Be Your Own Doctor: A Positive Guide to Natural Living*, Avery Publishing Co., Garden City Park NY, 1983.

BASIC CHEMICAL CONCEPTS

Your Body: The Ultimate Laboratory

Ten reasons to read this chapter:

1. It important to understand basic chemistry so you can fully understand what is going on in your body.

2. What are electrons and why are they so significant? (Hint: They are the root of the words electrolyte and electricity)

3. Why are there chemical groups anyway?

4. How does the charge on an atom determine how it reacts in the body?

5. How are metals, minerals, and electrolytes different?

6. Is a salt something more than what you sprinkle on food?

7. Now you can understand how mercury from your amalgam fillings can adversely affect your body.

8. What is the difference between a molecule, compound, and mixture?

9. Is organic more that just a health food term?

10. Is halogen more than just a type of light, and why are halogens toxic?

Why is it important to understand basic chemistry?

It is necessary to have an understanding of basic chemical concepts in order to make sense of some of the discussions in this book. Even if you don't understand the relevance of some of these concepts now, their importance will become clearer as the terms are discussed elsewhere in this book.

What are some of the terms you should know?

Terms such as these and their applications are discussed throughout this chapter:

- *Atom*
- *Metal*
- *Valence*
- *Acid*
- *Element*
- *Salt*
- *Electron*
- *pH*
- *Compound*
- *Organic*
- *Ion*
- *Molecule*
- *Mixture*
- *Inorganic*
- *Oxidant*
- *Isotope*

Why is the Periodic Table so important?

The Periodic Table of the Elements is probably familiar to those who have taken at least high school chemistry. If not, don't worry; the table and its relevance will be explained. The periodic table is only a simplified model of chemical relationships.

Understanding the components (elements), the ways they combine, and the relationships between them are the basis for understanding toxicology, or the reasons why some substances are poisonous.

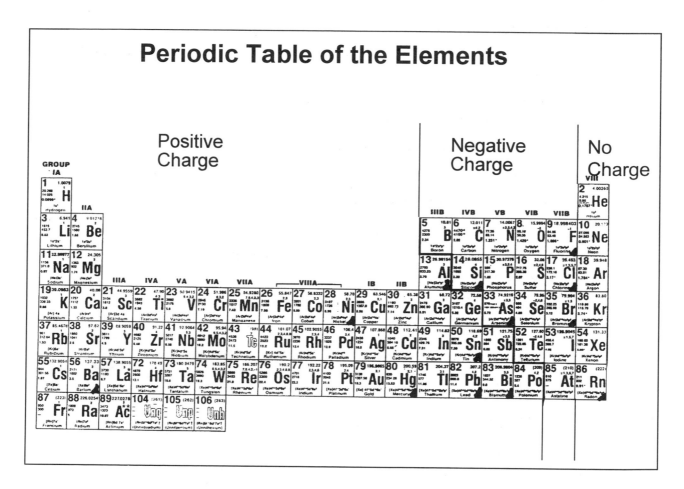

What are all the letters and numbers in the Periodic Table?

The chemical **elements**, each represented by one or two letters, are arranged so the atomic number, or atomic weight, gets progressively larger and heavier as one goes from left to right and from top to bottom on the table. In addition, these elements are arranged in groups (labeled IIA, IVB, etc. and defined later in the chapter) which form up-and-down columns. Each element has different properties - they look different, react differently, melt at different temperatures, and have different functions or toxic effects in the body.

An **atom** is a single unit of an element. Take, for example, the element carbon. One can have a carbon atom or a large number of carbon atoms which can form a charcoal briquette or a diamond depending on the arrangement of the atoms.

All atoms have three components according to current theory:

- *Protons*   *(positive charge)*
- *Neutrons*   *(no charge)*
- *Electrons* *(negative charge)*

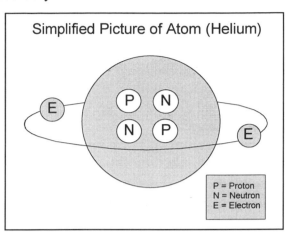

Simplified Picture of Atom (Helium)

P = Proton
N = Neutron
E = Electron

Protons are in the nucleus (center) of an atom. Each element in sequence has one more proton than the one before, and the number of protons determines which element it is. The **atomic number** is the number of protons in an atom of that element, and is shown in the upper left-hand corner of each element's box in the periodic table. For example, iron always has 26 protons; an element with other than 26 protons would not be iron. Protons have a positive charge. **Neutrons** are also in the nucleus, and the number of protons plus the number of neutrons equals the **atomic weight**, shown in the upper right-hand corner of each element box. Neutrons have no electrical charge.

Why are all of the atomic weights fractional numbers?

The atomic weight of any individual atom is a whole number, such as 12 or 35. However, a look at the periodic table shows atomic weights that are fractional, such as 35.453 for chlorine. Although most atoms, especially at the lower atomic weights, have a number of neutrons equal to the number of protons, some atoms of a particular element have a few more or less neutrons than this (usually more), and this changes their atomic weight. Atoms with such variations in numbers of neutrons are called **isotopes**. The fractional atomic weight given in the periodic table is calculated from the weights of the different isotopes and their relative abundance. Isotopes of an element often have slightly different properties, and those with relatively more neutrons tend to be less stable and even in some cases radioactive.

What are electrons, and how do they fit in?

Electrons surround the nucleus. Tiny compared to protons and neutrons, like the moon compared to the sun, they are so nearly weightless that they do not contribute to the atomic weight. Their purpose is to balance out the electrical charge of the atom.

Electron Rings

Nu = Nucleus (Positive Charge)
e = Electron (Negative Charge)

Although such a representation is not strictly accurate, for purposes of simplification it can be said that electrons are in concentric rings around the nucleus like planets around the sun. An optimal number of electrons fit into each ring: two in the first ring, eight each in the second and third rings, eighteen each in the fourth and fifth rings, and so on. The number of rings is determined by the number of electrons in the atom, which is in turn determined by the number of protons in the nucleus.

Electrons have a negative charge which cancels out the positive charge of the proton on a one-to-one basis. For example, carbon has an atomic number of six and an atomic weight of twelve. As an atom it is electrically neutral. This means that it has six protons (P), six neutrons (N); 6P + 6N = 12 = atomic weight. Six electrons (E) balance the six protons. The number of electrons in an atom is therefore equal to the atomic number. Test yourself: look at any element in the periodic table and its atomic weight and number, and figure out the number of protons, neutrons (average), and electrons.

Why are electrons so significant?

Electrons are especially important since the number of electrons in an atom relative to the number it would take to make a complete outer shell around the atom has a lot to do with the kinds of chemical reactions the atom enters into. Shells other than the outer shell (inside shells) are always complete and can be ignored for our purposes.

All element atoms want to have a full outer shell of electrons so they feel balanced. If they have too few or too many electrons to make a full outer shell, the atom will want to combine with other atoms so that each will have a complete outer shell. An atom with two extra electrons will combine most readily with an atom having two missing electrons, or with two atoms missing an electron each.

The passage of electrons down a wire is called electricity, a word with the same root as the word electron. Electricity and electromagnetic radiationhave adverse effects on the electrons and charged particles in our bodies.

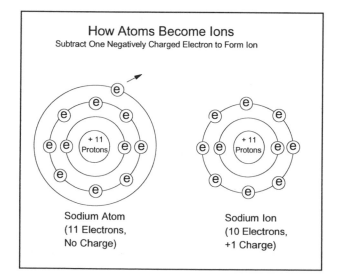

How Atoms Become Ions
Subtract One Negatively Charged Electron to Form Ion

Sodium Atom
(11 Electrons,
No Charge)

Sodium Ion
(10 Electrons,
+1 Charge)

What if atoms already have a complete outer shell of electrons?

The elements in the far right-hand column are called noble gases. They have complete outer shells, as determined by the numbers (2, 8, 8, 18...) given above. Helium (He), atomic number two, has two electrons, or a complete shell. Neon (Ne) has ten electrons, or 2 + 8, giving it a complete outer shell. The noble gases, for this reason, are stable just as they are and almost never react, since reactions have to do with electron exchange.

What is involved in electron exchange?

Much of chemistry, including the chemical reactions that go on inside your body and affect your health, have to do with electron exchange or bonded sharing. Let's look at some examples. Sodium has 11 protons and 11 electrons (atomic number 11). It wants to have a complete outer shell, which would make a total of ten electrons (two in the first shell, eight in the second). An atom which sacrifices electrical neutrality for a complete outer shell by either adding or subtracting electrons is called an **ion**.

Once sodium loses its extra electron it has a charge of +1 (11 pluses and 10 minuses = +1), and becomes a sodium ion. Chlorine has an atomic number of 17, with 17 each of protons and electrons. The electrons are arranged in rings of 2, 8, and 7 electrons for a total of 17. It wants 8 electrons in the outer shell, not 7, and so picks up an extra electron for a net charge of -1. Sodium (+1) combines with chlorine (-1) to make sodium chloride, which is electrically neutral (-1 + 1 = 0). A chemist would write this as:

$$Na^{+1} + Cl^- \rightarrow NaCl$$

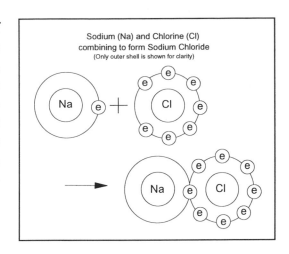

Sodium (Na) and Chlorine (Cl) combining to form Sodium Chloride
(Only outer shell is shown for clarity)

Why are there chemical groups anyway?

The chemical groups are the up-and-down columns in the periodic table, identified by Roman numerals and letters. Ions of group II elements have a +2 charge, an ion of a group III element such as aluminum has a +3 charge, and so on. As discussed previously, the charge is a reflection of the number of electrons, which in turn determines the reactions of the element. In the picture of the periodic table, groups are listed as IIA, IVB, and so on. The As and Bs can even be reversed in other versions of the periodic table, and have no significance for our purposes.

Some ions can have more than one charge, for reasons too complex to go into here. Mercury, for example, can exist as mercuric ion Hg^{+2} or mercurous ion Hg^+. Iron can be ferrous ion Fe^{+2} or ferric ion Fe^{+3}. If an element can have either of two different charges, the one with the higher charge ends in -ic and the lower ends in -ous. You may have encountered the word "ferrous" on a bottle of mineral supplements. The ferrous form of iron is more bioavailable (usable by the body) than the ferric form, since ions with a +2 charge are more natural to the body than those with a +3 charge.

The elements in each group have the same number of electrons too many or too few in their outer shell, so they will bind to cells or to other chemicals in a similar fashion. Their chemical action, however, is different. Examples such as the substitution of toxic mercury (Hg^{+2}) for necessary zinc (Zn^{+2}) are discussed later in this chapter.

What else should you know about charges?

The ionic forms of an element are said to have a **valence** of -1, -2, +1, +2, or +3. The valence is the same thing as electrical charge or electrical potential. In other books, the charge may be written differently: for example +2 can also be written as 2+ or ++, as in Ca^{+2}, Ca^{2+}, or Ca^{++}. In this book the +2 form is used for consistency. A -1 charge may simply be written as - (minus sign); this convention is used in this book, as in Cl^-. Similarly, a +1 charge is more simply written as + (plus sign), for example Na^+.

An electrically charged atom is an ion, but a group of atoms with an electrical charge is also an ion, or ionic group. For example, the ammonium group is NH_4^+, the phosphate group is PO_4^{-3}, the carbonate group is CO_3^{-2}, and the hydroxyl group is OH^-.

How are metals, minerals, and electrolytes different?

To a chemist, a **metal** is any element in the left-hand two-thirds of the periodic table, classified as such based on their positive charges and thus on the way these elements combine with other materials. Nearly any element with a plus charge (left side of table) can combine with nearly any element with a minus charge (right side of table).

The non-chemist, however, usually thinks of metals as the dozen or so shiny materials which could possibly be used to make a frying pan. A nutritionist might separate minerals from metals, defining a **mineral** as a metallic element which, in ionic (charged, or unbalanced) form, is necessary for bodily function. However, since minerals act as toxic metals in quantities significantly higher than what the body needs, a combination of these definitions will be used.

An **electrolyte** is a mineral necessary to the body, and the terms mineral and electrolyte are often used interchangeably. Both the electrolyte's identity (sodium, potassium) and its charge (-1, +2) are important. An electrolyte conducts electricity, as in a car battery where the sulfuric acid and water act as the electrolyte. In the body, it is very important to balance electrical charges, as these drive the nerves, muscles, and heart. If you go into shock or have a surgical operation, medical personnel may speak of the need for giving or balancing electrolytes.

Is a salt something you sprinkle on food?

Most people think of salt as table salt, or sodium chloride, but sodium chloride is only one of many salts. A **salt** is a combination of any positively charged ion (usually a metal) except hydrogen with any negatively charged ion (nearly always a nonmetal) other than hydroxyl (OH-). Salts are water soluble to a greater or lesser degree, and since the body is mostly water a salt form would be more **bioavailable**, or usable by the body.

How does all of this affect your body?

The lower the molecular weight, the more likely the element is to be found in the body. In their ionic form, such as Na^+ (sodium), K^+ (potassium), Ca^{+2} (calcium), and Cl^- (chloride), these elements are vital to the body and are least likely to be toxic. The higher the molecular weight, in general, the higher the toxicity. The lower molecular weight ions are usually minerals / electrolytes, and the higher weight ions, at least in the left-hand two thirds of the periodic table, are usually metals, thus the term heavy metals.

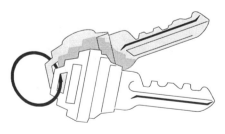

In replacement reactions, discussed in greater detail in the chapter on Chemical Toxicity, one ion can substitute for another of the same electrical charge, although the different ions have different effects. To say that one +2 ion can substitute for another is like saying that any key with two notches will fit into a particular lock but only the right one will open the door; the others will only plug up the lock.

What are some examples of replacement reactions in the body, and how can they kill you or make you sick?

The larger, more toxic ions will usually win if there is a competition for binding sites, like a 200 pound bully (mercury) picking on a 65 pound person (zinc). Within a group, for example group IIB, there is zinc (Zn), cadmium (Cd), and mercury (Hg), in order of increasing atomic weight.

IIB
30   65.38
Zn
Zinc
48   112.41
Cd
Cadmium
80   200.59
Hg
Mercury

Zinc in its ionic form, Zn^{+2}, is necessary for proper body function, and a deficiency of zinc can cause loss of smell and taste and immune function, among other things. Cadmium is toxic, and mercury even more so. Since cadmium and mercury in their more soluble ionized or salt forms Cd^{+2} and Hg^{+2} will attempt to participate in the same biochemical reactions as zinc, their presence will prevent some of the zinc from reacting. Although iron (Fe) is in a different group, it also has a +2 charge, and cadmium and mercury will also interfere with the action of oxygen-carrying iron, causing anemia and other disorders.

Similarly, sodium (Na) and potassium (K), both in group IA and both necessary in ionized form (Na^+ and K^+) for a number of bodily functions, must be in balance or one will try to take over the functions of the other. The sodium-potassium pump involves Na^+ on the outside of the cell and K^+ on the inside changing places to cause muscle contraction. This pump can be adversely affected by certain chemical reactions, so the proper exchange doesn't take place, causing weakness and other symptoms.

What is the difference between a molecule, a compound, and a mixture?

A **molecule** is an entity which can stand alone without immediately reacting and is electrically neutral. Molecules can be either single atoms or combinations such as sodium chloride. Elements in group VII, such as chlorine, exist in molecular form as groups of two, so molecular chlorine or iodine always exists as Cl_2 or I_2.

Molecular, or free, metals are those which have no ionic charge and generally have the characteristics one associates with metals, such as a characteristic metallic appearance, taste, and sound when struck. The **ionic** form of a metal is one in which there is an associated charge, or valence, usually +1, +2, or +3. A metal in the ionic form can combine with other elements or chemical groups with negative charges to form compounds. A **compound** results when two or more elements or groups combine to make a new material different from the molecular elements that formed them, just as two people marry to form a family that can be two people or several. A **mixture**, on the other hand, is a combination of two or more things whose characteristics do not change.

This can be confusing. Need some examples?

Some examples should help in understanding the difference between molecules, compounds, and mixtures. Molecular iron (Fe) looks and tastes typically metallic and can be picked up with a magnet. Iron in ionic form (Fe^{+2} or Fe^{+3}) can combine with other chemical entities to form a number of compounds, none of which look metallic or react to a magnet, as, for example, the iron pills on your vitamin shelf.

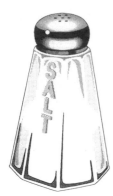

Another example is sodium chloride, or common table salt. Molecular sodium (Na) reacts violently with air and water, burns the skin, and is very toxic. Chlorine (Cl, found as Cl_2) is a poisonous greenish gas. Sodium chloride (NaCl), which is formed from these two elements, is a compound which is necessary for life and does not resemble either sodium or chlorine in any way. However, if you were to mix together sugar and salt, you would have a bowl full of something that still tasted and looked like sugar and salt, even if dissolved in water. This, then, would be a mixture.

Why are these distinctions important to you?

Metals may enter the body in either molecular (Hg) or ionic (Hg^{+2}) form, but the damage they cause is due to their chemically combining into compounds in the body. As discussed in greater detail in the section on replacement reactions in the next chapter on Chemical Toxicity, ions with the same electron valence, or charge, can substitute for each other in the chemical reactions that allow the body to function properly.

What are oxidizing and reducing agents, or oxidants and antioxidants?

The terms oxidant, oxidizer, and oxidizing agent all mean the same thing. They refer to a substance that causes a chemical reaction in which a material goes from a lower valence state to a higher one, such as Fe^{+2} to Fe^{+3}. A reducing agent does the opposite. Antioxidants, sometimes confused with reducing agents, are something different and have a protective function.

Substances which oxidize or reduce are sometimes grouped together and called **redox agents** (from the first letters of <u>red</u>ucing and <u>ox</u>idizing). Gunpowder, for example, combines oxidizing and reducing agents to cause a chemical reaction known as an explosion, or sudden release of energy.

What oxidation and reduction mean in plain English is that a reaction (energy production) is going on within the body (or outside the body to produce a toxic byproduct) which is not what the body is supposed to experience. Oxidants (like gunpowder) can be quite corrosive and damaging to tissues. Antioxidants, as the name implies, counteract the damaging effects of oxidants.

What are pH, acidity, and alkalinity?

A concept called **pH** is referred to in various parts of the book. pH is used to quantify the acidity or alkalinity of a solution (a solid dissolved in water, or a liquid mixed with water). pH refers to the percent of hydrogen in the solution, as greater hydrogen content means greater acidity. Percent is not quite accurate here, as pH is written in reverse logarithmic form. Simply put, this means that for each pH point lower, the hydrogen content (and acidity) is ten times higher. For example, a pH of 5.5 is ten times more acidic than, or has ten times as much hydrogen as, a pH of 6.5. The Richter scale, familiar to many California residents and used to measure the force of earthquakes, is also a logarithmic scale, so a 6 on the Richter scale (although not on the pH scale) is far more destructive than a 5 (about ten times more).

A pH of 7.0 is defined as neutral, and a pH below 7 is defined as acidic. The farther below 7, the more acidic, and the more acidic a solution, the more corrosive it is. A solution with a pH of 2 is generally more harmful than a solution with a pH of 4, as pH 2 is 100 times more acidic than pH 4. An **acid** is usually, but not always, formed from the hydrogen ion H^+ and a negative ion; some examples are:

- *HCl*   *hydrochloric acid, in the stomach for digestion*
- *H_2CO_3*   *carbonic acid, part of the body's buffer system*
- *H_2SO_4*   *sulfuric acid, in air pollution and acid rain*

A pH above 7 is considered to be alkaline. The higher the pH, the more alkaline, and the more corrosive. In general, the farther away from neutral pH 7 in *either* direction, the more damaging the solution is. A solution, or material to make a solution with a pH higher than 7 is an **alkali**. Most, but not all, alkalis (sometimes called **bases** in older textbooks) are made with the hydroxyl (-OH) ion. Some examples are sodium hydroxide or potassium hydroxide (NaOH or KOH), which are used in drain cleaners and used to be used in depilatories for removing body hair. Ammonia, which is written NH_3 (as gas) or NH_4OH (as water solution) is also alkaline.

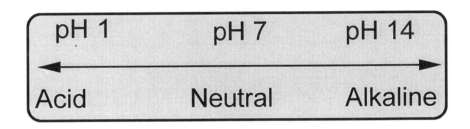

An acid and an alkali together form a salt plus water. For example:

$$HCl \text{ (acid)} + NaOH \text{ (alkali)} \rightarrow NaCl \text{ (salt)} + H_2O \text{ (water)}$$

How is your body like a swimming pool?

In most of the body and in the blood, the optimal pH is actually a bit higher than chemically neutral. A pH of about 7.4 is ideal and is maintained by buffer systems which are combinations of chemicals that keep the pH from fluctuating. Those readers with pools or hot tubs may recognize 7.4 as also being the optimal pH of the pool water. This is not coincidental. In a pool, the 7.4 pH is best for discouraging the growth of bacteria and fungus. This is true in the body as well.

Not all parts of the body function best at pH 7.4. A pH test strip can be used to monitor the pH of urine, which should ideally be between 6 and 6.5. A deviation from this range can indicate fermentation within the body (above pH 6), possible heavy metals or chemicals (below pH 6), or other problems.

Gastric juices (HCl) in the stomach should be around pH 2.0 to digest protein. A pH higher than this can lead to poor digestion of foods. There are tests available to determine your HCl levels.

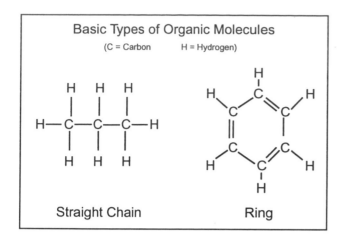

Basic Types of Organic Molecules
(C = Carbon   H = Hydrogen)

Straight Chain   Ring

Does the term organic refer to health food?
In some contexts, yes, but not in the chemical context being discussed here. An **organic** molecule is one that contains carbon. This definition has nothing to do with the idea of organically grown food (theoretically pesticide free). Organic molecules make up all life, and are found in every cell of our bodies and in most nutrients (some mineral forms are the only exception). Organic molecules are also found in nonliving things, including a large number of toxins.

Organic molecules always contain carbon by definition. They almost always contain hydrogen and often oxygen. Molecules containing only carbon (C), hydrogen (H), and oxygen (O) are called **carbohydrates** (note: sometimes referred to as CHOs from the component elements). Organic molecules can contain certain other elements in addition to these including sulfur (S), nitrogen (N), and phosphorus (P).

Organic molecules can be straight-chain, such as sugars and fatty acids. They can also form rings, usually six-sided, which can stand on their own, link together, or link with straight chains. They are electrically neutral.

What, then, are inorganic molecules?
Inorganic molecules do not contain carbon. These can be present as essential minerals in the body; however, many (but not all) inorganic molecules are toxic, in part because they are not compatible with our organic bodies. Inorganic molecules are usually salts. Elements most commonly found in inorganic compounds are the metals:

- *sodium*
- *calcium*
- *iron*
- *zinc*

- *magnesium*
- *chromium*
- *cobalt*

- *manganese*
- *nickel*
- *copper*

These combine with halogens or ions such as carbonate (CO_3^{-2}) or phosphate (PO_4^{-3}) to form different molecules with different properties.

What are halogen lights, and why are halogens toxic?
Halogens, also called halides, are discussed in detail in the chapter on Water Pollution, Fluoride and Chlorine. Halogens are the group VII elements fluorine (F), chlorine (Cl), bromine (Br), and iodine (I). These have a -1 charge and combine with metals to form salts or with organic structures to form halocarbons (organic molecules with carbon and at least one halogen) such as chlorofluorocarbons used in the manufacture of styrofoam. Halocarbons are usually quite toxic.

Many people have heard of halogen lights. Halogen lights contain a halogen gas, usually fluorine, so they can burn hotter. They are not toxic unless the glass bulb is broken.

Halogens such as chlorine and bromine are used in pools to kill microorganisms such as bacteria. It is not surprising that something fatal to bacteria, which are cells, can also have a toxic effect on our bodies, which are also made up of cells.

The thyroid gland requires iodine to function properly. Since the other halogens bind to the thyroid in a manner similar to iodine, they may reduce the amount of iodine available to the thyroid. For example, if you shower in chlorinated water, the chlorine is absorbed into your body through your skin. Symptoms of low thyroid function such as sluggishness and weight gain may result. You can purchase showerheads which filter chlorine out of the water.

A bit of controversy - are elements unchangeable?

Classical chemical theory states that elements, although they may combine infinitely to form compounds, do not become other elements. The number of protons in the nucleus, which determines the identity of the element, is thought to be constant. The only exception has been unstable radioactive elements which decay to more stable lower molecular weight elements, releasing a great deal of harmful (to us) energy in the process. Radium, for example, decays to become lead.

There is some evidence that elements can gain or lose protons in a biological system to form new elements. For example, sodium (11 protons) plus oxygen (8 protons) may be able to become potassium (19 protons) according to Louis Kervran in his book ***Biological Transmutations*** [1].

This may seem hard to believe, but much evidence of this exists [1]:

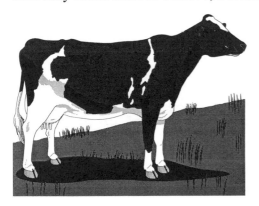

- Cows excrete more calcium in their milk than they take in from their vegetarian diet.

- If seeds are sprouted in distilled water (contains nothing but H_2O), the sprouts contain more of certain minerals than the original seed did.

- Hens take in little or no calcium on a natural diet, yet they lay eggs with a hard shell which is primarily calcium. However, if their diet is deficient in silicon, their egg shells will become soft, i.e. deficient in calcium.

There are many other examples of biological transmutation of elements in this reference source [1], including much data from laboratory studies.

What are the implications of biological transmutation?

There are many implications of the importance of the transmutation of elements in nutrition and medicine. Some applications of this principle include:

- A pregnant or lactating woman can correct her diet and supply enough calcium for herself and the baby by drinking horsetail tea (equisetum), which is rich in silica. This relationship is so well recognized that it is being applied commercially in France.

- Third world countries which have a limited supply of grain can multiply the nutritional yield by sprouting the grain seeds for a few days in water.

- In some cases of heart failure, the potassium level becomes dangerously high while the sodium level drops. The usual treatment involves restricting potassium intake while increasing sodium. This makes sense except for one small problem - it often doesn't work. The patient's potassium level goes higher still and death can result. An understanding of how sodium is transmuted to potassium could lead to more effective treatment.

- As in the previous example, the art of balancing electrolytes (charged mineral elements) could change with an understanding of this principle.

- Nails which break easily and fractured bones which are healing slowly, both signs of decalcification, could benefit from silica-containing horsetail tea. The principle of transmutation explains why.

- Bacteria, which are biological systems, have, at least in theory, the capability of breaking down radioactive wastes to less harmful elements.

- Some people with iron deficiency which is not helped by taking iron supplements can attain normal iron levels by taking manganese. There is only one proton's difference between manganese and iron.

In short, the principle of biological transmutation of elements, which has yet to gain wide acceptance, could revolutionize much of nutritional biochemistry and natural medicine.

Summary

An understanding of basic chemistry is the foundation for making sense of many bodily processes. The chemical components, the way they combine, their electrical charges, and the relationships between them are the basis for understanding toxicology, or why many substances are poisonous. A knowledge of toxicology can, in turn, lead to the application of ways to reverse the damage caused by the many toxic chemicals with which we come in contact.

References and Resources

- Kervran, C. Louis, ***Biological Transmutations***, Happiness Press, Magalia CA, 1966.

- *Many chemistry texts are available and geared to all levels of understanding.*

Primary Toxic Suppressors

-

Chemicals

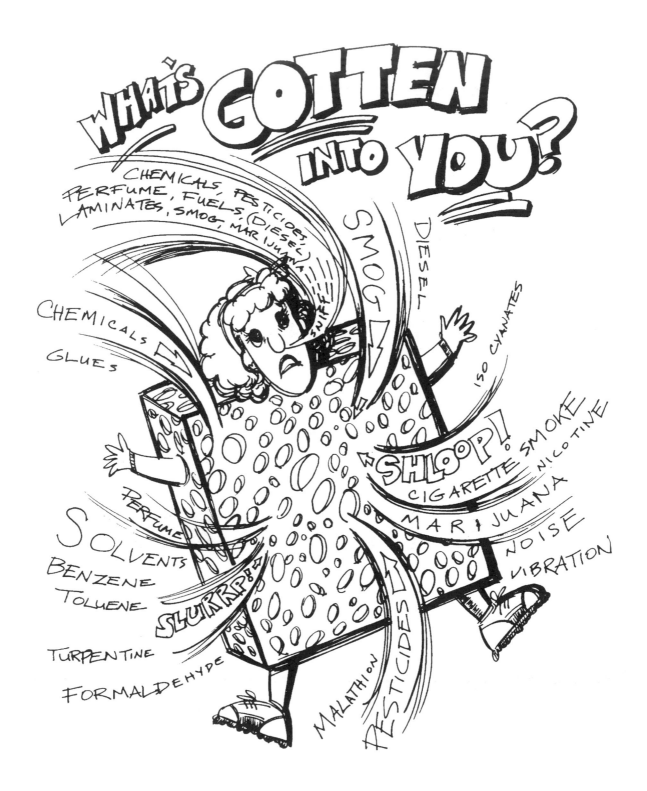

CHEMICAL TOXICITY

What's Gotten Into You?

In this chapter you can learn:
- *Why do some chemicals poison the body while others are necessary for health?*
- *What chemicals that we use every day can be hazardous to our health?*
- *What are some symptoms of chemical poisoning?*
- *Chemical exposure can cause learning disabilities, panic attacks, and fatigue.*
- *Why do people get more colds and flu at certain times of the year?*
- *What exactly is meant by "toxic"? How is the body affected?*
- *What effects do chemicals have on the immune system?*
- *How does long-term exposure to chemicals that we barely notice damage us?*
- *How does the body get rid of chemicals which are poisonous to it?*
- *Why do some people react to certain chemicals when others do not?*
- *Why do hospital personnel worry about balancing your electrolytes?*
- *What does erosion of the Pyramids in Egypt have to do with your health?*

WHY ARE CHEMICALS POISONOUS?

We are made of chemicals. So how can chemicals be poisonous?

All chemicals - elements and combinations of elements called compounds - are different in structure and properties, and affect the body in different ways. These basic chemical concepts were just discussed in the chapter on Basic Chemical Concepts. Some chemicals are necessary in order to maintain the many bodily functions, and are needed in specific amounts. But poisonous chemicals are toxic because they disrupt the proper functioning of the body. They do this by:

- **Damaging** the cells, like asbestos. Such damaged cells look like a porcupine under a microscope.

- **Interfering** in one or more of the complex biochemical processes that keep the body going, such as mercury binding with sulfur in proteins that keep your body detoxified.

- **Substituting** for a necessary substance, such as cadmium in tobacco smoke for zinc.

- Adversely **affecting** the body's **filters** which help to cleanse the body. These filters include the liver, kidneys, lungs, and lymph.

All of these are described with examples later in this chapter.

What determines how chemicals affect us?

Many things influence the way chemicals affect a particular person.. Some chemicals target a particular organ, while other effects are determined by individual genetic "weak links" in each person -- the Genetic Translator. The genetic translator is usually the determinant of symptoms, but some chemicals are so strong that they bypass the genetic translator and go directly to a targeted system.

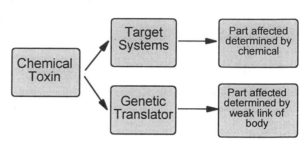

How many synthetic chemicals are there?

Each year the United States produces about 400 billion pounds of synthetic organic chemicals. This is equivalent to about eighty pounds of chemicals per year for each person on the planet. There are currently about 55,000 chemical compounds in production [1], and 48,000 chemicals listed by the Environmental Protection Agency (EPA). Of these, fewer than 1000 are tested for acute toxic effects, and only about 500 are tested for chronic effects. Every year 5-10 million poisonings are reported as a result of accidental exposure to toxic products in the home [2].

How are chemical toxins classified?

There are many types of chemicals which can be poisonous, including an excess of those chemicals necessary for life. These chemicals can be classified in a number of ways:

- By **principal effect** - caustic damage (i.e. tissue burning caused by drain cleaner), cytotoxicity (poisoning of cells), anoxia (lack of oxygen, as with carbon monoxide)

- By **body part** most affected - heart, liver, brain, kidneys

- By **place** found - industrial, household, medicine cabinet, outdoors, in the car

- By method of **ingestion** - inhaled, ingested (swallowed), topical (on skin)

- By **type or use** of product - insecticides, paints, solvents

- By **chemical class** - elements, salts, aromatics (ring-shaped compounds), halogenated hydrocarbons (compounds with halogen elements such as chlorine)

What are the two primary types of chemical exposure?

It is important to understand the difference between the two types of chemical exposure - acute and chronic.

Acute exposure is a one-time event in which the body is exposed all at once to more of a chemical than it can handle. With acute exposure, both the symptoms and the cause are usually readily apparent. Some types of acute exposure can cause death within a short period of time, depending on the type of poison and the dose. Some examples of acute exposure are:

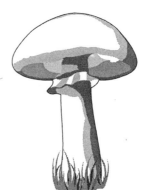

- Burns from corrosives such as drain cleaners and battery acids

- Overdose of narcotic or stimulant drugs

- Poisonous plants such as some mushrooms and mistletoe, which cause gastrointestinal and systemic effects, and poison ivy, which can cause an itchy rash

- Poisons from some insects, fish, and snakes can cause painful local or systemic effects

- Food poisoning from bacteria, molds, and their toxins can produce gastrointestinal and neurological symptoms

Chronic exposure occurs when a person is exposed to a toxin in small quantities over a long period of time, and the amount taken in is equal to or greater than the amount the body can metabolize and eliminate over time. Effects are cumulative and additive, and tend to worsen over time if the cause is not eliminated.

This book is concerned with chronic exposure to chemicals and other toxins. Chemicals from the list below and their sources and effects are discussed in greater detail in the next few chapters, as well as in the chapters on Metals, Drugs, Electromagnetic Radiation, and Food Additives.

What are some types of chronic chemical exposure?
Common sources of chronic chemical exposure are:

- **Insecticides**, rodenticides, fungicides, herbicides, repellents. These work by damaging the cells of the target animal or plant. But they can also damage our cells and penetrate our nervous system.

- **Nitrogen** in compounds such as petrochemical fertilizers affects communication to cells so they open up and take in toxins. However, nitrogen from natural sources such as compost is beneficial to plants and to humans, and helps the body to handle communications.

- **Halogenated hydrocarbons** like chloroform, which are liver and kidney toxins.

- **Alcohols and glycols** such as antifreeze can kill pets who are attracted to the sweet tasting antifreeze and lick it from the driveway or road. Children can also be attracted to the sweet taste and be similarly poisoned, and many children are killed each year in this way. Ethylene glycol is also found in brake fluids, as well as being a solvent for paints and inks. These compounds dissolve the fatty nerve sheaths, thereby stimulating and then depressing the central nervous system.

- **Aldehydes, ketones, ethers, and esters**, which are all types of chemical compounds. These include formaldehyde, found in wall paneling and many other products, and oil of wintergreen, found in some cleaning solutions. Oil of wintergreen smells like wintergreen candies and can be very tempting to children.

- **Paints and solvents** can damage the central nervous system by penetrating the fatty myelin nerve sheath.

- **Drugs**, both therapeutic and recreational, discussed in the chapter on Drugs.

- **Metals** and their salts, such as mercury and lead, discussed in the chapters in the Metals section.

- **Radioactive materials** start a chain reaction of cancer causing, free radical damage.

- **Soaps**, detergents, sanitizing agents, hair dyes, and deodorants. Detergents, which are formulated to dissolve oil, can also break down our lipid (fat) containing cell walls.

- **Cologne**, soaps, toilet articles and other scented products, which can be absorbed into the cells and are surprisingly toxic. These items are discussed in the chapter on Cologne and Personal Care Products.

- **Glues and laminants**, found in particle board and dental adhesives

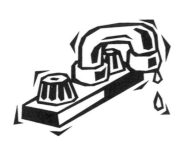

- **Halides**, also called halogens (as in halogen lights), which are chlorine, fluorine, bromine, and iodine. Some of these are deliberately added to our drinking water, although they are outlawed in Europe due to their toxicity. These chemicals are discussed in the chapter on Water Pollution, Fluoride and Chlorine.

- **Gases**, fumes, and air pollutants.

- **Inhaled fibers**, such as asbestos and silica, which are sharp and can puncture cells.

- **Aromatic** (ring shaped) hydrocarbons such as benzene and toluene, which dissolve cell membranes and nerve sheaths and can cause damage to the central nervous system..

- **Food additives**, discussed in more detail in a later chapter.

Most of these chemical substances can be found in use in the home.

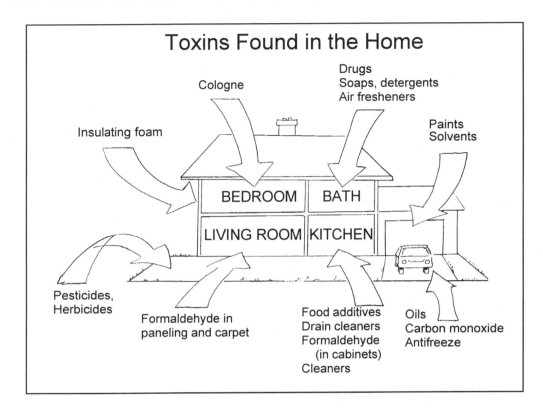

Toxins Found in the Home

Cologne

Drugs
Soaps, detergents
Air fresheners

Insulating foam

Paints
Solvents

BEDROOM | BATH

LIVING ROOM | KITCHEN

Pesticides,
Herbicides

Formaldehyde in
paneling and carpet

Food additives
Drain cleaners
Formaldehyde
(in cabinets)
Cleaners

Oils
Carbon monoxide
Antifreeze

Some items on this list, such as cologne, paint, drugs such as antibiotics, metals, deodorants, and fluoride may come as a surprise to you. Many people think of these things as harmless or even beneficial. But they are all chemicals which don't belong in the body and can have adverse, chronic effects such as fatigue or nerve damage.

Why is it sometimes hard to track down the cause of chemical toxicity?
With chronic exposure, it usually takes some detective work to find the cause. Even the symptoms may not be initially obvious. They may have existed for so long that you may wonder if this is a normal part of aging. Your symptoms may be due to exposure to more than one chemical, or to causes other than chemical exposure.

To further confuse matters, symptoms fluctuate in type and severity because the total body burden is in a state of constant flux. You will probably be more severely affected when the total body burden of toxins is highest. It may take careful observation over a period of time to figure out what is really going on.

One patient, a homemaker, found that a good high-energy day was almost invariably followed by a bad symptom-filled day. She finally realized that on good days she would get out the furniture polish, rug cleaner and brass polish, and energetically clean house. But the next day she suffered the effects of increased exposure to these toxins.

Clues to whether disease is chemically caused include clustering of disease in a specific group (i.e., workers in a factory or people in a particular neighborhood), or the appearance or disappearance of illness or symptoms with a change of occupation or environment [3].

What are some symptoms of chronic chemical exposure?
Some symptoms of chronic chemical exposure include:

- Sunlight sensitivity - Do you feel you can't go outside without sunglasses?

- Sensitivity to sounds - Do you feel that some noises are too loud, or that you experience difficulty concentrating with a radio playing?

- Sensitivity to certain penetrating smells - Cologne, diesel fumes, and paint seem to bother you more than they bother most people. Cologne may smell like bug spray, as a chemically overloaded person is often more sensitive to the penetrant used in both cologne and insecticide.

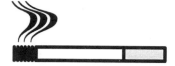

- Sensitivity to cigarette smoke, dust, or cut grass may indicate a fungus infection secondary to chemical exposure.

- Headache, head pressure, or stiff neck or back can be caused by chemicals affecting the meningeal system.

- Brain fog, a term that includes difficulty in completing projects, concentrating, making decisions, remembering appointments, or problem solving, or a feeling of spaciness.

It may come as a great relief to realize that symptoms which sound like mental problems actually may have a physical cause that can be reduced or eliminated. You are probably not going crazy or getting senile. You are slowly being poisoned.

Can chemical exposure cause learning and behavioral problems?
Chronic exposure to chemicals in school contribute to learning disabilities, hyperactivity, and absenteeism. These chemicals include:

- *Chemicals in carpets such as formaldehyde, dirt repellents, fire retardants, and cleaning solutions*

- *Pencil lead, ink, chalk, dust*

- *Formaldehyde in particle board and plywood used to make desks and cabinets*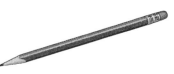

- *Cleaning materials such as rug cleaners and disinfectants*

- *Polyurethane insulating foam used in walls*

Behavior problems of many children are wholly or partially physiological. Physiological causes of behavior problems other than environmental chemical exposure include food additives, sugar, allergies, and fluorescent lights.

How early in life does chemical toxicity start?
A fetus can absorb toxins of many types from its mother's exposure. Then after birth, this baby, with its immature detoxification systems, is put into an environment that may be extremely toxic. The doting and well-meaning parents, who have outfitted the freshly painted nursery with new items, dress the baby in new permanent press clothing treated with a fire retardant compound, and lay it on a new mattress treated with fire retardant and pesticides, and covered with plastic mattress-protecting sheets. Then they wonder why baby cries and fusses all night [4].

Can chemical toxicity cause panic attacks?
Agoraphobia, a Greek word meaning "fear of the marketplace", is a disorder characterized by sudden panic attacks when in the store or mall, or driving in the car. It is considered by many to be a psychological disorder, but it may actually be caused by exposure to toxins in these places. Panic disorder has been linked to organic solvents found in the workplace [5]. Chemicals in the mall or store include formaldehyde in the carpets, sizing in new clothing, cologne, floor cleaner and floor wax. Fumes from cars and trucks on the highway include benzene, combustion products, and oils. This exposure overloads the body of a person who is already stressed by the many toxic stressors in their environment.

> **Agoraphobia may not be all in your mind - it may have a physical cause.**

In panic attacks, the body perceives a dangerous situation - the toxin - and the sympathetic nervous system signals the adrenal glands to secrete adrenaline to prepare for a fight-or-flight situation. This rush of adrenaline is perceived as a feeling of panic. After this happens a few times, the fear of having it happen again may be enough to trigger an attack on its own. Agoraphobic symptoms may also be brought about by non-chemical factors such as fluorescent lights or subsonic (below the level of hearing) vibrations from the ventilating system in a public place. Fluorescent lights flash on and off too fast to be consciously seen and can trigger a type of mild epileptic seizure.

Lowering the level of toxins in the body by reducing exposure or undergoing detoxification may eliminate agoraphobic symptoms without expensive and often ineffective psychotherapy. Many people with this disorder blame themselves. But it's probably the environment, not you!

One patient, a woman in her early 40s, couldn't get near the local mall and was diagnosed as agoraphobic. It turned out that she was extremely sensitive to the spray used to keep moths away, to perfume from department store counters and other shoppers, and to tailor's starch.

What is sick building syndrome (or new building syndrome)?
Newer buildings such as homes and offices may suffer from "sick building syndrome". Supposedly improved building materials and construction techniques have resulted in buildings with more laminants and other chemicals. But concern for energy efficiency has led to the building of comparatively airtight living and working spaces with windows that do not even open, so these

toxins are continually circulating and reentering the bodies of those who live and work there rather than being exhausted to the outside. Problems caused by tightly closed buildings are discussed in the chapter on Air Pollution.

Another type of sick building syndrome is found in older houses and workplaces. Chemical toxins such as lead and mercury in paint and asbestos in insulation, no longer used in new construction, are found in older buildings. Buildings that have been around awhile are also more likely to have been sprayed with pesticides, and to have a buildup of mold, mildew, and dust mites.

Where does the flu go when it's not going around?

Have you ever noticed an increase in the number of absences from colds, flu, and allergies in your workplace at the beginning of winter or summer? This is unlikely to be due to the change of seasons itself. In the spring and fall, while ventilating systems and heating/cooling ductwork are not in use, they become a storage and breeding space for viruses, bacteria, fungi, and dust mites. All of these are released into the air when the heat or air conditioning is turned on, particularly for the first time of the season. The problem can be reduced by installing and using an ozonator in the ventilating system, or by having the ducts cleaned by a professional specializing in this type of work. Even vacuuming the ducts and vents can be helpful.

What makes some chemicals more toxic than others?

There are a number of factors which influence toxicity, in addition to whether exposure is acute (short term) or chronic (long term). The type of chemical dictates what parts of the body will be affected and how severely. Other factors which are discussed on the next pages are:

- *The dose (how much)*
- *Length of time of exposure*
- *Route of exposure (entry into body)*
- *Travel through body*
- *Metabolic byproducts*
- *Excretion*
- *Individual susceptibility*
- *Potency (how toxic)*

How much is too much?

The dose is the amount of chemical relative to body weight that enters the body. All chemicals, including essential substances such as oxygen, or salt (sodium chloride) can produce toxic effects if consumed in large enough quantities.

The dose is usually measured per unit of body weight, as a specific amount of chemical would be more toxic to a small, thin, person than to a larger one, everything else being equal.

How long is too long?
Smaller doses over a longer period of time will have less of an effect than the same dose all at once. For example, beverage alcohol (ethanol - yes, it's poisonous - why do you think they call it in<u>toxic</u>ation?) is metabolized by the liver at a rate of about one ounce per hour. Drinking one ounce per hour for four hours will therefore have far less effect than four ounces at once.

On the other hand, a small exposure every day will add up to a higher total of toxic accumulation the longer you are exposed.

How can poisons get into the body?
The three major routes of exposure are:

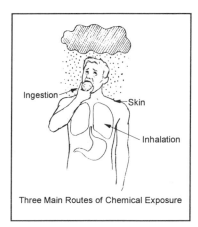

- *Inhalation - into the lungs*
- *Ingestion - into the stomach*
- *Topical   - through the skin*

The most serious route of exposure is generally the lungs if the substance can be vaporized (changed from liquid to gas, like steam), or the stomach if it cannot.

Three Main Routes of Chemical Exposure

How important is travel through the body?
In order to be toxic to the system, a poison must travel through the system. For example, a caustic substance will not usually travel through the bloodstream (unless injected), and so will not damage any part of the body not directly exposed to it.

As an example, barium is very toxic to cells, but it seems to be tolerated as a radiopaque contrast medium in the taking of x-rays with only slight toxicity because it is nearly insoluble in water. It can therefore be excreted without being absorbed by the body, which is mostly water. In theory, this is true, but many people with chronic health problems have a syndrome known as "leaky gut". As the name implies, substances which should not be absorbed from the digestive system into the bloodstream are in fact absorbed due to malfunction. Once in the bloodstream the barium cannot be easily excreted and must be chelated out like any other heavy metal, as described in the Metal Detoxification chapter.

How does the body prepare poisons for excretion?
Once a chemical is in the body it is metabolized, or broken down, into byproducts that can either be used by the body or be more easily excreted. The process of changing the ingested chemical to other products in the body is called biotransformation. Detoxification systems within the body such as cytochrome P-450 and the sulfur-containing compounds glutathione and metallothionein aid in this process, which is necessary for eventual elimination of the toxic substance.

Nutrition plays an important role in the effectiveness of these systems. Like any other systems in the body, the detoxification systems work best with the right kind of food, just as your car runs best with the right kind of fuel.

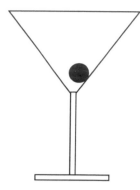

In some cases, the new byproduct is more toxic than the original. Methanol, for example, is metabolized into the more toxic formaldehyde. Ethanol, or beverage alcohol, is metabolized into acetaldehyde (also called acetyl aldehyde). Acetaldehyde, although less toxic than formaldehyde, is responsible for the hangover, related to oxygen deficiency, and some of the other toxic side effects that are attributed to alcohol. Methanol is actually found in beverage alcohol in small amounts (up to 10%), and the formaldehyde produced can cause symptoms such as the delirium tremens (DTs) of withdrawal.

Formaldehyde, interestingly, is the same substance found in carpets, plywood, and many other building materials. It can contribute to the difficulty in thinking and mood swings sometimes experienced by workers in new buildings. People who live in trailers can be exposed to the formaldehyde which outgasses from the plywood in interior paneling.

How does the body get rid of poisons?

Some chemicals are rapidly excreted, limiting their toxic effects. Those that are excreted more slowly can do more damage and have more long-term effects because they are in the body longer. Many substances are stored in the body, primarily in fat but sometimes in bone. They can therefore circulate for a long time, and chronic or repeated exposure can cause a higher and increasingly more toxic level to accumulate in the body. Like a bank account, the more you deposit, the greater is your balance. If more of a poison goes in than comes out, the total in the body goes up, leading to toxic overload and Toxic Immune Syndrome.

The body has a number of detoxification pathways, including:

- *The liver*
- *The kidneys (urinary excretion)*
- *Sulfur-based amino acids such as glutathione and metallothionein*
- *Breathing out from the lungs*
- *Sweat and excretion through skin pores*

Are all people created equal with respect to reactivity?

Personal susceptibility, and therefore the toxic dose, varies widely among individuals for several reasons:

- **Age** - The very young and the very old are more vulnerable.

- **Gender** - Women are more likely than men to collect larger amounts of fat-soluble toxins due to their greater amount of body fat. An example of this is PCBs, found in burning plastics, which accumulate in a woman's breast tissue and have been implicated in breast cancer. Nickel has also been linked to breast cancer. Alcohol also affects women more than men even when body weight is taken into consideration.

- **Other stresses** - A person whose body is stressed by other burdens is more likely to be affected by a toxin since the body systems that deal with the toxin are already overloaded.

- **Gallbladder problems** - These are a major factor in chemical toxicity. About 35% of the population has had their gallbladder removed, making this the most common surgery. Microorganisms in the gallbladder (giardia, helicobacter, fungus, and roundworm) block the hepatic bile duct, which slows down oil digestion, which causes increased absorption of oil soluble chemicals. A body deficient in necessary oils will soak up oil-based chemicals much as a dry sponge soaks up more liquid than a wet one. On the other hand, a body with sufficient beneficial oils can repel toxins like a duck's oil-soaked feathers repel water. Mercury from dental fillings is a major cause of gallbladder suppression, as bile adheres to mercury causing clogging sludge.

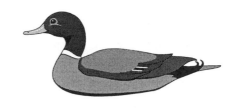

- **Insufficient dietary oils** - An insufficient intake of essential fatty acids found in good non-rancid cold-pressed or expeller-pressed oils (see Oils and Fats chapter in *Thriving In A Toxic World*) can also cause the dry sponge effect.

Are some poisons more poisonous than others?

Some substances are more potent than others. Potency is inversely proportional to the lethal dose. In other words, if it takes less of chemical A to kill an organism than of chemical B, then chemical A is said to be more potent than chemical B.

The usual measurement of potency is LD50, which stands for the Lethal Dose for 50% of test animals. Unfortunately the LD50 is calculated based on acute reactions (under 120 days) rather than chronic effects. Only those animals which die right away are counted. If chronic effects were examined, the LD50, or the maximum safe dose for most substances would likely be lower than it is.

Relative toxicity is difficult to quantify when measures other than death are used as criteria. For example, which is more toxic: a chemical which causes cancer, one which causes nerve damage, or one which causes lung scarring? In these cases the issues of toxicity and potency are not simple ones.

Doesn't the government protect us against toxic chemicals?

There are so many chemicals that there is no way they can all be tested thoroughly for both short-term and long-term (chronic) toxicity. Four million distinct chemical compounds have been reported in literature since 1965, with about 6000 new compounds added to the list each year. Of these as many as 70,000 are currently in commercial production. Over 700 have been identified in drinking water alone [6]. A National Research Council study found that complete health hazard evaluations were available for only 10% of pesticides and 18% of drugs used in the U.S. [7].

TYPES OF CHEMICAL TOXICITY

How do poisons do their damage?

There are many ways in which a chemical can be toxic, i.e. a number of different mechanisms by which a substance can cause its damage to bodily functions. As with the types of poisons, there are several ways that these effects can be characterized:

- *By main target organ - liver, brain, heart*

- *By type of effect - central nervous system depression, anoxia (lack of oxygen to tissues), lung edema (accumulation of fluid)*

- *By biochemical process interrupted - acetylcholine cycle, adrenaline/ epinephrine system. These are described later in this chapter.*

A combination of these classification systems is used here.

What happens when the body gets too little oxygen?

Oxygen is necessary for a number of vital functions in the body. The brain and central nervous system are particularly sensitive to a lack of oxygen, which will cause reversible and then irreversible damage. Reversible damage is correctable when the source of poisoning stops, while irreversible damage is permanent. This lack of oxygen is called **anoxia**.

There are two types of anoxia that can be caused by poisons: mechanical and chemical. Mechanical (physical) anoxia occurs when a gas, not dangerous in itself, is inhaled instead of oxygen. Molecular nitrogen (N_2) makes up about 75% of the air, but in itself has no biological activity, good or bad; yet inhaling pure nitrogen can be deadly because it blocks oxygen from getting to the lungs. This effect is comparable to a group of gang members keeping you from walking down a street simply by standing there and physically blocking your way.

Chemical anoxia is more complex. Using the previous analogy, chemical anoxia is like gang members not just blocking your way, but jumping you and beating you up. The effects of chemical anoxia are more difficult to reverse than those of physical anoxia due to chemical interaction with the cells and the resulting cellular changes.

Why is a running car in a closed garage deadly?

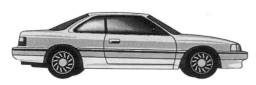

Ordinarily, oxygen is transported by the erythrocytes, or red blood cells, from the lung capillaries (tiny blood vessels) to the cells that need it. Oxygen binds with the hemoglobin in the red blood cells to form oxyhemoglobin, which gives up its oxygen to body cells before making the return trip to the lungs via the veins. If carbon monoxide (CO), found in car exhaust, is present, it latches onto the hemoglobin so tightly that there is no room for the oxygen to be bound and transported. If red blood cells are compared to taxicabs, then carbon monoxide fills the seats of the taxicabs so no other passengers can be transported.

In fact, the affinity of hemoglobin for carbon monoxide is so great that if only one part of carbon monoxide is diluted in 2000 parts of air, fully half of the hemoglobin in the body would bind to the carbon monoxide and thus be unavailable for oxygen transport [2]. Carbon monoxide is created by incomplete combustion, and is found in car exhaust or comes from a leaky, inefficient furnace. Exposure can be acute enough that death can result from a single high dose, or it can be chronic, as from a furnace or exhaust pipe with a very small leak. Since the brain is the first organ to be affected by lack of oxygen, central nervous system symptoms such as stupor, giddiness, weakness, and headache will be the first to show, with coma and death following in time. Deeply flushed or cherry-red skin can also be characteristic of acute carbon monoxide poisoning.

Many of us live in cities or in areas with considerable vehicular traffic. We are thus exposed to low levels of carbon monoxide on a long-term basis, potentially causing chronic symptoms such as depression, poor judgment, headache, and weakness.

Why is cyanide so poisonous?

Another type of chemical anoxia is caused by hydrogen cyanide (HCN), a gas which may be released in a number of industrial processes, especially those involving plastics. The cyanide group (CN⁻) does not interfere in oxygen transport, but causes problems at the intracellular level by blocking or inactivating respiratory enzymes, most likely an enzyme called cytochrome oxidase. Just as respiration means breathing, respiratory enzymes are involved in reactions that get oxygen to where it is needed. Thus the blood may be rich in oxygen, unlike the case with carbon monoxide, but the cells themselves may die of asphyxia (lack of oxygen) because the oxygen can't get into them [8].

What happens when atoms trade places?

Just as carbon monoxide replaces essential oxygen, other elements and compounds cause their toxic effect by replacing chemicals essential to body functions. These reactions are called **replacement reactions**. The chapter on Basic Chemical Concepts explains the groups of the Periodic Table of the Elements and why elements of each group (up-and-down column) will bind in a similar fashion.

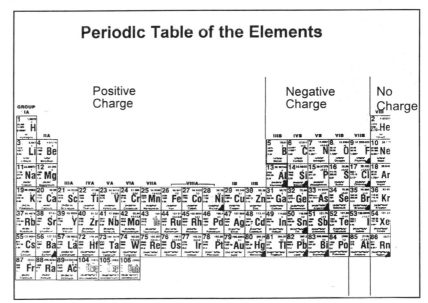

The elements in each group have the same number of electrons too many or too few in their outer shell, so they will bind to cells or to other chemicals in a similar fashion. Their chemical action, however, is different.

The lower the molecular weight, the more likely the element is to be found in the body. The higher the molecular weight, in general, the higher the toxicity. In their ionic form, such as Na^+ (sodium), K^+ (potassium), Ca^{+2} (calcium), and Cl^- (chloride), these elements are vital to the body and are least likely to be toxic. The pluses and minuses after the element symbols refer to the ionic form, or the loss or gain of electrons upon combining. Those elements needing electrons to complete their outer shell have minuses, and those with extra electrons have pluses. The numbers (-2, +3) indicate the number of electrons needed (minus sign) or extra (plus sign). A simple + or - means +1 or -1.

Within a group, for example group II (II refers to the number of extra electrons), there is zinc (Zn), cadmium (Cd), and mercury (Hg), in order of increasing atomic weight (65, 112, and 200 respectively). Zinc in its ionic form, Zn^{+2}, is necessary for proper body function, although an excess is toxic. Cadmium, found in paints, cigarettes, tires and brakes, is toxic. Mercury, found in amalgam fillings, paints, and some industrial processes, has no known use in the body and is even more poisonous.

Since cadmium and mercury, in their more soluble ionized or salt forms, will attempt to participate in the same biochemical reactions as zinc, their presence will prevent some of the zinc from reacting and performing its functions in the body. This is like a 65 pound person (zinc) competing unsuccessfully with 112 pound (cadmium) and 200 pound (mercury) people in a game of musical chairs. As a result, mercury leaching into the body from silver-mercury amalgam fillings will cause symptoms of zinc deficiency such as fatigue and loss of smell and taste, even if there is plenty of zinc available. Since cigarettes are a significant source of cadmium, quitting smoking usually increases the sense of taste by increasing the availability of zinc in the body without extra zinc intake.

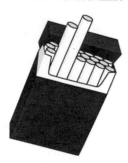

Cadmium from cigarettes may fool the body into thinking zinc is present, but the energy boost is temporary and the resulting energy drop is one of the factors which causes the smoker to crave another cigarette.

Replacement reactions are like putting the wrong type of battery in a toy; it may fit, but it won't work well and may damage the toy with too much or too little voltage.

Why is it so important to balance electrolytes?

Another example of a replacement reaction is sodium (Na) and potassium (K). Both are necessary in ionized form for a number of bodily functions and must be in balance or one will try to take over the functions of the other. A deficiency of sodium (or excess of potassium) can cause :

- *fatigue*
- *nausea*
- *lowered blood pressure*
- *cold hands and feet*

A deficiency of potassium (or excess of sodium) can cause:

- *water retention*
- *mind racing*
- *sleeplessness*
- *tiredness*
- *muscle tightness, cramps or twitching*
- *heart pounding, fast pulse*
- *anxiety*
- *pain in kidney area*

These symptoms are not absolutes, however. It is fairly well known that too much sodium can cause water retention and raise blood pressure, but few people realize that too little sodium can have the same effect.

One patient, a health care practitioner, was considerably overweight at 260 pounds and had a dangerously high bloodpressure reading of 230/140; 120/80 is normal. He had been on a severely salt-restricted diet for years without any positive effect before being treated by a practitioner who understood electrolytes and *increased* his sodium intake. He lost sixty pounds of water weight in six weeks. His blood pressure also dropped to nearly normal (130/85) within a relatively short period of time.

Calcium (Ca) and magnesium (Mg), both in group II, have to be kept in balance for the same reason. Fortunately, the body does a pretty good job of balancing out essential elements as long as there is not a deficiency or large excess of one or the other. The heavier elements, on the other hand, will preferentially bind over the lighter corresponding vital elements, like the larger person grabbing the chair in a game of musical chairs and not giving it up. The minerals, or lighter metals, eventually lose out to the heavy metals, which makes the metals quite toxic. Heavy metals can be compared to aptly-named "heavy metal" music. When it is playing loudly it will drown out softer classical music.

What are caustics and how do they do their damage?
Causticity, or corrosive effect, is usually seen in acute cases of toxicity. The most common caustics are the strong acids, such as battery acid, and the strong alkalis, such as drain cleaner. These rarely get into the bloodstream, but work their damaging effects by chemical destruction of the tissues with which they come in contact. The destruction they cause is comparable to a burn caused by fire.

How does chronic exposure to caustics occur?
Perhaps you have read about the way in which certain very ancient stone structures are eroding rapidly, worldwide. The Sphinx and Pyramids in Egypt, the Coliseum in Rome, and the Notre Dame cathedral in Paris have experienced erosion of stone to a greater extent in the past fifty years than in their entire previous existence. The famous Aqueduct in Segovia, Spain, built by the Romans 1900 years ago, is crumbling, a process that started comparatively recently. Officials in Spain are taking steps to reroute traffic away from it in an attempt to slow down further damage [9].

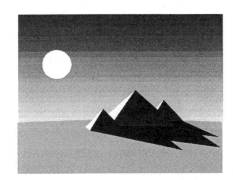

What does traffic have to do with stone erosion, and what does stone erosion have to do with chronic human exposure to caustics?

The culprit in this worldwide erosion of stone monuments and historic marvels is air pollutionmost notably acids in the air. One of the primary causes of this type of pollution is motor vehicle exhaust, added to emissions from industrial processes and other sources. Sulfur and nitrogen compounds, ozone, chlorinated hydrocarbons, and other pollutants combine with each other and with moisture in the air to make sulfuric, nitric, and hydrochloric acids, which is also the cause of "acid rain". These air pollutants and acids, heaviest in areas of dense vehicle traffic and industry, will etch stone in a fairly short time.

The smog in Los Angeles will eat away the rubber windshield gaskets of some foreign cars over time. Special gaskets have been developed for the U.S. market for this reason.

If acids in the air can eat away stone, what must they be doing to the tender tissues of the lungs as they are breathed in? Carbonyl chloride, better known as Phosgene gas during the war and still a byproduct of the chemical industry, causes its damage by corroding deep respiratory passages as it is breathed in. Since one of the body's responses to injury is to cause fluid to collect at the site of the injury, fluid pools in the lungs as a response to the irritation. This massing of fluid in the lungs, called edema, floods the alveoli, which are tiny bulblike structures in the lungs whose purpose is to transfer oxygen to the red blood cells in the capillaries. This alveolar flooding causes asphyxia. The person, in effect, ends up drowning from within.

Malathion, best known for the Medfly extermination program in California, is an insecticide in common use. It can eat away the paint and finish on cars, just as acids in the air erode stone. Peeling paint on cars in California seems to be more prevalent than on the East coast. Malathion and other chemicals in the air may be a reason for this. The damage to tender lung tissues from Malathion and other chemicals is not hard to imagine.

What is one possible cause of asthma and bronchitis?

Corrosives in the air cause an effect similar to that of Phosgene gas. Since they are much more dilute than Phosgene gas, the result is not instant death but rather a constant, cumulative irritation, such as bronchitis and asthma. The partial flooding of the alveoli reduces the amount of oxygen available to the cells. In addition, eroded lung tissue puts up less of a barrier to harmful chemicals and infectious agents than healthy lung tissue, much as abraded skin is more likely to let in bacteria and chemicals than intact skin. Remember the warning labels on deodorants and other personal-care products which say "Do not apply to broken or irritated skin"? This principle, for the same reason, applies to lung damage caused by air pollution. Abraded skin is roughed up, causing more surface area to be exposed to irritants. Damaged lung tissue is wrinkled and puckered, increasing the surface area and creating crevices for toxins.

Tobacco smoking also irritates the lungs. Smoking, discussed in the chapter on Drugs, is rather like inhaling concentrated fumes high in cadmium, nickel, and resins from your own personal chemical factory many times daily.

How can chemical exposure affect the central nervous system?

The central nervous system (CNS) consists of the brain, spinal cord, and peripheral nerves. Lack of oxygen (anoxia or asphyxia) will affect the oxygen-hungry CNS before any other organ systems.

CNS depression is marked by lowered responsiveness to stimuli. If severe enough it can lead to coma, respiratory and circulatory failure, and death. CNS depression results from a number of drugs, especially:

- *General anesthetics such as ether, chloroform, cyclopropane, and ethylene*
- *Barbiturates such as phenobarbital and pentobarbital*
- *Opium alkaloids such as morphine and codeine*
- *Alcohol*
- *Many other toxins (less commonly)*

CNS overstimulation can cause nerve irritability, hypersensitivity to stimuli, and convulsions that can be severe enough to be fatal. Toxins likely to cause CNS overstimulation include:

- *Atropine, found in preanesthetic medications and prescription eye drops. Atropine can cause dry mouth, blurred vision, agitation, and delirium.*

- *Strychnine, used in pesticides*

- *Ergot, derived from a rye fungus and used in migraine medications and in the manufacture of the hallucinogen LSD*

- *Cocaine, previously used as a dental anesthetic and now used primarily as a recreational drug*

The central nervous system is similar to the electrical system in a house. CNS depression is analogous to insufficient current or brownout, resulting in dimmer lights, impaired appliance performance, and possible damage to the appliance over time. In the body, there may not be enough power to work well, with resulting atrophy. CNS overstimulation is comparable to a power surge, which can burn out a TV tube or computer immediately or over time.

Another nervous system effect occurs whereby cerebral blood flow and spinal fluid is diminished in patients exposed to chemicals such as pesticides, glues and solvents. This can result in fatigue and brain fog and general diminished brain function [10].

How do toxins affect the transmission of nerve impulses?

In the central nervous system, nerve impulses such as pain, instructions to muscles, and messages to internal organs and systems pass from one nerve cell to the next in their path from the brain to their destination like electricity from an outlet through a wire to a light. In the case of pain, the direction of transmission is reversed and the impulse travels <u>to</u> the brain. Nerve cells don't touch each other. The impulse is passed from one nerve cell to another across a gap called a synaptic junction, or synapse, like a baton passed between runners. Chemicals in the nervous system called neurotransmitters exist for the purpose of sending these impulses across the synaptic junction. Two of these neurotransmitters are acetylcholine and norepinephrine, also called noradrenaline.

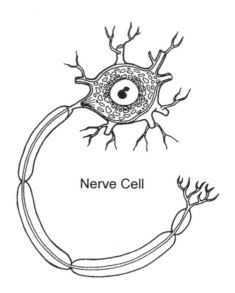

Nerve Cell

Some medically significant toxic agents reduce or exaggerate effective transmission of the nerve impulse across synaptic junctions. These toxic agents either mimic or block the effects of acetylcholine or norepinephrine, or hinder the making or release of these neurotransmitters. A neurotransmitter problem is like a frayed electrical cord. Such a cord leaks current where it shouldn't in the form of sparks (shorts) and prevents current from getting where it should. Multiple Sclerosis (MS), for example, is caused by leaks in the myelin sheath surrounding the nerve cells, with effects similar to those of a neurotransmitter problem.

Poisons that exaggerate the effects produced by acetylcholine release are called cholinergics. These include

- *Muscarine, which is mushroom toxin found in hallucinogenic mushrooms*
- *Pilocarpine, found in glaucoma medications*
- *Neostigmine, found in veterinary medications*

These compounds slow the heart, lower blood pressure, and increase fluid secretion into the respiratory tract. Toxic doses may lead to death by suffocation or circulatory failure.

Heightened neurotransmitter effects can be compared to an electrical circuit that is receiving too much electricity at once. While a large surge of electricity can blow out your appliances, a small but fairly constant increase over the optimal amount of electricity can strain the electrical system of the appliance, resulting in poorer performance and earlier appliance failure.

Toxins which exaggerate the normal effects of noradrenaline / norepinephrine produce disturbances of heart rhythm and high blood pressure, which are effects that can be fatal. Adrenaline is related to noradrenaline and is sometimes confusingly called epinephrine in the U.S.; the term adrenaline makes more sense as it comes from the adrenal glands. Adrenaline is the substance which causes a fight-or-flight response to life-threatening or stressful stimuli. Too much adrenaline will deplete glycogen and overload your system, the way too much electricity will overload the system of an appliance.

Blockers of the neurotransmitter acetylcholine include curare (used to temporarily paralyze muscles during surgery) and some compounds used in anesthesia such as succinylcholine. These drugs cause muscle weakness and can lead to death through paralysis of respiratory muscles. Botulinus and dinoflagellate toxins from food poisoning hinder synthesis and release of acetylcholine. Since not enough acetylcholine is available, the effects are similar to those of acetylcholine blockers.

How do some poisons affect the liver?

The liver is the largest organ in the body, weighing about three pounds in an adult. It is also the major detoxifying organ in the body and has several important functions [11]:

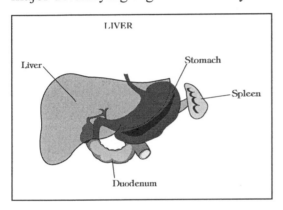

- It receives essential nutrients from the intestine, storing and secreting them as needed.

- It detoxifies a large number of toxic substances, rendering them less harmful.

- The liver produces bile from cholesterol and lecithin. Bile contains bile salts which are very important in the digestion of fats.

- Along with the pancreas, the liver helps to regulate blood sugar levels by storing and releasing sugar as glycogen, which is the body's primary energy source.

- The liver produces about 400 enzymes which facilitate many body functions, including but not limited to digestion.

Liver injury with accompanying jaundice, also called toxic hepatitis, usually occurs as a result of a number of toxins, including:

- Chlorinated hydrocarbons such as cleaning solvents

- Certain heavy metals such as arsenic found in some anti-protozoal medications, barium from gastrointestinal testing, copper and lead from old pipes, and antimony and tin from metal alloy manufacture and fireworks

- A variety of organic compounds.

Two major types of liver injury are liver cell necrosis (cell death), and fatty liver. With fatty liver, one cannot process fats and oils properly, so they build up in the liver, as well as in the arteries. High blood pressure, or hypertension, can result.

Liver cell necrosis causes sclerosis (hardening) and scarring, which in turn causes dry liver. Indications of this are cholesterol levels of under 135 and an LDH (lactose dehydrogenase - don't confuse this with HDL or LDL cholesterol) of less than 110. Dry liver is a condition in which the fatsoluble vitamins A, D, E, and K are not processed for use by the body, causing deficiency symptoms and free radical damage due to loss of the antioxidant effects of vitamins A and E. Dry liver is like a car engine that is allowed to run with insufficient oil. Sooner or later the engine is going to seize up. Both conditions are prevented or remedied by the ingestion of healthy emulsified oils, choline, and lecithin.

Some chemicals which produce cell necrosis are [12]:

- *Acetaminophen (one brand name is Tylenol), in large amounts over time*
- *Beryllium metal, a product of coal combustion*
- *Bromobenzene, a carcinogenic solvent and motor oil additive*

Producers of lipid (fat) accumulation in the liver include:

- *Cerium, a metallic element used as spark metal for gas lighters*
- *Cycloheximide, a fungicide and plant growth regulator*
- *Ethanol, or beverage alcohol*
- *Methotrexate, a cancer drug*
- *Tetracycline, an antibiotic*

Some toxins that produce both effects are:

- *Aflatoxin, from mold that grows on peanuts and potatoes*
- *Bromotrichloromethane, a solvent*
- *Carbon tetrachloride, cleaning fluid and solvent*
- *Chloroform, anesthetic and solvent*
- *Tannic acid, found in tea and used in dyeing fabric and tanning leather*
- *Tetrachloroethane, a solvent*
- *Trichloroethylene, solvent used in dry cleaning and degreasing metals*

How can chemical poisons damage the kidneys?
The kidneys are two bean-shaped organs found just above the waist and towards the back of the body. The kidneys' main function is to filter out certain waste materials from the blood and excrete them in the form of urine.

Many toxic chemicals focus on the kidney as their target organ: [12]

- Halogenated hydrocarbons
  - chloroform, a solvent and anesthetic
  - carbon tetrachloride, used as cleaning fluid
  - bromobenzene, a solvent and motor oil additive
  - hexachlorobutadiene, a widespread environmental pollutant

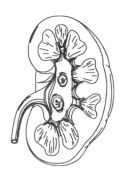

Kidney
(cross section)

- Most heavy metals
  - mercury and mercuric salts in particular

- Some drugs
  - aspirin (prolonged heavy use)
  - some anesthetics, especially halogenated hydrocarbons such as
  - methoxyflurane
  - some antibiotics, especially the mycins (neomycin, gentamicin, streptomycin), cephalosporins, and to a lesser extent tetracycline

- Pesticides and herbicides

- Ethylene glycol, used as antifreeze and as a solvent for paints and inks

Not all substances that influence kidney function will produce symptoms that appear to directly involve the kidneys. Altered renal (kidney) function may cause changes in blood pressure, blood volume, hormonal changes, neurological symptoms, and other systemic effects in some cases related to lowered potassium levels. Kidney problems can affect the levels of the hormone aldosterone, leading to high blood pressure. In some cases the producer of these effects is a metabolic byproduct of the original toxin that is formed within the kidneys in an attempt to eliminate the toxin.

Symptoms of kidney involvement due to heavy metal exposure include sugar in the urine and increased urination, followed if untreated by insufficient urination, kidney failure, and ultimately death. Mercury in particular causes renal damage, and is in fact used by animal experimenters to induce acute kidney failure in test animals by drastically lowering their body potassium levels.

It is suspected that a metabolite of halogenated hydrocarbons is the cause of kidney damage, rather than the solvents themselves. Experimental rats show early signs of kidney damage long after carbon tetrachloride (cleaning fluid) has been eliminated.

Occasionally, chemicals reach such high concentrations in the urine that they exceed their solubilities and precipitate out as crystals. To picture this, imagine adding more and more salt or sugar to a glass of water until no more will dissolve and solid crystals will be visible. The chemical crystals in the kidneys may be eliminated or deposited as sediment or stones, which can block the urine-transporting tubules causing considerable damage and pain. Some women have described the pain as being worse than that of childbirth. Calcium may also crystallize out of the blood, plaquing on the blood vessels. This leads to the narrowing of the interior blood vessel diameter which can eventually result in heart attack or stroke.

How can the heart and blood vessels be damaged by toxins?
The cardiovascular system consists of the heart and blood vessels. Most cardiovascular damage is caused by acute chemical exposure, for example by cocaine or by overdoses of cardiac drugs such as digitalis, a synthetic derivative of the herb foxglove.

Cardiovascular diseases such as hypertension (high blood pressure) and atherosclerosis (hardening of the blood vessels) are more prevalent now than in the past and are found primarily in industrialized societies. Fifty percent of today's mortality rates are due, at least in part, to cardiovascular disease, as compared to one in seven at the turn of the century. The role of low level chronic exposure to industrial chemicals and heavy metals in the development of cardiovascular diseases is strongly suspected.

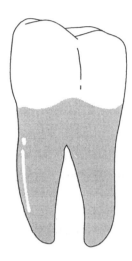

Nickel from dental crowns and root canals or other sources can cause inflammation of the arteries from allergy/sensitivity reactions. This inflammation can lead to plaque accumulation, hypertension, and osteoporosis. This is the "save the teeth but lose the body" approach.

> **Root canals - the "save the teeth but lose the body" approach.**

Inflamed arteries provide rough surfaces inside the arteries upon which calcium-containing plaque can build up just as mineral deposits build up in household plumbing or in showerheads. The openings in the blood vessels get smaller and the blood pressure rises. This is a consistent high blood pressure, as compared with an allergic blood pressure that fluctuates.

The body, in its desperation to find somewhere to store the toxins until it can deal with them, may even deposit them in blood vessels as plaque. Analysis of coronary artery plaque has shown that it can contain pesticides, BHT, toluene, aromatic hydrocarbons and other toxic organic chemical compounds [4].

In addition to the direct contribution of chemicals to plaque, there is an indirect effect. Chemicals cause inflammation, promoting the release of calcium and cholesterol to buffer the inflammation. When the inflammation is in the arteries, the calcium-cholesterol plaque can build up, in some cases completely blocking the blood vessel.

What are the ways in which the immune system is affected by chemicals?
Chronic low levels of exposure to a large number of environmental chemicals including pesticides and herbicides, solvents, and combustion products have been shown to affect, or can potentially affect, the immune system. There are three major types of immune system disturbances:

- *Hypersensitivity responses such as allergy*
- *Immune activation, which can lead to autoimmune disease*
- *Immune suppression, leading to long term infections such as pneumonia, and cancers*

Briefly summarized here, they are discussed in greater detail in the chapter on the Immune System in *Thriving In A Toxic World*.

Hypersensitivity - Some chemicals can cause allergic reactions, either a hypersensitivity to that material when exposed to it in the future, or a predisposition to allergic reaction to other substances. Allergy is a hypersensitivity to an external substance.

Immune activation - Allergy is an overly aggressive response to an external stimulus in the form of a chemical. Immune activation, or autoimmunity, is an overly aggressive response to one's own system and tissues. Chemicals that can cause immune activation include:

- Polycyclic aromatic hydrocarbons (PAH), such as formaldehyde isocyanate, trimellitic anhydride (used in the preparation of adhesives, dyes, and inks), benzene (in gasoline, varnishes, and used in the manufacture of some medications) and other solvents. PAH compounds are formed from many burning plastic materials.

- Mercurials such as mercurochrome antiseptic and thimerosal, a preservative in eyedrops

- Some drugs

Immune suppression - The immune system's purpose is to produce antibodies to outside invaders. Immune suppression causes the immune system to be less efficient at this than it should be. PAH compounds relating to combustion, such as benzo(a)pyrene and methylcholanthrene from exhaust emissions, cigarette smoke, and charcoal-broiled food have immunosuppressive effects, and are known carcinogens, or cancer causing agents. The state of Louisiana has a higher digestive system cancer rate than most other states, possibly due to dietary factors such as the consumption of blackened meats, a staple of Cajun cooking. Other immunosuppressive chemical effects are caused by:

- *7,12-dimethylbenz(a)anthracene, from incomplete burning of fossil fuels*

- *Tetrachloroazoxybenzene, from the manufacture and degradation of herbicides; such chemicals seep into our ground water.*

- *Fly ash, from coal combustion*

- *Toxaphene, carbofuran, diazinon, chlordane, and pentachlorophenol, which are insecticides and pesticides used in households by pest control companies*

- *Formaldehyde, found in laminants and other sources such as carpets and particle board*

- *Cigarette smoke*

- *Various air pollutants*

- *Some metals, including nickel, mercury, tin and lead*

- *Direct flame contact with fat from barbecued meats*

In short, chemical toxins can affect nearly every part of the body in numerous ways.

What Can You Do?

Avoid exposure to hazardous chemicals as much as possible. Chemicals to avoid and how to identify them and their sources are discussed throughout the chapters in this book section. Suggestions for chemical detoxification specific to the type of chemical are also made in the chapters in this section.

In general, sauna therapy is very helpful in eliminating almost any types of chemicals from the body. Many chemicals become stored in fat cells and only come out through the use of heat and exercise. Sauna therapy makes use of high heat (140-160 degrees F) to accelerate the elimination of toxins from the body. It is important to have a specially equipped sauna, with non-treated or safely treated wood walls and seats, oxygen piped in to reduce fatigue, and ventilation to the outside to keep you from reabsorbing eliminated toxins from the air. The average sauna in a health club does not fit these criteria.

It is also important to have medical support staff available to monitor your progress and take care of any adverse reactions. It is vital to see that you have replacement minerals and other nutrients, as minerals are lost through sweat. Fatigue and other uncomfortable and even dangerous symptoms may occur when minerals are depleted and not replaced.

It is important to open up the body's detoxification system by taking niacin, which dilates the capillaries and causes a histamine reaction which releases toxins. Ginger and large quantities of water promote sweating. These are like opening up the freeways before the city can be evacuated.

Hyperthermia (sauna) is the only detoxification program that we have seen to be consistently successful in ridding the body of fat-stored toxins such as DDE, PCBs and dioxin [13,14].

Therapies such as chelation (see Metal Detoxification chapter) and colonics are also useful, either by themselves or as an adjunct to sauna detoxification. Although chelation is mainly for removing metals, their removal or reduction can free up detoxification pathways in the body to more effectively deal with chemical toxins.

In the sauna, metal is released from the body at about 120 degrees while chemicals release at about 135 degrees. This is why metal detoxification optimally comes first.

Like any other major stressor, chemicals can permit secondary suppressors such as the various opportunistic microorganisms to gain a foothold in your weakened system. On the other hand, microorganisms such as giardia can prevent the gallbladder from processing good oils for your cells, which become oil deficient and start absorbing things like petrochemicals from the environment. You may need to take measures to treat the microorganisms and cleanse and support the gallbladder, as well as get the chemicals out.

It is a good idea to check for these microorganisms, as they may well be present. Microorganisms, and the treatments for them, are discussed in their own section of this book.

Other supportive therapies include:

- Detoxification diet

- Liver / Gallbladder flush helps optimize liver function, since the liver is a major organ of detoxification.

- Lymph massage and exercises help to move toxins from storage in the lymph glands into the bloodstream for elimination.

- Homeopathics

- Constitutional hydrotherapy allows the elimination of toxin-laden fluids [15]. Hydrotherapy includes whirlpool baths and hot and cold packs which stimulate and increase blood and lymph circulation.

- Glutathione complex helps in detoxification, especially of metals.

- Sulfur is necessary for the sulfur-based amino acids which aid detoxification.

- Kyolic garlic

- Sun Chlorella

- ACES antioxidants (Carlson Labs) act against free radical damage.

- Allergy treatment such as NAET, discussed in the Toxic Immune Syndrome chapter in *Thriving In A Toxic World* [16,17]. This can help desensitize a person to particular chemicals, but is not a substitute for eliminating the chemical from the environment and the body.

Summary

There are a large number of chemical toxins, and we are not aware of many of these.

Chronic exposure to these chemicals can cause a multitude of symptoms, including some you may have thought you just have to endure. A recognition of the sources of chemical toxicity can enable you to avoid them and lower the prevalence of symptoms caused by them.

Poisons do their damage in a number of ways, including anoxia (oxygen starvation), replacement reactions, and corrosiveness.

References and Resources

- Arena, Jay M., *Poisoning: Toxicology, Symptoms, Treatments*, Charles C. Thomas (publisher), 1974, 3rd ed.

- Ashford, Nicholas A. and Claudia S. Miller, *Chemical Exposures: Low Levels and High Stakes*, Van Nostrand Reinhold, NY, 1990.

- Bodin, F., and C.F. Chernisse, *Poisons*, McGraw-Hill Book Co., New York, 1970.

- Boyle, Wade, and Andre Saine, *Lectures in Naturopathic Hydrotherapy*, Buckeye Naturopathic Press, Palestine OH, 1988. *Discusses hydrotherapy and hyperthermia (sauna) in connection with chemical detoxification.*

- The Burton Goldberg Group, *Alternative Medicine: The Definitive Guide*, Future Medicine Publishing, Puyallup WA, 1994. *A number of chapters deal with methods that support chemical detoxification:*

Chelation Therapy	*pp. 126-133*	*Chelation*
Colon Therapy	*pp. 143-148*	*Colonics*
Detoxification Therapy	*pp. 156-165*	*Detoxification in general*
Environmental Medicine	*pp. 205-214*	*Environmental illness, chemical sensitivities*
Homeopathy	*pp. 272-280*	*Homeopathy*
Hydrotherapy	*pp. 281-298*	*Also called constitutional hydrotherapy*
Hyperthermia	*pp. 299-305*	*Another word for sauna therapy*

- Casaret and Doull, *Toxicology*, Macmillan Publishing Co., New York, 1986, 3rd ed. *Technical but very thorough. Considered a classic in the field.*

- Randolph, Theron G., *Human Ecology and Susceptibility to the Chemical Environment*, Charles C. Thomas Publishers, 1981.

- Rogers, Sherry A., *Tired or Toxic?*, Prestige Publishing, Syracuse NY, 1990.

- Rousseau, D., Rea, W.J and J. Enwright, *Your Home, Your Health and Well Being*, Hartley and Marks, Vancouver B.C., 1988. *How to build or renovate a non-toxic home.*

- Saifer, P. and M. Zellerbach, *Detox*, Jeremy P. Tarcher Inc., Los Angeles CA, 1984.

- Sherman, Janette D., *Chemical Exposure and Disease*, Princeton Scientific Publishing Co., Princeton NJ.

- Steinman, David and Samuel Epstein, *The Safe Shopper's Bible*, Macmillan, NY, 1994.

- Williams, Roger J., *Nutrition Against Disease: Environmental Protection*, Bantam Books, NY, 1971.

Human Ecology Action League (HEAL), P.O. Box 49126, Atlanta GA 30359, phone 404-248-1898. *They can refer you to support groups around the country that help patients with Environmental Illness.*

ORGANIC COMPOUNDS AND SOLVENTS

How To Dissolve Your Health

Do you have any of the these symptoms? They could be due to exposure to organic chemicals and solvents:

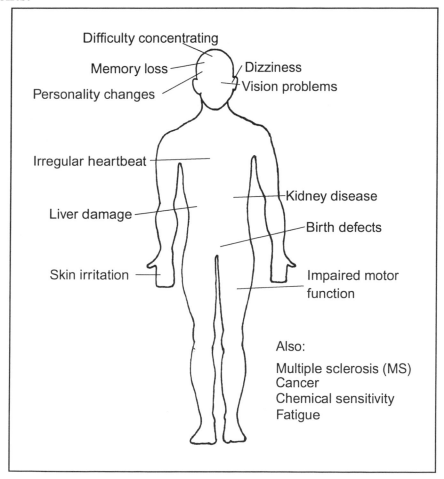

Difficulty concentrating
Memory loss
Personality changes
Dizziness
Vision problems
Irregular heartbeat
Kidney disease
Liver damage
Birth defects
Skin irritation
Impaired motor function

Also:

Multiple sclerosis (MS)
Cancer
Chemical sensitivity
Fatigue

In this chapter you can learn:

- *What does organic really mean?*
- *What are solvents and how do they do their damage?*

What does organic really mean?

Organic compounds are those compounds containing carbon. They usually also contain hydrogen, sometimes oxygen, and sometimes other elements. Organic, in this case, is not to be confused with organic health food produce.

Halocarbons contain halides, which are the elements chlorine, fluorine, bromine, or iodine, in place of one or more hydrogen atoms. Chlorinated compounds are the most common halocarbons.

H	H
|	|
H — C — H	Cl — C — Cl
|	|
H	H
Methane	**Dichloromethane**
(Not Chlorinated)	(Chlorinated)
	(Di = 2, Chloro = Chlorinated, Methane = Methane Base)

The organics under discussion here are generally

- *lipophilic (oil soluble)*
- *used as solvents, glues, paints, or in similar products*
- *toxic to varying degrees*

Toxic organics can be taken into the body by inhalation, absorption through the skin, and sometimes by drinking contaminated water.

Who is most susceptible to damage by organic chemicals?

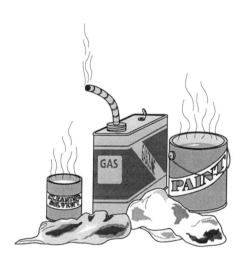

The oil solubility of organics poses a particular problem to people. The oil solubility causes them to collect in fatty tissues, where they are released slowly into the bloodstream to cause long-lasting toxic symptoms, rather than being excreted quickly. People who are oil-deficient, such as dieters and those with gallbladder problems, are at particular risk since the oil-starved body will latch onto oily substances such as diesel exhaust, in much the same way a dry sponge soaks up water.

By contrast, a person with enough good oil in their body will be more like a duck than a sponge; water rolls off a duck's back because of the oil in the duck's feathers.

What are solvents and how do they do their damage?

Industrial solvents are intended to be solvents of fats, or degreasers. In the body, they are especially attracted to the fatty sheaths of nerve fibers and the lipid (fatty) membranes of cells. The partial dissolving of these nerve fiber sheaths leads to nervous system effects such as:

- *Memory loss*
- *Difficulty concentrating*
- *Impaired dexterity*
- *Reduced motor function*
- *Altered personality*
- *Multiple sclerosis (MS)*

Carbon disulfide, used in rubber vulcanization, is an example of a chemical which can cause psychiatric disturbances. It is, in fact, very possible that many psychiatric problems have chemical toxicity as their root cause.

Nerve fibers conduct impulses from the brain, acting as both a relay and an amplifier, both passing on and speeding up the message. The myelin sheath acts like the outer insulation of an electrical cord. The erosion of the myelin sheath is like the fraying of an electrical cord, and nerve impulses can dissipate by shorting into nearby tissue rather than speeding up and reaching their destination. This leakage of the body's "electricity" can cause muscle and meningeal contraction, with resulting pain and deformity. Multiple sclerosis (MS) is a disease of the myelin sheath, and may be linked to solvents as well as to mercury and nickel.

Aspartic acid, an amino acid found in certain supplements and in the artificial sweetener aspartame (NutriSweet), has a similar detergent (oil dissolving) effect on the myelin sheaths. Although a necessary nutrient in small quantities, consistent doses of supplemental aspartic acid can also have this detrimental effect, especially in people with low body fat. (Aspartic acid as an additive may be listed as calcium aspartate).

What other problems do solvents cause?
Other solvent effects include: [1,2]

- **Carcinogenicity** - Many solvents are linked to the development of cancer, since they can penetrate the lipid (fat) membrane around the cells and damage the DNA (blueprint for reproduction). Vinyl chloride from plastics [3] and benzene from gasoline and room deodorizers [4] are some organics that can cause this kind of damage.

- **Skin irritations** due to skin contact with liquid or vapor are caused by removal of oil from the skin. A different type of skin effect was experienced by a patient who used to work on cars and would clean his hands with whatever solvent was available such as gasoline or transmission fluid. Years later his hands are still slightly numb, as if he were wearing gloves. It is possible that the fatty myelin sheaths of the nerves in his hands were damaged by the solvents, resulting in a garbled message when sensations such as touch are relayed from the hands to the brain.

- **Liver** - The liver is damaged by chloroform, ethanol (beverage alcohol, also a solvent), and other alcohols. Cirrhosis (drying, scarring, and hardening) of the liver is a well-known effect of chronic alcoholism for this reason. Alcohol also increases liver damage from other solvents.

- **Immune system** - Solvents suppress lymphocyte (white blood cell) function, adversely affecting the body's ability to fight off disease organisms.

- **Cardiac effects** - Fluorocarbons and other halogenated (containing halogen) elements such as chlorine or bromine) alkanes (straight-chain molecules) can cause cardiac arrhythmias (irregular heartbeat). These arrhythmias can be brought on by wearing a newly dry-cleaned suit or working with white typewriter correction fluid [5,6]. Teenagers have died from cardiac arrhythmias caused by the deliberate inhalation of correction fluid to get "high" [7].

- **Kidney** - Glomerulonephritis, a life-threatening kidney disease affecting the tubules of the kidney, can result from solvent exposure [8,9]. The condition can lead to dependence on kidney dialysis.

- **Panic attacks** have been linked to organic solvents common in the workplace [10].

What are some examples of solvents and their effects?

Trichloroethylene (TCE) - TCE is used as an industrial degreaser, dry cleaning fluid, and paint thinner. It is found in photocopy machines, correction fluid, carpet cleaning solution and floor polishes, and so is in many if not most office environments. It used to be used as a surgical anesthetic because it was so effective in causing loss of brain function. Health affects include [11]:

- *Headache*
- *CNS depression*
- *Poor coordination*
- *Nausea*
- *Burning eyes*
- *Mental confusion*
- *Cancer*
- *Irritability*
- *Disturbed vision*
- *Tremors*
- *Prenatal damage*
- *Loss of facial sensation*
- *Fatigue*
- *Muscle cramps*
- *Numbness and tingling in hands and feet*

Toluene - Toluene is used as a manufacturing intermediate for rubber, plastics, and is a component of gasoline. It is also found in:

- *The food preservative BHT - T stands for Toluene*
- *Tires*
- *Fragrances in perfumes*
- *Furniture wax*
- *Rug cleaning solutions*
- *Ink*
- *Plastic garbage bags*
- *Kitty litter*
- *Hairspray and hair gel*
- *Guitar string cleaner*

Points of attack are the central nervous system, liver, kidneys, and skin. Toluene can cause a number of symptoms including [12]:

- *Cancer*
- *Myelin disease such as MS*
- *Birth defects*
- *Asthma attacks*
- *Fatigue*
- *Headaches, seizures*
- *Brain fog, inability to concentrate, depression*

How can new carpeting kill mice and harm babies?

Formaldehyde is used primarily as a bonding material, and it has many diverse uses. Products that it can be found in include [13]:

- *Paints*
- *Pesticides*
- *Cleaning supplies*
- *Nail polish*
- *Air fresheners*
- *Foam insulation*

- *Glues*
- *Fuels*
- *Plywood*
- *Plastics*
- *Textiles*

- *Paper products*
- *Antiperspirants*
- *Fertilizers*
- *Cosmetics*
- *Mattresses, couches, cushions*

- *Tobacco smoke*
- *Carpeting, carpet pads*
- *Ceiling tile*
- *Particle board*

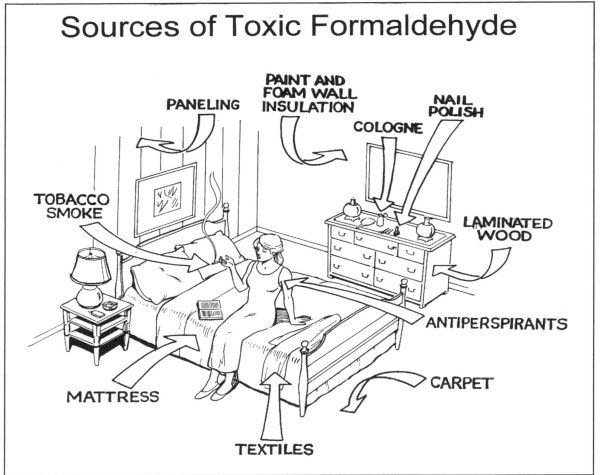

Particle board is made from wood waste (chips and sawdust) and 7% by weight of urea-formaldehyde. Particle board outgasses formaldehyde, especially when new and during hot, humid weather [14]. Formaldehyde is especially prevalent in mobile homes, which generally have a lot of particle board wood paneling and a small enclosed space.

One study showed that the addition of furniture to an otherwise empty house tripled formaldehyde levels [15].

Formaldehyde and other chemicals found in carpeting have been found in tests to kill mice that are kept in newly carpeted cages. Babies that crawl around on carpet, especially new carpet, can absorb considerable amounts of these chemicals due to the closeness of their nose and mouth to the carpet, and due to the comparatively large amount of skin contact with the carpet. One patient, a baby who was exposed to formaldehyde in this way, was red, puffy, blotchy, irritable and in pain, and had to be detoxified of the chemical by sauna therapy.

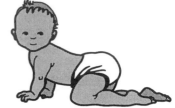

Do you think you have to die before you have embalming fluid in your body?

Formaldehyde is the primary ingredient in and has a characteristic odor of embalming fluid, unpleasantly familiar to Biology students and those who have visited mortuaries. Formaldehyde or embalming fluid suffocates the cells, or prevents oxygen from reaching them, so they don't decay. Unfortunately the cells of your body are also suffocated by formaldehyde. The characteristic smell of many dental offices is due to chemicals that include formaldehyde.

You can be affected by formaldehyde without being aware of the odor. Formaldehyde enters the body primarily through inhalation. It is also a metabolite of methanol (wood alcohol), which can be a contaminant (up to 10%) of ethanol (grain, or beverage, alcohol). The formaldehyde from the methanol may be partially responsible for the DTs suffered by alcoholics during withdrawal. Methanol is also a breakdown product of aspartame, the artificial sweetener.

A sensitivity to formaldehyde may be due to cross-reactivity with acetaldehyde, a byproduct of alcohol.

Health effects from chronic exposure to formaldehyde include [16, 17]:

- *Headaches*
- *Fatigue*
- *Arthritis*
- *Depression*
- *Nausea*
- *Immune system suppression*
- *Chronic cough, asthma*
- *Brain fog, inability to concentrate*
- *Chemical and food sensitivities*
- *Eye, nose, and throat irritation, burning*
- *Cancer, especially lung, pharynx, nose sinus, kidney, and brain [18]*

How much formaldehyde does it take to be a problem?

Even short-term exposure to formaldehyde can cause the following symptoms at levels as low as these, expressed in parts per million (ppm) [19]:

Symptoms	Concentration, ppm	Exposure time, minutes
Eye irritation	0.01	5
Able to smell it	0.05	1
Runny nose	0.05	5
Sore throat	0.5	5
Cough	0.8	5
Headache, disoriented	0.8-1.0	10-30

If a one to thirty minute exposure can cause symptoms, imagine the damage that can be caused with years of exposure!

To put these amounts in ppm into perspective, consider the amounts that are found in the following places [17]:

Normal house	0.03 ppm
House with UFFI*	0.12
Energy efficient home, even w/o UFFI*	0.10
Mobile home	0.40
Office building	0.44
Hospital	0.55
Shopping mall	1.50
Permanent press fabrics	0.70
Paper products	1.00
Biology lab	8.50

*UFFI = urea formaldehyde foam insulation

Studies have also shown that formaldehyde can cause damage to genetic material which can initiate cancer [4], while other studies have shown adverse effects at 0.12 to 1.6 ppm [20]. Formaldehyde is also a major contributor to Multiple Chemical Sensitivity (MCS), also known as Environmental Illness (EI).

In spite of this and other evidence, the government agency OSHA, which establishes regulations pertaining to chemical toxicity, feels that 3 ppm is a reasonable long-term exposure limit [21].

What are some other organic chemicals to watch out for?

- **Carbon disulfide**, used in rubber vulcanization, can cause nerve damage in the hands and feet, and psychosis.

- **Methyl chloride**, used in rubber and plastics, can cause nerve damage in the hands and feet, blurred vision, and short-term memory loss.

- **Acetone**, a common solvent used in nail polish remover and in cellulose production, can cause vertigo (dizziness) and weakness.

- **Methylene chloride**, a solvent with multiple uses including decaffeinating coffee, can cause delusions and hallucinations.

What Can You Do?

How can a buildup of organic chemicals in the body be treated?
Sauna detoxification, discussed in the Chemical Toxicity chapter, is very useful for ridding the body of organic compounds. The heat allows the toxins to be released from storage depots in the fat, liver and elsewhere, and then eliminated.

Oral glutathione, best known as a metal chelator, contains sulfur compounds which are part of the body's chemical detoxification system. Using chelation to remove metals from the body also frees up the body's own detoxification mechanisms to go after chemicals more effectively. Chelation is discussed in the Metal Detoxification chapter.

Supplements and other therapies useful in the elimination of chemicals from the body are discussed in the Chemical Toxicity chapter.

References and Resources

- Bodin, F., and C.F. Chernisse, *Poisons*, McGraw-Hill Book Co., New York, 1970.

- The Burton Goldberg Group, "Detoxification Therapy", pp. 156-165, *Alternative Medicine: The Definitive Guide*, Future Medicine Publishing, Puyallup WA, 1994.

- Dadd, Debra Lynn, *Nontoxic and Natural*, Jeremy P. Tarcher Inc., Los Angeles CA, 1984.

- Kaura, S.R., *Understanding and Preventing Cancer*, Health Press, Santa Fe NM, 1991.

- Meyer, Beat, *Indoor Air Quality*, Addison-Wesley Publishing Co., Reading MA, 1983.

- Rogers, Sherry A., *Tired or Toxic?*, Prestige Publishing, Syracuse NY, 1990.

- Rogers, Sherry A., *The E.I. Syndrome*, Prestige Publishing, Syracuse NY, 1986.

- Thrasher, Jack and Alan Broughton, *The Poisoning Of Our Homes and Workplaces*, Seadora, Inc., 1989. *Focuses on indoor formaldehyde toxicity.*

PESTICIDES

Is There That Much Difference Between you and a Bug?

Do you have any of the following symptoms? They could be due to exposure to pesticides:

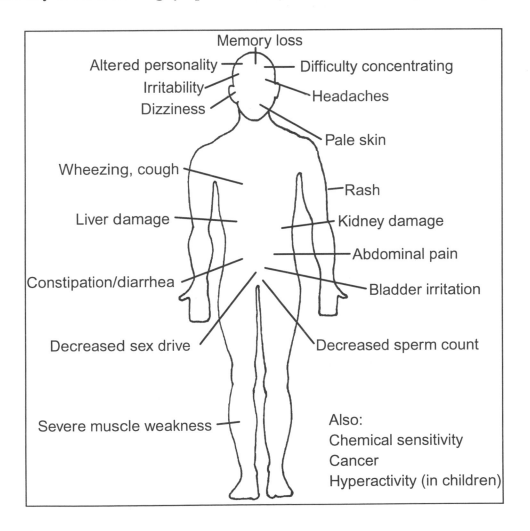

Memory loss
Altered personality
Difficulty concentrating
Irritability
Dizziness
Headaches
Pale skin
Wheezing, cough
Rash
Liver damage
Kidney damage
Abdominal pain
Constipation/diarrhea
Bladder irritation
Decreased sex drive
Decreased sperm count
Severe muscle weakness
Also:
Chemical sensitivity
Cancer
Hyperactivity (in children)

In this chapter you can learn:

- *Why are pesticides so toxic to us?*
- *How can you protect yourself from pesticide toxicity through diet?*
- *How can you be exposed to pesticides other than by deliberately spraying them?*
- *Why are progressively stronger and more toxic pesticides needed?*

- *Are the "inert" ingredients on the pesticide label harmless to us?*
- *What are some safe and effective alternatives to chemical pesticides?*

What are pesticides?

Pesticide is a generic term for chemicals which are made deliberately toxic to kill various types of pests. These include:

- *Insecticides*   *for insects*
- *Rodenticides*   *for rodents and vermin*
- *Herbicides*   *for weeds and unwanted plants*
- *Fungicides*   *for fungi and molds*

How many pesticides are there?

There are about 1500 different chemical pesticides [1], each of which can have many trade names. Thiram, for example, a common carbamate fungicide, had 26 trade names [2].

What is the difference between humans and bugs?

Pesticides are toxic to both bugs and people. People have fat in their bodies, and since pesticides are oil soluble they are stored in our fat. Bugs have no fat in their bodies, and so the pesticide attacks their nervous systems directly. The effect on bugs is acute, or short term. The effect on people is chronic, or long term, because the pesticide is stored in our fat and elsewhere in our bodies and released slowly rather than affecting us all at once [3]. However, when our fat is loaded with toxins, we lose this advantage.

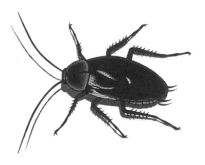

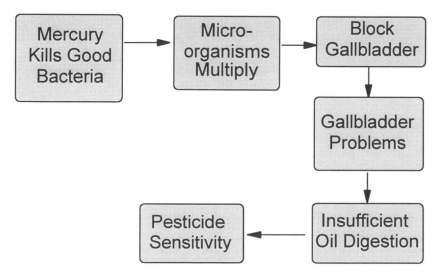

Some people are oil deficient, so this causes them to react more like a bug, i.e. suffer from more severe (acute) symptoms. Even an overweight person can be oil deficient. Oil deficiency can result from an insufficient intake of beneficial cis oils. It can also result from gallbladder problems, since the gallbladder digests and processes oils. Parasites such as giardia, which themselves may be secondary to mercury amalgam fillings due to the antibiotic (killing) action of mercury on the beneficial bacteria which protect us from parasites, can cause gallbladder problems.

How can people be exposed to pesticides?
People can be exposed to pesticides in a number of ways.

- *Inhaling sprayed pesticides*
- *Drinking water contaminated by runoff from sprayed fields.*
- *Eating meat and poultry which has been fed pesticide-sprayed grain*

Eating fruits, vegetables, and grains that have been sprayed is another way to be exposed to pesticides. The EPA has identified 66 cancer-causing pesticides that may leave residues in foods [4]. It is possible to ingest pesticides that have been banned in this country by eating imported foods. Ironically, pesticides banned from domestic use can be manufactured in this country. These pesticides are shipped to foreign countries, which use them on produce that they then ship back to the United States.

Organic produce is legally defined in California as that which is grown without chemical pesticides or non-natural fertilizers. Although organic produce is often more expensive, the extra cost may be worth it if you want to avoid exposure to these toxic substances.

It is significant that 25-50% of pesticides sprayed or dropped from the air miss the field that is their intended target. Over half of these enter the surrounding environment. 98% of the pesticides are ineffective against the insects they were originally meant to kill [5].

The use of lindane, a pesticide, on carrot crops caused a 15-50% decrease in the nutrient carotene, a vitamin A precursor [6].

Ron, a lawyer in his early 40s, developed kidney and liver problems; he lived in an agricultural, produce growing area that used pesticide sprays .

Another patient, an interior decorator in her 50s, lived in the agricultural San Joaquin Valley. She developed a number of symptoms which kept her from working, including brain fog, fibromyalgia (whole body pain) and fatigue. Diesel fumes, pesticides and perfumes brought on headaches. After sauna and other detoxification procedures, she recovered.

A possible cause of the problems both of these patients experienced is the high level of pesticides present in these areas.

How long are pesticides toxic?
Pesticides are long-lived and fat-soluble, so they can remain in the soil and in our bodies for decades, leaching out slowly and causing chronic damage. Release of these fat stored chemicals could explain why some people get sick when they lose weight. The fat acts as storage barrels for toxic waste, and when the fat/ storage barrel is removed, the toxins enter the body systems via the bloodstream, causing symptoms.

> **Pesticides can stay in the body for decades, causing trouble during that time.**

It is not uncommon for a person undergoing sauna therapy to release pesticides and other organic chemicals in their sweat to such an extent that a person nearby can smell the chemicals. This can happen even if the initial exposure was years or decades ago.

Nearly all Americans have residues of the pesticides DDT, chlordane, heptachlor, aldrin, and dieldrin in their bodies in spite of the fact that these chemicals have been banned for agricultural use for up to two decades. At least 46 pesticides have been found in ground water, used by most Americans for drinking water, in at least 26 states [4].

What are the main categories of pesticides?
There have been three generations of pesticides throughout history:

- *Salts (metal compounds) of heavy metals such as arsenic, lead, copper, mercury, and zinc. These were in use up to World War II, and are extremely toxic.*

- *Chlorinated and petrochemical-based pesticides, the first of which was DDT, introduced shortly after World War II.*

- *Organic pesticides and botanicals (plant products), which are coming into wider use as the toxicity of the chemical pesticides becomes more widely known.*

The term "organic" may cause some confusion. It can be used to refer to any carbon based molecule, including toxic petrochemical pesticides, as differentiated from inorganics such as metal salts. "Organic" can also be used to describe products derived from nature and which are relatively safe, a definition which would exclude petrochemical pesticides.

Buyer Beware! Some pesticide companies take advantage of this confusion. Misleading advertising states, "we use only organic pesticides", a statement which is chemically accurate. They count on the average consumer's perception of the word "organic" as meaning natural and safe. The consumer, thus deliberately confused, signs up for the pesticide company's services and is exposed to highly toxic chemicals. Meanwhile the pesticide company is legally in the clear because they are technically telling the truth. Buyer beware!

What types of pesticides present the greatest threat?
We are primarily concerned with exposure to chlorinated and petrochemical pesticides, as the other two types represent an insignificant threat at present. There are three types of organic pesticides which account for over 90% of pesticide use [7]:

- *Carbamates, which poison essential cell and nerve functions, are found in ant, fly, and roach killers.*

- *Organophosphates such as malathion block nerve activity, and are found in products to control plant pests.*

- *Halogenated pesticides control agricultural pests by poisoning cell metabolism.*

Organophosphate pesticides such as malathion cause [8]:

- *Long term alteration in brain waves and brain electrical activity, resulting in insomnia and irritability, and altered learning patterns and behavior.*

- *Severe muscular weakness*

- *Memory loss*

- *Difficulty in concentrating*

- *Decreased libido*

Malathion spraying has been known to damage paint on cars. Imagine the damage to our lungs and bodies!

> **Malathion can damage paint on cars. Imagine the damage to your lungs and body!**

A number of people came into a progressive clinic with health problems following Malathion spraying in California. One of these, a female computer programmer and top athlete with low body fat, came in with brain fog and low energy related to pesticide exposure. Her low body fat may have worsened her symptoms, as body fat acts as a buffer.

Ethylene dibromide (EDB) may be the most toxic pesticide in use today. It has been banned recently but is still in our grains and flours, and in imported products such as fruits and vegetables.

Nearly 50,000 cases of pesticide poisoning are reported every year [5]. A National Research Council study found that complete health hazard evaluations were available for only 10% of pesticides [9].

Why are more toxic pesticides necessary?

Insects develop a resistance to pesticides, so ever stronger ones are necessary to have the same effect. Individual insects do not become more resistant, but the species as a whole does. For instance, if a colony of ants is sprayed with insecticide, most of them will die. The small percentage not killed are genetically stronger and survive the spraying. (This is analogous to the way some people historically have been able to survive many of our diseases and plagues, such as the Black Plague.) These resistant ants breed with each other, producing future ant generations which also have pesticide resistant genes, as do their offspring for generations. Spraying these resistant ants with the same amount and type of insecticide as before will have little or no effect, so larger amounts or stronger insecticides will be necessary. Within a few insect generations, these new insecticides will be likewise ineffective.

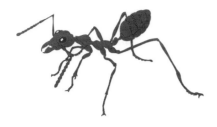

Some insects become so used to the insecticide that they live, eat, and breed in daily contact with the poison. One person's home was sprayed before he moved in years ago, but there is still an ant problem. If a number of these ants are killed manually, for example by stepping on a few dozen of them at once, their bodies release the distinctive odor of the insecticide. The poison no longer affects them at all.

The same type of resistance is developed by other pests such as mice, weeds, and the troublesome bacteria and fungi which live in our bodies. These "bugs" in our bodies have become resistant to antibiotics and fungicides so effective a few decades ago.

A bug that lives for, say, one year has 80 generations to adapt to pesticides, compared to our one 80-year lifespan. In a sense the risk to us is 80:1 compared to that of a bug. Since many bugs live less than a year, the risk ratio would then be even more than 80:1.

Why are pesticides more of a threat to us than to pests?

If many of us were to die off from the poisoning before breeding, within a number of generations our offspring might hypothetically become resistant to pesticides presently in use. This knowledge is of no use to those of us alive today. This is why pesticides, designed to be more toxic to pests than to us, actually end up doing more damage to us than to the ants happily swarming in our kitchens.

Why are people with ulcers more susceptible to poisoning by pesticides and other toxins?

Primary toxic suppressors such as metals, chemicals (including pesticides), or radiation can start a vicious cycle:

1. Primary suppressors lower immune function, kill protective bacteria, and lower resistance to destructive bacteria.

2. Bacteria such as helicobacter pylori gain a foothold in your body.

3. Bacteria put off toxic byproducts.

4. These byproducts adversely affect the gallbladder, blocking the hepatic bile duct.

5. Reduced gallbladder function reduces oil digestion and absorption. Symptoms of poor gallbladder function include

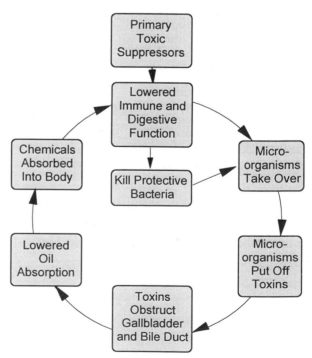

    tight shoulders, stiff neck and head pressure

6. Oil soluble chemicals, including pesticides, are absorbed into the body to a greater extent - the dry sponge effect.

7. These chemicals lower immune function further, leading to environmental illness (EI) and autoimmune diseases.

Pesticides can cause or worsen adverse reactions to other substances, or vice versa. A person taking the anti-ulcer medication Tagamet can be much more sensitive to pesticides, since Tagamet, as well as some other drugs, blocks the major liver detoxifying enzyme cytochrome P450 [10].

One patient, a man in his mid 30s who was very thin due to low body fat, was taking Tagamet and was exposed to pesticides. He became chemically overwhelmed. He couldn't be near chemicals or he would develop headaches and brain fog. He lost his job as a custodian due to his sensitivities.

Both Tagamet and helicobacter pylori (which can cause ulcers) affects the gallbladder, resulting in poor oil digestion and absorption, which in turn compromises a patient's ability to cope with chemicals. Working backwards from this reasoning, helicobacter pylori is often found in patients who have chemical toxicity or sensitivity problems.

There is also interaction between organophosphate pesticides and acetaminophen (Tylenol) [11].

What about insect repellents?
Insect repellents do not kill insects but merely set up an inhospitable environment for them. Repellents are the smelly oily substances you smear on your skin to avoid being bitten by mosquitoes or ticks. One of the most common insect repellents is N,N-diethyltoluamide, better known as Deet. It can be absorbed into the bloodstream through the skin, causing allergic reactions and nerve damage. Seizures have been linked to this compound [12]. And more recently, a case of death within two hours of absorption through the skin was cited in a TV documentary reporting on Deet.

Don't herbicides only harm plants?
Herbicides are formulated to kill plants. However, there is reason to believe that they are not harmless to humans.

Plants have chlorophyll, which give them their green color. Humans and other mammals have hemoglobin in their blood, which gives it a red color and is involved in oxygen transport. The chemical structures of chlorophyll and hemoglobin are startlingly similar, consisting in both cases of a structure called a porphyrin ring with a single metal atom in the middle - iron in the case of hemoglobin and magnesium in the case of chlorophyll. The metal atom gives the substance its characteristic color.

When a plant is sprayed with an herbicide, it goes from a healthy green color to a sickly brown color. Since hemoglobin is so chemically similar to plant chlorophyll, it seems reasonable that herbicides can also damage our hemoglobin, and thus adversely affect oxygen transport to our tissues. Lowered oxygen to the tissues and brain can lead to fatigue and impairment of mental function, depression and anxiety, among other symptoms.

What are some of the effects of chronic pesticide exposure?

There are many hundreds of chemical and trade names of pesticides, which will not be detailed here. Lists of these pesticides can be found in some of the books named as references for this chapter. Since the purpose of the various pesticides is the same - to kill life - the toxic effects of the various chemical pesticides are similar. Since bugs have cells, the function of which is the target of the pesticides, and we have cells, it is not surprising that our cells sustain damage as do those of the pests.

Fatigue and forgetfulness are some of the most common symptoms of pesticide exposure [13]. Other effects of chronic pesticide exposure are:

- **Carcinogenicity** - The cancer causing potential of pesticides is further discussed in the chapter on Carcinogens. A study of farmers in Italy who were licensed to use pesticides showed a significant increase in cancer, especially that of the stomach, kidney, rectum and pancreas [14]. Pesticides such as DDT, DDE, and PCBs affect the body the way too much estrogen does, and in this way can contribute to the development of estrogen-dependent breast cancer. A study cited with Archives of Environmental Health found 50-60% more DDE and PCBs in women with breast cancer than in women without cancer [15].

  Women working in the agricultural field have higher rates of cancer of the breast, ovary, and cervix as well as of the lung and bladder, and lymphoma and leukemia, as compared with women overall [16]. Pesticide exposure is the most likely risk factor.

- **Central nervous system** (CNS) effects - These include headaches, dizziness, loss of motor control, learning disabilities in children, CNS depression, behavioral disorders, frontal lobe (of the brain) impairment. In one study, Dieldrin was found in the brains of 6 out of 20 Parkinson's disease victims, but in none of the fourteen control samples [17]. This implicates Dieldrin and possibly other pesticides in the causation of, or at least contributing to, Parkinson's disease. Another study links pesticides to young-onset Parkinson's disease, which more usually affects the elderly [18].

- **Hyperactivity** in children [15].

- **Skin problems** of various types [19].

- **Gastrointestinal** symptoms - nausea, anorexia (loss of appetite), abdominal pains, excessive salivation.

- **Pancreas** effects - Pancreatitis (pancreas inflammation) and diabetes have been linked to pesticide exposure [20].

- **Liver** effects - jaundice, fatty liver, necrosis (cell death), increased susceptibility to viral hepatitis.

- **Kidney** effects - albumin or protein in urine, tubular necrosis (tissue death of the tubules in the kidneys, which help filter out toxins). A study of 1249 people living in a rural environment, with pesticide exposure, showed that the frequency of infectious inflammatory kidney lesions was 7.9-13.4% as compared with 1.5% in the controls [21].

- **Endocrine / Reproductive** - Pesticides and herbicides are associated with disruption in endocrine, reproductive and sexual function [22].

- **Respiratory** effects - pulmonary edema, chest tightness, bronchial constriction or spasm, wheezing, cough.

- **Other** effects - muscle weakness, pallor.

Some of these effects, especially nerve damage, are irreversible, as stated in a medical journal article as early as 1958 [23].

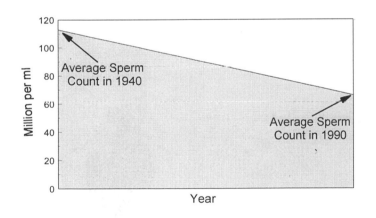

Aberrations relating to hormonal levels, especially in males, have been linked to prenatal pesticide exposure. Sperm counts have fallen in the last two generations. In an international study of almost 15,000 men, average sperm counts have dropped from 113 million per ml in 1940 to 66 million per ml in 1990 [24].

Undescended testicles in young boys have also increased in incidence.

Head lice? Think twice before you use that special shampoo.
Shampoo formulated to kill head lice usually contains Lindane or other pesticides. These toxic substances are rubbed into the scalp and left on for a while, using warm water that will increase penetration through the skin. Neurological and other health problems have been associated with the use of these pesticide-containing shampoos [25].

One patient, a woman in her mid 30s, was treated for lice and had brain and central nervous system damage, including anxiety and seizures. Sauna detoxification helped her regain her health.

Pets as well as people can be adversely affected by these pesticides. In one case, a dog washed in flea shampoo but not rinsed well started shaking and getting sick. A thorough rinsing in the shower reversed these symptoms. Otherwise the dog might have died for no apparent reason.

Are ingredients labeled "inert" on the pesticide label safe?

A warning when label reading - ingredients are listed as active or inert. Active ingredients are those which, in the case of pesticides, kill pests. Inert ingredients are those that do not kill pests, but the name is misleading in that they are not necessarily inert in the body. Some of them may in fact be more toxic than the "active" ingredients. The terms active and inert refer only to those ingredients which do, or do not, have the effect suggested by the label. Potential harm to humans is not considered when calling an ingredient "inert". Such ingredients need not be listed at all.

Forty "inert" ingredients are actually toxic by EPA (Environmental Protection Agency) standards and may cause cancer, brain and nervous system poisoning, and birth defects. Another sixty are classified as potentially toxic due to similarity to known harmful compounds. For example, the herbicide Roundup contains the "inert" ingredient POEA, which is more toxic to humans than "active" ingredient glyphosate [26].

What are some alternatives to chemical pesticides?

Alternatives to petrochemical and toxic pesticides include [15,24,27]:

- Plants such as marigolds repel certain harmful insect species.

- Chrysanthemums are another plant that can repel and even kill insects. Pesticides made from chrysanthemums are called pyrethrins. They are much less toxic than commercial pesticides and their toxicity to humans vanishes within a day of spraying.

- Helpful insects such as ladybugs which eat aphids, and praying mantises. These can be obtained from stores that supply organic gardeners.

- Attract birds by putting up bird feeders, since birds eat insects.

- An invasion of ants in the house can be controlled by keeping food where they can't get at it. If they find it, they touch feelers to communicate with the rest of the nest that there is a party going on at your house.

- If ants still get out of hand, they can be vacuumed up using the crevice tool on a vacuum cleaner.

- Orange and lemon peels repel some insects such as ants.

- Mint sprinkled or planted near ant nests repels them.

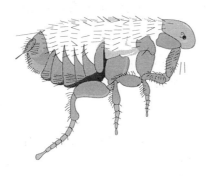

- Daily thorough vacuuming is somewhat useful in keeping the flea population down.

- Brewers yeast and B vitamins fed to your pets will make them less attractive to fleas.

- A product made by Avon called Skin-So-Soft, when applied to a dog's coat, has been said to repel fleas.

- Garlic and bay leaves repel cockroaches.

- Another method which is sometimes successful against certain pests is heat. Close all windows, remove pets and plants, plan to stay elsewhere for a few days, and crank up every safe source of heat you have. This can also help burn off toxic paint and carpet fumes.

- Boric acid, a granular white solid often sold as a laundry cleaner, repels pests such as ants. It is not entirely nontoxic, but is safer than most insecticides.

- Some companies now use liquid nitrogen, which is much colder than your household freezer, to freeze a wide variety of pests. Nitrogen is nontoxic if not breathed directly when cold, and leaves no residue. Nitrogen also kills by substituting for oxygen, needed by termites for life.

- In addition to nitrogen, termites can be killed using microwaves or an electro-gun. Like nitrogen, these leave no lingering chemicals.

- Tobacco water, made by soaking cigarette or pipe tobacco in water, can be used to water plants to kill some insects that infest plants. It makes sense that tobacco is harmful to both ourselves and insects.

- Cloves and clove oil repel some insects, including flies and ants.

- Rubbing alcohol can be wiped, or detergent solution can be sprayed, on plant leaves to kill plant pests.

How can the right type of fertilizer discourage plant pests?

It is helpful to fertilize plants using natural materials. Just as our bodies are stronger on natural and healthful foods, so do plants respond better with natural fertilizers such as manure and compost. In an experiment with fertilizers, tomato plants were divided into two groups: those fertilized naturally and those fertilized with synthetic sources of nitrogen such as ammonium sulfate. The naturally fertilized plants grew tastier - and probably more nutrient-rich - tomatoes. It came as a surprise to find that bugs strongly preferred the artificially fertilized plants.

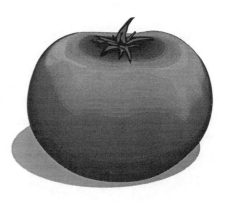

It seems that plants produce their own natural bug and disease repellent when fed as intended by divine creation.

The natural nitrogen controls the intake and communication of the cells so they take in only nutritious and not toxic things. This is true for both plants and people.

Are there any tests for pesticides in the body?

A technique called gas chromatography can measure pesticides in a body fat sample. In addition, an IgG test can determine whether your blood cells are reacting to pesticides. This test determines reactivity rather than the direct presence of pesticides. Pesticides are rarely found in high levels in the blood or urine because they are stored in the fat.

Did you know that pesticides can contribute to overweight?

Pesticides are stored primarily in fat but also in the liver. One of the causes of overweight is the body's retention of water and fat to try to dilute pesticides and other poisons. These stored toxins will be released slowly, causing symptoms, until they are excreted.

> **Did you know that pesticides can contribute to overweight?**

One patient, a woman in her 50's, sprayed for ants and then had a rapid weight gain of 20 pounds. She also began experiencing nausea, brain fog, mood swings and allergies. She continues struggling with an escalating weight gain, even though she didn't have a weight problem prior to the spraying.

What Can Be Done?

Are there treatments for pesticide exposure?

Sauna therapy, discussed in the chapter on Chemical Toxicity, allows pesticides and other chemicals to be released from storage and eliminated much more quickly. Some people who have absorbed a high level of pesticides can excrete so much of the chemical through their pores during sauna therapy that the air in the sauna smells of pesticides.

Other therapies and supplements as listed in the chapter on Chemical Toxicity are also of benefit.

Summary

Pesticides are chemicals which are made deliberately toxic to poison the cells of pests. Since we are also made of cells, these chemicals are toxic to us as well. A deficiency of beneficial oils in our diet can increase the absorption of and the harm from pesticides and other chemicals. It is not necessary to personally spray pesticides to be exposed to them. Generations of bugs develop a resistance to pesticides so ever more toxic (to us) ones are needed. "Inert" ingredients in the

Pesticides

pesticide formulation are often quite harmful to us. Fortunately, there are safe and reasonably effective alternatives to chemical pesticides.

References and Resources

- The Burton Goldberg Group, "Detoxification Therapy", pp. 156-165, *Alternative Medicine: The Definitive Guide*, Future Medicine Publishing, Puyallup WA, 1994.

- Dadd, Debra Lynn, *Nontoxic and Natural*, Jeremy P. Tarcher Inc., Los Angeles CA, 1984.

- Hallenbeck, W.H., and K.M. Cunningham-Burns, *Pesticides and Human Health*, Springer-Verlag, New York, 1985.

- Mott, Lawrie, and Karen Snyder, *Pesticide Alert: A Guide to Pesticides in Fruits and Vegetables*, Sierra Club Books, San Francisco CA, 1987.

- Regenstein, Lewis, *America the Poisoned*, Acropolis, 1982.

- Rogers, Sherry A., *The E.I. Syndrome*, Prestige Publishers, Syracuse NY, 1986.

- Rogers, Sherry A., *Tired or Toxic?*, Prestige Publishers, Syracuse NY, 1990.

- Van Strum, C., *A Bitter Fog: Herbicides and Human Rights*, Sierra Club Books, San Francisco CA, 1983.

- Wier, D. and M. Shapiro, *Circle of Poison*, Institute for Food and Development Policy, San Francisco CA, 1981.

- **Pesticide Hotline**, U.S. Environmental Protection Agency, NPTN Texas Tech University, Thompson Hall, Room S129, Lubbock TX 79430. Phone 800-858-7378. *Telephone hotline open M-F, 8 AM to 6 PM EST to answer questions on pesticides.*

COLOGNE AND PERSONAL CARE PRODUCTS

Smelling May Be Hazardous To Your Health

Do you wear cologne or use other personal care products? Do you have the following symptoms? There could be a connection.

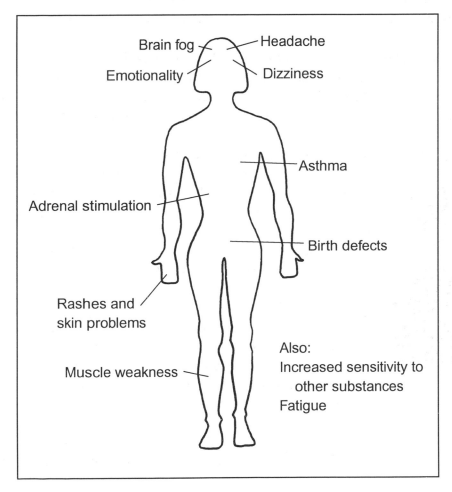

In this chapter you can learn:

- *What personal care products can cause problems.*
- *Why cologne is so toxic to both yourself and others who inhale it.*
- *Why some people wear too much cologne without being aware of it.*
- *What are some symptoms of cologne and cosmetic allergy?*
- *Can cosmetics contribute to cancer?*
- *What psychological damage is being done by the promotion of these products.*

What personal care products can cause problems?
Colognes and personal care products are in such common use and contain so many toxic chemicals that they deserve a chapter of their own. Personal care products include:

- *Colognes, perfumes*
- *Cosmetics, makeup*
- *Acne medications*
- *Powders*
- *Nail products*
- *Creams and lotions*

- *Other scented products*
- *Deodorants*
- *Hair removal products*
- *Hair dyes, sprays, shampoos*
- *Toothpaste, mouthwash*
- *Sanitary pads and tampons*

Colognes are particularly harmful. Unlike the other products listed which expose only the user, colognes and other scented products expose other people, by design, to their odor and therefore to the toxic penetrating chemicals causing the odor. These are particularly toxic for the user, however, since s/he is both inhaling it and absorbing it through the skin almost continuously.

What is the difference between cologne, perfume and essential oils?

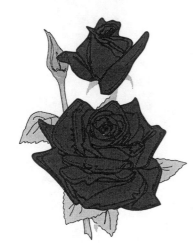

At one time, perfumes were made by carefully pressing the essential oils out of flower petals, spices, fruit rinds, and other natural aromatic substances. These were then combined into pleasant-smelling mixtures. True natural perfumes were then, as now, prohibitively expensive and out of the financial reach of most people. Today's perfumes are likely to be a combination of natural and synthetic fragrances.

Today's much cheaper colognes are made mostly or wholly of synthetic ingredients in a laboratory. There are very few commercial scented products available today that ever saw a flower. Instead, scents are created which bear as much resemblance to flowers as orange-flavored chewable aspirin bears to a freshly picked orange. Even some so-called essential oils, worn by health-minded people, contain synthetics or they would be unaffordable. Nothing costing a few dollars or so per half ounce can be made solely from pressed flower petals. These essential oils may be better than commercial colognes, but not by much.

Why are colognes and scented products so toxic?
Up to 5000 different chemicals are used in various combinations in scented products, and 84% of these have had little or no human toxicology testing [1]. 95% of chemicals used in fragrances are synthetic compounds derived from petroleum, including many toxins and sensitizers that are capable of causing cancer, birth defects, central nervous system disorders and allergic reactions [2]. Methylene chloride, a known carcinogen that can also cause autoimmune diseases, is one of the 20 chemicals most commonly found in fragrance products in 1991, even though the FDA banned

the chemical in all cosmetic and fragrance products is 1989. The FDA is unable to police the fragrance industry since it is exempt from listing product ingredients [3].

A single brand of cologne contains dozens of chemicals, none of which belong in the human body. These chemicals include:

- **Petrochemicals**, which are waste products of the oil industry. These are doctored up to smell like something that some people in industrialized societies are conditioned to find pleasant.

- **Alcohol** as a solvent for these chemicals. Alcohol is also a solvent for the lipid (fat) layer of our cells and the myelin sheath of our nerve cells. Nerve damage including multiple sclerosis (MS) can result. The damage caused by solvents is discussed in the chapter on Organics.

- **Penetrants** for staying power. The penetrants used are the same ones used in insecticides. In fact, one sign of chemical toxicity is a hypersensitivity to these penetrants, which causes cologne to smell like bug spray to many people.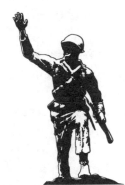

  During the Vietnam war, the enemy soldiers could often find our soldiers by the cologne smell, even when no cologne had been worn for a while, due to the staying power of the penetrants.

- **Musks**, especially Musk AETT and Musk Ambrette, are commonly used in fragrances. They have shown potent neurotoxic effects. Nerve cells and their myelin sheaths can break down with chronic exposure to these synthetic musks [4]. This breakdown can cause nerve cell atrophy, tremors, and symptoms similar to multiple sclerosis (MS) and Parkinson's disease.

Toxic effects have been reported for many of the volatile organic compounds in cologne and fragrance, including benzaldehyde, alpha-terpineol, benzyl acetate and ethanol, even at relatively low dose levels [5].

A well-known actress became puffy and fatigued around the time her new cologne line was released for sale. Her symptoms may have been due to exposure to the chemicals in the cologne.

Toluene, also discussed in the Organics chapter, is in most colognes. Effects of toluene in fragrances include [6]:

- *Headaches*
- *Confusion*
- *Anxiety*
- *Birth defects*
- *Mood swings*

- *Seizures*
- *Disorientation*
- *Depression*
- *Cancer*
- *Inability to concentrate*

- *Fatigue*
- *Brain fog*
- *Restlessness*
- *Asthma attacks*

Toluene is so effective at dissolving grease that it is used to clean body oils from fingers off guitar strings. It dissolves body oils in the body in the same way.

Overall, there are hundreds of mostly untested ingredients, 95% of which are synthetic, in colognes and scented products. These are absorbed not only through the skin of the wearer, but also through the olfactory nerves in the noses of both the wearer and those who are in the vicinity and are exposed against their will. The olfactory nerves are a direct route to the brain, as users of inhaled cocaine and methamphetamine know.

A number of patients have been know to go into seizures as soon as they were exposed to cologne. Such people often have something wrong with their gallbladders. The parasites helicobacter pylori and giardia can interfere with gallbladder function, which in turn can cause poor oil absorption and the resulting sensitivity to chemicals, including cologne.

Studies show that 72% of asthma patients had adverse reactions to perfume [7]. Perfume in kitty litter gravel is a major cause of asthma in humans [8].

Doesn't everyone like cologne?

Some people find the smell of cologne to be extremely unpleasant. For this reason, and because of chemical toxicity and allergies to cologne components, it is the opinion of some people that wearing cologne in public can be, like smoking, an invasion of personal space. It is similar to entering a room with a blaring radio tuned to a station you like but most others would rather not listen to, or lighting up a cigarette and exposing others to the odor and health hazards.

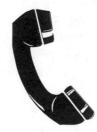

Cologne wearers also leave their signature on the earpieces of public telephones, the hand nozzle at the gas station, the hands of others after a handshake, and the shoulders and hair of those who are hugged by them in greeting. The unfortunate recipients of the secondhand cologne must then scrub their skin, hair, or clothes, or put up with a smell they would not have chosen.

> It is our hope that this discussion will help cologne users, who are probably otherwise quite considerate, to be aware of how their personal decision to wear scented products may be adversely affecting the comfort and health of many others around them.

Some restaurants in Northern California have No-Cologne Zones similar to nonsmoking areas. This is in response to consumer demand. More people are recognizing that we have enough indoor air pollution and that they don't have to tolerate unwanted cologne in their lungs and bodies any more than they have to tolerate unwanted smoke. It would be a good idea to suggest the setting up of No-Cologne Zones at restaurants that you go to - many restaurants supply comment cards. Such a change would not infringe on anyone's rights but would give all patrons a choice of whether or not they want to risk absorbing chemicals from cologne into their bodies.

> No-Cologne Zones - An idea whose time has come

Why do some people wear so much cologne?
We have probably all encountered people who appear to have bathed in cologne, wearing an amount that gags even those who otherwise like cologne. Why do they wear so much? There are physiological reasons for the overuse of cologne, including:

- *Nose fatigue*
- *Allergic addiction*
- *Zinc deficiency*
- *Fear of body odor*

There is a phenomenon sometimes referred to as **nose fatigue**, in which an odor ceases to be noticed once the person is used to it. For example, both authors used to work in chemistry laboratories, not noticing a characteristic smell that visitors would notice immediately. Workers in a dental office rarely notice the characteristic smell that is part of their work environment. A person used to the smell of cologne will slowly increase the amount that s/he puts on in order to be able to smell it.

By way of analogy, a frog dropped into hot water will hop out immediately. However, if the frog is put into cool water which is then gradually heated, the frog will complacently sit there until it has been boiled alive, not noticing the gradual increase in temperature. Similarly, a person who gradually increases the amount of cologne used will not notice the increase, while the passerby may notice the strong smell immediately.

Zinc deficiency, common in those who have mercury amalgam tooth fillings or smoke cigarettes, often causes a lack of smell and taste. This is due to the competition for biological binding sites in the body by the mercury or the nickel and cadmium in the cigarettes. Again, the person puts on more cologne to compensate for the fact that they can't smell it very well. Smokers sometimes use cologne to try (usually unsuccessfully) to cover up the smoke smell.

Some people are allergic to components in cologne, and addiction and allergy are strongly linked. In fact, allergists will often ask if there is a food the patient feels s/he can't live without. That is usually the allergen. The person who wears cologne every day may have an **allergic addiction**. When asked not to wear their fragrance, they may experience some anxiety and even symptoms suspiciously similar to withdrawal symptoms. One patient had to give up his daily application of cologne when he moved into a new household with an Environmental Illness (EI) sufferer. He found this surprisingly difficult to

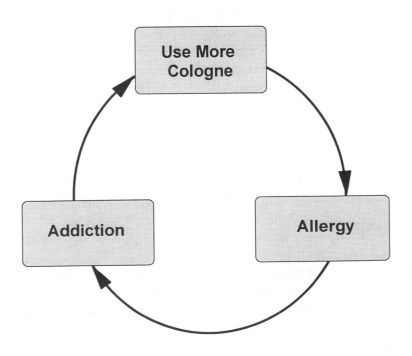

do. It was as if there were a hole in his life where the chemical odor and addiction had been.

Indulgences become habits, and habits become addictions. This is the case both in general, and for some wearers of cologne. The rule of frequency: the more you do or use something, the more likely you will become allergic to it.

There are also social reasons why people wear too much cologne: an abhorrence and **fear of natural body odors**, which must be covered up. Much of this self- consciousness about odors is created by Madison Avenue advertisers who have much to gain by talking people into purchasing anti-odor products such as deodorants and mouthwash. There are natural products that accomplish the same thing, without the chemicals found in most commercial preparations.

There is also a strong social taboo against informing someone that they smell bad, even if the unpleasant odor is caused by something synthetic that the person has applied. Therefore, the person may never know that s/he is offending.

Is allergy to cologne common?
Sensitivity to cologne components, as mentioned, is quite common. The allergy sufferer may or may not be aware of the allergy or the cause, or that the allergy may be self- induced. As with all allergies, symptoms vary according to individual predisposition, but some common ones are:

- **Brain fog** - This may be slight and chronic for a perfume wearer, or can be sudden and severe. A person with this reaction may be in conversation when a cologne wearer walks by, and will immediately lose track of the content of the conversation and appear confused. CNS effects can increase in severity all the way to brain seizures.

- **Emotional** - The sympathetic nervous system reacts to what it correctly perceives to be a dangerous invader, and signals the adrenal glands to secrete adrenaline to prepare for a confrontation. The rush of adrenaline (the fight-or-flight hormone) can cause a sudden feeling of anxiety, anger, or depression. Some cologne users may be getting a short term adrenaline high from the cologne, although they are probably not aware of it. The short-term high is then followed by a long-term low. This was probably the case with the aforementioned patient who had to give up cologne. Depression and anger can be caused both by cologne exposure and withdrawal.

- **Rashes** and increased sunlight sensitivity (called photosensitivity) can occur on the part of the skin of an allergic user where the scented product was applied.

- **Fatigue** and muscle weakness

- **Increased sensitivity** to other toxins or allergens as the body is overloaded with more than it can cope with.

- **Meningeal system contraction** similar to that caused by other toxic chemicals. Structural misalignments can then occur from the pressure, with a multitude of accompanying symptoms such as headaches and light sensitivity as discussed in the chapter on Structural Problems.

A program aired on 20/20 News on December 22, 1995 discussed the subject of colognes, and found that many people who interviewed job applicants were bothered by strong cologne, but only 1 out of 25 were willing to talk about it to the applicant. There are several conclusions that can be drawn from this:

- For every person who is willing to tell you that your cologne bothers them for any reason, there are probably at least 25 who are suffering in silence.

- In most job interviewing situations, there are typically many qualified applicants, and interviewers may look for the tiniest things to help weed out applicants so their choice can be narrowed down. A person who *doesn't* wear cologne to an interview may end up winning the job race by a nose (pardon the pun).

What other scented products may be toxic?

Cologne is one of the strongest scented products, but there are many scented products that contain lesser amounts of these chemicals. Penetrants in the products are especially hazardous. These scented products include other personal care products such as:

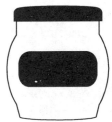

- *Deodorants, makeup, lotion, and bath salts*
- *Soaps and detergents, clothes-dryer sheets*
- *Household cleaning products*
- *So-called air fresheners*
- *Baby powders and oils*

What are the risks of personal care products other than cologne?

Other personal care products affect only, or primarily, the user. The following information is presented not to convince people to give up these products entirely, but rather to help users of these products to make informed decisions, and in some cases to be aware of alternatives. In most cases a side by side comparison of a commercial product and the corresponding health store product will show the "health" product to be less toxic. This is, however, not always the case.

Cologne and other personal care products containing toxins may cause acute (immediate) symptoms if a person is allergic to one of the components. These symptoms may include sneezing, asthma attacks, rashes, and others. More often the symptoms, listed in previous pages, come on slowly after long-time use of the product, becoming chronic (long term). Severity of symptoms, as with exposure to other toxins, is related to the amount and duration of exposure, as well as to the person's overall toxic load.

Can cosmetics cause cancer?

Several ingredients which are found in a number of cosmetic products are known to be carcinogenic. These include

- *Talc*   *found in powders*
- *Coal tars*   *found in eye makeup*
- *Mineral oil*   *found in lipstick*
- *Saccharin*   *found in toothpaste*

These ingredients may be found in other products as well. Read the labels.

Why else should you read the labels?

Buyer Beware!   Many health-conscious consumers are attracted to beauty aids with natural-sounding ingredients such as honey, jojoba oil, vitamin E, or herbs. Manufacturers who want to attract more such consumers add a small amount of a heavily promoted natural ingredient to a product which is still filled with artificial colors, fragrances, and preservatives. Buyer beware!

The FDA requires a complete listing of ingredients on all domestic cosmetics packaged after April 1977, in decreasing order and using standardized language. However, any product which alters or claims to alter bodily functions is considered to be an over-the-counter drug and is exempt from such labeling. Examples of such products include [9]:

- *Deodorant soaps*   *Fluoridated toothpaste*
- *Dandruff shampoos*   *Antiperspirants*
- *Sunscreens*

Don't cosmetics remain harmlessly on the surface of the face?

Cosmetics, also called makeup, are made up of petrochemicals, metal salts, fragrance, penetrants, and other chemicals which do not belong in or on the body. These chemicals are both absorbed through the skin and inhaled. In response to public demand for "natural" cosmetics, some products overpromote the small amount of vitamin E, collagen, cucumber, or whatever which is added more for the purpose of labeling and sales than for true effectiveness.

Metal salts, which are compounds made from metals, are commonly used to color cosmetics. Most compounds, such as table salt, are white or colorless. The colored compounds are almost exclusively made from metals, such as the paint colors cobalt blue and cadmium yellow. Many of the metals are toxic, as discussed in the chapters on Metals.

Nearly all cosmetics contain oil-based petrochemicals, which accounts for their greasy feel and staying power. Penetrants also increase staying power. Fragrance is usually added to cover up the oil-refinery smell that would otherwise be noticeable.

A woman in her 50s had skin cancer which was very likely caused by the cosmetics she used and/or her sunblock/tanning lotion.. She stopped using them, and did sauna and chemical detoxification and took flax oil as part of her treatment. She regained her health. She now uses only CA Botana natural cosmetic products.

Where does lipstick go when it goes away?

Lipstick, as wearers know, must be frequently reapplied throughout the day. Where does it go? It is ingested as the wearer licks her lips, eats, or drinks. The oils and metals in the lipstick vary by product, but it is safe to say that they do not belong in the human digestive tract.

Foundation may be oil-based or water-based. Because it is applied to a larger area of skin, it can clog pores and interfere with the skin's role in elimination of toxins.

Mascara and eyeliner sometimes have lead or coal-tar dyes for intense color. They are necessarily applied very close to the eye, a very sensitive part of the body that can absorb chemicals from its immediate surroundings and send them elsewhere in the body via the tiny eye capillaries. Mascara wands and eyeliner brushes can harbor infection and for this reason should never be used by another person or kept for very long (2-3 months). The mascara or eyeliner itself can become contaminated with bacteria from the brush.

What about hair care products?

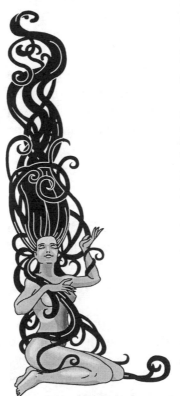

Hair dye, like mascara, contains coal-tar dyes and metals. They also contain aniline dyes, known to cause cancer in animals. Even the dark colors have bleaching agents to allow the color to penetrate the hair shaft. These chemicals do not simply sit on the hair but are absorbed to a certain extent by the scalp.

One study suggests that women over the age of fifty who have used hair dyes for ten or more years have an increased risk of breast cancer. Medical consultants for *Consumer Reports* magazine recommend that hair dyes be avoided by pregnant women due to possible fetal damage [9].

Women who used synthetic hair dyes had a 50% greater chance of developing non- Hodgkin's lymphoma, a type of cancer of the lymph system, than women who never dyed their hair. Hair dyes were also implicated in leukemia and multiple myeloma [10].

Permanent wave solutions and hair straighteners contain potent caustic (burning) chemicals which change the structure of the protein of the hair. As with hair dye, these chemicals are absorbed by the scalp, and are also inhaled during the actual procedure.

Safer natural hair dyes include henna (red/brown), chamomile or lemon juice to brighten blonde hair, and walnut husks (dark brown).

Hairsprays are essentially varnish, held in liquid form by solvents and sprayed using chemical propellants. All of these are not only inhaled in large quantities while the product is sprayed on the hair but inhaled and absorbed in lesser quantities for a while afterwards. These chemicals can also be inhaled by people near or in contact with the hairspray user.

Shampoos contain dozens of chemicals with unfamiliar and unpronounceable names, most of which are listed on the bottle. Shampoo components may not be as dangerous as those in other hair care products, but they are deliberately scrubbed into the scalp and can be absorbed into the bloodstream from there.

Are nail products harmful too?

Nail polish is lacquer, similar to that used to lacquer furniture. Used habitually, it can keep the nail bed (where the nail meets the finger, and where new nail growth is generated) from breathing properly. If the nail and nail bed get too little oxygen, this may set up conditions conducive to fungus growth. Nail polish remover and nail polish contain acetone, a strong solvent which is strong enough to dissolve lacquer so it certainly dissolves lipids in the body, the cells, and nerves.

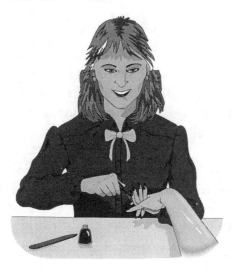

Acrylic nails expose the wearer - and cosmetologist - to some potent chemicals when the nails are put on. The procedure is not a one-time thing, but requires frequent filling of the gap exposed as the nail grows, resulting in consequent frequent chemical exposure. Acrylic nails prevent proper circulation and exposure to oxygen in the covered area, including the nail bed. Fungus infections under the nails are not uncommon, and permanently deformed or discolored nails can result from lack of blood circulation to the nail bed. A person whose nails have been thus disfigured may end up wearing acrylic nails indefinitely to cover up the damage, perpetuating the problem.

A chronic illness clinic used to have its office next to a beauty salon that worked with acrylic nails. One of the reasons that they ended up moving is complaints from patients who couldn't come to the clinic because of the toxic fumes from next door.

Body odor and deodorants - a new approach

Underarm deodorants usually contain aluminum, a toxic metal used for its drying properties. An excess of aluminum has been linked to Alzheimer's disease. Antiperspirants, usually combined with deodorants in a commercial product, deliberately clog up the sweat glands under the arms. Sweat is one of the body's ways to eliminate toxins, and antiperspirants interfere with this. Some substances such as alcohol, rancid oils in meat, fungus food such as sugar and vinegar, and various toxins can cause increased odor in some people. Removing the offending substance from the diet or environment may solve the odor problem.

Other causes of body odor include zinc deficiency, liver disease, diabetes, and parasites. Recommended measures for body odor include: Drink more fluids, colonics or other bowel cleansing, vitamin B complex, vitamin A (25,000 IU daily for a few weeks), vitamin C, chlorophyll, magnesium, zinc, liver glandulars, the homeopathics hepar. sulph. and sulfur. Skin brushing - scrub the body in gentle circular motions to remove dead skin and improve circulation. Apply baking soda under arms and/or between toes [11].

A person who is well past puberty may not even have underarm odor, but habitually uses deodorants every day for years just in case. Try going without deodorant on a weekend or day when you will be alone - you may find that you can do without it.

If you still feel you need deodorizing, there are alternatives to commercial deodorants:

- In many cases simple hygiene such as a daily shower is all that is needed.

- Rubbing alcohol will kill the bacteria that cause odor, and a once a day wipe with alcohol may do the trick. Alcohol is not harmless, since it is a solvent that can damage fatty cell walls and is implicated in cancer development. However, once it dries it is gone, unlike deodorants and antiperspirants.

- Magnesium is less harmful than aluminum, and magnesium based deodorants such as deodorant crystals are available in health stores.

- Tea tree oil (melaleuca) and oils of pine, lavender, geranium and peppermint fight bacteria and can be used as deodorants.

- Dry baking soda, which is often used to deodorize refrigerators and sink drains, can also be applied to the underarm area.

Vaginal deodorants were created by companies looking to make money from women's insecurities by peddling a useless if not harmful product. Most commercial vaginal deodorants contain only chemical scents, and have no antibacterial action. These deodorants are the cause of many allergic reactions, rashes, and irritations. They can also set up an environment for fungal growth. In addition, a man may have an allergic reaction to these products from contact during intercourse.

Vaginal odor is usually a sign of an underlying problem such as a parasitic infection (trichomonas, yeast). As with all symptoms, identification and treatment of the root cause is indicated, rather than simply masking the symptom.

Women's sanitary products, made of plain cotton, should be safe, right?
Tampons are made of a combination of cotton and synthetic fibers designed to be absorbent. Cotton is usually heavily sprayed with insecticides, and the super-absorbent synthetics have been implicated in a rare and sometimes fatal condition called toxic shock syndrome. Information on this infection is included in most tampon boxes.

Deodorant tampons contain a scent which may cause irritation. Since a tampon in use does not smell, the deodorant has no function other than to allay a woman's advertiser-created insecurities.

Some women say that tampon use increases cramping and/or amount of flow. Tampons, especially the new super-absorbent ones, act like a wick and draw more blood out of the body than would naturally flow out. The increased bleeding, in turn, depletes iron, calcium and potassium, increasing cramps and fatigue.

Sanitary pads are also made of cotton and synthetics, but pads are in much less contact with a woman's mucous membranes, so there is little risk. Washable menstrual pads are available from some health-oriented stores. A few washings will remove most of the pesticide residues from the cotton. The pads are surprisingly easy to use and wash, and are kinder to the environment than disposable products.

What about mouth care products?

Toothpaste usually contains fluoride, a poisonous chemical discussed in the chapter on Water Pollution, Fluoride and Chlorine. Almost all commercial toothpastes and some health store toothpastes contain fluoride. Fluoride is the active ingredient in most toothpastes formulated for sensitive teeth.

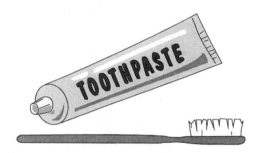

Tooth whitening products sold for home use usually contain a fine scouring powder for their whitening action. Scouring powder used in the kitchen sink will remove stains in the short run but will wear off the enamel in the long run. The same is true of tooth whitening products. Some tooth staining is caused by coffee and tea. Eliminating these will benefit the teeth and the rest of the body.

Can mouthwash be deadly?

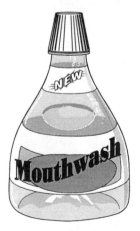

Mouthwashes contain artificial flavors, typically something strong like mint or cinnamon, sometimes a sweetener to make it more palatable, artificial color, and enough alcohol to kill a small child who, attracted by the taste, drinks enough of it. There may be enough alcohol in mouthwash to set up an alcohol craving in a recovering alcoholic.

Severe mouth odor is generally caused by an infection (bacterial, fungal, or parasitic) of the sinuses, gums, or digestive tract. The cause (what sets up the toxic microbiological environment) should be explored rather than covering up the symptom. Mouth odor may be largely imaginary; again the advertisers are playing to our insecurities. Mild breath odor is easily managed with ordinary oral hygiene and by avoiding offending substances such as garlic, alcohol, and tobacco. A mouthwash containing aloe vera and potassium sorbate is available. It is safe and beneficial and is made to be swished in the mouth and then swallowed.

What other personal care products can be harmful?

Hair removal creams, or depilatories, used to contain a caustic substance, potassium or sodium hydroxide. Liquid and granular drain openers, a drop of which can cause blindness or gastrointestinal scarring, contain the same chemical! This is not surprising when you consider that drain openers are made to dissolve hair clogs. Even though new hair-dissolving chemicals are now used and depilatories have a cream base, they often irritate skin.

Acne medications are usually not very helpful, as the cause of acne and pimples is usually internal. Acne may also be caused by an allergic systemic or skin reaction, in which case identifying and eliminating the offending substance will do more good than putting something on your skin. Acne medications can themselves cause allergic reactions, including a worsening of your skin condition.

Benzoyl peroxide is an acne medication which actually seems to be effective in many cases. It works by temporarily drying and sterilizing the skin. A pamphlet put out by a carpet company lists remedies for household carpet stains; benzoyl peroxide is one stain having no remedy as it is considered to be permanent. Would you want something that permanently damages carpet on your face? It is better to wash your face with plain water, using a safe hand and face dip to keep microorganisms off of your face and the hands that touch your face.

Powders - face, body, talcum, and baby powder are made of tiny particles of talc or other substance. This fine powder is inhaled when used, and the particles can lodge in the lungs, causing scarring of delicate lung tissues.

Are personal care products only harmful physically?

This chapter has focused on the deleterious physical effects of personal care products. However, the advertisers' messages which sell these products can be emotionally devastating over time. Primarily aimed at women, these messages convey the idea that the Real You is foul-smelling and unattractive, and that you are offensive to others if you appear in public without covering your hair, face, skin, armpits, and teeth with purchased products.

Advertisers and manufacturers are in business to make money, and they are not overly concerned about any insecurities they may create in the process. They are not deliberately insensitive, but the main focus is selling their product and the profit margin.

An awareness of any "you're-not-okay" messages in personal care product advertising can be a signal to remind you that you have a choice in making an informed decision regarding the use of these products, rather than blindly following the recommendations of those whose main objective is getting you to spend your money on their product.

What You Can Do

What are the alternatives?
You have several choices in the area of personal care products. You can look at the pros and cons of any particular product and:

- Make an informed decision, based on the risks described in this chapter versus the perceived benefit to yourself, to continue using a particular product.

- Evaluate society's messages and the risks associated with the products, and give up at least some of them.

- Substitute less harmful alternatives as mentioned throughout this chapter.

- Treat the root causes of any problem that may be contributing to unhealthy-looking skin, body odor, bad breath or other cosmetic or aesthetic problem.

References and Resources

- Buchman, Diane Dincin, *The Complete Herbal Guide to Natural Health and Beauty*, Keats Publishing Inc., New Canaan CT, 1995.

- The Burton Goldberg Group, "Body Odor", pp. 890-1, *Alternative Medicine: The Definitive Guide*, Future Medicine Publishing Inc., Puyallup WA, 1994. *This chapter discusses some natural alternatives to commercial deodorants.*

- Dadd, Debra Lynn, *Nontoxic and Natural*, Jeremy P. Tarcher Inc., Los Angeles CA, 1984. *Discusses relatively nontoxic alternatives to personal care products as well as other household products.*

- Hampton, Aubrey, *What's In Your Cosmetics?*, Odonian Press, Tucson AZ, 1995.

- **Citizens for A Toxic-Free Marin**, P.O. Box 2785, San Rafael CA 94912-2785. Phone 415-485-0647 or 415-485-6870. *Activist and information group in Marin County, California seeking to protect people from fragrances in public places via information and legislation.*

AIR POLLUTION

What You Can't See Can Kill You

Do you have the following symptoms? Air pollution may be one of your problems.

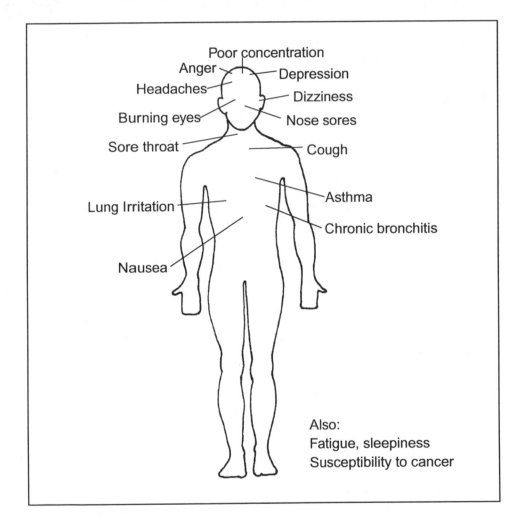

In this chapter you can learn:

- *What is in air?*
- *Does pollution affect everyone equally?*
- *There is both outdoor and indoor air pollution, and the indoor type may be worse.*
- *How do buildings breathe, and why does it matter to us?*

- *What can be done about indoor air pollution?*
- *Is ozone bad or good?*
- *What is acid rain?*

What is air made of?

Air typically is composed of about 78% nitrogen (N_2), 21% oxygen (O_2), and 1% everything else, including water vapor, trace elements and gases, and pollutants. We take about 10,000 breaths of air per day, bringing in 1.5 pounds of oxygen and releasing one pound of carbon dioxide and up to 200 chemicals. Although pollutants comprise less than 1% of the total volume of the air we breathe, they are capable of doing a great deal of damage.

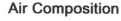

Air Composition

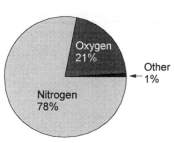

What affects the amount of pollution in the air?

The amount and type of pollution in the air is dependent on:

- *Whether you live in a city or small town*

- *Amount and type of nearby industry*

- *Wind direction - wind can blow pollution towards you or away from you*

- *Time of day, since some toxic gases are formed from reactions catalyzed by sunlight*

- *Altitude where you live, since heavier toxins are concentrated at lower altitudes*

- *Location of mountains and natural features - the well-known smog in Los Angeles is due in part to the chain of mountains east of the city, which traps pollutants rather than allowing them to blow east away from the city.*

Are humans responsible for all air pollution?

Not all pollutants come from industry. Many pollutants come from natural sources, such as volcanoes (particulates and gases), some hot springs (sulfur compounds responsible for the rotten-egg smell), biological decay (methane), and plant material (pollen and spores).

Does pollution affect everyone equally?

The sensitivity of the individual to different pollutants varies depending on:

- *Age - the old and very young are most susceptible*
- *Preexisting conditions such as asthma*
- *Amount taken in*
- *Duration of exposure*
- *Other toxic burdens*
- *Immune system and other body weaknesses*

What are some symptoms of air pollution exposure?
One of the symptoms of air pollution exposure is death. Some estimates by health officials attribute up to 20,000 deaths per year in the U.S. to effects of pollutants in the air [1]. Some general symptoms of chronic pollution exposure include:

- *Pulmonary (lung) irritation and cough*
- *Burning eyes*
- *Throat and nose sores*
- *Asthma and chronic bronchitis*
- *Increased susceptibility to cancer.*

> **One of the symptoms of air pollution exposure is death!**

Other symptoms depend on the pollutant and individual sensitivity.

Exposure to auto and industrial exhaust can also cause hidden mineral deficiencies which can affect any and every organ [2].

What are some basic types of air pollutants?
There are a number of types of pollutants, listed here with examples:

- *Gases*   *carbon monoxide, nitrogen oxides*
- *Inorganics*   *hydrogen fluoride*
- *Organics*   *mercaptans, pesticides*
- *Particulates*   *smoke, aerosols, asbestos*
- *Reducing agents*   *oxides of sulfur and nitrogen*
- *Oxidizing agents*   *ozone*
- *Radioactives*   *iodine 131*
- *Thermal*   *heat from nuclear and industrial plants*

Air pollution sources can be either

- *Primary, or emitted directly from sources, such as carbon monoxide and sulfur dioxide*

- *Secondary, from reactions of primary pollutants with other atmospheric components and pollutants. Examples are sulfates and ozone.*

Is all air pollution outdoors?
The air indoors is often more toxic than the air outdoors. This is especially true in newer, tightly sealed buildings which seal in the pollutants generated indoors. However, old buildings have their dangers, especially mold and mildew spores, and chemicals and materials such as asbestos insulation and lead paint which are banned from use in newer construction.

Most people in industrialized countries spend nearly all of their time indoors. The term "indoors" refers to any enclosed space, including:

- *Car*
- *Airplane*
- *Train*
- *Theater*

- *Home*
- *Laboratory*
- *Sports arena*
- *Office*

- *Subway tunnel*
- *School, classroom*
- *Doctor/dental office*
- *Restaurant*

How do buildings breathe and why is it significant to you?

The ventilation rate refers to the rate at which air in an indoor space is replaced by outside air. This is determined by construction methods and whether windows and vents are open. Building standards have varied over the years in their requirements for air exchange. These requirements tend to go up when airborne disease is a threat, and go down during energy crises because more tightly sealed buildings use less energy to heat and cool.

Is ventilation rate connected to disease?

Ventilation rate is expressed in units of cubic feet per minute per person (cfm). In 1824, the requirement was 4.5 cfm, which was increased to 30 cfm in 1895 as a response to the tuberculosis epidemic. Tuberculosis, an often fatal lung disease, is spread through the air. The requirement was lowered to 10 cfm in 1936, and lowered even further in 1973 to 5 cfm as a response to the energy crisis [3].

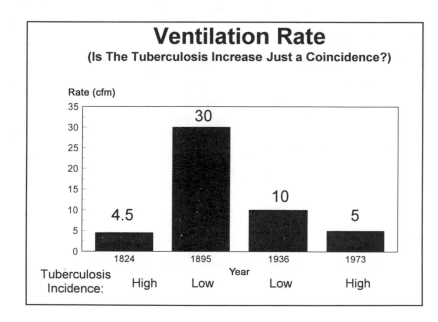

Interestingly, and perhaps not coincidentally, now that the ventilation rate is back to where it was in 1824, the incidence of tuberculosis (TB) is once again on the rise. There is some concern for the spread of TB through air travel with the recirculation of air in an enclosed system.

Another measure of ventilation rate is the number of complete air exchanges per hour. Modern buildings have an air exchange rate of 0.4 to 10 air exchanges per hour. By contrast, a mild 5 mph breeze can replace air on an open porch about once per second, or 3600 air exchanges per hour. It is easier and cheaper to build a tighter building than to add more insulation, and we can, in theory, build structures in which the air is 100% recycled, i.e. zero air exchanges per hour.

Since air inside buildings is nearly always more concentrated in pollutants than outside air, the higher the ventilation rate, the better for our health.

What happens in poorly ventilated buildings?

Pollutants generated indoors are concentrated and inhaled by those who live or work in the buildings. Some of the more immediate symptoms of this chemical exposure include:

- *Sleepiness*
- *Anger*
- *Nausea*
- *Fatigue*
- *Dizziness*
- *Joint and muscle aches*
- *Depression*
- *Poor concentration*
- *Headaches*
- *Eye irritation*

Chronic (long term) problems can develop after years of exposure to indoor pollution.

Many patients develop problems, including chronic fatigue, chemical sensitivities, and autoimmune disease as a result of years of exposure in chemistry laboratories, among other causes.

In one case a whole family got sick from formaldehyde exposure in a new house. The child had rashes and inability to concentrate. The mother and child underwent sauna detoxification, and the child's rashes and problems studying went away.

What are some types of indoor air pollutants?

Types of indoor air pollutants include:

- **Formaldehyde** from urea-formaldehyde foam insulation, plywood, hardwood paneling, carpet, and fabric. Other sources and the effects of formaldehyde are discussed in the chapter on Organic Chemicals. Emission of formaldehyde is at its worst when the building is tightly sealed, when the product is new, and when the air is humid.

- **Aerosol spray products**, including cleaners, hairspray, deodorants, paints, and insecticides. Aerosol sprays contain the active ingredient (deodorant, paint, etc.), a solvent to keep it in solution, and a propellant to make it spray out of the can. All of these are chemicals with potential for harm, especially when held inside an enclosed space.

- **Air "fresheners"**, an ironic name, work by covering up one odor with another chemically created one, by coating the nasal passages with an undetectable film of oil, or by chemically deadening the nerves in your nose which are odor receptors [1].

  - **Microbes and mold spores** in the air come from breathing, sneezing, air filters, air ducts, humidifiers and dehumidifiers, vacuum cleaner exhaust, and human and animal skin scales.

  - **Asbestos**, consisting of tiny sharp particles which pierce lung cells and cause irreversible lung disease, is found in insulation of old buildings, appliance insulation, building tiles, roofing shingles, and brake linings in cars.

- **Carbon dioxide** (CO_2) is a metabolic waste product that can accumulate in the air of a crowded, poorly ventilated building. It is not very toxic in itself, but a person who is breathing more CO_2 is getting proportionately less oxygen, and is likely to be sleepy and think less clearly.

- **House dust** varies greatly in composition according to location (urban, rural, near road) and indoor activities. It can contain animal hair and scales, aerosol spray components, dust mites, mold spores, and other pollutants.

- **Cooking gas** and carbon monoxide (CO) from furnaces and water heaters can rob the body of oxygen. Some patients are so sensitive to cooking gas that they need to switch to electric appliances in order to get their health back.

- **Colognes** and other scented products, discussed in the chapter on Colognes, contain many harmful chemicals which enter the body of anyone who wears or smells them.

- Many **cleaning products** are toxic. A 15-year study in Oregon showed that women who stayed at home during the day had a 54% higher cancer death rate than women who worked outside the home. The study suggests that chemicals in household products might be a causative factor [1]. Ammonia in vapors from cleaning liquids can cause permanent visual damage, including cataracts [3].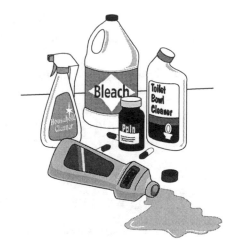

One patient who did domestic work, a woman in her late 50s, got sick from her cleaning products. She started getting better after she switched to less toxic products in addition to doing sauna detoxification, taking glutathione (an oral chelator), and being on a good support supplementation program, as well as other treatments.

How can you reduce indoor air pollution?
Many things can be done to reduce exposure to indoor air pollutants, particularly in your home where you have some control over ventilation and creation of new pollution.

- Open windows to increase ventilation. Ventilation, especially in the kitchen and bathroom, reduces humidity, which in turn reduces mold and mildew growth and the release of formaldehyde.

- Clean and maintain heating ducts, air filters, air conditioners, humidifiers, and dehumidifiers.

- Filters for vacuum cleaners are available, as are central vacuum systems which exhaust vacuumed air to the outside, but they can be expensive.

- Green plants absorb carbon dioxide and some pollutants.

- Keep use of aerosol sprays to a minimum.

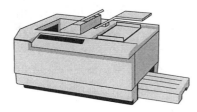

- Photocopy machines, which contain harmful toners and chemicals, can be vented to the outdoors or kept in a room in which nobody works regularly.

- Furnaces, water heaters, and gas stoves should be cleaned and maintained regularly to reduce gas leaks and carbon monoxide emissions.

- Air cleaners of various types can be used, as discussed in the Other Needs chapter in the Supporters section in *Thriving In A Toxic World*.

Due to the increasing frequency of illness and symptoms related to materials in new office buildings and workplaces, some states are starting to pass legislation that sets guidelines for indoor air quality [4].

What is a gas?
All matter is either gas, liquid, or solid. A gas is a material which has no definite shape like a solid or definite volume like a liquid. Gases are usually colorless, but can have color. Chlorine gas (Cl_2), for example, is yellow-green. Gases may or may not have an odor; the amount of odor does not correlate to the amount of toxicity. Steam, or water vapor, is a gas.

What are some pollutant gases that affect us?
Pollutant gases tend to be primarily from combustion products, such as the burning of gasoline (and sometimes oil) in motor vehicles, and from some industries. These gases include oxides of nitrogen, carbon, and sulfur. All of these can be toxic.

Nitrogen oxide, also called nitric oxide (NO) is produced by all high temperature combustion (burning) processes involving air. It is quickly oxidized (chemically changed) to nitrogen dioxide (NO_2) in sunlight. NO_2 is a red-brown poisonous gas which acts as an oxidizing agent within the body. Oxidizing agents can be corrosive and can cause undesirable reactions in the body. The lungs are especially affected, and nitrogen oxides can cause respiratory disease, bronchitis, and pulmonary edema (water in the lungs). The edema is the body's retention of water in an attempt to dilute toxins.

Carbon monoxide (CO), discussed in greater detail in the chapter on Chemical Toxicity, is a product of incomplete combustion (burning). It interferes with oxygen transport. In fact, carbon monoxide binds hemoglobin, the oxygen-carrying component of blood, 250 times more efficiently than oxygen, so oxygen hardly has a chance. Carbon dioxide (CO_2) is far less toxic, but can be an asphyxiant (prevent breathing of oxygen) and blood acidifier in large quantities. It also contributes to global warming, also called the "greenhouse effect".

Sulfur dioxide (SO_2) and sulfur trioxide (SO_3) are the major air polluting forms of sulfur, along with small amounts of sulfides and mercaptans, which are other sulfur compounds. Until forty years ago, sulfur dioxide was the most noxious air pollutant in urban and industrial areas due to the use of coal burning for heat and electric power.

SO_2 has a characteristic taste rather than smell when inhaled, and can cause coughing and difficulty breathing. Sulfur dioxide and water combine to form sulfuric acid (H_2SO_4), a strong acid that can eat away stone and so can do a lot of damage within the body. SO_2, when breathed in, is changed in the moist environment of the lungs to sulfuric acid, which irritates the delicate lung structures. Other toxic sulfur compounds include hydrogen sulfide (H_2S), which smells like rotten eggs and is more toxic than carbon monoxide.

What is in air that can corrode your body?

The terms oxidant, oxidizer, and oxidizing agent all mean the same thing. They refer to a substance that causes a chemical reaction in which a material goes from a lower valence state (charge) to a higher one, such as Fe^{+2} to Fe^{+3}. A reducing agent (erroneously called an antioxidant) or free radical scavenger does the opposite. The chapter on Basic Chemical Concepts covers these ideas in detail, but what this means in plain English is that a reaction is going on within the body (or outside the body to produce a toxic byproduct that then enters the body) that is not what the body is supposed to experience. Oxidants can be quite corrosive to tissues.

The skin and other body tissues are fuel for oxidative reactions much like wood is fuel for a fire. An example of a strong oxidant is food grade 35% hydrogen peroxide, which will bubble and cause the skin to turn white and then painfully red. However, 3% hydrogen peroxide, the concentration sold in drugstores, is much more dilute and can kill bacteria while rarely being harmful to body tissues. It is painful only on open cuts.

Is ozone bad or good?

You have probably heard that ozone (O_3) is nasty stuff that is a major constituent of smog. You may also have heard that ozone protects us from harmful ultraviolet (UV) radiation from the sun, and that its rapid depletion is cause for concern, as with the ozone hole over Antarctica. Let's sort this out - is it bad stuff that is on the rise, or good stuff that is being depleted?

Ozone as an inhaled air pollutant can be quite toxic. Ozone and water forms oxidant hydrogen peroxide:

$$O_3 + 3H_2O \rightarrow 3H_2O_2$$

Ozone has a characteristic odor/taste that can be detected in the air immediately around high energy electrical equipment, especially that which produces sparks. Ozone, produced naturally, is responsible, along with negative ions, for the clean fresh smell of rain and waterfalls. It can be used to improve the freshness of water in hot tubs and pools. Ozone is used in Europe and in Los Angeles to purify the municipal water supply.

While "purify" has a nice sound to it, the purification process involves ozone's capacity to kill microorganisms which can cause disease. These microorganisms are cells, and our bodies are made up of cells, so it follows that a substance which kills one type of cell can also damage another type - ours. However, ozone is less toxic than other chemicals such as chlorine which are used for this purpose. Chlorine can leave residues in the pool or hot tub as it combines with other compounds present in the water. Ozone is so reactive that it changes to harmless oxygen and is gone, leaving no residue.

Ozone acts primarily as an oxidizing agent that forms hydroxyl radicals (OH). Radicals, also called free radicals, can cause cancer and other cell damage by stealing electrons from molecules. Ozone can also be irritating to mucous membranes. OSHA sets a maximum limit of 0.1 part per million (ppm) for chronic exposure, and 0.3 ppm for short term exposure [5].

How can ozone protect you from sunburn?

Ozone in the upper stratosphere, miles from Earth's surface, has a beneficial effect. It protects us from short-wave ultraviolet (UV) rays from the sun. A greater exposure to UV rays can do harm in two ways:

- The danger of skin cancer increases. Each 1% ozone loss correlates to a 3-6% increase in the skin cancer rate [5].

- Many reactions that form toxic byproducts in the atmosphere (secondary pollution) are catalyzed by UV radiation; the more UV that gets through, the more toxic byproducts are produced.

Chlorofluorocarbons, chemicals found in aerosol sprays and refrigerants and used in the manufacture of styrofoam products, release chlorine into the upper atmosphere. One chlorine atom can destroy several ozone molecules. Environmentally hazardous styrofoam and refrigerants are being, and should be, reduced.

How can the sun worsen pollution?

Ultraviolet (UV) energy from the sun combines with primary emissions nitrogen oxide and reactive hydrocarbons from auto exhaust. Nitrogen dioxide and ozone are formed by this photo-chemical reaction, along with peroxyacetalnitrate, a chemical which causes eye irritation.

What exactly is smog?

Smog is air pollution made visible. The word smog was originally coined to combine the words smoke and fog. Today, smog is a mixture of smoke, water vapor, particulates, and primary and secondary pollutants. Motor vehicle exhaust is the largest source, followed by industrial emissions. Over 69 million people live in areas that exceed smog standards [6].

Many people who get sick in smoggy places like Southern California regain their health when they move to a place with comparatively clear air such as Montana. One patient, a nurse in her 30s from Ohio, became environmentally ill (EI) after she moved to San Diego, California. She also developed brain fog, fatigue and seizures. Moving away from San Diego was what she needed to do to get better, which took about three months in her new environment. She still had allergies but they were not nearly as severe.

What causes acid rain?

Sulfur dioxide and nitrogen oxide from industry combine with other compounds in complex chemical processes that form acids (sulfuric and nitric). These contribute to what is known as acid rain. Acidity is measured by pH, where a pH below 7.0 is acid and a pH above 7.0 is alkaline. The farther a substance gets from pH 7.0, either higher or lower, the more caustic the substance is.

Acid rain plagues especially the eastern United States, where much heavy industry and traffic is concentrated and the prevailing winds, which blow from west to east, carry pollutants from elsewhere in the country. The average pH of rain in the absence of industry related pollution sources is 5.6. In the eastern U.S., rain has a pH of less than 5.0, and as little as 4.2 in wide areas, Since pH is logarithmic, a pH difference of 1.0 translates to ten times as acidic, which is a huge difference indeed. A sample of acid rain in the northeast consists of 65% dilute sulfuric acid (H_2SO_4), 30% dilute nitric acid (HNO_3), and 5% other dilute acids.

A bit of irony to ponder

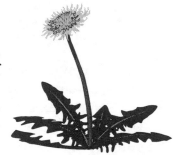

Plant seeds grow better in soil that is slightly alkaline (pH 6.2 to 7.2), and acid rain contributes to conditions which do not favor the growth of seeds. Seeds don't even want to open in the hostile acid environment. Plants such as fungi and yeast also grow best in an alkaline environment in the body. Many of us are making our bodies more alkaline by eating fermenting foods such as sugar.

The acid keeps the fungus, which are spores (similar to seeds), under control by keeping them in a dormant state. The irony here is that we are making our soil more acidic, resulting in the undesirable condition of less plant growth. At the same time, we are making our bodies more alkaline, resulting in the undesirable condition of more fungus and yeast growth.

What is in the air other than gases?

The category of particulate matter includes anything in the air that is not a gas. Matter exists in three states - solid, liquid, or gas. A material becomes a gas only when its boiling point is reached, and even a very fine mist of a solid or liquid substance is still not a gas, but is a particulate.

The largest sources of particulates are coal-fired electric power plants and paper mills.

There is a very large variety of particulates, with widely varying effects. Most of these major categories are discussed elsewhere in this book section.

- *Smoke from industrial processes, fires, tobacco*

- *Aerosol sprays of all types, such as paints and air fresheners*

- *Pesticides*

- *Fly ash from some industrial processes*

- *Pollen, molds, and spores*

- *Asbestos and other fibers*

- *Dust, which contains dust mites*

- *Soot, which is carcinogenic (cancer causing)*

- *Printers' ink and pencils*

- *Metals - Among those identified in urban air are iron, lead, zinc, cadmium, copper, aluminum, arsenic, potassium, sodium, vanadium, molybdenum, and manganese [7]. These tend to occur in concentrations of over 0.1 micrograms per cubic meter, or in concentrations large enough to have a noticeable effect on the body.*

What are the dangers of particulates?

Particle sizes vary; the smallest are not heavy enough to settle and remain airborne indefinitely. The smaller particles are exhaled and do not remain in the body, while the largest are usually trapped in the larynx or bronchial tubes before reaching the lungs. The medium sized particles, of sizes 0.5 to 5 microns, are the most dangerous as they can enter the lungs and cause their damage there.

Particulates act synergistically with other pollutants because they have large surface areas on which reactions can take place. For example, sulfur dioxide gas has a more toxic effect in the presence of sulfate particles, soot, coal dust, tobacco smoke, and asbestos.

The average cigarette emits about 30 mg (1/1000 ounce) of breathable particulates.

What Can You Do?

There are a number of things that can be done to reduce the effects of air pollution:

- *Glutathione to detoxify chemicals in the body*

- *Redox / antioxidants - ACES, bioflavonoids, pycnogenol, quercetin, rutin, lipoic acid, Mitochondrial Resuscitate (Metagenics)*

- *Toxi-Cleanse, a detoxification product by Metagenics*

- *Kyolic garlic*

- *CoQ_{10}*

- *Boswellia*

- *Single cell algae, Sun Chlorella*

- *Sauna as described in the Chemical Toxicity chapter*

- *Lymph clearing, Enzymatic Therapy*

- *Lymph cleansing - Voder, constitutional hydrotherapy, red root tea*

- *Herbal wraps*

- *Colonics can help remove chemicals that have been dumped into the digestive tract.*

- *Tai Chi*

The Alpine Air Cleaner (Alpine Industries, Blaine MN), discussed in the Other Needs chapter in **Thriving In A Toxic World**, can help clean indoor air of a number of pollutants.

Summary

Air pollution, especially indoor air pollution which is to a certain extent under our control, is a significant source of toxins which can cause short-term and long-term health problems. However, there are things you can do to make at least indoor air more breathable, as discussed throughout this chapter.

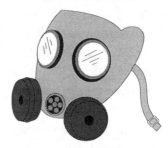

References and Resources

- Dadd, Debra Lynn, **Nontoxic and Natural**, Jeremy P. Tarcher Inc., Los Angeles CA, 1984.

- Gammage, RB and SV Kaye, **Indoor Air and Human Health**, Lewis Publishers, Chelsea MI, 1985.

- Meyer, Beat, **Indoor Air Quality**, Addison-Wesley Publishing Co., Reading MA, 1983.

- Rogers, Sherry A., **Tired or Toxic?**, Prestige Publishing, Syracuse NY, 1990.

- Rousseau, D., W.J. Rea and J. Enwright, **Your Home, Your Health and Well Being,** Hartley and Marks, Vancouver BC, 1988. *How to build or renovate a non-toxic home.*

- Thrasher, Jack and Alan Broughton, **The Poisoning Of Our Homes and Workplaces**, Seadora, Inc., 1989. *Focuses on indoor formaldehyde toxicity.*

- Turiel, I., **Indoor Air Quality and Human Health**, Stanford University Press, Stanford CA, 1985.

WATER POLLUTION, FLUORIDE AND CHLORINE

Water Treatment Ideas Are All Wet

Do you have the following symptoms? There may be something in your water besides water, and these contaminants may be responsible.

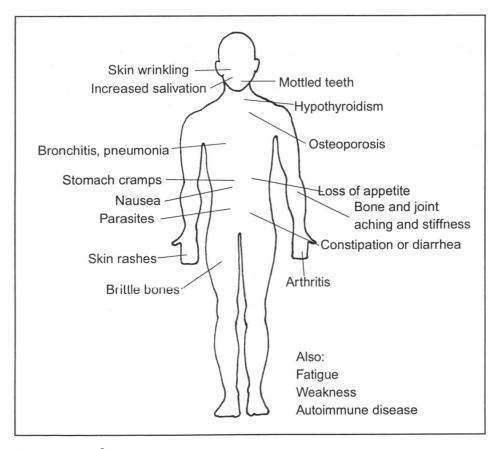

In this chapter you can learn:

- *What contaminants can be found in water?*

- *How can you have your water tested?*

- *What are halogen lights, and what do they have to do with water pollution?*

- *If you are unwilling to drink your tap water, you shouldn't be showering in it.*

- *Chlorine from pools can lead to pneumonia and bronchitis and can worsen arthritis.*

- *Fluoride, which is found in toothpaste and in children's dental treatments, and is often deliberately added to water supplies, has been shown to cause premature aging and cancer.*

- *What do white or brown spots on the teeth mean?*

- *Fluoride, contrary to popular belief, has not been shown to reduce tooth decay.*

What is in water?

Water in its pure form is simply H_2O, or molecules formed by two hydrogen atoms and one oxygen atom. Water you encounter in real life, however, may contain much more than just H_2O. Like air, water is usually full of contaminants.

According to recent surveys, most drinking water contains over 700 chemicals [1,2]. The tap water of 30 million people in the U.S. contains potentially hazardous levels of lead [3]. One of every four municipal water systems has violated federal tap water standards [4]. The water coming into 80 million American homes contains significant levels of cancer-causing chemicals [5].

What contaminants might be in water?

Many contaminants can be found in water. These include:

- **Chlorine** *added as a disinfectant*

- **Fluoride** *added for the dubious purpose of preventing dental cavities*

- **Organic molecules**, *most of which are harmful. These include gasoline and solvents, and are discussed in the chapter on Organics.*

- **Chlorocarbons**, *formed from the reaction of chlorine and organics. These may be more harmful than either of the original constituents.*

- **PVCs**, *which are plastics from water piping*

- **Copper** *from piping in older houses, discussed in the chapter on Other Metals*

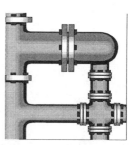

- **Lead** *from pipe solder in older homes, also discussed in the chapter on Other Metals*

- **Other harmful metals**

- *A wide variety of* **microorganisms**, *including bacteria, parasites, fungi, and algae. These are discussed in the section on Microorganisms.*

- **Pesticides** *(see Pesticide chapter) and fertilizers that seep into underground water supplies and end up in the water system by percolating through the ground*

- ***Minerals***, *including sodium chloride (salt), which can be beneficial but can adversely affect the taste*

- ***Radon*** *from natural radioactivity*

- ***Nitrates*** *from fertilizers and decomposing plants*

- ***Dirt***

Most of these are discussed in other chapters as referenced. The halogen elements fluorine, found as fluoride, chlorine, bromine and iodine are explored in this chapter. Non-water sources of the halogens are also discussed here.

Is there a legal limit to the amount of harmful substances in the water?

The Environmental Protection Agency (EPA) sets guidelines limiting the amounts of the above contaminants which can be found in any water that is used for drinking, including tap water and bottled water. The water is tested regularly at the reservoir or water plant, assuming you have municipal water and not a private well. The Safe Water Drinking Act requires utilities to test their water for an EPA-published list of 38 contaminants, including bacteria and solvents [6]. If the water exceeds EPA standards for any contaminant, the water utility is required to remedy the problem.

Even if you have municipal water which passes inspection, it can pick up an unacceptable level of contaminants from the piping in your house.

How can you tell if your water is acceptable?

If you have a private well or an older house, it may be wise to have your water tested at your tap, rather than at the source to pick up contamination from household pipes. There are private companies which do this for a fee. It may be possible to have your water tested free by a company that would like to sell you an expensive water treatment system. However, their results may be biased towards finding problems - correctable, of course, by their product.

The best testing laboratory is one that is independent and state certified. State or local health departments sometimes test for bacteria free of charge. The American Council of Independent Laboratories (phone 202-887-5872) and The American Association for Laboratory Accreditation (phone 301-670-1377) can direct you to testing labs in your area [6].

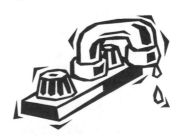

What are some of the problems with tap water?

Green stains in the sink are usually from copper salts leaching from copper pipes in older homes. This may not be harmful, although high copper levels have been linked to sociopathic behavior and allergy. However, copper stains can be an indirect indication of harmful lead contamination, since lead was usually used to solder copper pipes.

Water with a reddish brown stain is usually rusty from iron deposits from your pipes. Let it run until clear before using it.

If your water smells like rotten eggs, this is the gas hydrogen sulfide, which is a product of bacterial growth. The bacteria involved rarely cause anything more serious than diarrhea. The sulfur compounds themselves grab onto both heavy metals and minerals, and can both carry metals into your body and deplete necessary minerals.

Cloudy water can be due to dirt, iron particles, or bacteria, or to something as harmless as tiny air bubbles that dissipate quickly. Cloudiness is most likely to be a problem when it appears suddenly, such as contamination from flooding or a broken pipe.

Halogens

What are halogens?
Halogens are the elements in the second to last column of the periodic table (see the chapter on Basic Chemical Concepts). They are on the right side just before the inert gases which have a complete outer ring of electrons. The halogens all need one more electron to complete their outer ring, i.e. have a valence of -1, and so have similar characteristics. The halogen elements are, from lightest to heaviest, fluorine, chlorine, bromine, iodine, and astatine. Astatine is so rarely encountered that for the purposes of this discussion only the first four elements will be considered.

What are halogen lights?
You may have heard of halogens in the context of halogen lights. Lights with halogen gases inside them are called halogen lights. Halogens are so reactive that they burn brighter than ordinary lights in a vacuum. Inside a bulb this reactivity is okay. Inside your body it's not.

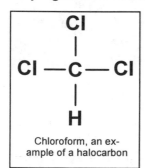

Chloroform, an example of a halocarbon

The name game
Understanding the naming system of halogens is useful in figuring out some of the unfamiliar chemical names you may encounter in your reading. To confuse matters, halogens are sometimes called halides. The combining form is hal- or halo-, referring to a compound with at least one atom of any halogen compound. For example, a halocarbon is a carbon-containing (organic) compound with one or more halogen atoms.

In their elemental form, halogen elements end with -ne. When combined with metals to form salts, they change their name so that they end with -de. Thus elemental chlorine becomes chloride, as in sodium chloride (table salt), and so on. Any chemical compound with fluor, chlor, bromo, or iodo anywhere in its name contains fluorine, chlorine, bromine, or iodine respectively. A compound may contain more than one halogen atom of one or several types.

Why are halogens so dangerous?
The halogens readily combine with nearly anything with at least one extra electron, making them quite reactive, especially the lower weight elements fluorine and chlorine. This reactivity is important in understanding why there are so many halogenated compounds, and even more impor-

tant in understanding what makes them so toxic. Any element which does not belong in the body and is quick to combine with the many compounds in the body will cause trouble. Just as an overactive child or school bully will interact with the other children and disrupt the classroom, so do halogens react and stir up the body in the form of free radical damage.

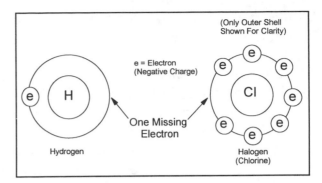

There are thousands of organic, or carbon containing, chemicals. Nearly all of these contain hydrogen. Hydrogen, with one electron, needs one more electron to complete its shell which needs two electrons. Halogens are also short one electron, and thus have similar binding characteristics to hydrogen.

Halogens will therefore easily take the place of one or more hydrogen atoms in a compound, and the number of halogenated organic compounds is very large for this reason. Halogenating an organic compound will usually make it more toxic. For example, methane, CH_4, contains one carbon atom and four hydrogen atoms. When progressively more chlorine atoms substitute for the hydrogen atoms, the compound becomes progressively more toxic:

- CH_4 *Methane*   *Natural gas*
- CH_2Cl_2 *Dichloromethane*   *Solvent*
- $CHCl_3$ *Chloroform*   *Anesthetic*
- CCl_4 *Carbon tetrachloride*   *Cleaning fluid*

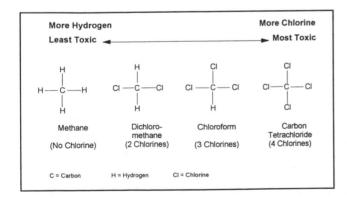

Dichloromethane, also called methylene chloride, is used for decaffeinating coffee. This is something that drinkers of this beverage may want to think about, as residues of this chemical may be left in the coffee.

Dry cleaned garments give off toxic gases in your closet for some time after cleaning. These can be carbon tetrachloride or some other dry cleaning agent.

Which halogens and halogen compounds cause most concern?

This chapter is primarily concerned with the salt forms of the halogens, as organic compounds are covered elsewhere (chapters on Organics, Pesticides). Equal space has not been given to all four halogens. Rather, they are discussed in a depth proportionate to their danger to the population, both in toxicity and in likelihood of exposure. Fluorine, which is highly reactive, is not needed in the body, and is routinely added to our water supplies, is the greatest hazard and is covered in depth. Chlorine is a necessary element in the body and is thus less toxic than fluorine, even though it is also routinely added to drinking water and found elsewhere. Iodine is needed by the body, and iodine and bromine are less likely to be encountered at toxic levels than are fluorine and chlorine.

Where is iodine found?

Iodine is a reddish-brown crystalline solid in elemental form at room temperature. In its iodide form, it is needed, along with copper, zinc, and other minerals, for proper thyroid function. The safest form of dietary iodine is seaweed or liquid dulse, derived from a type of seaweed.

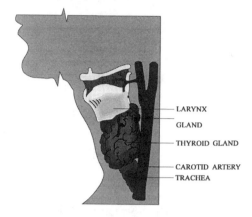

LARYNX
GLAND
THYROID GLAND
CAROTID ARTERY
TRACHEA

Excess iodine can build up in the thyroid gland over time. Too much iodide will actually depress thyroid function, which can lead to depression of other endocrine gland functions. It is added to some table salt - the label will say "iodized" - to help prevent goiter, a thyroid condition caused by insufficient dietary iodide. Goiter is essentially an enlarged thyroid looking for iodine. Goiter is especially prevalent in the midwestern United States, an area far from the ocean and from natural sources of iodine.

A form of iodine, ammonium iodide, is used as a disinfectant cleaner. Potassium iodide is sometimes used for killing parasites, particularly in the upper respiratory system, and for bringing up phlegm and waste matter from the lungs. It is safer than many other anti-parasite medications, but should be taken for no longer than ten days to prevent excess iodine buildup. Iodine is sometimes used as a skin antiseptic in the form of povidone iodine. This is the stuff they paint you orange with in the hospital before surgery, and one of the best known brands is Betadine, made by Purdue Frederick.

Allergy to iodine is fairly common. Iodine is the heaviest and least reactive of the halogens, and a toxic dose is encountered less often than with fluorine and chlorine.

Is it true that bromine was used as a war gas?

In World War I, bromine and chlorine gas was used to kill soldiers in the trenches. In World War II, it was one of the poisonous gases used in the gas chambers. Bromine's lethal nature has been known for some time.

Bromine is a brownish liquid in elemental form. In its salt form, bromide is sometimes used to disinfect pools and especially hot tubs, since it tends to be less irritating than chlorine which is also used for this purpose. If too much bromide is added, or the pool water is too acidic, bromine gas will be released. This is more likely in hot tubs, since bromine is more apt to become a gas at higher temperatures. The inhalation of bromine gas will often cause immediate coughing, and the person so affected will usually exit the tub quickly, so chronic or toxic exposure is rare.

Ozone, a much safer alternative for disinfecting pools and tubs, is widely used in Europe for this purpose. After killing bacteria, ozone breaks down into harmless oxygen and water. Europeans may be more aware of the toxic nature of bromine due to their war experiences.

Chlorine

Is chlorine toxic too?

Chlorine is often added to public water supplies for disinfectant purposes, since it is toxic to potentially infectious microorganisms. Since all cells, whether bacterial or our own, have much in common, it is not surprising that chlorine is toxic to us as well.

What are some sources of chlorine?

Other sources of chlorine (molecule) or chloride (salt) include:

- Table salt, which is sodium chloride. Potassium chloride (sometimes called light salt or lite salt) is a dietary substitute for those who are advised to restrict sodium.

- Laundry bleach is sodium hypochlorite, which releases chlorine. Chlorine is a bleaching agent.

- The pulp and paper industries also use chlorine for its bleaching properties.

- Chlorine is usually used in pools and hot tubs as a disinfectant. It helps to keep out odors and cloudiness caused by microorganisms.

- Many organic chemicals enter our water from industrial wastes, underground gasoline storage tanks, and sewage purification processes. Many of these become chlorinated by the chlorine added to our drinking water. Ironically, a process intended to make our water safer by killing germs may actually be making it more deadly by increasing the toxicity of organic pollutants. Nearly all chlorinated hydrocarbons (organics) are quite toxic [7]. Trihalomethanes formed from the reaction of organic compoundsand chlorine added to the water are carcinogenic in the liver, kidney and intestines [8].

- Many solvents such as carbon tetrachloride and dichloromethane mentioned above contain chlorine.

- Some drugs (note the Chlor- prefix):

Chlordiazepoxide	*(Librium, a sedative)*
Chlorpromazine	*(Thorazine, used on mental patients)*
Chloroquine	*(Antimalarial and for arthritis)*

Why is chlorine gas toxic?

Chlorine is a greenish gas at room temperature. It is extremely irritating to the lungs, since chlorine added to the water in our bodies forms hydrochloric acid, which is very corrosive. Severe acute (short term) exposure to chlorine gas, as in a chemical spill, can be fatal. The acid-burned lung tissues will allow fluid to pool in the lungs, a condition called edema. This fluid makes it difficult to get enough oxygen and death by asphyxiation can result, like drowning from within.

How can exposure to chlorine gas occur?

Chronic exposure to chlorine gas can occur when one swims regularly in a chlorinated pool or works in an industry which uses or produces chlorine. An estimated 15,000 workers are exposed to chlorine from industrial processes [9]. Chronic exposure causes symptoms similar to those of acute exposure, but they are longer lasting and less severe. These effects may not be consciously noticed if mild and long lasting, but they are causing damage just the same. Slight lung edema can result in less oxygen being taken in, hindering the development of good aerobic (oxygen using) cells and favoring the development of anaerobic, or fermenting, cells such as yeast and cancer cells. A fermenting environment from insufficient oxygen raises the alkalinity in the body and provides a good environment for fungi and parasites.

Chlorine exposure over a long time can lead to bronchitis and pneumonia, again because of lung irritation. The irritation to mucous membranes is most often noticed as eye irritation from swimming in chlorinated pools.

What is chlorine's connection with allergy, arthritis and cancer?

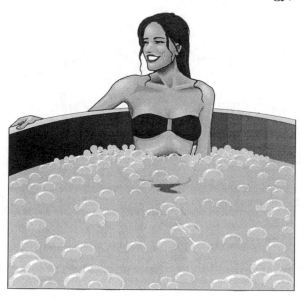

Allergy to chlorine is not uncommon. As is often the case with allergies, symptoms are varied according to the individual's genetic weakest link, and the cause may be difficult to track down. It is not uncommon for swimmers to develop arthritis and other immune system problems, resulting at least in part from constant exposure to chlorine in chlorinated pools. Soaking arthritic joints in hot chlorinated water may ease the symptoms temporarily but make the arthritis worse in the long run. The heat eases the stiffness but more chlorine will be absorbed through the skin, worsening the stiffness.

Hot tubs which are often heavily chlorinated pose a particular risk as the heat opens up the pores, thus allowing even more chlorine to enter the body.

One patient, a man who was an Olympic gold medalist swimmer and who was exposed to a lot of chlorine from pools and as a result, may have developed ankylosing spondylitis, an autoimmune disease related to spinal arthritis. His illness improved when he later switched to using pools disinfected with filters, ozone, copper and enzymes rather than chlorine. He also changed his diet to one with fewer sweets and more healthful omega-3 oils, and made general lifestyle changes.

The consumption of chlorinated water accounts for 15% of all rectal cancers and 9% of all bladder cancers in the U.S. People drinking chlorinated water over a long period of time have a 38% increase in rectal cancer risk and a 21% increase in bladder cancer risk [10].

Is showering safe?

> **If you are unwilling to drink your tap water, you should not be showering in it.**

It is possible to absorb more chlorine into the body from showering in chlorinated water than from drinking it. The largest organ in the body is the skin, which contains many pores that are opened wider when exposed to warm or hot water. The pores that have been opened from the shower or bath will then let in more chlorine.

A 40 year old woman switched from tap water to bottled water and used a shower filter, and lost 20 pounds. Chlorine toxicity and sensitivity was causing her weight gain, as her body retained water to try to dilute the toxin. There was also improvement in her energy level and joint pains.

How can chlorine be removed from the body?

Chlorine can be cleared from the body through a supervised sauna program, as chlorine can exit through the pores when sweating. Care must then be taken not to then absorb more chlorine; a filter should be used on your after-sauna shower. One such filter is made by Nigra enterprises. Exercise also helps to clear chlorine by working the lymphatic detoxification system and by inducing sweating.

Fluoride

Why is fluorine so dangerous?

Fluorine is routinely added to drinking water in the form of sodium fluoride, fluositic acid, or sodium silicofluoride for the highly dubious purpose of preventing dental cavities in children. Fluorine is very toxic, causing deaths from acute exposure and many types of chronic health problems in a large number of people. An estimated 100 million people suffer from fluoride's effects and 30,000 to 50,000 people die from fluoride-related illness each year, including 10,000 to 20,000 who die yearly from fluoride-induced cancer [11]. Fluorine is so reactive that it is rarely found in nature.

How much fluoride is usually added to water?

One part per million (ppm) is the amount usually considered to be effective for the reduction of cavities. As you will see later in this chapter, this amount is both ineffective and toxic. Fluoride is more poisonous than lead and slightly less poisonous than arsenic [12].

What happens if the 1 ppm limit is exceeded?

There is an area of Turkey called Kizilcaoern where the people all seem to age much faster than others. Nearly everyone in the village looks, acts, and feels older than his/her chronological age. Even those in their thirties are wrinkled, tired, and suffer from arthritis, brittle bones, and impotence. The water in the village is naturally fluoridated at a level of 5.4 parts per million (ppm). Parts of India which have a

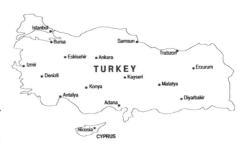

comparable high level of fluoride have a large portion of the population with similar problems [13]. Bone and tooth disorders related to fluoride have been found in other parts of India where levels are a much lower 0.7 to 2.5 ppm. Recall that American cities and municipalities which add fluoride to their water do so at a level of 1 ppm.

Water in some parts of the world such as Kizilcaoern, Turkey is naturally fluoridated, as fluoride salts occur in the earth's crust in varying quantities. Water in many parts of the United States and other parts of the industrialized world is artificially fluoridated at the 1 ppm level.

What are some of the sources of fluoride?
Fluoride can be taken into the body from a number of sources. Given the toxicity of fluoride, it is important to recognize and eliminate exposure to the greatest extent possible. The total from all sources is what affects the body. Some sources are listed below and explained immediately afterward:

- *Pesticides*
- *Toothpaste and mouthwash*
- *Industrial processes*
- *Foods and beverages*
- *Naturally fluoridated water*
- *Drugs such as the tranquilizer trifluoperazine*
- *Artificially fluoridated water*
- *Fluoride-containing tablets and vitamins*
- *Dental fluoride treatment paste*
- *Coal and high octane gasoline*
- *Nonstick coatings on pots and pans*

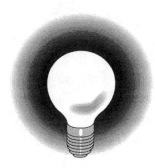

Fluoride is a byproduct of industrial processes, including the manufacture of fertilizer, the smelting of aluminum, the extraction of phosphate, and the making of steel. The generating of power from coal and high octane gasoline also produces fluoride compounds [14]. Fluoride in the form of hydrogen fluoride gas or water solution is used in the decorative etching of glass, or on a much larger scale, to frost the insides of light bulbs. Workers in all of these industries are at particular risk, but those living in areas near such plants are also exposed.

Is fluoride found in food and beverages other than water?
Some beers, wines, and soft drinks are manufactured in fluoridated areas. Many canned foods such as soups, beans and pasta dishes are made with water which may be fluoridated. When dining out in a fluoridated area, be aware that foods cooked with water such as rice and pasta, as well as coffee or tea, will probably contain fluoride. Some tea leaves are naturally high in fluoride, and such a tea can contain 1-2 ppm even when brewed in pure water. Produce irrigated with water from fluoridated areas absorbs fluoride, and some low-grade phosphate fertilizers contain fluoride as part of their manufacturing process which is also absorbed by the plants.

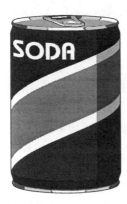

The amount of fluoride in Coke Classic and Diet Coke, bottled in fluoridated Chicago IL, is 2.56 ppm and 2.96 ppm respectively. Beers and wines vary in fluoride content depending on where they are manufactured; this location must be listed on the bottle or can. Tea other than herb tea contains 1.2 to 2.4 ppm fluoride even if brewed in fluoride-free water. Chamomile tea is one herb tea with a high natural fluoride concentration. Buy fruit juice that hasn't been reconstituted (if reconstituted, or "from concentrate", this should be listed on the label). Mother's milk, the beverage of choice for babies, has only 0.01 to 0.05 ppm of fluoride [15]. In a study of 43 ready-to-drink fruit juices, 42% had more than 1 ppm of fluoride [16].

The Teflon non-stick coating on pots and pans is a fluoride-containing compound. Some of this compound can enter the food you eat which has been cooked in this type of cookware if it erodes and wears off. One well known manufacturer issues warnings with their newest coated cookware to not heat the cookwear empty for longer than three minutes or it can give off toxic fumes, which could be "fatal to pets." Can this also be toxic to people? They also warn you not to scratch the surface, either in the cooking process, or by placing it in your dishwasher against sharp prongs. If this coated cookware can visibly lose its coating over time - where do you think it goes?

What about dental sources?

Some dental offices treat children's teeth with a concentrated fluoride compound that supposedly prevents decay. The logic of using fluoride for this purpose is that fluoride binds calcium, which is the

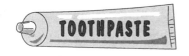

base mineral in plaque. Plaque is a sticky substance that can adhere to teeth and harbor bacteria that can contribute to dental cavities.

Even if the child spits out the fluoride paste, s/he is taking in fluoride. Many children swallow it because it is flavored and tastes good. Acute cases of fluoride poisoning, in some cases ending in death, have resulted from swallowing this paste.

Fluoride treatment, applied either at the dentist's office or at home, is sometimes used for symptomatic treatment of sensitive teeth. Sodium fluoride is listed as the active ingredient in toothpastes formulated for sensitive teeth.

Nearly all commercial toothpaste and even some health-store toothpaste contain fluoride. If present, it must be listed on the label, usually as sodium fluoride or stannous (tin) fluoride. Trade names such as Fluoristan (Crest toothpaste) are a giveaway to the presence of fluoride. Keep in mind that children often swallow toothpaste when brushing or even eat it out of the tube due to the added flavoring and sweetening, thus getting much more fluoride than the manufacturer intended. Acne-like eruptions around the mouth have been linked to the use of fluoridated toothpaste [17,18].

Some mouthwashes also contain fluoride, although most do not - read the label.

Children's vitamins such as Tri-Vi-Flor contain fluoride, as do prescription fluoride tablets that children are supposed to chew on a regular basis.

Both toothpaste and insecticide - where's the logic?

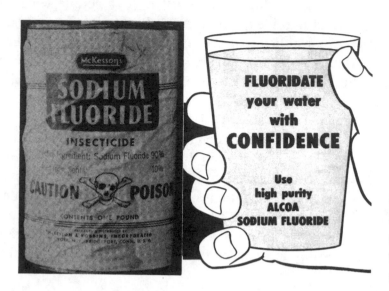

Sodium fluoride itself - the same compound found in toothpaste - is sold as an insecticide. Like all agents whose purpose is to destroy life, it is very toxic when used for this purpose - or any other [photographs from source 11].

What are some of the symptoms of fluoride exposure?

Symptoms of fluoride exposure are varied, depending in part on the genetic weak link of the person affected. Since certain parts of the body are more affected, most notably the skeletal system and collagen, certain symptoms show up predictably with chronic or acute exposure. These are explained in greater detail following this list:

- *Gastrointestinal - nausea, stomach cramps, increased salivation, constipation, loss of appetite*
- *Collagen - bone and joint aching, stiffness*
- *Skin - wrinkling, rashes, mouth and lip sores*
- *Skeletal - dental fluorosis (mottling of teeth)*
- *Tiredness, weakness*
- *Neurological*

This list sounds a lot like premature aging. For this reason, fluoride has been called the Aging Factor [11].

Most of these symptoms are known to the same medical establishment and regulatory agencies that promote the use of fluoride. The U.S. Pharmacopoeia lists these symptoms as occurring when 1-2 pints (2-4 glasses) of water fluoridated at 1 ppm is ingested daily. The Physician's Desk Reference (PDR) is also quite familiar with the symptoms of fluoride toxicity. Both of these reference works are well known and well used by many allopathic physicians.

Fluoride's toxic effects are so well known that its use has been banned in ten European countries as of 1984 [19].

What are the acute effects, and why are they relevant?
Studies of acute (severe short term) effects give quick insight into the sort of damage which might occur with longer term but lower level exposure to a chemical. Inadvertent opportunities for such study occurred during accidents involving fluoridation plants, in which much more than 1 ppm was dumped into the water supply.

During such an accident, which occurred Nov. 11, 1979, in Annapolis, MD, the water contained 50 ppm of fluoride. Neurological symptoms occurred in 65% of 10,000 people who suffered acute fluoride poisoning following the accident [20]. In another accident, a fluoride pump malfunction in Hooper's Bay, Alaska caused too much fluoride to enter the water. One death and over thirty cases of illness resulted, including nausea and vomiting, fatigue, and neurological symptoms such as tingling hands and arms [21].

How can fluoride cause skin wrinkling and arthritis?
Collagen, described in greater detail in the chapter on Body Systems in *Thriving In A Toxic World*, forms muscles, skin, tendons, and parts of certain organs such as the lungs and kidneys. When mineralized, it is also part of the skeletal system.

Fluoride levels as low as 1 ppm in drinking water have been shown to cause an increase in the urinary excretion of chemicals such as hydroxyproline that indicate a breakdown of collagen. Collagen synthesis is disrupted and collagen is broken down in skin, lung, bone, tendon, and elsewhere in amounts as little as 1 ppm [22-25]. 1 ppm, as you recall, is the usual amount added to drinking water, so the purported therapeutic level is the same as the toxic level.

Fluoride also interferes with proper collagen formation, and this plus the premature breakdown of collagen leads to wrinkling. The body apparently tries to compensate for the decrease in the body's ability to produce intact collagen by making more imperfect collagen and/or non-collagen protein [26-30].

A healthy body knows which collagen tissues need to be mineralized and which do not. Both aging and fluoride cause the body to pull calcium out of the bones and begin to mineralize soft tissue such as ligaments and muscles, causing inflammation, arthritis and stiffness. Arteries start to become calcified, a process known as arteriosclerosis, or hardening of the arteries. Bones and teeth, which should be mineralized, are mineralized insufficiently and begin to soften.

Early stages of fluoride-induced damage to bones and cartilage are pain in the spinal bones, progressing to spine stiffness and limitation of movement, followed by the development of a characteristic hunchback (kyphosis). These symptoms are often labeled rheumatoid or arthritic [31-33].

Fluoride: an osteoporosis treatment?

Osteoporosis is a condition in which the bones become porous and brittle, leading to easily broken bones, loss of height, and an upper back hump. It is so common in industrialized societies that it is almost considered a normal part of aging, especially for women, who have less bone mass than men to begin with. An accumulation of fluoride is indicated as one of the causes of osteoporosis.

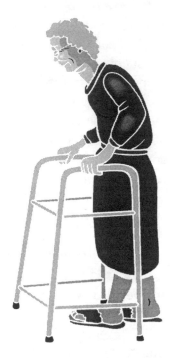

Several studies, including one which examined over 540,000 records of cases of osteoporosis, showed that the incidence of hip fracture increased by 27-41% in areas fluoridated at the 1 ppm level as compared with nonfluoridated areas. These studies were written up in the *Journal of the American Medical Association* [34-39].

Osteoporosis is increased and bone density is decreased with exposure to fluoride. Ironically, fluoride is being promoted as an osteoporosis *treatment*, which goes against common sense and study results [40-47].

Before fluoride and similar toxins were introduced into the environment, women went through menopause without being given synthetic estrogen for thousands of years. Estrogen is now routinely given to postmenopausal women to prevent osteoporosis and other disorders. It would be better to eliminate the causes of osteoporosis rather than dealing with the symptoms.

What do spots on the teeth mean?

Skeletal effects of fluoride begin with dental fluorosis, a condition in which the teeth first show opaque white mottled areas, and then brown staining. Proponents of fluoridation claim that this is merely a cosmetic problem, but it is unlikely that a chemical consumed systemically would affect only the teeth and nothing else. Teeth and bone are similar, so bone is affected soon after the teeth show signs of fluoride toxicity.

Children from areas with 1.0-1.4 ppm flouridation had a dental fluorosis rate 30-35% higher than children with 0.3-0.4 ppm fluoride [48]. 30% of children who were given fluoride supplements show dental fluorosis [49]. Fluoride supplements are the leading cause of dental fluorosis in children in nonfluoridated areas [50]. 74% of children in Amsterdam, Holland developed dental fluorosis as a result of the consumption of fluoride tablets [51].

Skeletal fluorosis occurs when fluoride disrupts the proper mineralization of bone. Osteoporosis and osteoarthritis result, as well as bone spurs and other anomalies. Calcification of the cartilage between the disks of the spine leads to fused vertebrae, with stiffness and loss of motion resulting.

How does fluoride affect the immune system?

Fluoride weakens the cells which attack foreign invaders, opening the door to increased infections. Fluorine confuses the immune system's ability to distinguish between self and non-self by combining with the body's tissues, leading to autoimmune diseases such as rheumatoid arthritis, lupus, and skin conditions.

Does fluoridation lead to cancer?

Cellular mutations occur more or less regularly in even a healthy body. DNA is the genetic component of the cell that is the blueprint for the development of new cells, and the cell has a built-in repair system to repair genetic damage so that mutations are not passed on. Researchers have found that 1 ppm of fluoride inhibits DNA repair enzyme activity by 50%. Both genetic abnormalities such as birth defects and cancer would be expected to increase as a result. A number of experiments on animals, insects, and plants [9] have demonstrated this to be the case.

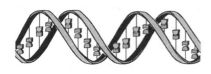

Fluoride has been associated with DNA malformations, genetic damage, and birth defects [52-58].

In a study done in 1975 by Drs. John Yiamouyiannis and Dean Burk, the cancer death rate of the ten largest fluoridated cities was compared with the cancer death rate of the ten largest nonfluoridated cities. The cancer death rates were comparable from 1940-1952, before artificial fluoridation was introduced. By 1969, the nonfluoridated cities averaged 195-200 cancer deaths per 100,000 people, while the fluoridated cities averaged 220-225. There was no other difference between the cities that could account for this 10% difference in only one generation. Are you comfortable with having a chemical added to the water supply that could increase your chances of developing cancer by 10%?

In another study, it was found that the bone cancer rate among 10-19 year old males was 6.9 times higher in fluoridated than in nonfluoridated areas of New Jersey [59]. Fluoride in drinking water at the 0.5 to 1 ppm level increased tumor growth rate in cancer-prone mice by 15-25%, most likely by inhibiting the immune system's effectiveness [60].

What about endocrine glandular system effects?

According to the **Merck Index**, fluoride was at one time used medically to depress thyroid activity. As little as 5 mg. (1/6000 ounce), the amount consumed daily by the average person drinking fluoridated water, has a thyroid lowering effect, with associated symptoms including fatigue [61]. Fluoride can lower thyroid activity by blocking iodine, another halogen and thus chemically similar, and binding to calcium. It is probably not coincidental that lowered thyroid function is common in those suffering from chronic fatigue and environmental illness.

Symptoms of lowered thyroid function include cold hands and feet and a lower body temperature than normal (98.6 degrees F orally).

Since the endocrine glands are tied together in a complicated feedback loop, lowered thyroid function can lead to disordered functioning of the rest of the endocrine system.

Is fluoride necessary?

Proponents of fluoridation claim that fluoride is an essential trace mineral, but evidence of this has not been found. In one study [4], rats were raised through four generations on double-distilled water and a carefully selected and purified diet to virtually eliminate any fluoride. No deficiency symptoms were found. Another rat study supported these results.

Is fluoride useful?

Studies done in the 1930s showing a correlation between fluoridation and lowered tooth decay have since been thoroughly discredited. Many other studies, both human and animal, have shown no link between fluoridation levels and tooth decay. In fact, the Center for Disease Control and the British Ministry of Health both admit that no credible study has shown fluoride to be of any benefit whatsoever. Studies have repeatedly shown, however, that there is a definite link between the amount of fluoride in the water and the incidence of dental fluorosis and other anomalies.

So why fluoridate?

Okay, so it has been shown beyond doubt that:

- *Fluoride provides no benefit, and*
- *Fluoride is very toxic.*

It seems reasonable that it should not be added to our water, right? Yet water fluoridation continues. The reasons for this are the same reasons that other toxins of questionable benefit such as chemotherapeutic drugs are still used: greed for profit and political expediency. Fluoride is used by some dentists and doctors who believe the party line. They may be well meaning but are kept in ignorance.

Details of the politics involved, the various governmental cover-ups, and the major corporations which stand to benefit from continued fluoridation are found in Dr. John Yiamouyiannis' book listed in the Reference section for this chapter. Dr. Yiamouyiannis is one of America's foremost biochemists.

What Can Be Done?

What can you do?

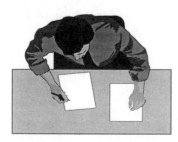

Various political actions and letter writing campaigns might help to end fluoridation. If you are not sure whether your water is fluoridated, a call to the water department of your city may provide that information.

A more practical and immediate approach would be to drink and cook with only bottled water, a good idea whether or not your water is fluoridated due to the other pollutants in most tap water. Fluoride at 1 ppm has no detectable taste, unlike chlorine added as a disinfectant. Boiling water does not reduce the fluoride content.

Some Guidelines

An awareness of other sources of fluoride as listed earlier in this chapter and a determination to avoid these sources will help considerably in avoiding fluoride. You should be able to find a non-fluoridated toothpaste at your local healthfood store, or you can use either plain baking soda alone, or a baking soda/salt combination. Even hydrogen peroxide can work just as well for brushing your teeth, provided that you don't have mercury amalgam fillings. Do not allow your child's teeth to be fluoridated. Avoid nonstick cookware coatings; glass pots are best overall.

References and Resources

- Yiamouyiannis, John, *Fluoride: The Aging Factor*, Health Action Press, Delaware OH, 3rd ed., 1993. *This book talks about the negative health effects and the politics of fluoridation.*

- Waldbott, George et al, *Fluoridation: The Great Dilemma*, Coronado Press, Lawrence KS, 1978.

- Dadd, Debra Lynn, *Nontoxic and Natural*, Jeremy P. Tarcher Inc., Los Angeles CA, 1984.

- **The Safe Water Coalition**, West 5615 Lyons Court, Spokane WA 99208, phone 509-328-6704. *This organization educates legislators and the public about the hazards of water fluoridation.*

- **National Testing Laboratories**, 6555 Wilson Mills Road, Cleveland OH 44143, Phone 800-458-3330 or 216-449-2525. *A certified water testing facility.*

CARCINOGENS

How To Kill And Mutate A Cell

Have you been exposed to any of these toxins? They have been associated with the following cancers:

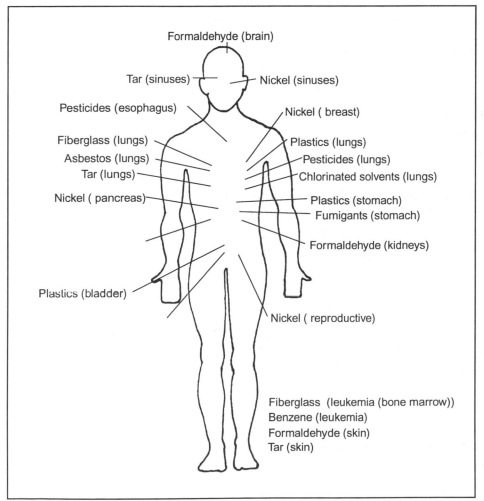

Formaldehyde (brain)

Tar (sinuses) — Nickel (sinuses)

Pesticides (esophagus) — Nickel (breast)

Fiberglass (lungs) — Plastics (lungs)

Asbestos (lungs) — Pesticides (lungs)

Tar (lungs) — Chlorinated solvents (lungs)

Nickel (pancreas) — Plastics (stomach)

Fumigants (stomach)

Formaldehyde (kidneys)

Plastics (bladder)

Nickel (reproductive)

Fiberglass (leukemia (bone marrow))
Benzene (leukemia)
Formaldehyde (skin)
Tar (skin)

In this chapter you can learn:

- *How carcinogens enter the body*
- *What are some of the chemical carcinogens?*
- *Where are these carcinogens found?*
- *Food and other dyes do not leave the body*

What types of carcinogens are there?

Carcinogens are cancer causing agents. The primary carcinogens are chemicals, radiation, and viruses, as well as heat and other mechanical irritation. This chapter is concerned with chemical carcinogens.

About 70% to 80% of human cancers may be caused by synthetic chemicals which are not themselves carcinogenic but which become so through interaction with other environmental or genetic factors [1].

How do chemical carcinogens enter the body?

Chemical carcinogens are introduced into the body in a number of ways:

- *By breathing polluted air in cities and industrial environments*
- *By eating food with contaminants or certain additives*
- *By drinking contaminated water*
- *By taking carcinogenic drugs*
- *By smoking tobacco or marijuana*
- *By repeated skin contact*

What parts of the body are affected by carcinogens?

Although any carcinogen can affect any body cell, carcinogens often predictably attack certain parts of the body, as shown in the diagram at the beginning of this chapter.

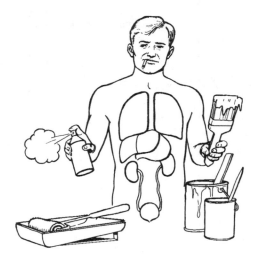

What are some chemical carcinogens?

There are various types of cancer-producing chemicals. In some cases, combinations of these are considerably more dangerous than the sum of the individual chemicals; one plus one sometimes equals three or more.

Some chemical carcinogens, discussed in the following pages, are:

- *Asbestos*
- *Fiberglass*
- *Carbon monoxide*
- *Pesticides*
- *Fumigants*
- *Benzene*
- *Dyes*

- *Some cosmetic materials*
- *Mineral and other oils, tars*
- *Chlorinated solvents*
- *Plastics and rubbers*
- *Fungicides*
- *Formaldehyde*
- *Metals such as nickel*

Asbestos - Asbestos is a fibrous, naturally occurring mineral widely used until recently in construction and other applications due to its fire retardant and insulating qualities. The fine asbestos dust contains needle-like crystals which look like a bur or sticker from a plant. The crystals lodge in the lungs, attaching like a plant bur, causing scarring of the lungs, lung cancer, and mesothelioma, which is a cancer of the lining of the chest wall and abdominal cavity. These fine crystals can puncture cell walls, letting in other carcinogens. Asbestos workers are ten times as likely as the general population to develop lung cancer. If they smoke, the risk becomes 90 times greater.

Fiberglass - A fibrous material like asbestos, fiberglass is used as a construction and insulating material. Exposure leads to higher rates of both lung cancer and leukemia. An adverse effect on the immune system is suspected.

Cosmetics and toilet articles - Carcinogens are found in some common toilet articles. The primary ingestion routes are skin contact and inhalation. Some carcinogens and the products in which they are found are:

- *Saccharin*   *toothpaste sweetener (as well as diet drinks and food)*
- *Toluene*   *solvent in nail polish and polish remover*
- *Talc*   *talcum powder and feminine deodorants*
- *Dyes*   *hair dyes, cosmetics (especially oil-based)*
- *BHT*   *preservative used in skin care products*
- *Coal tar*   *dandruff shampoos*
- *Formaldehyde*   *nail polish, hairspray, mouthwash*

Oils, tars, soot - Cancers of the scrotum were found to be prevalent among chimney sweepers over 200 years ago. The primary carcinogen in soot is benzopyrene. Soot, coal tar products, road tar, waxes, benzene (a coal tar byproduct), and creosote (a wood preservative used on telephone poles) are linked to cancers of the skin, lungs, and sinuses.

Pesticides - 27 pesticides are suspected or known carcinogens according to the EPA. DDT, Aldrin, and Dieldrin were removed from the market in 1972, but may still be responsible for present and future cancers. Chlordane and Heptachlor, used mostly for termites, can cause brain tumors and leukemia. Toxaphene is carcinogenic in lab animals. Chlorinated pesticides are responsible for an increased rate of lymphomas, leukemia, lung cancer, and esophageal cancer.

Fumigants and sterilizing agents - Ethylenedibromide (EDB) is found in pesticides and fumigants. It is also found in automobile emissions since it is used as a gasoline anti-knock agent, replacing lead. EDB is an unusually fast-acting carcinogen. Ethylene oxide, a fumigant and hospital sterilizing gas, is linked to leukemia and stomach cancer.

Fungicides and wood preservatives - Creosote, pentachlorophenol, and hexachlorobenzene are carcinogenic, especially when treated wood is burned and the fumes are inhaled. Creosote is sometimes used as a cheap dark furniture stain, especially on inexpensive furniture made in Mexico.

A patient became ill after slicing up creosote-coated telephone poles with a chain saw to make wooden stepping stones. The creosote was released as a mist when the wood was cut, and the toxic mist was inhaled. The creosote, made to penetrate telephone pole wood, penetrated the patient's clothes and skin and gave him third degree (very serious) burns and caused vomiting. His quote: "Like the worst sunburn you can imagine!" This patient, who had ankylosing spondylitis, feels that this exposure may have contributed to his illness.

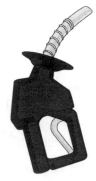

Benzene - Benzene is a solvent and a gasoline component, as well as having many other uses. Benzene and isocyanates have replaced lead in gasoline, and these toxins, as well as benz(a)pyrene, are coming out of every tailpipe in America. Contact with benzene can be made by inhaling fumes, inhaling resultant exhaust, and by skin contact. Benzene is linked especially to leukemia; workers exposed to it for over ten years have 33 times the leukemia risk of the general population. Most people have been exposed to benzene for thirteen years since catalytic converters and benzene have replaced lead in gasoline.

Dyes - Dyes are used in industry, foods, and hair coloring. They can lead to bladder and urinary tract cancers. Unlike many other toxins that are collected and eliminated by the lymph glands, dyes do not leave the lymph glands but instead simply collect there. Eating or drinking highly colored foods such as soft drinks does not change the color of the urine, indicating that these dyes are not excreted.

Formaldehyde - Formaldehyde is used as a plywood and carpet adhesive and laminant, and is found elsewhere in the home as well as a number of other places. Largely responsible for the typical new house smell, it is found especially in mobile homes. Formaldehyde is linked to skin cancers, especially squamous cell carcinoma and kidney and brain cancers. Formaldehyde has been associated with cancers of the pharynx, sinus and nasal cavity [2]. Formaldehyde is also linked to environmental illness and chronic fatigue, as discussed in the chapter on Organics and Solvents.

Formaldehyde is used as an embalming fluid because it keeps out oxygen and thus prevents decay from aerobic (oxygen using) bacteria and organisms. In a living person, formaldehyde exposure can also cause an oxygen deficiency and a type of suffocation.

Formaldehyde is used as a cleaner in dental offices and is partially responsible for the characteristic dental office smell. It can cause headaches and nausea in some people.

Chlorinated solvents - These have many applications in consumer products and industry. The primary routes of entry are skin contact and inhalation. Trichloroethylene, used as a dry cleaning agent, is one of the many chlorinated solvents; many glues and plastics fall into the same category. Their carcinogenic effects focus mostly on liver cancer, with the lungs a secondary target. Dichloromethane, also called methylene chloride, is used to remove caffeine from coffee, residues of which may remain in the brewed coffee. This toxic product moves a 5% caffeinated product down to 2-3% caffeine so it can be called decaffeinated.

Plastics and artificial rubbers - Workers using these substances have increased risk of lung, stomach, and bladder cancer, as well as leukemia. Polymer bags used for breast implants caused as many problems as silicone, and were banned for this use before silicone was.

Metals - Some carcinogenic metals and their related cancers are:

Nickel is one of the most carcinogenic of metals, damaging the body's RNA needed for cell replication. Nickel's cancer causing potential is well known to research scientists, who routinely inject laboratory animals with nickel when they want to induce cancer. Yet nickel is used in dental materials, such as stainless steel braces and caps, as discussed in the chapter on Nickel and Root Canals.

Nickel has never passed ADA-41 dental safety standards but sneaks in as part of stainless steel. 33% of women and 12%

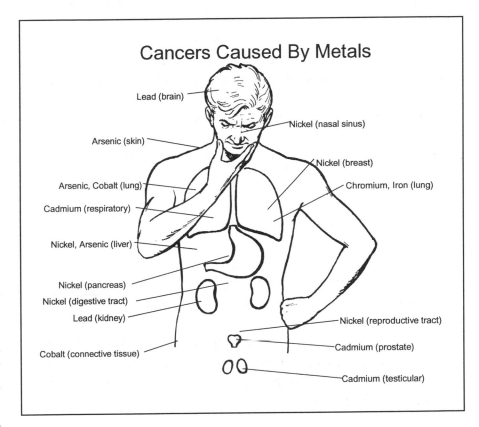

Cancers Caused By Metals

Lead (brain)
Nickel (nasal sinus)
Arsenic (skin)
Nickel (breast)
Arsenic, Cobalt (lung)
Chromium, Iron (lung)
Cadmium (respiratory)
Nickel, Arsenic (liver)
Nickel (pancreas)
Nickel (digestive tract)
Lead (kidney)
Nickel (reproductive tract)
Cadmium (prostate)
Cobalt (connective tissue)
Cadmium (testicular)

of men are allergic to nickel, but allergy is not necessary for cancer to form.

Carbon monoxide is well-known to be toxic but is not generally thought of as a carcinogen. As described in the chapter on Chemical Toxicity, carbon monoxide (CO) lowers the amount of oxygen in the blood. Smoggy air, especially in cities, contains CO in amounts small enough not to cause acute symptoms. However, a lowered blood oxygen level over a long period of time would tend to suppress the growth of good aerobic (respiratory, or oxygen consuming) cells and favor the growth of anaerobic, or fermenting, cells. Fermenting cells are the precursors to cancer. In this way carbon monoxide, although not directly carcinogenic, can set up conditions in the body conducive to the development of cancer. Carbon monoxide, produced by a burning cigarette, may be partially responsible for cancers caused by smoking.

What Can You Do?

First, identify carcinogens and then remove them or reduce your exposure to them. Then follow suggestions in the Cancer chapters of both *Thriving In A Toxic World* and *Alternative Medicine: The Definitive Guide* (see References and Resources).

Summary

A great many chemicals taken into the body in a number of different ways can cause or favor the development of cancer. Recognizing these chemicals and their sources and avoiding them whenever possible will very likely reduce your chances of developing cancer.

If you have cancer, just killing the cancer without stopping the cause may be the tip of the iceberg. 1/3 of us will get cancer and 80% will die from it. With over 500 known carcinogens, it makes sense to stop the source and detoxify your body while treating the tumor.

References and Resources

- The Burton Goldberg Group, *Alternative Medicine: The Definitive Guide*, Future Medicine Publishing, Puyallup WA, 1994, *especially the chapter on "Cancer", pp. 556-586. Pages 584-586 list many useful books and research and support groups, including resources for specific therapies.*

- Dreher, Henry, *The Complete Guide to Cancer Prevention*, Harper and Row, NY, 1988.

- Epstein, Samuel S. and David Steinman, *New Hope: Everything You Wanted to Know About Breast Cancer Prevention But The Cancer Establishment Never Told You: A Guide For Dramatically Reducing Your Risk*, Macmillan Publishing Group, NY, 1993.

- Kaura, S.R., *Understanding and Preventing Cancer*, Health Press, Santa Fe NM, 1991.

- Levitt, Paul M. and Elissa S. Guralnick, *The Cancer Reference Book*, Facts on File Inc., New York, 1983, 2nd ed.

- Tobe, John H., *How To Prevent and Gain Remission From Cancer*, Provoker Press, St. Catharines, Ontario Canada, 1975. *Toxins that can contribute to cancer and natural methods that can help heal it.*

DRUGS

Getting Well This Way Can Make You Sick

Do you have the following symptoms? Do you use any drugs or medications, including over-the counter drugs, prescription drugs, alcohol, caffeine, or tobacco? These substances may be causing some of your health problems.

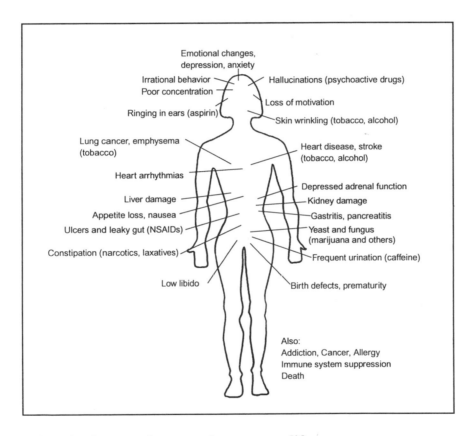

Fourteen things in this chapter that can change your life:

1. What is a drug, and what are some difficulties in defining the term "drug"?

2. How do all drugs damage the immune system?

3. What drugs are against life?

4. Cancer-fighting drugs can cause cancer.

5. Why does chemotherapy often cause one's hair to fall out, and cause vomiting and diarrhea?

6. Most drugs are symptom-suppressing, not curative.

7. *What are some alternatives to drugs?*

8. *Is there any difference between legal and illegal drugs?*

9. *If you took drugs in the 1960's, residues of these drugs may still be in your body.*

10. *Tobacco is as addictive as crack cocaine, and nearly all smokers are addicted.*

11. *How can you quit smoking, or at least reduce the risks of smoking?*

12. *What is alcoholism? - the answer may be less obvious than you think.*

13. *Caffeine in coffee, tea and cola is a drug.*

14. *How can you tell if you are addicted to a substance?*

What are some definitions of a drug?

If you ask ten people what substances are included in or excluded from the definition of the word "drug", you are likely to come up with ten different answers. Some people think of a drug only in terms of street drugs, or prescription medications. Others include activities such as working hard, shopping, or gambling because of the addictive hold they have on some people. Health food purists may call sugar a drug, while fast-food junkies may consider vitamins drugs. The Physicians' Desk Reference (PDR), a guide to pharmaceuticals, also considers vitamins to be drugs. Users of alcohol, tobacco, and coffee may vehemently deny that these substances are drugs, since the word has a stigma and these substances are legal.

The word root pharmaco, used in such terms as pharmacology (the study of drugs) and pharmacist (dispenser of drugs) is taken from the Greek word *pharmakos*, meaning *poison* [1]. It seems that the ancient Greeks knew something about medications that we are just rediscovering.

Interestingly enough, another Greek word, *pharmikia*, translates "sorcery", which in turn usually means weaving a spell - this can correlate with tricking one into a life dependent on drugs, whether prescription (some people become addicted), legal (alcohol, tobacco) or street drugs.

What is the legal definition of a drug?

The legal definition of a drug used to be a substance that might be deliberately taken into the body and can be harmful. **This definition has recently been expanded for regulatory purposes by the FDA to include those substances which are beneficial and have curative properties**. This reclassification allows the government's regulation and suppression of natural healing substances and necessary nutrients such as amino acids, vitamins, and herbs, whether or not there is any risk of harm from them. This subtle shift in definition can jeopardize your freedom to have easy access to your choice of supplements. The Centers for Disease Control (CDC) states that lifestyle and prevention are the keys to health - perhaps the CDC and the FDA should talk to each other.

So what, exactly, is a drug?

For the purposes of this chapter, a drug is defined as a chemical substance with all of the following characteristics:

- It is not naturally found in the body.

- It overrides and does not support or enhance the body's natural healing mechanisms, and may interfere with them.

- It is deliberately taken into the body by any route.

- It is taken for the purpose of changing the way one feels, for alleviating symptoms, or for curing disease.

- It produces some functional change within the body.

- Many drugs are synthesized isolates from natural sources such as herbs. A synthesized isolate is a laboratory-produced copy of an individual component of a natural source.

Drugs include substances that do at least one of the following:

- Attack a disease causing agent, such as an antibiotic which kills bacteria.

- Artificially change one's mood or energy level as does coffee, alcohol, Prozac, or Valium.

- Relieve symptoms. Prednisone, for example, acts as an anti-inflammatory drug by turning down the immune system - inflammation is part of the way a healthy immune system works even though it is sometimes painful.

- Affect the function of an organ or system, such as the heart (rhythm regulators) or kidneys (diuretics). In most cases these drugs are simply another type of symptom suppressing medication which does not deal with the root cause of the problem.

Drugs as defined here do not include safe vitamins and other nutrients, herbs, homeopathic remedies, or activities. **Since drugs override the body's natural mechanisms for healing, they are the opposite of homeopathic remedies, which support the body's own natural healing mechanisms.**

What are side effects and what is their significance?

Side effects have been defined as unwanted effects of a drug, such as the tendency of aspirin to promote stomach ulcers. In actuality, drugs have only effects, which we designate as actions (good) and side effects (bad). Aspirin's ulcer-promoting effect is as much a part of its character by the same mechanism as its headache relieving effect.

All drugs have so-called side effects, or the strong potential for side effects. It is therefore important to understand what drugs can and cannot accomplish and what their side effects are. When the negative effects are greater than the intended effects and you can't stop taking the medication, this is called addiction, another type of side effect.

One of the many side effects is the loss of nutrients caused by most drugs [2]. Nutrient deficiencies can then cause many symptoms of their own, as discussed in the Supporters section of *Thriving In A Toxic World.*

Prescribed medications have altered many diseases and lives for the worse. One article cites over seventy examples of this, taken from medical journals and representing a wide spectrum of drugs and their effects. Maybe things haven't changed much since the 17th century French playwright Moliere made the observation that "nearly all men [sic] die of their medicines, not of their diseases" [3].

There are about 130,000 deaths per year, or about 356 per day, that are directly related to the use of legal prescription and OTC drugs [4].

According to the *Physician's Desk Reference*, certain drugs are associated with the side effect of mental confusion. Some of the more common ones are [5]:

- *Anestecon solution*
- *IFEX*
- *Marplan tablets*
- *Duragesic Transdermal (pain relief)*
- *Xylocaine with epinephrine injections (local dental anesthesia)*

- *Dilantin (anticonvulsant)*
- *Xanax (antidepressant)*
- *Wellbutrin tablets*

What are the different types of drugs?

There are many different classes and subclasses of drugs. Drugs can be classified by organ system affected (cardiovascular drugs, for example), by major action (antibiotics), or by method of ingestion or application (dermatologicals). A mixture of classifications is used here, and some drugs fall into more than one category.

The following is a brief list of the types of drugs, with some examples. A complete listing would take up many pages, so only the main categories and most commonly used drugs are listed here. Brand names of examples have capitalized first letters.

- **Psychoactive drugs**
    - Antianxiety   -   Librium, Valium, Xanax
    - Antidepressants   -   Elavil, Prozac
    - Stimulants   -   cocaine, amphetamines, caffeine
    - Narcotics   -   codeine, morphine, heroin
    - Sedative/hypnotics -   barbiturates, sleep aids
    - Antipsychotics   -   Thorazine

- **Cardiovascular drugs**
    - Anticoagulants   -   coumadin, warfarin
    - Heart rhythm regulators -   verapamil, propranolol (Inderal)
    - Diuretics   -   Lasix

- Antihypertensives - Lopressor, Captopril

- **Antibiotics**
  - Antibacterials - penicillin, cephalosporin
  - Antifungals - Nystatin, Diflucan, Amphotericin B, Sporinex
  - Antiparasitics - Vermox (for worms), Flagyl (metronidazole, for amoebas)

- **Cancer chemotherapeutic agents** - Adriamycin, 5-fluorouracil

- **Dermatologicals** (skin products)
  - Acne medication - Retinol, tetracycline
  - Antiperspirants - many commercial brands
  - Psoriasis medication - Diprolone
  - Topical antibiotics, fungicides - Neosporin, Lotrisone
  - Analgesics - Solarcaine
  - Cleansers, lotions - many commercial brands

- **Anti-inflammatories and analgesics**
  - Steroids - cortisone, Prednisone
  - Aspirin, ibuprofen, acetaminophen - Tylenol, Bayer
  - Non-steroidal anti-inflammatory drugs (NSAIDs) - Anaprox, Naprosyn

- **Digestive aids**
  - Antacids - Rolaids, Maalox, Tums
  - Laxatives - Ex-Lax

- **Anticonvulsants** - Dilantin

- **Antihistamines and respiratory medications**
  - Cold medications, antihistamines, decongestants
  - Nasal sprays - benadryl, Afrin
  - Bronchodilators - theophylline

- **Reproductive**
  - Contraceptives - oral, diaphragm, foam, condom, IUD
  - Fertility promoters - Pergonyl

- **Hormones**
  - Estrogen replacement - Premarin
  - Thyroid hormone - Synthroid
  - Testosterone - Android
  - Oxytocics (for childbirth) - Pitocin

- **Diabetes agents** - insulin, Glucotrol

- **Muscle relaxants** - Flexeril, Robaxin, Quaaludes

- **Antiemetics** (anti-nausea medications) - Compazine, Tigan

- **Ophthalmic preparations** (for use in the eyes)
  - Antiglaucoma   -   Pilocarpine
  - Topical anti-inflammatory -   Visine
  - Antibiotic ointments or drops -   Sulfacetamide
  - Lubricants   -   commercial brands

What drugs are against life?

Drugs that actually attack a disease-causing agent are relatively few and include antibiotics and cancer-fighting drugs. The purpose of these drugs is to kill cells (bacterial or cancer). In doing so, they inevitably also kill necessary, useful cells and protective microorganisms in our bodies.

Antibiotics - The word comes from the roots "anti", meaning against, and "bios", meaning life (as in biology, the study of life). Antibiotics, therefore, are drugs against life. Marketers like the word "medication", but the actual effect is poison because they kill.

Antibiotics can be broad-spectrum or narrow-spectrum. Broad-spectrum antibiotics have a shotgun effect and kill a wide variety of bacteria, and are generally used if the infective agent is not known. Narrow-spectrum antibiotics, like a rifle shot, targets specific bacteria and usually pack a bigger wallop than the broad-spectrum antibiotics, provided the bacteria's identity is known and the right antibiotic is matched to it. The difference between the two can be understood by comparing the effects of firing a sawed-off shotgun into a crowd, versus firing a .38 into a crowd.

How can you avoid the shotgun effect?

When an infection is suspected, the AMA recommends that it is best to take a culture, as for example a throat culture if strep throat is suspected. Once the specific bacterium is identified through the culture, a narrow spectrum antibiotic for that type of bacteria should be prescribed (like a .38 gun). However, many doctors simply prescribe an antibiotic based on what might be causing the infection without taking a culture (the "shotgun approach"). This approach might also be called "Ready, Fire, Aim".

Ideally, the culture should also involve placing a drop each of several likely antibiotics on the bacterial culture to see which one kills the bacteria most effectively. Slightly different strains of bacteria may be present in different people, each needing a slightly different antibiotic.

The usual method of prescription is to use <u>you</u> as the "culture dish", prescribing one antibiotic after another until they find one that works. Doesn't it make more sense to find out what the target is first, rather than using a "broadside approach" and just hoping you hit the target? Random stomping rarely kills many cockroaches - it's best to turn the lights on. Similarly, it's best to see what type of bacteria one is trying to eliminate.

Although antibiotics can be useful and even lifesaving in managing an acute bacterial infection, they have a number of drawbacks:

- They can suppress the immune system in the long term.

- They are ineffective against viruses, yeasts, worms, and non-bacterial parasites. In fact, they promote the proliferation of yeasts and other parasites by killing the beneficial bacteria that keep these pathogens in check.

- They can cause allergic reactions that can be serious or even fatal. Anaphylactic shock, which can be fatal, is often caused by penicillin.

- They kill the good protective bacteria along with the bad. This is rather like spraying your garden with herbicides which kill the flowers along with the weeds. The protective bacteria keep yeast under control and help with digestion, as well as having other functions such as B vitamin production. Biotin, a B vitamin thus produced, is antifungal. Acidophilus, a type of beneficial bacteria, produce acid which helps to kill the eggs of parasites. Protective bacteria are 99% of the total bacteria, and are your body's first line of defense.

- They must be taken for the full course, as prescribed. This period is usually ten days. If discontinued sooner, there is a strong likelihood that the bacteria most resistant to the antibiotic will survive, mutate, and breed, producing a new infection caused by bacteria that will not be easily killed. This can happen even if the full course of antibiotics is taken. In other words, the more often antibiotics are taken, the greater the likelihood that they won't work when they are really needed. New antibiotic-resistant strains of syphilis and tuberculosis have been surfacing recently, decades after these diseases were thought to have been conquered.

- They can inhibit the effectiveness of the immune system's T-cells and reduce their efficiency in fighting viral infections [6]. Some viruses are becoming pandemic (world-wide epidemic) due to the use of antibiotics.

A large percentage of adults with Chronic Fatigue Syndrome have a history of frequent and recurrent antibiotic treatment in childhood or teen years [7].

A nationwide survey of children between the ages of one and twelve years who have taken over 20 cycles of antibiotics are 50% more likely to have developmental delays, including speech and language problems and multisystem developmental disorders [8].

It is sometimes a good idea to take protective bacteria (sometimes called probiotics) such as acidophilus (preferably) or bifidus two hours after each antibiotic dose. These are sold in capsules or found in good quality yogurt. They help to replenish those protective bacteria which are killed by the antibiotic. Most acidophilus is derived from milk, so use caution if you are allergic to dairy products. There are dairy free brands of acidophilus, such as Kyodophilus, Megadophilus, and Ultradophilus, as well as Ultrabifidus and Replenz. Be sure to check the label to get the product that is right for you.

Why are anti-cancer drugs so toxic?

Anti-cancer drugs can be very potent and toxic. They can suppress the immune system so that it can no longer fight the cancer on its own, and therefore must be strong enough to kill all of the cancer cells and not just most of them. Cancer cells are mutated fermenting body cells rather than foreign invaders, and therefore drugs that kill fermenting cancer cells will also damage normal respiratory cells.

What are some of the side effects of cancer drugs?

Drugs that target fast-growing cancer cells can especially damage fast-growing normal cells such as hair follicles. This explains why many people on chemotherapy lose their hair. When the body detects a strong poison, the liver reacts by trying to expel it. Violent nausea, vomiting, and diarrhea usually accompany chemotherapy for this reason. Most anticancer drugs, including painkillers such as morphine and prednisone (not strictly anticancer, but often used to control pain in cancer patients), suppress the immune system at a time when a stronger immune system is most necessary, and opportunistic infections such as fungus overgrowth and mouth sores are common during chemotherapy. Some deleterious effects of chemotherapy are permanent. Drugs given to suppress side effects often have side effects of their own. Amazingly, most anti-cancer drugs are carcinogenic (cancer causing) in themselves, as discussed in the Cancer chapter in *Thriving In A Toxic World*.

Is there another approach to supporting the body in fighting cancer?

Allopathic medicine tends to look at cancer as something to kill or fight. Accordingly, drugs for this purpose focus on killing, inactivating, or shrinking the cancer.

It is known that the body successfully dispatches mutated cells, technically cancer cells, all the time before a tumor can form, as described in the Cancer chapter in *Thriving In A Toxic World*. This happens when the immune system is strong and working optimally. Supporting the body in doing what it is designed to do seems preferable to bombarding the body with drugs which weaken the body's immune system when it's needed at its strongest to fight the cancer.

Does this mean that cancer chemotherapy always does more harm than good?

Certainly not. While building up the immune system naturally so that it can fight the cancer would be the ideal, this takes time, and time is something that one may not have if one is dealing with a fast-growing cancer. Some cancers, such as Hodgkin's lymphoma, respond well to chemotherapy.

Integrated therapies - Some natural cancer remedies exist, such as shark cartilage, which limits the blood vessel supply to the tumor and in effect starves it. These remedies are discussed in the chapter on Cancer in *Thriving In A Toxic World*. An important part of cancer treatment is the identification and elimination of the cause of the cancer.

What types of drugs are most often used?

Symptom-suppressing drugs make up the bulk of the different types of drugs. These are called symptom-suppressing because they do not get to the root cause of the problem but rather alleviate

> **Even symptom-suppressing drugs can save your life.**

the symptoms. While most symptom-suppressing drugs do nothing but make the patient feel temporarily better, some of them can be life-saving in their symptom relief. Examples are inhalers for asthma attacks, drugs to control potentially life-threatening heart arrhythmias, drugs such as epinephrine to control often-fatal anaphylactic shock, and drugs to stop severe electrolyte-depleting diarrhea in a baby. Rule of thumb: If the symptom can kill you, then symptom-suppressing drugs can be a real life saver. Drugs can be used to buy you time until you get to the root cause of your health problems; solving and treating the root cause can often free you from dependence on the drug.

How does advertising contribute to drug use?

We are conditioned by advertising and by Western culture to believe that if something is less than optimal, or doesn't feel good, then something is wrong and needs to be fixed. This works to the good if you delve into the cause of your fatigue, say, rather than simply accepting it. Too often, though, this ethic translates into a strong desire to do whatever is necessary to make unpleasant symptoms go away, within minutes if possible. This approach can be referred to as "Dr. Feelgood vs. Dr. Getwell".

What can be wrong with taking symptom suppressing drugs?

In general, the problems involved in taking symptom-suppressing medications are:

- **Masking a serious underlying problem** - Pain is a signal that something is wrong, and masking the symptoms may cause one to delay finding out what is really causing the problem. This delay can be serious or even fatal. A headache may be a stroke victim's only warning, and masking it with aspirin can be deadly.

- **The rebound effect** - With regular use, many symptom-suppressing drugs cause the very symptoms that they are used to treat. This is the flip side of the principle of homeopathy, in which a substance that can cause symptoms in large amounts can tell the body that it's out of balance so the body can correct itself when the substance is given in small amounts. Aspirin can cause rebound headaches; nose drops can cause greater nasal congestion than what was originally present; laxatives condition the bowel to become dependent on them, leading to constipation; sleep aids can ultimately worsen insomnia. Prozac, the sleep aid and anti-anxiety drug, which initially calms people, has been linked to violent behavior, murders and suicides.

- **Side effects and/or allergic reactions** are possible with any drug.

- **Interaction with other drugs and even foods can occur, with serious effects or inactivation of the drug**. The antibiotic tetracycline, for example, is rendered less effective by taking it with milk. Barbiturates and alcohol, which are both depressants, work together to form a combination which is much stronger than either one alone; this combination can kill you.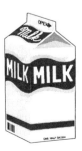

- **They can pose a danger to a developing fetus**, in spite of pre-release drug testing. The Thalidomide disaster, in which the sleep aid Thalidomide was given to pregnant women, resulted in babies with deformed limbs.

- "Inert" ingredients in these medications, such as alcohol and sugar in syrups, propellants in inhalers and aerosols, artificial colors and flavors, and tablet binders can cause problems in susceptible individuals. **Allergy to these inert ingredients is possible.** Some of these "inert" ingredients can be toxic, especially in large amounts, even if one is not allergic.

- **Children seeing their parents take medication for every little thing are more likely to self-medicate.** This can take the form of a young child getting into the baby aspirin and eating them like candy, or the teenager who turns to alcohol or other drugs as a quick fix for emotional pain.

- **Many symptom-suppressing drugs suppress the body's mechanisms for dealing with the underlying problem**. Coughing, running nose, and mild diarrhea are the body's way of expelling undesirable matter, and drugs to control these symptoms also thwart the body's best intentions. Fever helps the body to fight infection sooner (see the Immune System chapter in *Thriving In A Toxic World*), so fever reducers such as aspirin can cause the infection to linger.

What are some common symptom suppressing drugs?

In addition to the above general drawbacks, some common symptom-suppressing drugs and their effects are:

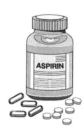

Aspirin - Aspirin relieves fever, pain, and inflammation. In large doses or in sensitive individuals it can cause ringing in the ears (tinnitus), reduce the blood's ability to clot, cause kidney damage, and cause gastrointestinal bleeding. Anaphylactic shock, an often fatal allergic reaction, is more likely with aspirin than with most other drugs.

Pain relievers - Narcotic pain relievers, available only by prescription or illegally, can be addictive if used improperly or for too long. Their effect can be dangerously strong if mixed with alcohol, since both are depressant drugs.

Cold and allergy medications - These include oral or nasal decongestants, cough suppressants, painkillers, and fever reducers. None of these actually help to cure the cold or allergy, and may retard the body's efforts. Histamines, which attack pathogens, are produced by the immune system in response to an invader, and antihistamines, used to reduce nasal congestion and dripping, work against this natural mechanism. The use of antihistamines is like removing the police from the scene of a riot, allowing burning and looting to take over.

Steroids - Steroids, including cortisone and prednisone, are anti-inflammatory drugs. They can reduce joint swelling and itching skin, among other symptoms. They do this by turning off the immune system's normal inflammatory response, reducing discomfort but in the process making the immune system less effective by design.

Synthetic steroids also depress adrenal function by imitating real steroids and turning off the body's feedback system. Withdrawing from these drugs often results in low energy due to the underfunctioning of the adrenals. They also steal calcium from the bones and body, possibly leading to osteoporosis after long-term use. Lower calcium can lead to lower bone mass, and in severe cases death from the stopping of a calcium depleted heart.

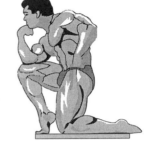

A 70 year old man was taking prednisone. His doctor wanted to wean him from the drug by one daily tablet per month, down from nine daily tablets. A progressive clinic said that at the rate he was losing calcium he would be in danger within two months. His heart stopped from lack of calcium after 1 1/2 months. In this way the drug indirectly killed him.

Anabolic steroids are sometimes used in excess by body-builders, with dangerous consequences. Steroids can combine with anticoagulants or anticholinergics to cause serious side effects including cardiac and respiratory arrest [6].

Steroids can contribute to cancer formation

Anabolic steroids work by causing cell growth and buildup. This may be what you want if muscle cells are being built up, but dangerous if mutated cells are being stimulated to grow into cancer and the steroids themselves are suppressing immune function. Also, muscle growth occurs at the expense of other organs.

Sports medicine - Analgesics and anesthetics, such as cortisone, Lidocaine, and Demerol, are sometimes used to keep an injured athlete on the playing field a bit longer. The injured tissue is then subject to further injury, which may be permanent.

Nonsteroidal anti-inflammatory drugs (NSAIDs) also reduce pain and inflammation. They inhibit prostaglandin E2 (PGE2), an eicosanoid, or hormone, which is part of the inflammation cycle. PGE2 has beneficial effects such as rebuilding tissues such as the intestinal lining. Artificially suppressing PGE2 will reduce pain but will also reduce the benefits, leading to ulcers and leaky gut, which in turn leads to allergy and then more inflammation in a vicious cycle.

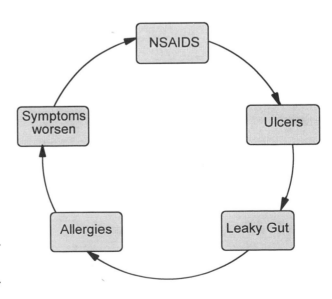

NSAIDs, often taken for symptomatic relief of the pain of osteoarthritis, can actually make it worse. They can increase the rate of cartilage deterioration and joint damage [9-11].

It is better to increase PGE1 and to a lesser extent PGE3, related hormones which regulate PGE2 naturally. A number of natural substances are useful in raising PGE1 and PGE3 levels and controlling free radical damage caused with inflammation:

- *Fish and flax oils, and in some cases small amounts of borage oil, evening primrose oil, and black currant seed oil*
- *Bioflavonoids quercetin, rutin, pycnogenol*
- *Vitamins E and C (Carlsons brand)*
- *Garlic (Kyolic)*
- *Life Solubles (Integris)*

This knowledge has led to a whole new industry of medical foods such as Eicosanoid balancing bars, which have a proportionate balance of carbohydrates, protein and fat that promotes the release of fat-burning energy from the cells and prevents hypoglycemic ups and downs.

Laxatives, especially phenolphthalein and other stimulant laxatives, can cause mineral depletion, side effects and allergies. The allergies come from "leaky bowel", which lets potentially allergenic waste products enter the bloodstream due to the harsh reaction that causes the colon to essentially vomit. As the colon is forcibly emptied, valuable minerals are also expelled. Even natural herbal laxatives such as cascara sagrada are stronger than what the body was designed to tolerate. With regular usage, laxatives can lead to the bowel's becoming "lazy" and refusing to work on its own; the result is constipation. Laxative abuse can lead to severe and even life-threatening renal (kidney) failure [12]. Losing potassium and calcium through bowel purging can lower energy and can cause muscle cramps, insomnia, anxiety and fatigue.

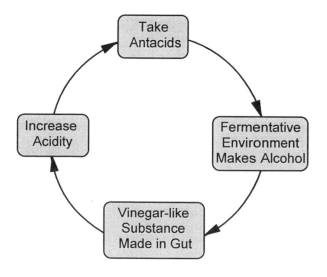

Antacids can help relieve the burning sensation known as heartburn, or the stuffed feeling from eating too much. Many OTC antacids contain aluminum, a toxic metal which is suspected in causing problems such as Alzheimer's disease in large amounts. Some heart problems and stomach ulcers cause a burning sensation similar to indigestion; masking the symptoms with antacids can delay getting needed medical assistance. Antacids set up a fermentative environment, making acidic vinegar in the gut and increasing acidity and worsening the problem in the long run. Antacids also set up conditions conducive to yeast and fungus growth.

Diet aids often contain phenylpropanolamine (OTC) or amphetamines (prescription), which kill the appetite and artificially and temporarily raise the energy level. Diet aids, however, actually diminish energy by depleting the adrenals and lowering DHEA and cortisol, as well as progesterone levels and prematurely using up the brain's neurotransmitters. This is analogous to using credit cards which can temporarily increase your standard of living, but their indiscriminate use can cause long term financial collapse.

Weight loss resulting from the use of these drugs is rarely maintained, since healthy eating habits and lifestyle changes have not been learned, and there may be a rebound effect of increased appetite when the drugs are discontinued. Eating less by any means can reduce levels of nutrients in the body, and increased hunger is the body's way of attempting to get sufficient nutrients.

Heart arrhythmias and high blood pressure can result from the use of these stimulant drugs as well as herbs such as Ma Huang.

Psychotropic drugs - Antidepressants, sedatives, hypnotics, and anti-anxiety drugs are prescribed, most often by psychiatrists, to reduce depression or anxiety, smooth out the highs and lows of bipolar depression, and make mental patients easier to handle. These are powerful drugs with a number of side effects such as sluggishness and difficulty thinking, although they have their uses if a patient is otherwise nonfunctional.

Tricyclic antidepressants and other psychotropic drugs raise serotonin, the brain's pleasure-producing, relaxation- and sleep-inducing chemical, in the short term but lower it long-term. These drugs can have a speed-like effect along with a feeling of disconnection from one's emotions and from the outside world. Your brain compensates by lowering your serotonin receptors. For this reason, the use of these drugs has been linked to homicides and suicides, and over thirty mass murder court cases have tried to use psychotropic drugs, mostly prescription, as a defense.

Do symptom suppressing drugs have any value?

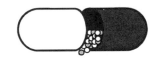

There are other drugs as well in the symptom-suppressing category. Apart from the few life-saving drugs mentioned, the others have little or no value other than temporary symptom relief, and also have the potential for undesirable side effects. Does this mean that they should never be used? Ideally not, although in real life the relief from occasionally using a drug as directed may outweigh the slight risk from such use. Now you are probably more aware that the underlying condition is not being helped, and that there is some risk in these drugs, however small. At this point you and/or your doctor can make the decision regarding the use of such drugs, ideally while solving the real root cause.

What are some of the alternatives?

The choice is not necessarily between toughing it out and taking risks. There are safe, non-drug alternatives for most of the symptoms mentioned.

Pain relief - Massage of sore muscles, or massage of the back of the neck or temples can help to relieve a headache. Biofeedback and hypnosis can be used for chronic pain of all types, as can TENS (transcutaneous electronic nerve stimulators), oxygenation of painful areas, judicious use of lasers, acupuncture and acupressure, and "superfoods" such as Life Solubles and Sun

Chlorella. The omega-3 oils, bioflavonoids such as quercetin and pycnogenol, and other substances listed above for balancing the eicosanoids are useful for pain relief. The amino acids tryptophan and DL-phenylalanine and the herb turmeric have anti-inflammatory actions. Vitamins B5, B6, and C (refer to the Supporters section in *Thriving In A Toxic World* for recommended dosages of these and other supplements) support the adrenal glands in making cortisol, a powerful anti-inflammatory substance. Homeopathic remedies for pain and inflammation may also be useful.

Colds - Your mother was right - chicken soup helps reduce nasal congestion. So does breathing steam, by itself or with peppermint oil or Vicks Vapo-Rub, but be careful of scalding. Liquid germanium may also be useful, especially in a nebulizer which converts the germanium to a mist to be breathed, releasing oxygen.

Laxatives - A daily bowel movement is ideal, and 2-3 times daily is even better. If your bowels move only once every two or three days, or longer, this is a sign that your body is not working optimally or your diet is deficient in fiber, oils, enzymes, or protective bacteria. These deficiencies can lower bile flow and peristaltic action, the contractions by which food is moved down the digestive tract.

Elimination less than once a day can cause toxins to build up in the bowel, and putrefaction can occur. If you are not in distress, however, it may be better to simply let nature take its course, rather than using harsh laxatives. Here are some natural ways to promote effective bowel action and help nature take its course:

- Take Ultrabifidus or Mega Bifidus to increase bowel movement.

- High fiber foods such as whole grains and raw vegetables, or natural laxatives such as psyllium seed will provide bulk.

- Prunes and figs are gentle natural laxatives.

- Flax, olive, and other oils help to increase the outflow of waste through the colon.

- Enzymes can improve digestion and clear bowel impaction

- Colonics can improve peristalsis (movement of food through the digestive tract), as can bifidus and acidophilus (beneficial bacteria), either orally or as an implant after a colonic.

- Vitamin B6, taurine (an amino acid), ox bile, lecithin, inositol, and choline increase bile

- Lipotropic Plus (by Ethical Nutrients), Lipogen (by Metagenics), and Liver-Tox (by Enzymatic Therapy) can increase bile flow and help cleanse the liver.

- Boldo (an herb), magnesium, and homeopathics such as LGB 414 are also beneficial in aiding digestion. Magnesium helps the bowel to retain water.

- Garlic (Kyolic brand recommended) can kill parasites and fungus which can interfere with digestion.

- Kill fungal or bacterial infection that can cause water retention in the higher bowel and dry hard stools in the low bowel.

As with all symptoms, it is better to look for and treat the root cause of constipation rather than subjecting your colon to violent contractions induced by harsh, habit-forming laxatives.

Diet aids - Overweight is a symptom, rather than a primary problem. It can be due to the retention of water or fat to dilute toxins and allergens, or to imbalances in thyroid hormone or insulin. Overweight can be due to taking in too many calories, but surprisingly this is usually not the main cause of overweight. As always, it is important to recognize and treat the cause, not just the symptom. For example, low blood triglycerides (less than 100) usually correlates with a weight problem that is **not** due to excess fat or calories. Weight control and calories are discussed in the Weight Control chapter in **Thriving In A Toxic World**, along with the primary problems leading to overweight and their remedies.

If your adrenals and DHEA are depleted due to the use of diet drugs or other causes, adrenal function can be supported using wild yam cream, tyrosine, pancreatic acid, B6, PABA, and GLA oils.

Recreational Drugs

What are recreational drugs?
The term refers to self-medication used to artificially change one's mood, raise one's energy level, lift one's spirits, cope with problems by dulling the associated feelings, or let down inhibitions. The use of substances for this purpose goes back to the beginnings of recorded history, and include illegal "street drugs" like marijuana, heroin, barbiturates, cocaine, and LSD, as well as legal substances such as alcohol, tobacco, and caffeine.

What are street drugs?
"Street drugs" is another term for illegal drugs. Major categories include depressants, stimulants, and hallucinogens. These drugs are usually injected into a vein or muscle, smoked, swallowed, sniffed (snorted), or taken in combination.

Depressant drugs

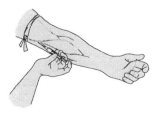

Heroin, which is usually injected intravenously, is a depressant drug which causes a false feeling of well-being and total relaxation. It is strongly addictive, and withdrawal symptoms can be severe but generally not life-threatening. Overdose can be fatal; depressant drugs can slow and stop the heart and respiratory functions. Unintentional overdose usually results when the drug is more concentrated than what the user is used to, since there is no quality control on the streets. Use of heroin, like medical use of morphine (heroin is diacetyl morphine, a close cousin to morphine) can suppress the immune system and can slow down the body's detoxification pathways, allowing toxins to build up in the body. The constipation that results from the use of depressant drugs is an example of this.

Acupuncture has a nearly 100% success rate in alleviating symptoms of heroin and opium withdrawal [13].

Barbiturates (pronounced bar-bit-choo-rits, not bar-bit-choo-its), also known as downers, may be purchased illegally or by prescription. They are depressant, addictive drugs. Unlike heroin withdrawal, in which you may wish you were dead, barbiturate withdrawal can be fatal and should be done gradually under medical supervision.

Stimulant drugs

Stimulant drugs, which are used for a feeling of increased energy and alertness, include cocaine and amphetamines. Cocaine hydrochloride is a white powder that is inhaled (snorted), while cocaine base, also called "crack", is smoked. Amphetamine, also called "crystal" or "meth", can be swallowed, snorted, or injected. A "speedball" is a stimulant and a 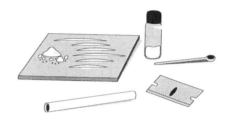 depressant drug taken together, usually heroin and cocaine by injection. Stimulant drugs are addictive, especially crack cocaine. Overdose can be fatal due to cardiac (heart) overstimulation. Sudden death from cocaine use, even with the first dose and unrelated to overdose, has been known to occur. Celtics number one pick basketball star Len Bias died of a heart attack believed to be related to cocaine. His first (as some say) cocaine experience was death.

Withdrawal can be unpleasant, and brings to mind Newton's Law: **"What goes up must come down"**. Coming down can bring fatigue and depression as the drug brought energy and elation.

Hallucinogens

Hallucinogens include LSD, STP, DMT, mescaline, peyote, and others. LSD, or d-lysergic acid diethylamide, is derived from the rye fungus ergot. It is so powerful that an average dose is about 200 micrograms (mcg). A microgram is a millionth of a gram; a gram is 1/28 ounce; 200 mcg would be a barely visible speck of powder. The effects are primarily mental, rather than physical and mental both as with depressants and stimulants. Users report hallucinations, mystical experiences, and supernatural understanding.

Hallucinogens are not thought to be physically addictive and are rarely psychologically addictive, although they are far from harmless. Overdose of naturally-occurring psychedelics (hallucinogens), such as mescaline and peyote, can cause vomiting which eliminates the excess. Death from overdosing on hallucinogens is not the direct result of using hallucinogens, but fatalities that have been directly related to their use were caused by behavior and perception changes (e.g. trying to fly, or driving while under the influence), or by adulterants. "Bad trips" or psychotic episodes have been reported, with both short (hours) or long (months) duration. Tragically, some people never fully return.

All drugs are stored in the body tissues to some extent, and hallucinogens have been known to cause "flashbacks", or episodes of hallucination, months or even years afterward. People who used psychedelics (hallucinogens) in the 1960s may experience flashbacks while undergoing sauna detoxification decades later as the drugs are released into the bloodstream from storage sites in the fat and elsewhere. Chromosome abnormalities are possible, especially with long-term use, along with the risk of birth defects.

Timothy Leary, a prominent advocate of LSD use in the 1960's, appeared in the 1990's to have disjointed thoughts and was spacey and hard to follow in conversation when he appeared on talk shows. This may be the result of too many acid (LSD) trips.

Marijuana

What about marijuana?
Marijuana is also called pot, grass, or reefer. A marijuana cigarette is called a joint. Although illegal, it is almost as much a mainstream drug as it is a street drug. It is used recreationally by 12 to 30 million Americans [14], including many who are otherwise conservative. Marijuana, a leafy material, is usually smoked, but has been known to be eaten by itself or put in food such as brownies.

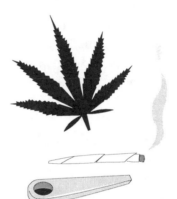

What are the effects of marijuana?
Reported subjective effects vary, with users reporting euphoria, relaxation, enhanced creativity (not proven), and other positive effects. Users often report a heightened sense of whatever they are feeling at the time of smoking, whether good or bad: sociable, paranoid, depressed, tired, excited. Appetite, especially for sweets, is usually triggered, as marijuana sets up conditions favorable to yeast growth which then depletes blood sugar. Yeast overgrowth can occur fast enough to cause sugar cravings within hours of smoking, followed by drowsiness and sleepiness.

Marijuana has not been proven to be physically addictive, although it may be psychologically addictive for some users. It can be used as an escape from taking responsibility and dealing with the problems of maturity. There is no such thing as a marijuana overdose; the drug itself has not been reported to have caused a death as a direct drug effect, although driving while impaired by any drug can be dangerous.

Marijuana is considered by some to be a stepping stone to more dangerous drugs.

Can marijuana be useful medically, and how?
Marijuana research has shown that cannabinoids, the active chemicals in marijuana, are medically useful. Medical benefits include [15]:

- *Relief of nausea, as from chemotherapy*

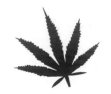

- *Dilating air passages in the lungs, useful to asthmatics*
- *Combating convulsions*
- *Decreasing eye pressure, or glaucoma*
- *Killing pain*
- *Lowering blood pressure*

About 50% of post-chemotherapy patients who tried marijuana or oral THC in any form reported that it relieved their therapy-associated nausea [16].

The value of marijuana in relieving the side effects of cancer chemotherapy is so well recognized that more than 70% of cancer specialists in a Harvard University survey stated that they would prescribe marijuana for this purpose if it were legally available. Nearly half of these specialists have advised patients to break the law if necessary to obtain marijuana [17].

Because of the stigma of recreational use, legal and public acceptance of any possible beneficial effects of cannabinoids, even in pharmaceutical use, is probably a long way off in most of the country. However, in the 1996 election, Californians passed Proposition 215 which allows people to grow or use marijuana for medical use when recommended by a physician. It will be interesting to watch the interpretation and execution of this legal change.

What are marijuana's negative effects?

Marijuana, unlike tobacco and alcohol, does not cause death by overdose and is not considered by most to be physically addictive. However, it is far from harmless. The active ingredient, tetrahydrocannabinol (THC) is fat soluble and is stored in body fat, unlike alcohol, which is rapidly metabolized and excreted. For this reason, marijuana (THC) can be detected in small quantities in the blood 2-4 weeks after the last use.

Its slow release into the blood also means that its effects are present for a while, although not to a debilitating degree. A regular user has an ever-increasing amount being stored in the body. It can take months to get back to normal after quitting since the drug is released from the fat cells and excreted very slowly. Feelings of being "stoned" have been reported by ex-marijuana users who undergo sauna detoxification, even years after the drug use.

Psychological effects of marijuana, other than the immediate high, include:

- *Loss of concentration, short term memory lapses, brain fog*
- *Mood changes such as depression and paranoia*
- *Decline in motivation and increase in procrastination*
- *After prolonged use, depression, apathy, and even suicidal thoughts*

Will marijuana-associated impairment clear up after quitting its use?

Much cognitive function, such as the ability to focus attention, concentrate, remember and filter out irrelevant information, and the speed of information processing, were both adversely affected by marijuana smoking, with effects worsening with increased frequency and duration of use [18]. An additional problem is the development of an on-going yeast infection. [19]

The ability to focus attention and filter out irrelevant information, and the speed of information processing, were both adversely affected by marijuana smoking, with effects worsening with increased frequency and duration of use [18]. It can take a long time to return to normal even after quitting. Cognitive impairments, although minor, can continue for a long time and perhaps permanently after stopping the smoking of marijuana [19,20].

Physical effects include lung damage caused by the inhalation of any kind of smoke, made worse by the fact that marijuana smokers usually inhale deeply and hold the smoke in their lungs as long as possible. Because of this smoking pattern, smoking one joint causes a marijuana user to absorb five times the amount of carbon monoxide and four times the amount of tar as does a tobacco smoker after one cigarette [21]. A few joints per day can therefore cause as much lung damage, including cancer, as a pack of cigarettes per day, smoked for the same length of time. Immune system damage is likely from heavy use, as are birth defects. A tendency towards DNA damage from marijuana smoking has been shown [22].

Other adverse physical and mental effects include [23]:

- *Disrupts all phases of gonadal or reproductive function.*
- *Harmful to fetal development*
- *Symptoms of airway obstruction*
- *Squamous metaplasia - abnormal and precancerous changes in the airway tissues*
- *Cancer of the mouth, jaw and tongue*
- *Non-lymphoblastic leukemia in children of marijuana smoking mothers*
- *Neurobehavioral toxicity*
- *Long-term impairment of memory in adolescents*
- *Prolonged impairment of psychomotor performance*
- *A six-fold increase in the incidence of schizophrenia*
- *Genetic damage can be caused by marijuana [24,25]*

Marijuana grows best in areas such as Hawaii, Mexico, Colombia, and Viet Nam, which have heavy volcanic and geothermal activity. Nearby soil is likely to contain mercury, which enters the plant and is then inhaled when smoked [26]. Other contaminants include herbicides such as Paraquat (used by government agents to kill marijuana plants in the fields and often causing more damage than marijuana itself), other drugs such as phencyclidine (PCP, or Angel Dust) and others, and other leafy material (which may or may not be toxic) to increase the weight before sale. All of these adulterants are, or can be, toxic, and may account for many of the side effects attributed to marijuana.

Marijuana's use can lower the level of hydrochloric acid in the stomach, which allows fungus and helicobacter pylori to proliferate. Fungal growth can cause craving for sweets (referred to as "the marijuana munchies"), fatigue, brain fog, and other symptoms often associated with marijuana use. Fungal overgrowth, or ongoing yeast infection can continue long after the drug has been given up. Both marijuana and fungus can cause immune system suppression.

Tobacco

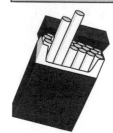

How addictive is tobacco?
Nicotine, the active ingredient in tobacco, is nearly as addictive as crack cocaine. Does this sound hard to believe? Let's look at the nature of addiction.

What exactly is addiction?
Addiction is present when all of the following elements are present:

- A substance (or activity) is not needed by the body to sustain life.

- There is a desire for, and use of, the substance every day, or several times a day (although addiction can be present without daily use).

- It is very difficult to stop using the substance even when there is a strong desire to stop.

- There are physical and emotional withdrawal symptoms when the substance is not available.

- There are strong cravings, anxiety, and difficulty thinking about anything other than the substance if it is not available.

- The person will resort to extreme measures to satisfy the craving such as spending the rent and grocery money on the substance, going through the trash for discarded bits of the substance, or going out to the store in a blizzard.

- It takes more and more of the substance to achieve less and less satisfaction. The need for ever increasing doses is called tolerance, although tolerance can be present without addiction.

It can safely be stated that a person who shows all of these reactions to a substance is definitely addicted to that substance.

What proportion of cigarette smokers are addicted?
Think of everyone you know or have known, including yourself, evaluate their smoking behavior, and separate them into three categories:

a) Nonsmoker

b) Addictive smoker by the above criteria, or quitting but going through withdrawal, craving, and obsessive thoughts about smoking.

c) Nonaddictive smoker. This person can truly take it or leave it, smokes maybe a few times a week, and has no problems if the supply runs out.

There's nobody or almost nobody in the last category, is there? In other words, nearly everybody you know, and by extension the general population, either doesn't smoke at all or is addicted. Smoking tobacco, like smoking crack cocaine, without addiction is almost impossible. Yet the power of self-delusion is such that even someone who has smoked a pack a day for years can insist that they smoke because they like the taste, and that they can quit whenever they want to.

Smokers say they like the relaxing effect of tobacco, but this relaxing effect is due to the alleviation of the withdrawal symptoms, which can start within 30 minutes to three hours after the last cigarette. Smoking is relaxing only in comparison to withdrawal, and a heavy smoker is either smoking or withdrawing almost constantly.

What is nicotine?

Nicotine is the active ingredient in tobacco. It is responsible for both the relaxing or stimulating effects of tobacco and the high addictiveness. Nicotine is a liquid, water soluble alkaloid with no medical therapeutic uses. It is so toxic that a single drop of pure nicotine placed on the skin can cause death within minutes!

> **A single drop of pure nicotine on the skin can cause almost-instant death!**

Nicotine constricts blood vessels, raises blood pressure, stimulates the heart rate, and stimulates brain neurotransmitters [27]. Nicotine initially causes stimulation, followed by depression. Like most other addictive drugs, it causes a phenomenon called tolerance, i.e. progressively more is needed to get the original effect. Nicotine is also found in chewing tobacco.

What other harmful components are in tobacco?

Another component of cigarette smoke is carbon monoxide, which can cause asphyxiation. At the levels typically experienced by smokers, carbon monoxide causes diminished oxygen in the body, so that less oxygen can get to the brain and cells.

Tar, the brownish-yellow stuff that can be seen on the cigarette filter, clogs the alveoli in the lungs and is carcinogenic (cancer causing). Sticky blackish deposits on the lungs, like road tar, can be seen at autopsy.

Nickel, a carcinogen and allergen, is found in cigarette smoke. Other heavy metals in tobacco are cadmium, lead, and arsenic. Cadmium lowers the levels of zinc, an essential mineral necessary for the senses of smell and taste. This is part of why appetite may increase along with the amount of zinc in the body after quitting smoking. Lowered zinc levels also lower anti-cancer immune enzymes, accounting in part for the cancer causing potential of tobacco. The sex hormones progesterone (female) and testosterone (male) are also reduced when a zinc deficiency is present.

Nitrogen oxides are found in both smog and cigarette smoke. They can damage throat and lung tissues and oxidize the body's fats, making them carcinogenic.

Acetaldehyde, also found in both cigarette smoke and smog, is a strong cross-linking agent. Cross-linking of skin causes premature wrinkling, and cross-linked arterial tissue toughens and leads to cardiovascular disease.

What are some of the effects of smoking?

Physical symptoms experienced by smokers include coughing, burning in the chest, dizziness, nausea and loss of appetite. Withdrawal symptoms include obsessive craving for cigarettes, extreme irritability, sleeplessness, depression, and inability to concentrate.

Long term effects of tobacco smoking include [27]:

- A higher death rate at all ages compared with nonsmokers. Men who smoke less than half a pack a day have a death rate 60% higher than nonsmokers at a given age; one to two packs a day, about 90% higher; two or more packs a day, 120% higher.

- Heart attacks and strokes

- Lung cancer is rare in nonsmokers but is the most frequent cause of death in smokers after heart attacks and strokes. About 85% of lung cancers are caused by smoking, for a total of about 100,000 deaths a year in the United States.

- Emphysema and chronic bronchitis. The smoker's risk of death from emphysema and chronic bronchitis is 6.5 to 15 times that of the nonsmoker.

- Other cancers are more prevalent in smokers than in nonsmokers:

    cancer of the mouth - 5 times more prevalent
    cancer of the larynx - 6 to 9 times more prevalent
    bladder cancer - 2 to 3 times; also pancreatic cancer

- 90% of lung cancers and 50 % of bladder cancers are in smokers [28]. Tobacco and alcohol are considered the main risk factors for oral cancer [29].

- Premature, low birth weight, and unhealthy newborns born to women who smoke.

- The risk of spontaneous abortion (miscarriage) in smokers of 11 or more cigarettes per day is 3.35 times that of nonsmoking controls [30].

- Cigarettes are the cause of more than one-third of all residential fire deaths, according to the United States Fire Administration.

- Decreased resistance to other toxins and microorganisms due to liver overload and overall immune system suppression.

The longer one smokes, and the more cigarettes smoked per day, the greater the health risk from any of these causes.

Chewing tobacco, the use of which is on the rise, can cause cancers of the mouth and throat.

How dangerous is smoking, statistically?

In 1994, substance abuse killed about 200,000 women, four times as many as died from breast cancer. About 75% of these deaths were related to tobacco, 20% to alcohol, and 3-5% to other drugs. The fastest growing group of smokers are women younger than 23 years old [31].

The *Lancet*, a mainstream medical journal, published results of an American Cancer Society study of over one million Americans from 1982 to 1988. Smoking attributable deaths are going up in men, and going up even more sharply in women. One in four to one in three people die from a cause directly attributable to smoking.

Smoking attributable deaths in the United States, in thousands [32]:

Year:	1965	1975	1985	1995 (est.)
Male	183	240	277	318
Female	14	56	132	240

Stopping smoking can reduce heart attack risk 50-70%. In one study, the death rate from heart disease in men under age 65 was 427 per 100,000 compared with 166 per 100,000 for those who never smoked [33], or nearly three times as high.

Cigarettes cause two million preventable deaths, including cancers, heart attacks, vascular disease and emphysema. About one thousand Americans die of these per day. **Smoking will kill more Americans than AIDS, heroin, crack cocaine, alcohol, car accidents, fire, and murder combined** [34].

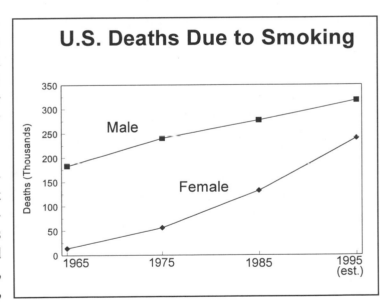

If smoking is so dangerous, why isn't it illegal?

The reasons why some less harmful drugs are illegal and some more harmful drugs are legal have much more to do with politics than with public health or common sense. The tobacco lobby is wealthy and powerful, and has the power to defeat anti-smoking legislation. The well-financed tobacco lobby teams up with Madison Avenue to addict new generations through advertising. "Political science" often overrules science when a lot of money is involved.

What is passive smoking?

Passive smoking is also a danger. The term refers to the smoke inhaled by a nonsmoker who is in the vicinity of a smoker. Studies have shown that children of smokers have more respiratory infections than do children of nonsmokers. People with allergies or asthma are at particular risk from passive smoking.

Children exposed regularly to passive smoke were 38% more likely to develop new incidences of otitis media (ear infection), and the episodes lasted longer, as compared with nonexposed children [35]. The EPA has officially linked passive smoking and increased risk of lung cancer [36].

In one study, 191 nonsmoking patients with primary lung cancer were compared with 191 nonsmoking controls without cancer [37]. It was found that more than 25 smoker-years (number of household smokers times number of years of exposure) doubled the lung cancer risk.

What can be done to protect yourself against passive smoking?

Fortunately, the nonsmokers' rights movement is gaining momentum, especially in California. If you are concerned about your health and if you are tired of being forced to inhale smoke from the cigarettes of inconsiderate smokers, there are actions you can take. Confront the inconsiderate smokers - politely - if you are comfortable doing so. Many smokers are decent people who won't resent the reminder that they are endangering your health and well-being.

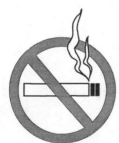

Make use of restaurant comment cards. These are valuable to restaurant managers. If one patron in 100 fills out a comment card, then management assumes that your comment represents the views of 100 people! Good business owners will pay close attention to the views of 100 people. Praise restaurants with nonsmoking policies. A few comments such as the following may generate a change in policy: "We planned on dining at your establishment, but on finding that we would have to wait in/pass through a smoke-filled lobby/bar/dining section, we decided to take our business elsewhere." Try it. This beats getting the government involved.

What about smokeless tobacco?

Smokeless tobacco, sold as chewing tobacco or snuff, contains nicotine which makes these products nearly as addictive as smoked tobacco. Although smokeless tobacco is less likely to cause lung cancer than cigarettes, it is associated with a high incidence of mouth and throat cancers. Chewing tobacco and snuff can raise blood pressure due to its nicotine and sodium content [38].

How can you quit smoking?

If you don't smoke, don't start! There are many drawbacks and no advantages. If you smoke but would like to quit, there are a number of approaches. Almost all smokers have tried to quit at least once but didn't succeed for long, as this is a powerful addiction. Don't give up. You may need to try a different approach. Some approaches include:

146

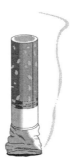

- Cutting down gradually

- Aversion therapy

- Hypnosis

- Different types of formal stop-smoking programs

- Cutting cigarettes out altogether, also called "going cold turkey". This is usually more effective than gradual withdrawal.

- Nicotine patches or gum, available by prescription. These relieve the worst of the physical withdrawal symptoms while you deal with the psychological withdrawal.

- A support group of would-be quitters, including twelve step programs modeled after those used by Alcoholics Anonymous.

- Nutritional support, including vitamin and herbal support for the adrenals, minerals such as zinc and chromium, and amino acids such as glutamine to stabilize blood sugar. Zinc, by replacing the toxic cadmium from cigarettes (they have similar binding sites) can reduce cravings and withdrawal symptoms.

We wish you success! Take the first step and find the approach that works for you, and with the support of a knowledgeable practitioner you can overcome.

Is there anything to do to reduce risks before, during, and after quitting smoking?
It is not uncommon for a long-term smoker to develop smoking-related health complications, especially cancer, several years after quitting. There are several things that can be done while or after quitting smoking to reduce these health risks:

- Chelate out cadmium (reduces beneficial zinc) and nickel (carcinogen and allergen), both of which are in tobacco smoke. Chelation is discussed in the chapter on Metal Detoxification.

- Take beneficial minerals, especially zinc.

- Have the Adrenal Stress Index (ASI) test done to determine whether additional adrenal support is needed (such as the hormone DHEA or pregnenolone).

- Take vitamins, especially vitamin B5 (pantothenic acid) to support adrenal gland function.

- Take omega-3 oils such as flax oil to increase levels of hormones such as adrenaline, which are usually diminished from smoking.

- Take antioxidants such as vitamins A, C, E, bioflavonoids, and selenium to counteract smoking damage.

- Life Solubles and Kona minerals contain many of the above nutrients.

This is where a knowledgeable practitioner can best support you by putting together a support program that encompasses these measures, individually tailored to your needs.

Alcohol

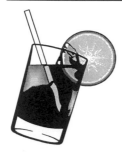

Is alcohol also a drug?

Beverage alcohol, or ethanol, is a powerful and toxic drug disguised as a social beverage. Industrially, it is used as a solvent and degreaser. You can "dress up" alcohol with mixers, fruits, fancy glassware, little umbrellas, swizzle sticks, and cute names, but the fact remains that alcohol is a dangerous, addictive drug.

What are some effects of alcohol?

Although it may initially appear to be a stimulant, alcohol is actually a depressant drug. Seemingly positive subjective effects include euphoria and relaxation of inhibitions. Negative effects include irrational and violent behavior, dizziness, lack of coordination, poor reflexes, and nausea and vomiting. Driving ability is impaired, but so is the ability to judge the degree of impairment, a dangerous combination. This is why many people who are obviously drunk insist that they are able to drive. The consequences of this misjudgment are often fatal.

How much is a "drink"?

One "drink" is usually taken to mean one ounce of pure alcohol, which has the same effect regardless of what form it is in. One ounce of pure alcohol is equivalent to:

- *12 ounces of beer,*
- *5 ounces of wine,*
- *1 1/2 ounces of whiskey, or*
- *An average (not double) cocktail.*

Alcohol is also found in mouthwash (Listerine has 26.9% alcohol [39]), medications such as Nyquil (25%, or 1/4 ounce per dose), and cough syrup. The alcohol in mouthwash, if used for years, can contribute to the development of mouth cancer. Find a brand with natural ingredients, such as Oxyfresh, which actually releases oxygen and does the job without the detrimental effects of alcohol.

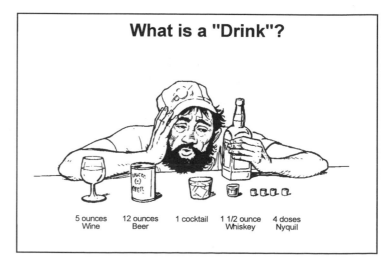

What is a "Drink"?

| 5 ounces Wine | 12 ounces Beer | 1 cocktail | 1 1/2 ounce Whiskey | 4 doses Nyquil |

What is alcoholism?

Alcohol is addictive, as defined in the previous section on tobacco. However, it is not as addictive as tobacco, as it is possible to be a nonaddicted occasional drinker. The line between nonaddicted and addicted is not clear cut. Alcoholics Anonymous has a checklist to determine whether alcohol is a free choice or a problem for you.

There are a number of myths about alcoholism, such as the image that an alcoholic is a filthy, unshaven, staggering drunk lying in the gutter. There are several different patterns of alcoholism, most of which are not stereotypical, but all of which are alcoholism:

- The person who gets drunk every day - this is the stereotype.

- The person who has alcohol with lunch and/or after work every day, without becoming visibly drunk.

- The person who keeps a bottle in the desk drawer, the car, and the clothes hamper, but is functional.

- The person who can go for days without alcohol, but goes on a drunken bender every weekend or every payday.

- The person who rarely or never drinks distilled liquor, but consumes a lot of beer or wine regularly.

Most alcoholics don't accept that they are alcoholics as long as they are still drinking alcohol. They are attempting to judge their degree of impairment or addiction with a mind which is itself impaired.

Personal growth slows nearly to a standstill once the use of alcohol or other mind-altering drugs starts. A person who starts drinking alcohol in his or her teens and stops at the age of forty is basically still a teenager in an adult's body, and often needs to have counseling to move ahead with their life. Alcoholics Anonymous provides this kind of support, as well as support through Alanon for the other family members.

What are the toxic effects of alcohol?

Whether or not one is addicted, alcohol is toxic. The amount of toxic effect depends, as with cigarettes, on the amount of alcohol consumed and the length of time that it has been used. The body will detoxify alcohol at a rate of one ounce every 60 to 90 minutes but although the drug is gone the toxic effects linger and are cumulative. These long-term effects include [40]:

- Cell death, especially in the brain.

- Hepatitis and cirrhosis of the liver (dry or scarred liver); also fatty liver.

- Cancers of the liver, mouth, larynx, pharynx, and esophagus. Breast cancer risk is shown to be increased by 39% with one drink per day average lifetime consumption, by 69% with two drinks per day, and by 130% (more than double) with three drinks per day, as compared with nondrinking controls [41].

- Alcohol and tobacco are the main risk factors for oral (mouth) cancer [29]. Evidence of a causal relationship between alcohol consumption and cancers of the head and neck is increasing [42].

- Gastritis, pancreatitis

- Cardiovascular disease, stroke, hypertension.

- Hypoglycemia, hyperlipidemia

- Fetal alcohol syndrome in babies whose mothers are heavy alcohol users - low birth weight, learning difficulties, facial and cranial deformities.

- Depression, anxiety, amnesia, blackouts.

- Irrational, aggressive and violent behavior is shown, even in placebo-controlled trials done to rule out effects of expectation [43].

- Nutritional deficiencies. B vitamins, especially vitamin B1, are often depleted, as are minerals. Alcohol dilutes, dissolves, and takes nutrients out of the body. Since alcohol is an oil solvent (and is used as such industrially), it can carry out fatty acids and the oil-soluble vitamins A, D, E, and K as well.

- 94% of alcoholics tested showed impaired verbal and nonverbal performance, memory deficits and perceptual motor skills [44].

- Heavy alcohol consumption can contribute to male infertility [45,46], although there is usually at least a partial recovery when alcohol is given up [47].

- Excessive alcohol consumption has been linked to osteoporosis, decreased bone formation, and defective bone mineralization [48,49], as well as bone marrow damage [50].

- Alcohol intake, including and even especially beer, is linked to higher cancer rates [51-53]. This is likely due to the fermenting yeast in beer being similar to fermenting cancer cells.

- Anemia related to folic acid deficiency is common in alcoholics and heavy users of alcohol [54].

- Even moderate alcohol use can raise blood pressure, and chronic alcohol intake is one of the strongest predictors of high blood pressure [55,56].

Alcohol interacts with a wide variety of other drugs, especially other depressants, sometimes with fatal results.

Alcohol increases cancer risk. Alcohol and cigarettes together multiply cancer risk; the risk is not just additive. 90% of cancers of the mouth, larynx, esophagus, and liver are in those who both smoke and drink alcohol. Acetaldehyde, a carcinogen, is found in smoke and is a metabolite of alcohol [28].

The typical alcoholic has a large belly and spindly arms and legs - the same body proportions as seen in pictures of starving children. Although the alcoholic may (or may not) be overweight, the body proportions in both cases are generally the result of severe malnutrition. Not only do alcoholics usually not eat properly, their bodies do not absorb all the nutrients they do take in. Alcohol dissolves and carries out the beneficial oils which themselves aid in the absorption and utilization of nutrients.

One patient, a 55 year old man who had been drinking alcohol nearly all of his adult life, developed autoimmune problems, arthritis, gallbladder problems, and liver damage. He was diagnosed with ankylosing spondylitis, an arthritis-related autoimmune disease. He was put on a program to keep his dry liver moist, including cod liver oil, oil soluble vitamins A, D, E and K, a liver detoxification protocol, and amino acids and protein powder. His health has returned.

What about those studies which claim that alcohol is beneficial?
There have been a few studies which claim that moderate alcohol use actually lowers the risk of heart disease. There are a couple of possible reasons for this apparent effect [57].

Glucose Tolerance Factor (GTF) may have a protective effect. GTF is a fermentation product of alcohol, but it is also found in nutritional sources such as the brewer's yeast itself which is far less toxic.

It may be that the slightly higher incidence of heart disease in nondrinkers is the cause rather than the effect of abstaining. In other words, some people who do not drink alcohol abstain because of preexisting heart disease.

Many of these studies were done in France, where alcohol, especially wine, is consumed regularly. However, the French live a lifestyle that is healthier in some ways than ours. They eat far less sugar, use fewer antibiotics, have fewer C-section births, and have fewer mercury fillings in their teeth, among other differences. The independent nature of the French gives them some resistance to our so-called scientific advances. These lifestyle differences, and not their alcohol consumption, may be responsible for the perceived benefits. Recall the discussion in the Testing Methods and Bias chapter in *Thriving In A Toxic World* on the lack of validity of studies with more than one variable.

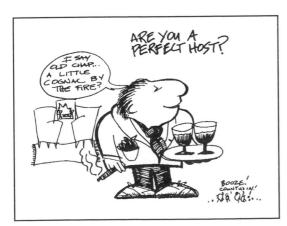

What else is in alcoholic beverages besides alcohol?

Alcoholic beverages are made from fruits or grains; these sources are called congeners. Many of these cause allergic reactions, including an **allergic addiction** or gluten intolerance which may account for some cases of alcoholism, especially where only one type of alcoholic beverage appears to fill the addictive need. Some types of alcohol and their congeners are:

- *Whiskey*   *Rye, barley*
- *Beer*   *Malt, hops*
- *Wine*   *Grapes, other fruit*
- *Bourbon*   *Corn*

Other ingredients which have been found in beverage alcohol include [58]:

- *Plastic (PVP)*
- *Mineral oil*
- *Glycerin*
- *Ammonia*
- *Methylene chloride (solvent)*
- *Artificial flavors*
- *Sulfur compounds*
- *Asbestos residues*
- *Lead residues*
- *Hydrogen peroxide*
- *Artificial colors*
- *Pesticide residues*

Fermenting yeast byproducts are also found in alcohol. These additives or contaminants are toxic to even a healthy person. A long term alcohol user would likely be affected by these to a much greater extent, since his detoxification systems have been weakened by alcohol and his cells have been made more permeable by alcohol's solvent effects.

Distillation, which concentrates the alcohol to an extent greater than that naturally produced by fermentation, also concentrates pesticides and some other contaminants.

What happens when you overdose?

Effects of overdose include unconsciousness, coma, and death. Chug-a-lugging alcohol, or drinking as much and as fast as possible, is a common fraternity hazing stunt which has led to a number of deaths. Alcohol is certainly not an innocuous drug, and its legality and social acceptance does not negate the dangers.

What happens when an addicted person quits drinking?

Withdrawal symptoms in an addicted person include delirium tremens (DTs), or hallucinations; shaking and tremors; and depression. The morning-after hangover is similar to withdrawal in that more alcohol will temporarily alleviate the symptoms. Alcoholics sometimes refer to this effect as "the hair of the dog that bit you". The hangover effects, including a pounding headache and hypersensitivity to stimuli, are caused by the metabolism of a large amount of alcohol to acetaldehyde, a substance that may be more toxic than alcohol itself. Methanol, or wood alcohol, can comprise up to 10% of the alcohol in beverage alcohol. Methanol and its metabolite formaldehyde (embalming fluid) are more toxic than ethanol and contribute to DTs.

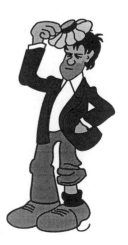

Recovery from alcohol use or abuse depends on the extent of alcohol use. A light or moderate non-addicted user may only need to realize the dangers involved, make up his or her mind to give it up, and do so with minimal discomfort. An alcoholic can make use of Alcoholics Anonymous or other programs. Before therapy can begin, however, the body must be physically detoxified of alcohol, a process sometimes called drying out which may require hospitalization and medication. After drying out, the body should be fully detoxified, including getting rid of the fungus overgrowth which commonly is found in those who use alcohol. Alcohol craving can continue if the fungus is not eliminated. These cravings are the fungus clamoring to be fed.

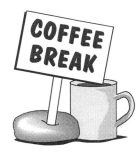

It is common for those in alcohol recovery to be addicted to sugar. After a typical Alcoholics Anonymous meeting, members can often be found in the back of the room with a cup of heavily sugared coffee and a couple of donuts. Sugar cravings will continue until fungus or bacteria are eliminated. Also, alcohol is made from sugar, yeast (a fungus), moisture, and warmth, conditions that exist in the body of a sugar-eating recovering alcoholic. Such a person will be making alcohol in his/her body, a phenomenon called the **auto-brewery syndrome** or a dry drunk.

Quitting isn't easy, but it is much easier when the body is detoxified of fungus. A sober, drug-free life is worth it!

Caffeine

Caffeine can't be a drug, can it?

Coffee is the most commonly used drug in the United States [59]. Caffeine is a drug used primarily for its stimulant effects, although many people who drink caffeinated beverages do so for the taste. A cup of coffee or its equivalent in the morning makes the user feel more alert, with improved concentration and greater energy. In actuality, the habitual caffeine user is simply canceling out the withdrawal symptoms of lethargy and brain fog to attain the state that would be normal if the person were not a caffeine user.

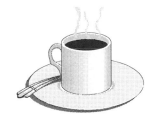

Caffeine pushes the adrenal glands to produce more adrenaline, raising energy short term but depleting the adrenals and lowering overall energy over the long term.

Caffeine is a member of a chemical family called the methylxanthines, which include caffeine, theobromine (found in chocolate), and theophylline (asthma medication; also found in tea). These are all addictive and cross-reactive.

Caffeine is addictive, with increasing tolerance and withdrawal symptoms. Unlike addiction to the other drugs, however, caffeine addiction is not disabling (in fact, caffeine can be "abling" in the short term), and a person can drink several cups of coffee a day for years with no ill effects that are readily apparent. However, caffeine use can cause fungus growth, constricted arteries, constipation, and faster blood clotting which can in turn lead to stroke, heart attack, or phlebitis. The faster clotting time is visible under the microscope during the Live Blood Analysis (LBA) test, discussed in the chapter on A Visit To The Doctor in *Thriving In A Toxic World*.

Where is caffeine found?

It takes 50 to 100 milligrams (mg) of caffeine to produce the characteristic pharmacologic actions of the drug. A milligram is 1/30,000 of an ounce. Some sources of caffeine and the amount contained are in this chart [27].

The amount of caffeine in coffee depends on method of preparation. Brewed coffee usually contains more caffeine than instant. The amount of caffeine in tea depends on brewing time. Colas differ depending on brand.

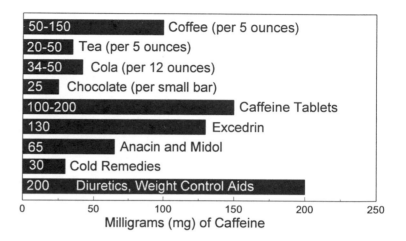

Caffeine in Common Products

Milligrams (mg) of Caffeine	
50-150	Coffee (per 5 ounces)
20-50	Tea (per 5 ounces)
34-50	Cola (per 12 ounces)
25	Chocolate (per small bar)
100-200	Caffeine Tablets
130	Excedrin
65	Anacin and Midol
30	Cold Remedies
200	Diuretics, Weight Control Aids

In addition to the above sources, caffeine is found in:

- *Dr. Pepper soda*
- *Other pain medications such as APC tablets*
- *Caffeine pills such as NoDoz and Vivarin*
- *Some cold remedies such as Dristan and Triaminicin*
- *Weight control aids such as Dexatrim, Dietac, and Prolamine*
- *Jolt cola, an especially high caffeine brand that is named for this characteristic*
- *Ma Huang, an herb*
- *Kola nut*
- *Guarana*
- *Green tea*

Coffee, tea, and colas come in decaffeinated versions, and most types of medications come in non-caffeinated brands. Decaffeinating coffee and tea, however, usually uses a chemical called methylene chloride, or dichloromethane. Residues of this toxic chemical may be left in the beverage. Decaffeinated coffee contains 2-3% caffeine, down from the usual 5%, and is not truly caffeine-free.

What are the adverse effects of caffeine?

Symptoms of usage, especially large amounts or long-term use, may be so subtle as to go nearly unnoticed, or may be quite uncomfortable. Many people don't think of caffeine as a drug and so may not make the connection between caffeine intake and symptoms. These symptoms include:

- CNS stimulation - irritability, nervousness, insomnia, headaches, ears ringing. Heavy caffeine use (4-5 cups of coffee) can cause an increase in headache risk by 30% for males and 20% for females [60]. Habitual caffeine use, when discontinued, can lead to a withdrawal headache that starts about 18 hours after the last caffeine and peaks 3-6 hours later [61]. Even low caffeine intake has been correlated with withdrawal headaches [62].

- Gastrointestinal - nausea, diarrhea, stomach pain

- Cardiovascular stimulation - tachycardia, heart arrhythmias, palpitations, high blood pressure. There is a direct correlation between the amount of coffee consumed and the raising of blood pressure [63].

- Cancer - basal cell carcinoma patients were studied, and it was found that caffeine consumption was higher in cancer patients than in controls [64]. A caffeine intake of over 3 cups of coffee per day is associated with higher cancer rates [65]. It can damage cellular DNA and interfere with its repair [66,67]. Caffeine also sets up a fermenting environment, preferred by cancer cells.

- Miscarriage - the increase in the miscarriage rate in women who drink coffee or caffeine in any form as compared with controls who didn't use caffeine ranged from more than double for those who drank 2-3 cups of coffee (141-280 mg/day) to a fifteen-fold increase when 421 or more mg of caffeine was consumed on a daily basis [30].

- Bone loss - Caffeine in amounts equivalent to two or more cups of coffee daily has been linked to increased bone loss, osteoporosis and hip fracture [59,68]. Those who drink more than three cups of coffee per day increase their risk of osteoporosis by 82% [69]. Caffeine acts as a chelate to remove calcium, causing inflammation which pulls calcium from the long bones.

- Heart attack - heavy coffee consumption (5 or more cups per day) has been shown to increase the risk of heart attack in a study done on women [70].

- A high intake of caffeine can decrease fertility in women [71].

- Other - frequent urination, flushing

Withdrawal symptoms include headache, irritability, lethargy, drowsiness and yawning, inability to concentrate, depression, restlessness, caffeinated beverage cravings, and runny nose. As with other stimulants, Newton's Law - **"What goes up must come down"** - is in effect here.

Caffeine may be one of the safer drugs and milder addictions, but it still has no place in the body of someone who is working towards better health. This is true for the other recreational drugs as well.

There are coffee substitutes, made from grains, which can provide an alternative social drink and the satisfaction of a warm, soothing cup for the daily "coffee break". This can be helpful during the transition phase as you take caffeine out of your diet.

To Think About

Are you addicted?

Most of the drugs discussed here are or can be addictive. Certain foods and substances such as sugar can also be addictive. **Indulgences lead to habits, and habits lead to addiction**. Are you addicted? Your judgment on the matter may be impaired by the drug(s) you are taking. **Try going without the substance for 90 days**. If you can't seem to do so, there's your answer. If you can and do give up the substance, look back and ask yourself whether you would like your life to be the way it was before. The answer will rarely be yes.

Some comment and questions to ponder

There are a wide range of opinions on which drugs should be legal and which should be illegal. Some questions and thoughts on the subject to consider:

- A drug will affect the body in a particular way independent of its legal status.
- Should drugs be left legal once they are discovered to be dangerous?
- Should anything effective that is not dangerous be classified as a drug?

Some drugs that have no medicinal value and are proven to be dangerous, such as alcohol and tobacco, are legal for reasons that have more to do with powerful political lobbies than public health concerns. Should we let classifications based on political considerations determine which drugs we see as okay? A blind acceptance of the status quo can lead to hypocrisy. It seems to be best to educate ourselves about any drug of any type that we might consume and make an informed decision about whether or not to use it, rather than depending on the government or special interest groups to protect us.

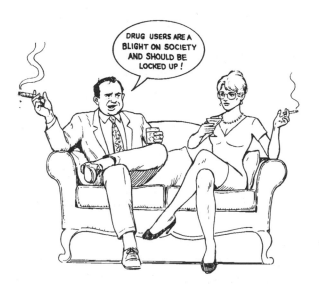

Are we hypocritical?

References and Resources

- The Burton Goldberg Group, "Addictions", pp. 485-493, *Alternative Medicine: The Definitive Guide*, Future Medicine Publishing, Puyallup WA, 1994.

- Cooley, Leland and Lee Morrison Cooley, *Pre-Medicated Murder?*, Chilton Book Co., Radnor PA, 1974.

- Dadd, Debra Lynn, *Nontoxic and Natural*, Jeremy P. Tarcher Inc., Los Angeles CA, 1984.

- Hoffer, Abram and Humphrey Osmond, *New Hope For Alcoholics*, University Books, NY, 1966.

- Krogh, David, *Smoking: The Artificial Passion*, W.H. Freeman and Co., New York, 1991.

- Levine, R., *Pharmacology: Drug Actions and Reactions*, Little, Brown and Co., 1978.

- Levy, Stephen J., *Managing the Drugs in Your Life*, McGraw-Hill Publishing Co., NY, 1983.

- Murray, Michael T., *Natural Alternatives to Over-The-Counter and Prescription Drugs*, William Morrow and Co. Inc., New York, 1994. *Discusses side effects of common medications and some natural alternatives, listed by medical condition. Good halfway measure - better than drugs but still symptom-suppressing rather than root-cause oriented.*

- Murray, Michael T., *Natural Alternatives to Prozac*, William Morrow, NY, 1996.

- Murray, Michael T., *The Healing Power of Herbs*, Prima Publishing, Rocklin CA, 1992, 1995. *Herbs listed alphabetically and how they can help common ailments, again providing an alternative to drugs.*

- Pearson, Durk, and Sandy Shaw, *Life Extension*, Warner Books, New York, 1982.

- *Physician's Desk Reference*, Medical Economics Co., Oradell NJ, 1993.

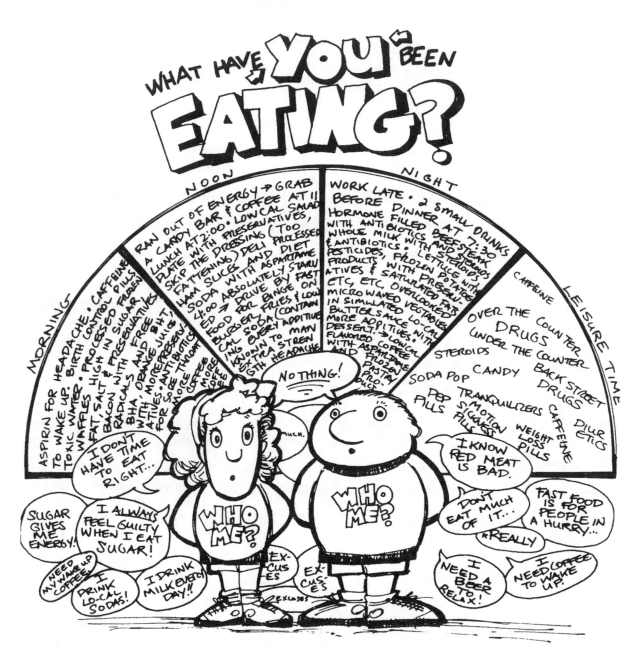

EAT IT NOW...PAY FOR IT LATER!

FOOD ADDITIVES

Why Does Food Need This Kind Of Help?

Do you have any of the following symptoms? They may be due to food additives.

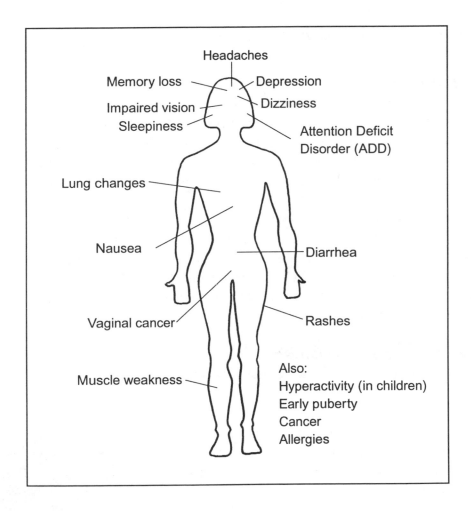

In this chapter you can learn:

- *What are food additives, and are all of them added intentionally?*

- *The average person eats about his or her own weight in food additives per year.*

- *The average meat-eating person consumes about a glassful of antibiotics per year from the meat.*

- *Why are additives used?*

- *Government regulations don't protect us from food additives. Most additives do not need to be on the label, but they are still in the food.*

- *What are the different types of food additives, what are their dangers, and where are they found?*

- *What do "natural" and "organic" mean when used to describe food?*

- *How are artificial flavors made? Are artificial sweeteners safe?*

- *Can additives cause hyperactivity in children?*

- *How can students be made smarter?*

- *The less a food is processed, the healthier it is.*

What are food additives?

Food additives are substances which do not occur naturally in foods. Additives can be intentional, or added for a purpose such as coloring or preservation. They may be unintentional; substances may enter the food during growing and processing. The FDA lists 2800 intentional food additives [1]. About 3000 chemicals are deliberately added to our food supply [2]. Many of these are not legal for use in other countries such as Canada and parts of Europe.

How much of these additives are consumed?

It is estimated that the average American consumes nearly 150 pounds, or about his or her own weight, in food additives per year, including 10-15 pounds of flavoring agents, preservatives, and dyes. More than 10,000 [3] to 15,000 [4] known chemicals may be involved in food production from ground to stomach. The average meat-eating American is consuming as much as a glassful of antibiotics yearly from meat.

What are some sources of food additives?

Additives of both types (intentional and unintentional) include:

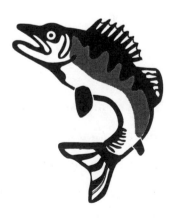

- Drugs given to cattle before slaughter that are in our beef

- Pesticides and chemical fertilizers used on produce and grains, which are then either consumed directly or taken in by animals that we eat

- Unintended environmental pollutants that enter the food chain, such as mercury in fish from polluted waters

- Colors, bleaches, flavors, textures, softeners, waxes

- Preservatives, artificial sweeteners

Why are additives used?

The bottom line for the food producer or manufacturer is profit - making as much money as possible in as little time as possible. To this end, those involved with food production and sale - farmers, processors, shippers - use whatever methods they can, within legal limits (usually). These methods include:

- Using hormones and antibiotics to shorten the length of time needed to fatten a steer to market weight

- Using preservatives to extend shelf life of food, since wasted food is wasted money

- Coloring oranges, waxing apples, and bleaching flour for consumer eye appeal

- Using pesticides on produce and grain to minimize losses and blemishes from pests

- Using cheaper ingredients, or synthetic rather than natural ingredients, to decrease product cost to attract consumers

- Developing and using artificial sweeteners and imitation oils to meet consumer demand for lower calorie products

- Raising vegetables for good shipping qualities to minimize expensive losses

The race to save money on production costs leads to flavorless non-aged beef which is full of drugs and hard pink tasteless tomatoes picked before they are ripe. Artificial flavors and colors are used to make up the difference whenever possible. Consumers have been conditioned to want picture-perfect devitalized produce and expensive, heavily advertised nonfoods. The end result is a marketplace full of unnatural chemicals and "foods" which may do the body more harm than good.

What's wrong with making food cheaper and more attractive?

The methods used to save money and attract consumers lead to our ingesting harmful chemicals in the form of intentional and unintentional additives. In the process, nutritional quality is often sacrificed.

What can you do to protect yourself from this unwanted chemical exposure?

The first line of defense is to be well informed about the various additives, including those not mentioned on the product label. This is the purpose of this chapter. Once you have this information, you will be better equipped to make food buying decisions.

Don't government regulations protect us?

Government labeling regulations state that certain information must be printed on the product label or container, and that the information must be accurate. Other information which we might find useful in order to protect ourselves from harmful ingredients need not be on the label.

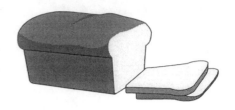

Ingredients must be listed in descending order by weight. Only intentional additives need to be listed, and only if they are added to the end product rather than to an intermediate product. For example, a loaf of bread may list flour as the first, or most plentiful, ingredient. The chlorine dioxide used to bleach the flour need not be listed, nor does the pesticide that was added to the grain.

Certain food colors must be listed due to their high allergic potential. Other colors can be lumped together and simply called "artificial colors". Flavors and spices can be grouped together and simply called "artificial and natural flavors" or "spices" without elaboration.

Another glitch in the labeling law allows omission of ingredients on the label where listing of ingredients might reveal a company's "secret formulas" to competitors. To protect trade secrets, which seems to be a higher priority than public health, a multitude of ingredients can be hidden by the terms seasonings, spices, and flavorings. Ingredients such as whey (a milk product) and peanuts can be hidden in this way. These ingredients can cause severe and even fatal allergic reactions in susceptible individuals [5].

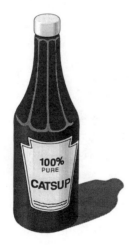

What are government standards of identity?

The government has minimum standards of identity for certain foods, such as mayonnaise, ice cream, catsup, margarine, and milk. Mayonnaise, for example, must contain a minimum amount of whole egg, and ice cream must contain a minimum amount of butterfat. These ingredients do not need to be listed on the label, since they are implied by the name "mayonnaise" or "ice cream". If a product resembles another product for which standards of identity have been set, but does not itself meet these standards, it must be called by another name. There are many cheaper look-alike products which, for this reason, are called "imitation" -- such as mayonnaise, frozen dairy dessert, ice milk, sandwich spread, process cheese food, and whipped topping.

What is the conflict faced by manufacturers?

Manufacturers must comply with these regulations, but they must also tempt consumers to buy their products. This conflict of interest can lead many of them into packaging practices that are, to put it euphemistically, creative. If a product has a commonly accepted word in its name such as fruit, milk, cheese, meat, or crab, the product must contain a certain minimum percentage of these foods. One way around this regulation is to put the word "flavored" after the word, as in "fruit flavored". Another common dodge is to use an alternative spelling. Thus there are cereals made of "froot", chips and spreads with "cheez", and dubious-looking seafood salads made of "krab". There is no legal standard of identity for froot, cheez, or krab. Manufacturers can therefore lure consumers with nonfoods that sound like foods, save money by using unnatural ingredients, and avoid government agency penalties. Pretty good deal - for them, not for us.

What do the terms "natural" and "organic" mean?

Other words that are commonly used in these health-conscious times are "organic" and "natural". The term "natural" is normally used to mean something made by nature, even though that may have been many processing steps ago. Refined sugar is therefore considered natural by this definition. "Natural" has only a loose legal definition, and in some states only 5% of the product may need to be from nature rather than from a laboratory to qualify as legally natural.

California is one of the few states that has a legal definition of "organically grown". Land used for growing organic produce must be free of pesticides and inorganic fertilizers for several years (the exact number varies by state) for the claim "organically grown" to be legally applied. In most states the term "organic" can mean practically anything.

What items are considered food in this society?

Food can be that which is easily recognizable and presumed healthful - fruits, vegetables, whole grains, meat, eggs, milk and milk products. At the other end of the spectrum are (non)foods which may or may not mimic something natural - sweetened cereals, meatless gravy mixes, marshmallow-filled desserts, dinner mixes consisting of white rice or pasta with a packet of chemicals. Many of these nonfoods are just mixtures of additives with white flour for bulk. The nutrient content may be close to zero, apart from calories.

Is real food always healthy?

Even the food in the recognizable and presumed healthful category can have an appalling number of unintentional additives. Although most of these additives are applied deliberately at some stage, it is not intended that they be in the finished product (as compared with, say, food colors or flavors). Regardless of intention, however, these chemicals **are** in the food, and after eating them the chemicals are in our bodies.

What's wrong with meat?

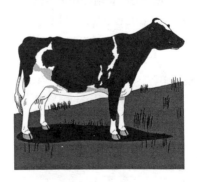

Take meat, for example. A hundred years ago, cattle roamed the range. They ate, slept, exercised, and mated as they chose, and matured at a rate determined by God. After about three years, they were slaughtered, and the meat was hung up to age naturally, resulting in meat that was tasty and free of unnatural drugs.

Cattle raising has changed drastically in the name of profit. The ideal beef steer, milk cow, calf, pig, lamb, or chicken is one that stands in one place, voluntarily or otherwise, and eats around the clock, reaching marketable weight in half the time it would take naturally. These ideal animals would not have desires that would conflict with this goal, such as wanting to exercise or mate or show their annoyance at this treatment. Sick or dying cattle cut into profits. To this end, i.e. making money quickly, [6]:

- Cattle are fed pesticide treated grain. Additional pesticides are often given to treat the parasitic infections that the weakened animals can't fight off themselves. The pesticides can be so concentrated that the animals' excrement will not attract flies. Pesticides are stored in the animal's liver, lymph, and fat. Animal livers contain more nutrients than muscle meat, but since they are the animal's detoxifying plant, the livers may now contain more harmful chemicals than does the rest of the animal.

- Cattle are given tranquilizers to keep them from wanting to do anything but eat. If you feel sleepy after eating a heavy meat-containing meal, this may have something to do with it.

- Antibiotics are used to prevent and treat infections. These antibiotics, ingested by humans, can cause allergic reactions in susceptible individuals, and are toxic in general over time. Bacterial infections are becoming antibiotic resistant due to misuse of antibiotics, including their use in meat. Since antibiotics kill the beneficial bacteria that keep yeast under control, the epidemic of recurrent yeast infections may be related to the eating of meat containing antibiotics.

- Diethylstilbestrol (DES), a drug which can cause otherwise rare vaginal cancers and breast problems, is used to pad the animal's body with moisture and fat.

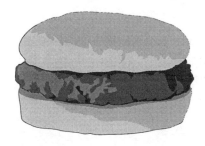

We are ingesting all these drugs with our steak. Conditions are similar in the mass producing and marketing of other animal products - milk and milk products, lamb, pork, eggs, and chicken.

A study reported in *Science News* found 75 different chemical compounds in the smoke from charcoal broiled hamburgers, including hydrocarbons, furans, steroids, and pesticide residues.

It has been noticed by parents and doctors throughout the country that the physical changes of puberty are occurring a year or two earlier on average than in the previous generation. The previous average age of puberty was in turn a year or two earlier than in the generation prior to that. Hormones are given to cattle and chickens to increase their growth rate so they mature and reach marketable weight faster. The resultant meat, milk, chicken, and eggs are consumed in large quantities by children. There may well be a connection between the growth hormones given to food animals and the earlier maturation of our younger generations.

Meat in itself can be a healthful product, but the additives are so harmful that meat as we know it can be hazardous to your health.

So we should all be vegetarians?
If you have chosen not to eat animal products, you are not home free. Produce and grains are nearly always sprayed with pesticides. Some of the pesticide residues can be removed by washing or by peeling off the vitamin-rich skin, or by washing the produce in a weak bleach solution, hydrogen peroxide, or vegetable washes sold in health food stores. Pesticides, however, are absorbed through the plant roots and permeate the cells of the fruits, vegetables, and grain.

How does pollution affect plants?

Water and air pollution is also absorbed into these plants. For example, Irvine, a city in Orange County, California was, until recently, primarily an agricultural community. As you drive north through Irvine on one of several eight-lane freeways heading towards nearby Los Angeles, you will notice the orange-brown sky up ahead, the smoke-belching diesel trucks, the new skyscrapers and industrial plants, and Irvine's recently expanded airport. You will notice air that you can almost taste as you rub your burning eyes. You will also notice, incongruously, acres and acres of farmland, with neat rows of produce stretching towards the horizon.

Since you are reading this book, you are probably health conscious and possibly chemically sensitive. How comfortable would you feel about eating this produce, which has absorbed the air and water in the area? Unfortunately, Irvine is not an isolated example. Such contaminated produce is sent to supermarkets all over the country. One solution would be to buy produce from local organic growers, or to grow your own whenever possible.

What are some kinds of intentional additives?

There are many types of intentional additives. These are classified here according to type and discussed following this list:

- *Waxes*
- *Bleaches*
- *Nutrients*
- *Sweeteners*
- *Humectants*
- *Preservatives*
- *Artificial colors*
- *Artificial flavors*
- *Anticaking agents*
- *Stabilizers and thickeners*

Are preservatives good or bad?

Some preservatives may also be called antioxidants. A product label may use the phrase "to retard spoilage" after the name of the preservative. Preservatives may be used to prevent the formation of toxic breakdown products such as aflatoxins from the mold on peanuts and potatoes. In this case they have a beneficial effect which outweighs the hazards. Unfortunately, preservatives are often used for the comparatively frivolous purpose of maintaining a fresh appearance. Preservatives include:

• Sodium sulfite	Used in salad bars, dried apples, fish. High allergic potential, including possibly fatal anaphylactic shock.
• Calcium propionate	Used in baked goods
• Sodium nitrate, nitrite	Used in cured meats, frankfurters, and bacon. Can form cancerous nitrosamines.
• Ascorbic acid	Used in fruits and acid foods. This is Vitamin C - harmless, beneficial
• Citric acid	Used in acidic foods, fruits. Safer than most.

- Tocopherols — Vitamin E - harmless, beneficial

- BHA and BHT — Used in baked goods, cereals, oils. Antioxidant. Can cause lung changes and hypersensitivity.

- EDTA — Chelating agent to remove minerals that may cause deterioration or discoloration.

Nitrates, which are often added to meats such as hot dogs and lunch meats, may cause headaches in susceptible people [7].

Why are stabilizers and thickeners used?

Stabilizers and thickeners are used to keep foods such as salad dressing from separating, and to improve "mouthfeel" (a self-explanatory food industry term). Although they are not necessary, they are for the most part relatively harmless. Most of these are natural products derived from seaweeds, gums, lecithin, pectin, and cellulose, and are safe to consume. Examples are:

- *agar*
- *guar gum*
- *alginate*
- *gum arabic*
- *methylcellulose*
- *carrageenan*
- *gum tragacanth*
- *sodium caseinate*
- *mono- and diglycerides*

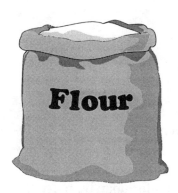

Do bleaches have any purpose other than cosmetic?

Bleaches whiten food, or remove color so that artificial color will look better. This is similar to the process of bleaching your hair so that even dark colors will penetrate better. Bleaches are primarily used on flour, oils, margarine, fruits, and maraschino cherries. Chemicals used include calcium bromate, potassium bromide, chlorine dioxide, and nitrogen peroxide, which are toxic. The use of these products is especially unacceptable considering the purely cosmetic benefit gained combined with the products' toxicity.

What are humectants, and where are they used?

Humectants, also call humefactants, keep food moist by absorbing and retaining water. They are used mainly in baked goods, cake mixes, meats, and marshmallows. Humectants include:

- Polyphosphates — Injected or rubbed into meat

- Propylene glycol — Used in your car in larger amounts as antifreeze; toxic

  Mannitol, sorbitol — Do double duty since they are also used as sweeteners. Not beneficial, but less harmful than other humectants and sweeteners.

- Glycerol, glycerine — Used in toaster foods, marshmallows, flaked coconut

Why are artificial colors used?

Artificial colors are used to color foods, either to impart color to candies and other nonfoods, or to enhance or disguise colors of natural foods such as oranges. Artificial colors can be divided into two categories - naturally derived and chemically created. Chemical colors usually go by names such as FD&C (Food, Drug, and Cosmetic) Red (or blue or yellow) No. such-and-such. Each number has a different formula, and these are periodically taken off the market and replaced as cancer-causing potential or other risk is discovered. Some of these colors are listed individually on labels due to their high allergic potential, while others are lumped together as "artificial colors".

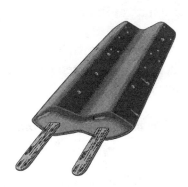

Food dyes are stored in the lymph nodes, essentially forever. For example, if you eat beets or take riboflavin (vitamin B2), your urine may temporarily and harmlessly turn red or bright yellow as your body eliminates the natural coloring agent. However, if you eat an artificially dyed food such as bright orange cheese puffs, fruit drinks or sodas, your urine does not change color. This means the dyes are not being excreted and are thus retained in the body.

Can additives cause hyperactivity in children?

Allergic reactions to tartrazine, also known as yellow dye #5, have been reported as early as the 1940s. In animal experiments red dye #3 applied to the nervous system caused rapid voltage changes. These changes are possibly related to hyperactivity and attention deficit disorder (ADD). Many hyperactive children show a startling behavioral improvement when these and other additives are removed from their diets. Animal studies show that certain food dyes interfere with chemical communication in the brain. In low doses the dyes enter the brain readily, inhibiting the uptake of neurotransmitters by the nerve cells [8].

Naturally derived colors are generally safe, and include:

- *Beta carotene*   *Vitamin A precursor, found in carrots. Orange-yellow color.*
- *Caramel*   *From cooked sugar, gives brownish color and characteristic flavor*
- *Beet juice*   *Reddish color*
- *Riboflavin*   *Yellowish color and nutrient (vitamin B2)*
- *Chlorophyll*   *From green plants. Green color*

How are artificial flavors made?

Artificial flavors are usually made by analyzing a real food flavor (such as vanilla, lemon, or ham) to determine the combination of chemicals that produce the flavor. Some of these chemicals - there may be dozens contributing to a single flavor - are then mixed in the laboratory to produce a flavor that bears some resemblance to the real thing. An example is vanillin, a crystalline phenolic aldehyde (a chemical group) which is the primary, but not the only, fragrant component found in the vanilla bean. Commercial vanillin, made in the laboratory, has never seen a vanilla bean.

Almost all artificial flavors are listed on the label simply as "artificial flavors". Their safety cannot be commented on since so many chemicals may be involved, but at least only small amounts are used.

How are shiny foods like the hood of your car?

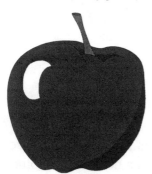

Waxes are used to give a shiny coating to jelly beans and other candies, and to both shine (for consumer appeal) and preserve fruits and vegetables such as apples, cucumbers, and peppers. Most of these waxes are petroleum derivatives such as paraffins, carnauba, and petroleum naphtha, and differ from the wax on your car only in quantity

Naphtha, an ingredient used in car finishes, is so toxic, it can destroy brain cells. It is a clear liquid similar to a solvent like paint remover or paint thinner. A visiting artist at a local state college used it as a special ingredient in a glazing mixture to achieve special affects. He cautioned students to use care in mixing the glaze "recipe". Curiously, this teacher, who had been mixing this toxic ingredient in his own art materials for many years, sounded, when he spoke, like a New Jersey boxer who had taken too many punches. Had the toxicity of the materials he warned his students of taken its toll to the point he no longer realized the damage done? Enamored of the special effects which were a hallmark of his style of painting, he seemed addicted to the use of this material which he seemed disinclined to give up, no matter the cost.

What keeps powdered foods from clumping?

Anticaking agents are used to prevent caking in powdered foods and table salt. Almost any additive with aluminum and/or silicate in the name, such as sodium aluminosilicate, calcium silicate, or silicon dioxide, is likely to be an anticaking agent. Silica is basically sand, and aluminum is a toxic metal in salt form which has been linked to Alzheimer's disease.

What is done about the great American sweet tooth?

We are born with a preference for sweet foods. Nearly all babies prefer a bottle of sugar water over plain water. Unfortunately, manufacturers exploit this by adding sweetener to even the most unlikely products. Some salad dressings contain more corn syrup than oil or vinegar - read the labels sometime. This use of sweetener in practically everything is only fueling the epidemic sugar addiction in this country. Sugar addiction is a vicious cycle. Sugar in any form feeds fungus (yeast), which multiplies and takes sugar from our blood, which in turn causes more of a sugar craving.

There are a number of different kinds of sweeteners used in products. These include:

- *Sugar*
- *Corn syrup*
- *Artificial sweeteners*
- *Sorbitol, mannitol*

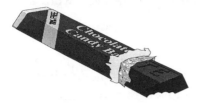

Sugar, its deleterious effects, and foods in which it is found are discussed in detail in the Carbohydrates chapter of ***Thriving In A Toxic World***. Corn syrup has the drawbacks of sugar, and is additionally an allergen for many people due to its source: highly allergenic corn. Sugar is indicated in words ending in "ose", such as lactose or fructose, as well as sucrose (table sugar).

Sorbitol and mannitol are absorbed more slowly than sugar, and are sometimes recommended for diabetics for this reason, but they are really no better than sugar.

Artificial sweeteners include cyclamates, banned in the 1960s for their cancer causing potential, saccharin, which has also been implicated in cancer formation, and aspartame (NutriSweet).

What are the problems with the sweetener aspartame?

Aspartame, a relatively recently introduced artificial sweetener, is made up of the amino acids phenylalanine and aspartic acid. It tastes more like sugar than either cyclamate or saccharin, and does not have the bitter or salty aftertaste associated with saccharin. It is the most prevalent artificial sweetener in use today, and is used in a wide variety of diet products, especially diet sodas. It cannot be used for cooked or baked goods since it will decompose with heat.

The manufacturers tout the fact that their product is made of these natural ingredients, the two amino acids. However, when chemically combined they are not the same as they would be individually, and their breakdown products, such as methanol and its metabolic byproduct formaldehyde, can be toxic.

There have been a number of health problems associated with aspartame use. About 6000 consumers have called the FDA and volunteered information on side effects, including hundreds of cases of convulsions. Other side effects reported include [9]:

• *Headaches*	• *Confusion*	• *Impaired vision*
• *Depression*	• *Dizziness*	• *Muscle weakness*
• *Hyperactivity*	• *Rashes*	• *Memory loss*
• *Nausea*	• *Insomnia*	• *Diarrhea*

Aspartame can, ironically, cause weight gain, the opposite of the reason most people use the additive. The sweet taste, although not due to sugar, can stimulate the release of insulin, which increases the appetite and leads to more food consumption. The insulin reaction can also cause control problems for diabetics and hypoglycemics.

> **Artificial sweeteners can actually lead to weight <u>gain</u>.**

Aspartame caused severe joint pain in 58 of 551 (10.5%) aspartame reactors [10]. This pain is sometimes mistaken for arthritis, but goes away when aspartame use is discontinued. Headaches

[11] and particular sensitivity to aspartame among those with mood disorders [12] were also linked to aspartame use under placebo-controlled clinical conditions.

Are added nutrients always a good thing?

Nutrients are added to enrich or fortify foods. "Enriched" refers to the few synthetic vitamins added, for example to flour, to replace the many natural nutrients removed in processing. The way they enrich foods is comparable to a thief stealing your wallet and then handing you back bus fare. The danger in consuming "enriched" foods lies in the deception involved in the use of the word. People are often misled into believing that such foods are actually healthful, and may be less likely to work at getting proper nutrition as a result.

"Fortified" refers to nutrients added to products where they would not be found normally, for example orange juice with added calcium. "Fortified" does not necessarily mean more nutritious, as the added nutrient may be in a form which is not well absorbed in the body. Fortification is done primarily to appeal to the health-conscious consumer.

Many intimidating multisyllabic terms on labels may merely be relatively harmless, beneficial vitamins. Thiamine mononitrate, sodium ascorbate, DL-alpha tocopherol acetate, and calcium pantothenate are simply forms of vitamins B1, C, E, and B5 respectively.

What is "Chinese Restaurant Syndrome"?

This syndrome is so named due to the effects of monosodium glutamate (MSG), commonly used by Chinese restaurants. MSG is widely used in almost all processed food. 25-30% of the population experiences one or more adverse reactions to it [13]. MSG enhances flavor by stimulating your taste buds - it doesn't change the food, it changes you.

MSG can cause many symptoms, including:

- *Flushing*
- *Fatigue*
- *Joint pain*
- *Nausea*
- *Hunger soon after eating*
- *Rashes*
- *Anxiety*
- *Asthma*
- *Irregular heartbeat*

MSG use can even be fatal to those who are very sensitive [14].

If you have problems with MSG (which may or may not be listed on the package label), there are other compounds which are similar to or contain MSG which should be avoided as well:

- *Sodium or calcium caseinate*
- *Hydrolyzed or textured vegetable protein*
- *Autolyzed yeast*
- *MSG may be part of "flavoring" or "natural flavoring"*

Many people have been cleared of a wide variety of symptoms when MSG is removed from their diet.

What can happen when food additives are discontinued or reduced? or: Why Johnny can't read or write - a second opinion

Many of the problems caused by food additives as discussed in this chapter can be reversed by the discontinuation of or sharp reduction in the ingestion of food additives. Improvement may come quickly.

In a study done in 803 New York City public schools, certain food additives were removed in stages. Standardized tests were given to the students and their percentile (%ile) rank (how they performed compared to other students in the country) were correlated to the reduction in food additives. The results [8] are revealing:

School term	Action taken	Date tested	%ile rank
Spring 1979	Start study	Spring 1979	39th
Fall 1979	Reduced sugar, banned 2 food colorings	Spring 1980	47th
Fall 1980	Banned all synthetic colorings and flavorings	Spring 1981	51st
Fall 1982	Removed BHT, BHA	Spring 1983	55th

The overall increase in test scores was 15.7%, which is certainly statistically significant.

Have all of the food additives been discussed?

The number of food additives discussed is necessarily limited, as there are about 2800 intentional additives currently in use, but the major categories have been covered. At this point you should be able to decide which food additives are acceptable to you, and what you need to look for to avoid those which are not. Unfortunately our planet is so polluted that even the most conscientious organic grower cannot guarantee produce or meat that is free of unwanted chemicals. The goal, therefore, is to aim for food that is as free as possible from the most harmful and least necessary ones. As with the chapter on Nutrition in *Thriving In A Toxic World*, the best advice is to eat food that is as close to natural as possible.

References and Resources

- Bland, Jeffrey, *Your Health Under Siege*, The Stephen Greene Press, Brattleboro VT, 1981.

- Buist, Robert, *Food Chemical Sensitivity*, Avery Publishing Group, Garden City Park, NY, 1988.

- The Burton Goldberg Group, "Diet", pp. 161-191, *Alternative Medicine: The Definitive Guide*, Future Medicine Publishing Inc., Puyallup WA, 1994. *This chapter discusses food additives among other topics. It has a listing of sources of additive-free meat and poultry at the end of the chapter.*

- *East West Journal*, editors of, *Shopper's Guide to Natural Foods*, Avery Publishing Group, Garden City Park, NY, 1988.

- Herbert, Victor, and Genell J. Subak-Sharpe (editors), *The Mount Sinai School of Medicine Complete Book of Nutrition*, St. Martin's Press, New York, 1990.

- Kilham, Christopher, *The Bread and Circus Whole Food Bible*, Addison-Wesley Publishing Co., Reading MA, 1991. *Discusses how to find relatively safe additive-free foods; includes some recipes.*

- Millichap, J. Gordon, *Environmental Poisons In Our Food*, PNB Publishers, Chicago IL, 1993. *Many types of unintentional food additives and contaminants are discussed, as well as intentional food additives, poisons that can enter the food from the packaging, and food irradiation.*

- Mindell, Earl, *Earl Mindell's Safe Eating*, Warner Books, New York, 1987.

- Null, Gary and Steve, *The New Vegetarian*, William Morrow and Co., New York, 1978.

- Steinman, David, *Diet For A Poisoned Planet*, Ballantine Books, NY, 1990. *In-depth consumer guide with listings of foods and their contaminant levels.*

- Winter, R., *A Consumer's Dictionary of Food Additives*, Crown Publishing, NY, 1984.

Primary Toxic Suppressors

-

Metals

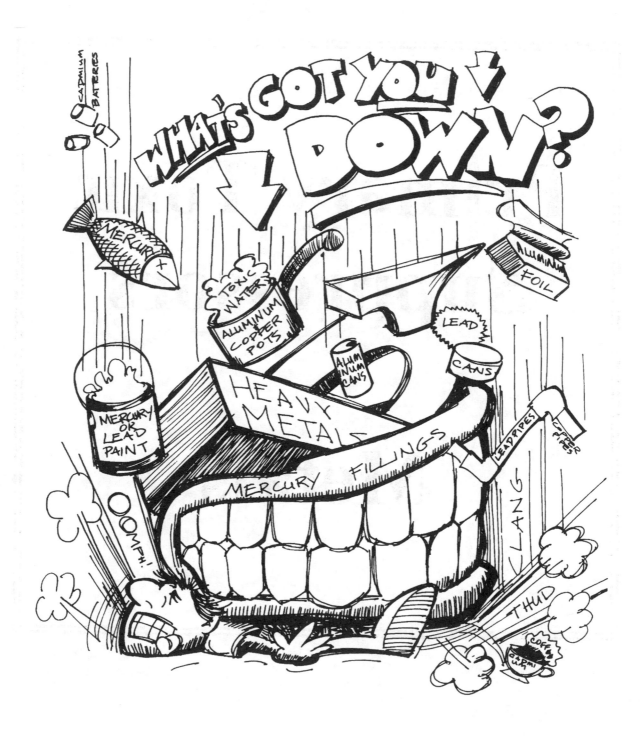

METAL TOXICITY

What's Got You Down?

In this chapter you can learn:

- *Can metals be toxic, and how do they do their damage?*
- *What is a metal?*
- *Where are toxic metals found?*
- *Why are some products colored?*

Can metals be toxic?

There are a number of metals which can cause chronic toxicity in humans. Mercury, which is 50-54% of the so-called "silver" amalgam fillings that the majority of Americans have in their mouths, is the most prevalent toxic metal in our society, in terms of the number of people adversely affected by it.

What are some of the important terms needed to discuss metals?

A few definitions are necessary in order to have a greater understanding of metals and their reactivity in the body. Definitions and examples aiding understanding are covered in greater detail in the chapter on Basic Chemical Concepts, but are reviewed briefly here.

What is a metal?

There are different definitions of a metal, depending on who you ask.

- To a chemist, a metal is anything in the left-hand two-thirds of the periodic table (found in the Basic Chemical Concepts chapter), classified as such based on the way these elements combine with other materials.

- The non-chemist, however, usually thinks of metals as the dozen or so materials that appear metallic, shiny and hard, such as iron, copper, or gold.

- A nutritionist might separate minerals from metals, defining a mineral as a metallic element which, in ionic (charged) form, is necessary for bodily function.

However, minerals can act as toxic metals if present in quantities significantly higher than what the body needs. Copper, for example, is necessary for the function of some enzyme systems but is poisonous in higher amounts. For this reason, a combination of these definitions of metals and minerals will be used.

What different metal forms are there?

- **Molecular**, or free, metals are those which have no ionic charge (defined shortly) and generally have the characteristics that one associates with metals - a characteristic metallic appearance, taste, and sound when struck.

- The **ionic** form of a metal is one in which there is an associated positive charge, or valence of +1, +2, or +3. A metal in the ionic form can combine with other elements or chemical groups to form compounds.

- A **compound** results when two or more elements or groups combine to make a new material that is different than the molecular elements which formed them. A **mixture**, on the other hand, is a combination of two or more things whose characteristics do not change.

- A **salt** is a compound formed from a metal (anything with a plus charge other than hydrogen) and a nonmetal (anything with a minus charge other than hydroxyl, OH^-).

Why is all of this significant?

Metals may enter the body in either molecular or ionic form, but the damage they cause is due to their combining into compounds chemically in the body in the ionic form.

How do metals do their damage?

Metals do their damage in one or more of these ways, described briefly after listing and in detail in these chapters on metals:

• *Fight for site*	• *Charge*
• *Antibiotic effect*	• *Steal necessary substances*
• *Genetic changes*	• *Bind metallothionein*
• *Free radicals*	• *Bind with self to cause allergy*

IIB

30	65.38
Zn	
Zinc	

48	112.41
Cd	
Cadmium	

80	200.59
Hg	
Mercury	

Fight for site - Ions with the same electron valence, or charge (such as +2), can substitute for each other in the chemical reactions which allow the body to function properly. For example, toxic ionic mercury (Hg^{+2}), if present, can take the place of necessary zinc (Zn^{+2}) or iron (Fe^{+2}) in biochemical reactions.

Charge - Two or more dissimilar metals in an electrically conductive medium called an electrolyte form a type of battery, as discussed in the chapter on The Battery Effect. Body fluids such as saliva or blood act as an electrolyte, and metals in the mouth from fillings, crowns, and root canal posts (combining mercury and nickel) complete the battery. Once the dissimilar metals form an anode and cathode, corrosion takes place as on the poles of a car battery and leaches into the mouth. The water-soluble toxic metal salts formed as corrosion products then enter the rest of the body.

Antibiotic - Mercury, in particular, has an antibiotic effect. Metal salts, in fact, were commonly used as pesticides in agriculture before the advent of organic (meaning, in this sense, carbon containing and toxic) pesticides. Mercury and other salts were used as antibiotics, ingested and topical (on the skin) before more modern antibiotics were developed. Mercury had replaced lead in paints to stop bacterial and fungal growth. About ten years ago, other fungicides replaced mercury since mercury was recognized as dangerous. Mercury in the mouth kills beneficial bacteria in the body.

Stealing substances - Iron transports oxygen to sites where it is needed in the body. If mercury substitutes for iron, oxygen will not be transported to as great an extent. Mercury will bind to the oxygen to form an oxide of mercury, which, unlike oxygen, is not useful to the body. Sulfur and selenium, essential materials, are "stolen" in similar ways.

Genetic - Nickel, in particular, adversely affects RNA, which is part of the process of cell duplication. Improper cell duplication leads to cell mutations which can then lead to cancer and birth defects.

Metallothionein is a natural sulfur containing substance in the body that clears heavy metals. A greater metal burden than the body is able to bear will clog this detox pathway. Mercury in the body can thus interfere with the removal of aluminum. A buildup of both mercury and aluminum has been linked to Alzheimer's disease.

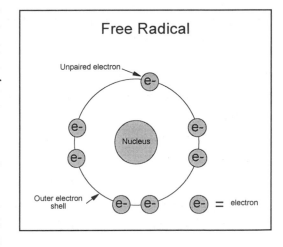

Free radicals involve an atom with an unpaired electron (an odd number of electrons in the outer shell). The unpaired electron wants to find a mate, and will rip an electron from the nearest atom it finds, creating a new free radical in a chain reaction. Free radicals can be compared to the lone male who enters the dance floor, cutting in on a couple and producing another lone male who cuts in on another couple, in a chain reaction.

Allergy - The immune system recognizes the body's own tissues as self and leaves them alone, while attacking anything non-self. Metal may bind with the protein in the body's tissues, causing the immune system to see these tissues as unfamiliar non-self. The immune system's resulting attack on parts of the body is known as autoimmune disease, which may also have causes other than metals.

Where are toxic metals found?
Sources of the various metals are described in detail in the following few chapters. Some of the sources and their metals include:

- *Amalgam fillings*   *mercury, silver*
- *Dental root canals*   *nickel*

- *Dental crowns*   *nickel*
- *Cooking utensils*   *iron, aluminum, stainless steel*
                                   containing nickel, copper

- *Old paint*   *lead, mercury*
- *Antiperspirants*   *aluminum*
- *Volcanic eruptions*   *mercury*
- *Inexpensive earrings*   *nickel*
- *Some glazed pottery*   *lead*
- *Cigarettes*   *cadmium, nickel*
- *Batteries*   *lead, cadmium, nickel*
- *Auto exhaust*   *lead, platinum, cadmium, aluminum*
- *Insecticides*   *arsenic, mercury*
- *Metronidazole (antifungal*   *arsenic*
  drug, trade name Flagyl)

What causes colors in some products?

Some metal salts are colored, and are the source of color in products such as paints (cobalt blue, cadmium yellow, and others), cosmetics, and colored flames in fire logs.

Fireworks are made with saltpeter, which initiates a redox reaction culminating in an explosion. Metals, which are responsible for the bright colors in fireworks, also enter into the reaction. For example:

- *Aluminum*   *sparks*
- *Copper*   *blue-green*
- *Strontium*   *red-orange*
- *Magnesium*   *bright white*
- *Sodium*   *yellow*

How are our bodies like fireworks?

Oxidation-reduction (redox) reactions, which occur to produce fireworks colors, also occur in the body.

Magnesium burns steadily while aluminum sparks. This relationship applies within the body as well. In the brains of Alzheimer's disease victims, aluminum has been shown to accumulate, and Alzheimer's disease is characterized by gaps in memory and function. These gaps are like sparks rather than magnesium's smooth flow. Magnesium in the body and brain can be suppressed by aluminum.

What are some of the most significant toxic metals?

Mercury (usually found in dental work) and nickel (dental work and stainless steel cookware) are two of the most toxic metals. They are also the ones most likely to be found in the bodies of people of industrialized countries. The majority of people have mercury amalgam fillings in their mouths, and millions of people also have nickel in their mouths in the form of stainless steel crowns, root canal posts, and braces. These two metals are so important that the next two chapters are devoted to them.

Other metals likely to cause problems are lead, cadmium, copper, aluminum, arsenic, and platinum. These are discussed in the chapter on Other Metals.

If metal poisoning is one of your health problems, the chapter on Metal Detoxification can explain how to remove metals from your body.

References and Resources

- The Burton Goldberg Group, *Alternative Medicine: The Definitive Guide*, "Heavy Metal Toxicity", pp. 927-8, Future Medicine Publishing, Puyallup WA, 1994.

"I don't feel comfortable using a substance designated by the Environmental Protection Agency to be a waste disposal hazard. I can't throw it in the trash, bury it in the ground, or put it in a landfill, but they say it's okay to put it in people's mouths. That doesn't make sense."

- Richard D. Fisher, DDS

"...both doctors and dentists have to be concerned with evaluating the clinical implications of using toxic metals in the human body."

- Theron Randolph, MD

WARNING: This office uses amalgam filling materials which contain and expose you to mercury, a chemical known to the State of California to cause birth defects and other reproductive harm. Please consult your dentist for more information.

MERCURY

Slippery As A Thief

Do you have - or have you had - mercury dental fillings (silver-to-black fillings)? Do you have any of the following symptoms? There may be a connection.

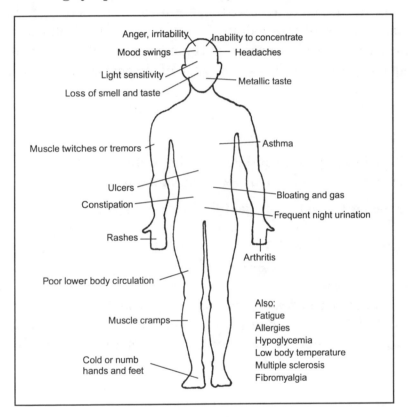

Anger, irritability
Mood swings
Light sensitivity
Loss of smell and taste
Inability to concentrate
Headaches
Metallic taste
Muscle twitches or tremors
Asthma
Ulcers
Constipation
Bloating and gas
Frequent night urination
Rashes
Arthritis
Poor lower body circulation
Muscle cramps
Cold or numb hands and feet

Also:
Fatigue
Allergies
Hypoglycemia
Low body temperature
Multiple sclerosis
Fibromyalgia

Ten things in this chapter that can change your health:

1. Mercury is very toxic in all forms, and this has been known for centuries.

2. Mercury is the main component in common "silver" dental fillings in the mouths of most Americans.

3. How is mercury absorbed into the body from fillings?

4. What are some symptoms of mercury poisoning?

5. How can mercury increase the toxicity of other poisons?

6. Why does the American Dental Association permit and encourage the placing of mercury fillings?

7. *Should fillings be removed and replaced, and how can this be done safely?*

8. *What are some other hazards faced in the dentist's office? What should you look for in a dentist for optimum health?*

9. *How can mercury in the body tissues and blood be removed?*

10. *What kind of health improvement can be expected after mercury amalgam removal?*

What is the problem with mercury?

It has been known for centuries that mercury in all forms is very poisonous. Hippocrates, sometimes called the father of medicine, remarked on the toxicity of mercury over 2000 years ago. Mercury has been used in a number of industrial processes and medications for over a thousand years. For example, neurological damage was common in people who worked with mercury compounds in hat-making plants. This was the origin of the phrase "mad as a hatter".

It is known that:

1. Mercury is very toxic.

2. Metal (silver-mercury amalgam) dental fillings are the greatest source of mercury in the bodies of nearly anyone who has or has had them [1].

3. Therefore mercury amalgam dental fillings represent a major hazard to health.

These allegations, especially # 2 and 3, are in dispute for reasons that are motivated more by politics and greed than by science and concern for public health. The reasons behind this are discussed later in this chapter. However, the dispute exists and many people still blindly trust their dentists, who have no training in toxicology and who themselves blindly trust what they are taught in dental school. For this reason this chapter is heavily referenced - over 200 references - with medical and scientific journal articles from the U.S. and throughout the world, and even some historical ones.

Dentists lead the list in suicide frequency as ranked by occupation. They have stresses similar to those of doctors, with mercury exposure as an added factor. Depression and divorce are also high among dentists, as is infertility among female dentists and hygienists. All of these problems among dental workers may be related to mercury exposure [2,3,4].

What are some of the properties of mercury?

Mercury is the only metal that is liquid at room temperature. The fact that it is liquid is significant in that liquids outgas (enter the air as vapor) more readily than solids and can therefore be inhaled and absorbed more easily. Mercury is a shiny, silver-colored liquid metal that rolls easily into a ball and is familiar to anyone who has ever broken a thermometer. It is used in thermometers because it expands and contracts readily with relatively small temperature changes.

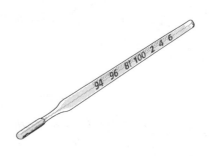

Mercury forms both inorganic and organic compounds. Inorganic compounds are those which do not contain carbon, and include both mercurous (valence of +1) and mercuric (valence of +2) salts (salts are compounds formed from a metal plus a nonmetal).

What are some sources of mercury compounds?

Mercuric and mercurous compounds have found medicinal use as external antiseptics because they kill cells, and the cell-killing ability accounts for some of their toxicity when ingested. Some examples of mercury-containing medicinal compounds are:

- *Mercurous chloride, or calomel*

- *Mercuric chloride*

- *Mercurochrome and merthiolate, reddish liquids dabbed onto cuts and scrapes*

- *Thimerosal, used as a preservative in personal care products, including eye drops*

If an ingredient has "mer" somewhere in its name, it probably contains mercury salts. Mercury salts are also widely used in industry, and are discharged into the air and water.

Organic compounds are those which contain carbon, and organic mercury compounds are even more toxic than the metallic or inorganic forms. When mercury in any form is taken into the body, it often undergoes a chemical change within the body, often aided by certain bacteria, into a more toxic organic compound. Types and sources of organic mercury compounds include:

- Methylmercury, found in some tuna and seafood. However, seafood also has selenium and sulfur, which provide a protective effect by binding the mercury to limit its ability to enter into damaging reactions.

- Phenyl mercuric propionate, used as an anti-mildew additive.

- Alkylmercury salts, widely used as fungicides. Mercury is used to kill fungus and mildew because it is poisonous to cells.

- Mercury compounds, expelled from burning coal, enter the air and rain.

- Mercury is a byproduct of the chlorine and alkali production industry.

Mercury is also found in nature. Mercury from volcanoes enters the air and oceans. A few years ago a volcanic eruption made sunsets worldwide more colorful. This reddish color was caused by mercury in the air, and an increase in mercury related health problems was noted.

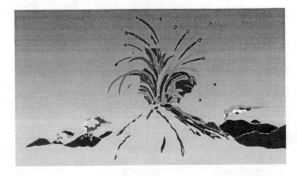

It is estimated that about 20 million pounds of mercury flow into the sea each year, about half each from industrial and natural sources. 250,000 pounds per year are used by dentists in the United States alone [5].

Why is mercury so toxic?

Mercury in all forms is particularly dangerous because it is so easily absorbed into the body, due in part to its being liquid. Metallic and organic mercury especially are very volatile, meaning they enter the air rapidly from the liquid state and are then inhaled. For this reason, a mercury spill from a broken thermometer or spilled fungicide should never be vacuumed up unless exhausted to the outside, as this would disperse the mercury into the air to be readily inhaled. Mercury is also easily absorbed through skin, lung tissue, and, if ingested, stomach and intestinal tissue. Chelators, discussed later in this chapter and in the Metal Detoxification chapter, can pull mercury out of these tissues.

Mercury and lead together are more toxic than either one separately, each amplifying the toxicity of the other. The metal detoxification systems of the body such as metallothionein, if saturated with one metal, will not be able to deal effectively with other metals.

What is the greatest source of mercury?

The greatest single source of mercury is from mercury amalgam tooth fillings [6,7], which are in the mouths of an estimated 85% of Americans.

How can you tell whether you have mercury fillings?

Mercury fillings are the dark dental fillings in the teeth, as compared with composite fillings which are tooth-colored. Mercury fillings range in color from silver (shiny or dull) to black. The silver color is usually seen for a few months after the filling is placed, after which it oxidizes, or changes, to a nearly-black color. Release of mercury from the fillings into the body is highest when they are new and silvery. Fillings placed in the armed services may retain their silvery color for years rather than darkening, as a different mixture of metals is sometimes used.

What is the difference between silver, mercury, and amalgam fillings?

These are all names for the same thing. The full name for these fillings is silver-mercury amalgam fillings, meaning a mixture of silver and mercury. Dentists often call them silver fillings, which sounds nicer and less toxic, but this book refers to them as mercury fillings to emphasize their toxic nature, which is due primarily to the mercury.

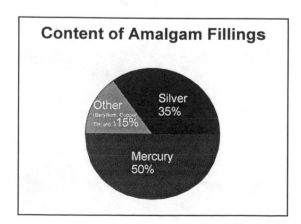

Content of Amalgam Fillings

Silver 35%

Other (Beryllium, Copper, Tin, etc) 15%

Mercury 50%

So-called "silver" fillings contain about 30-35% silver, 15% tin or tin and copper, a trace of zinc, and a full 50-54% of mercury [8], although the exact composition can vary between manufacturers. Since mercury is the greatest component of amalgam fillings by weight regardless of manufacturer, they should more accurately be called mercury fillings rather than silver.

What is one of the more toxic forms of mercury?
Methylmercury, 100 times more toxic than elemental mercury, is formed in our mouths by a bacterium called streptococcus mutans, which is in the mouths of everyone [9]. Methylmercury is detoxified in the body to the comparatively less toxic elemental mercury, but if this mercury is not eliminated, the mercury will remethylate back to methylmercury in a never ending cycle [10].

Both the elemental mercury from the amalgam and methylmercury formed from it in the body are toxic burdens affecting most of us.

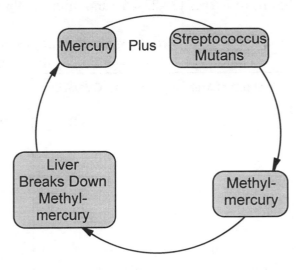

How is mercury absorbed from fillings?
Mercury is absorbed from our fillings in several ways:

- **Lungs** - Volatile mercury, vaporized from the surface of the fillings, is inhaled. 80% of the mercury vapor from fillings is absorbed by the lungs [6,11-14] and passed into the arterial blood.

- **Nose** - Some of this vapor enters the nasal pharynx in the nose and is absorbed by the nerve fibers there that lead directly to the brain. For this reason, this is the preferred route for ingestion of cocaine. Inhaled mercury reaches the brain just as quickly.

- **Roots** - Mercury is forced by expansion down through the tooth root, into the bones and gums and from there into the bloodstream. This is particularly true of teeth with crowns, as mercury expands and contracts with heat and cold (remember what thermometers contain, and why). With crowns over the fillings the expanding mercury has nowhere to go but toward the root. In addition, electron transfer causes mercury to travel electrically through the root into the bloodstream and along the nerve pathways (meridians). For these reasons the rate of mercury migration is increased if a gold crown is placed over a tooth filled with amalgam [15,16]. However, the strongest battery-driven migration is for nickel/stainless steel caps and posts.

- **Stomach** - Broken bits of fillings and minute amounts of corrosion products are worked loose through chewing and then swallowed. Expansion and contraction of the filling from eating hot and cold foods can crack teeth over time, releasing more mercury bits to be swallowed. The mercury is then absorbed from the stomach into the bloodstream [5,17,18].

- **Gums** - Mercury is absorbed through the gums and mucous membranes of the mouth. It then enters the bloodstream through the capillaries in these tissues.

Mercury is transported and absorbed primarily through the blood [19-21], lymph [20], and the axons of nerves [20,22-26], and migrates throughout the body [27-30].

Don't fillings eventually stop releasing mercury?

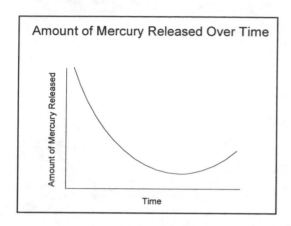

Amount of Mercury Released Over Time

Mercury leaves dental amalgam continuously throughout the lifetime of the filling [31]. The amount is greatest when the filling is new and then it oxidizes and turns greyish black. The oxidation forms a partial seal over the filling, and so the amount of released mercury drops rapidly to a relatively constant plateau level for years. After 7-30 years, the filling gradually cracks and disintegrates, releasing more mercury from freshly exposed surfaces.

Mercury enters the body at a rate of 3 to 17 mcg (micrograms) per day [7]. The mercury enters the body more quickly than the body's detoxification systems can dispose of it, resulting in a slow buildup of mercury and other metals such as aluminum in body tissues [20,32,33]. Mercury is stored principally in the kidneys, liver and brain [6,32,34].

When is mercury released from the fillings?

Mercury is released continuously even when at rest. An even greater amount of mercury is released, as shown by testing:

- During placement of fillings [35-43]

- During removal of fillings [44-49]

- When chewing [50-55]. Chewing removes some of the protective oxidative coating on the surface of the filling. Increases in both temperature and friction also play a part in the increase of released mercury [6,56]. After chewing, mercury vapor levels remain raised for up to 90 minutes [9,34,51,52,57].

- When swallowing [58-63], especially after chewing.

Should you rinse with hydrogen peroxide?

Rinsing of the mouth with bacteria-killing 3% hydrogen peroxide is usually a good idea, but only if there are no mercury fillings present. Hydrogen peroxide can oxidize the mercury in the fillings, causing higher levels to be ingested. A regular user of hydrogen peroxide may have fillings that are a shiny silver color rather than their usual nearly black state. The black state is a layer of oxidation similar to rust on iron which lowers but does not eliminate the reactivity of the amalgam surface. A fresh unoxidized mercury surface is being exposed with each rinse with hydrogen peroxide.

Hydrogen peroxide can both oxidize a metal surface and strip off the oxidized portion. By the same principle, certain oxidants can remove rust, an oxidation product, from an iron surface.

How does diet affect mercury release?

Sweets and fruits are acid and tend to chelate mercury faster, which can in turn increase microorganisms such as helicobacter pylori and yeast (discussed in the Microorganisms section.

What kinds of symptoms does mercury cause?

Symptoms of mercury toxicity are many and varied, since mercury can both reach and affect nearly every cell in the body. Systemic (overall) effects can occur [64-66] for this reason. The particular symptoms you experience first depend on your own genetic weakest links and on other toxic suppressors. These symptoms may include the following [11] and as shown in the diagram on the first page of this chapter. Many of these symptoms are explained in greater detail following this list:

- **Behavioral** - depression, emotional instability (mood swings), inability to concentrate, sleep disturbances, irritability, forgetfulness

- **Cardiovascular** - abnormal heartbeat, pressure and pain in chest, high or low blood pressure, anemia [67,68]. Mercury can damage blood vessels, reducing blood supply to the tissues [20]. Heart problems have been shown [69,70].

- **Blood** - adverse on red blood cells [71]. Mercury binds to hemoglobin in the red blood cells, thus reducing oxygen carrying capacity [21,22,33,34,57,72].

- **Central nervous system** [73-75] - light and sound sensitivity, headaches, convulsions, tremors [76-78], muscle twitches, numbness and tingling of extremities, dizziness, hearing or vision difficulty, black and white dreams (instead of color)

- **Detoxification systems** - By overloading the detoxification pathways, other toxins are eliminated less efficiently. The effects of these toxins are discussed throughout the chapters of this book.

- **Digestive** - constipation or diarrhea (by themselves or alternating), digestion problems, colitis, loss of appetite, ulcers, bloating and gas, loss of smell and taste

- **Endocrine** - thyroid dysfunction, low body temperature, cold hands and feet, decreased libido, frequent night urination, leg and muscle cramps, joint pain, kidney stones, slow healing

- **Energy** - Chronic fatigue, drowsiness, hypoglycemia, muscle weakness

- **Immune system** - allergies, asthma, environmental illness, Hodgkins' disease, swollen glands, susceptibility to colds and infection

- **Joints and muscles** - arthritis, fibromyalgia, lupus

- **Kidney problems** [79-84]

- **Oral cavity** - bad breath, bleeding gums, canker sores, bone loss, increased salivation (due to battery effect, discussed in the Battery Effect chapter), metallic taste, periodontal (gum and jawbone) disease, purple-black gum pigment near fillings (sometimes called mercury tattoo), leukoplakia (an oral precancerous condition caused by local metal irritation)

- **Reproductive** - infertility, miscarriage, premature birth

- **Skin** - acne, itching, skin flushing, rough skin, rashes

How does mercury toxicity affect the reproductive system?

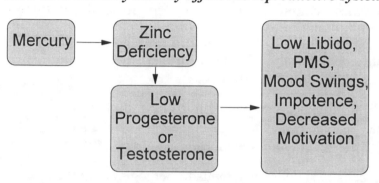

Reproductive effects can occur, such as infertility, miscarriage and prematurity. Mercury lowers zinc levels, which then lowers progesterone levels. Progesterone is needed to bring a pregnancy to term. Birth defects, especially involving the brain and learning ability, can be caused by mercury, as the metal can pass through both the placental barrier and the blood-brain barrier contrary to prior belief [85]. Low libido (sex drive) and premenstrual syndrome (PMS) are examples of a downward spiral of problems whose root cause is mercury toxicity.

Lowered progesterone levels can lead to infertility. PMS and infertility are common among many young female dental workers due at least in part to their mercury exposure. Male dental workers also suffer from infertility. Mercury lowers zinc levels, which in turn leads to lower testosterone (male hormone) levels.

Mercury can cause single strand breaks in the genetic material DNA [86,87], which can in turn lead to birth defects.

Severe reduction in reproductive function due to mercury has been well-documented [2,4,6,34, 85,86,88-101].

Can babies absorb mercury from their mothers?
Mercury can cross the placental barrier [6,52], which screens out many harmful substances. This has been shown in both human [102-105] and animal [106-111] studies. Mercury is, in fact, stored in the fetus and infant before the mother [32].

Mercury can also be transmitted to the infant via breast milk [6,52,105,111]. Mercury from amalgam is stored in the breast milk and in the fetus at levels up to eight times that in the mother's tissues [19,52].

How is the immune system affected?

It has been shown that mercury rapidly depletes the immune system [1,9,15,20,21,87,112-128]. Mercury has been shown to induce auto-immune diseases [15,20,21,87,112,113].

Mercury can cause an increase in the number and severity of allergies [20,34,117,129-131].

T-cell counts can be adversely affected by mercury [126]. T-cells are the communicators of the immune system, and so a defect in this area can affect total immune system functioning.

What other types of symptoms are caused by mercury?

Candida (yeast) overgrowth that is difficult to get rid of is also associated with mercury in the mouth [11,132]. Mercury acts as an antibiotic, and, like medicinal antibiotics, it kills the friendly bacteria which help control yeast overgrowth.

Any of these symptoms can affect almost anyone with amalgam fillings. Some people, however, are especially sensitive, or allergic. Even one filling can cause susceptible people to be totally debilitated or have seizures.

Replacement reactions, also called fight for site, occur when mercury (usually with a +2 charge) grabs the biological spaces which should be filled by necessary minerals. Symptoms that can be caused by a deficiency of minerals displaced by mercury include:

- *Magnesium*   *irregular heartbeat, receding gums*
- *Iron*   *anemia*
- *Copper*   *anemia, thyroid dysfunction, impaired digestion*
- *Zinc*   *anorexia nervosa, loss of taste and smell [133], loss of appetite, low libido, PMS*
- *Iodine*   *thyroid dysfunction*

Some digestive problems can be caused by parasite or bacterial infection such as helicobacter secondary to immune system suppression by mercury. Mercury, in effect, opens the door like the Trojan horse so that undesirables can come in. Mercury combines with bile and can cause bile from the gallbladder to become more alkaline, providing a favorable environment for parasites. These parasites can plug up the hepatic or bile duct so that needed digestive and other enzymes from the gallbladder, liver, and pancreas are not released. Gallbladder function then suffers.

Mercury acts as an antibiotic, and was used in some medicines until safer alternatives came along for this purpose. In the body mercury also acts as an antibiotic, and like medicinal antibiotics it kills off the beneficial bacteria which repel parasites and aid in digestion. Yeast overgrowth with its attendant symptoms of fatigue, sweets cravings and vaginal infections is often traced to the antibiotic effect of dental mercury. Suspect this as a root cause when yeast is a continuing problem in spite of repeated treatment. The symptom (yeast overgrowth) will not likely go away until the root cause (mercury) is dealt with. The effect of dental mercury on normal gut flora is well documented [134,135].

Alzheimer's disease has been linked to mercury and Alzheimer's disease patients commonly have sweets cravings due to the mercury-yeast connection.

Thyroid problems or mercury toxicity?

Endocrine problems such as low body temperature often improve rapidly when amalgam is removed, a sure sign that the amalgam was causing the problem in the first place. Normal body temperature is about 98.6 F orally. People reacting to amalgam components often have a temperature range of 96.2 to 97.6 degrees, which can rise to 98.2 in as little as one day after amalgam removal and to 98.6 soon afterward [136]. A low body temperature is a sign of low thyroid function, and many people have mistakenly been given thyroid hormone to remedy a symptom caused by amalgam fillings.

Synthetic thyroid hormone (thyroxin) can shut down the natural feedback cycle of the pituitary gland and its production of Thyroid Stimulating Hormone (TSH). This shutdown then adversely affects the rest of the endocrine system. It would be far better to correct the cause of the apparent thyroid malfunction by removing the fillings that are responsible for the low body temperature, rather than prescribing supplemental thyroid hormone.

What are the mental symptoms of mercury toxicity?

Since mercury is so soluble, it can be absorbed through the roof of the mouth, which is less than an inch from the posterior pituitary gland. The posterior pituitary gland (master gland), a regulator of the lower (below the waist) endocrine system, has much to do with reproductive hormones and therefore mood and outlook on life. Mercury would tend to have a suppressant effect on the posterior pituitary. Mental symptoms of toxicity affecting the posterior pituitary include: [137]

- *Depression*
- *Timidity*
- *Rage*
- *Phobias*
- *Anxiety*

- *Lowered libido*
- *Indecisiveness*
- *Lack of self confidence*
- *Compulsions*
- *Mood swings*

Mercury tends to accumulate in all tissues, but especially in the brain [20]. It is one of the substances that can cross the blood-brain barrier. Brain levels of mercury are directly proportional to the number of amalgam filling surfaces in the mouth [19,34,138]. Within the brain, mercury is stored preferentially in the pituitary gland and hypothalamus [20,32].

Accumulation in the brain leads to mental and nervous system effects such as brain fog, depression, vision difficulties, and others as listed above. Mental effects are among the most common due to mercury's special affinity for the brain. Mercury inhibits the effects of certain neurotransmitters:

- *Dopamine*   *controls pain, well-being*
- *Serotonin*   *relaxation, sleep, well-being*

- *Adrenaline*   *energy and stamina*

- *Noradrenaline,*   *sleep cycles*
  melatonin

Inhibition of these neurotransmitters by mercury can account in part for the feelings of depression and loss of motivation.

Other mental/neurological symptoms include:

- General neurological symptoms [139-142]

- Mental illness [143-145]

- Demyelinization, which can lead to such diseases as multiple sclerosis (MS) [71,146-148].

- Developmental problems [103]

- Cerebral palsy [149]

- ALS (Amyotrophic lateral sclerosis, or Lou Gehrig's disease) [150-153]

- Alzheimer's disease [154-160]

- Psychological problems, including loss of function and memory, anger and emotionality, and timidity [144,145,161]

How does mercury cause fatigue and lack of energy?

Mercury binds to nitrogen and sulfur in proteins, oxygen from the lungs, sulfur from the liver's detoxification systems, and selenium from the colon. Lower levels of body tissue oxygen due to mercury's binding it may lead to:

- Fatigue caused by low blood sugar secondary to low blood oxygen

- Parasite infestation by setting up an anaerobic (less oxygen) environment, and by lowering the level of the good bacteria which fight off parasites

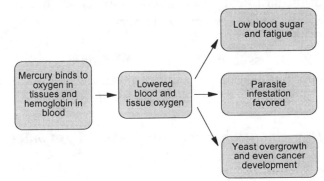

- An anaerobic environment also favors the development of yeast infections and cancer, since yeast is a fermenting spore and cancer is a fermenting cell rather than a normal respiratory (oxygen using) cell.

Mercury binds with hemoglobin, which is responsible for oxygen transport to the tissues. This results in less oxygen reaching the tissues. The body attempts to compensate for this by increasing the amount of hemoglobin in the blood. A normal or increased hemoglobin (oxygen carrying) level combined with symptoms usually associated with low hemoglobin such as anemia are often indicative of mercury toxicity. Copper is also required to prevent anemia, and mercury can compete for copper's binding sites. A lowered hematocrit (red blood cell count) can be indicative of lowered blood copper levels.

The terms hematocrit and hemoglobin, found routinely on blood test printouts, can be confusing. If blood is compared to a train carrying oxygen to where it is needed, hematocrit is a measure of the number of boxcars on the train (red blood cells), while hemoglobin is a measure of the carrying capacity of each boxcar, or red blood cell.

Other mineral levels can be lowered by mercury's tendency to fight for site. A deficiency of any of these minerals can lead to fatigue and other symptoms:

- Cobalt, calcium, magnesium, potassium, and sodium are all required for energy.

- Zinc is needed for the manufacture of adrenaline.

- A deficiency of zinc, copper, or potassium can lower adrenal activity.

- Cobalt, usually obtained from vitamin B12 (cyanocobalamin) prevents pernicious anemia, a cause of fatigue.

- Mercury blocks magnesium and manganese transport required for memory, resulting in lowered ability to concentrate.

These mineral deficiencies may be primarily due to dietary deficiencies. However, deficiencies may also be secondary. The mineral may be in the body but cannot get to where it is needed because mercury has blocked the way. This is like putting a too-large battery in a toy - it won't fit in the slot made for a smaller battery, both denying power to the toy and blocking the slot from receiving the correct size battery.

Fatigue associated with mercury toxicity can be due to several of mercury's effects, including reducing adrenaline and neurotransmitter effects, reducing oxygen to tissues, and interfering with coenzyme A, which converts sugar to energy.

How can mercury increase the toxicity of other poisons?

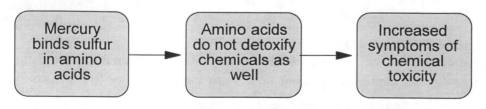

Mercuric ion (Hg^{+2}) binds to sulfhydryl groups (-SH) in proteins and disulfide groups (-SS) in amino acids. These sulfur containing groups have an important detoxification function in the body. Increased toxicity from chemicals and metals other than mercury can result from mercury binding these sulfur groups and preventing them from detoxifying the chemicals.

Mercury binding the bile lowers the ability of the body to absorb fat, leading to increased absorption of toxic oil-soluble chemicals such as solvents and pesticides like a dry sponge.

Selenium is an antioxidant which binds in place of oxygen and which protects against free radical damage from chemicals which can lead to cancer. Mercury can bind to selenium, making it useless for this protective purpose.

What else can mercury do?

Mercurous ion (Hg^{+1}) pushes out Na^{+1} (sodium), K^{+1} (potassium), and Li^{+1} (lithium). Sodium and potassium are part of the cellular sodium/potassium pump which causes muscle movement. Interference with sodium and potassium can lead to muscle weakness for this reason. Leg and muscle cramps may be due to potassium deficiency.

Lithium is sometimes given as lithium carbonate to patients suffering from bipolar depression (manic depressive illness) since lack of lithium is one of the causes of the disease. Lack of lithium may itself be caused by mercury preventing lithium from working as it should in the brain. Mercury is like the 200 pound bully attacking a 7 pound baby; the small baby doesn't have much of a chance. 200 and 7 are the molecular weights of mercury (the bully) and lithium (the baby) respectively. If you have been diagnosed with bipolar depression, maybe what you need is less mercury, not more lithium pills.

Mercury fights for binding sites in the kidney, another organ for which it has a special affinity. A mineral and electrolyte balance is needed in order for the kidney to perform its functions, and a poorly functioning kidney can lead to edema (fluid buildup in the body). These minerals are prevented from entering into their reactions when mercury is there to interfere. Suppression of potassium by mercury also affects the kidneys which takes you from making adrenaline to maintaining electrolyte balance, and the lowered adrenaline level can lead to lower energy.

Detoxification systems such as metallothionein, cytochrome P-450, and bile are adversely affected by mercury. Metallothionein binds toxic metals in the body to prepare them for excretion. Mercury ties up this material so it cannot clear out other metals such as lead, cadmium, and aluminum.

Mercury from amalgam binds to -SH (sulfhydryl) groups, which are used in almost every enzymatic process in the body. Mercury therefore has the potential to disturb all metabolic processes [162].

Some people appear to be allergic to whatever food they eat. No matter what they eat, at least one thing in common is ingested - mercury (or nickel). Mercury released from amalgam during chewing may be the cause of most of the symptoms which seem to be caused by the food. If a mercury vapor test, described later in this chapter, is done, it may show a low to moderate level of mercury initially, but a sharply increased level after chewing gum. This is also what happens when

> **Do you seem to be allergic to most foods? Check what you're eating them with.**

food is chewed. Such a test result combined with apparent allergy to most food points to mercury as a probable culprit. Nickel, which may also be contributing to the problem, is in stainless steel posts and braces.

The four top front teeth drain upward through the nose into the brain. Mercury or nickel in these teeth can cause nasal polyps and subsequent difficulty breathing through the nose. Ankylosing spondylitis, an autoimmune disease causing fusing of the spine and considerable pain, can sometimes be traced to metal in the four top front teeth.

What is the dispute about mercury?

Mercury's poisonous nature is not in dispute. One of the issues of dispute is the fact that mercury comes out of amalgam. The ADA admits mercury comes out of amalgam, reversing its previous position that it does not. However, the primary dispute involves the toxicity of the mercury which comes out of the amalgam.

How do we know mercury comes out of amalgam in toxic form, despite claims by some dentists to the contrary?

- Amalgam is a mixture, not a true compound. Mercury, therefore, does not change its toxic nature by definition of a mixture.

- It has been argued that amalgam, because it hardens (changes), is characteristic of a compound. Even if this were so, there is no mercury compound that is not toxic. Why should amalgam be the exception?

- The mercury content of fillings declines as a direct reflection of the age of the filling. After five years, fillings have lost half of their surface mercury content, and after 20 years, most of the surface mercury has been lost [11]. This lost mercury has nowhere to go except into and through your body. About half of mercury fillings need to be replaced after 11 years, and most mercury fillings need to be replaced before 20 years, as they tend to fracture, corrode, and crumble around the edges. The likely cause of this crumbling is the evaporation of the only highly volatile (vaporizing) component, mercury. Another likely cause involves the thermodynamic properties of a metal mixture which is heated and cooled (hot soup, ice cream) repeatedly; this is called metal fatigue. Fillings are designed to corrode. The ADA claims that oxidation forms a coating which prevents mercury from outgassing. This claim does not stand up to testing.

- Cadavers with amalgam fillings have higher levels of mercury in the lungs, kidneys, brain, and liver tissue than cadavers without amalgam fillings [11]. In fact, certain countries prohibit the cremation of cadavers with mercury fillings because of the toxicity.

- An instrument, the Jerome Mercury Vapor Analyzer, can detect mercury vapor in the mouth. After chewing gum or food, average mercury levels are 20 to 50 micrograms per cubic meter (mcg/m^3). Levels as high as 400 mcg/m^3

have been reported. By contrast, the occupational Safety and Health Agency (OSHA) has set 50 mcg/m^3 as the highest level allowed in the workplace (based on 40 hours per week exposure, even very short-term), and is considering lowering this to 20 mcg/m^3 [11]. Many people have higher levels of mercury vapor in their mouth, on an ongoing basis, than OSHA allows in a working environment.

- There is considerable anecdotal and statistical evidence of symptom improvement when amalgam is removed [5,9,11,136].

Science or political science?
Despite all the evidence that mercury in amalgam is toxic, the ADA persists in saying it is not. Why? The ADA is a powerful political entity which exists, like any union, to protect its own financial and other interests and to support their average to poor performing members. It would be detrimental to the ADA to admit that they have been making a colossal mistake for the past 165 years that silver-mercury amalgam has been in use. The lawsuits alone would probably bankrupt them.

They are not eager to do extensive and expensive scientific testing on the matter when they have much to lose and nothing to gain from the results. In fact, if they really believed that amalgam was harmless, they would be happy to fund such research to silence their critics, but this is not happening. They appear to be more interested in justifying their position than in finding the truth, similar to the position of the tobacco industry. Therefore, don't count on the ADA to fairly represent public health or your interests.

Dentists must attend ADA accredited dental schools and pass tests administered by the Board of Dental Examiners, a group which is greatly influenced if not controlled by the ADA, in order to practice dentistry. The information learned by even the most conscientious dentist - and passed on to patients - is therefore strongly biased.

Monopolistic advertising practices, the dissemination of wrong information, and information suppression are all illegal, or at least they would be if practiced by a party with less political clout. In 1995, the Federal Trade Commission (FTC) found the California Dental Association guilty of suppressing information and also of trying to enforce their views without having the legal power to do so.

Most state dental boards forbid dentists to tell their patients about the toxicity of the mercury in their amalgam fillings. If your dentist tells you that mercury is nothing to worry about, this may be a response to the fear of losing his/her license for being honest about the risks, rather than a belief that mercury is harmless [162a].

How did the ADA get started?
The history of dental amalgam and the ADA and its predecessor, the American Society of Dental Surgeons (ASDS) is an interesting one. In the early 1800s, silver mercury amalgam was developed because a dental filling material was needed which would mold to the tooth cavity and then

harden to a usable surface. Plastics were essentially unknown then, and amalgam was the only material available other than gold foil, which was prohibitively expensive for most people.

The ASDS was formed in 1840. In recognition of the fact that mercury was toxic - this was known even then - members were required to sign a pledge stating they would not use mercury fillings. Breaking this pledge meant expulsion from the ASDS. Soon there was much dissension within the ASDS among those who opposed mercury fillings, those who supported them, and those who didn't care about mercury but resented being made to sign a pledge. Because of this dissension, the ASDS disbanded in 1855. The ADA, which supported amalgam fillings, was formed at about this same time. It has continued to grow ever more powerful until at this point its primary purpose for existence seems to be to support itself.

What are the legal limits of mercury exposure?

The pressure of the ADA is such that the most incredible illogic is allowed to persist. The

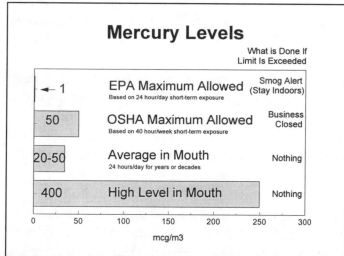

OSHA limit for mercury exposure in the workplace, as mentioned previously, is 50 mcg/m^3, assuming a 40 hour per week exposure. Scientific testing of mercury toxicity has caused them to reevaluate the safety of this amount, with the result that the new safe limit may soon be 20 mcg/m^3. NIOSH (National Institute of Occupational Safety and Health) sets an even stricter limit of 20 mcg/m^3, again based on a 40 hour per week exposure. The Environmental Protection Agency (EPA) has a limit of only 1 mcg/m^3, based on continuous exposure, even if short-term. These limits, illogically, apply anywhere but in the mouth, where measurements may be 20 to 400 mcg/m^3 24 hours a day for years.

Mercury amalgam is treated as a toxic material, with clearly defined protocols for safe handling and disposal, since it is considered to be both dangerous before insertion and toxic waste after removal [163].

Mercury-containing camera batteries have recently been outlawed in California due to concerns over toxicity. Tennis shoes which contain a battery to make them blink are now not allowed to be sold due to the mercury content of the battery. The amount of mercury in the battery is about equivalent to the amount in one average amalgam filling. It's banned in your shoe but safe in your mouth?

> **Mercury - Banned in your shoes but safe in your mouth?**

On August 10, 1990, the FDA announced that [164]:

"In light of emerging scientific data, the FDA needs to re-examine the use of amalgam. It may be necessary to reclassify amalgam and take various regulatory actions."

Yet to date, several years later, nothing has been done. The FDA seems to move more decisively to remove amino acids like tryptophan and herbs like comfrey and chaparral from health food store shelves. On June 29, 1990, the EPA announced a ban on mercury in interior latex paint products due to the deaths of children from the mercury in the paint. This ban took effect August 27, 1990; however, mercury can still be released from older paint on walls during remodeling. The maximum allowable limit for mercury in paint had been 200 parts per million (ppm). Amalgam typically contains 500,000 ppm.

In late 1993, the courts in California finally acknowledged that dental mercury is a poison, and stipulated that a warning would be posted as of early 1994 on packages of amalgam material and in some dental offices:

> **WARNING: This office uses amalgam filling materials which contain and expose you to mercury, a chemical known to the State of California to cause birth defects and other reproductive harm. Please consult your dentist for more information.**

Later in 1994 the courts overruled this decision, an example of the power of political influence. In 1996, the decision was again reversed: the warning sign should be posted. However, this is probably not the last word on the subject. The warning is also incomplete, as mercury can cause far more than reproductive harm, but this is at least a step in the right direction.

Daily exposure to mercury concentrations of 10-20 mcg/m^3 during a 40 hour work week produces physical and mental symptoms in most employees. Allowable mercury in workplace air, as mentioned, is 50 mcg/m^3 in the U.S., but only 10 mcg/m^3 in the ex-Soviet Union and Switzerland. A patient with twelve or more occlusal surfaces in his/her mouth (one filling may have several such surfaces) gets about 29 mcg of mercury per day, based on many intraoral measurements. A mouth with many fillings can release up to 560 <u>mg</u> (560,000 mcg) of mercury over several years [165].

What are some of the tests for mercury?
No single test can diagnose mercury toxicity for certain. Mercury is not usually found in body fluids because it tends to bind to the sulfur in the body's tissues. A combination of symptom observations and laboratory testing helps to indicate the effects of mercury and monitor a patient's progress upon removal. Laboratory tests include:

- **Blood tests** - These are not generally done for mercury itself [33], as the level of mercury in the blood represents only recent exposure, and is not indicative of the tissue mercury level. Tests measuring the oxygen-carrying ability of the blood (hemoglobin), or iron and other mineral levels, is more useful.

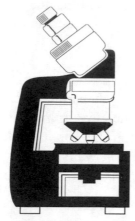

- **Live blood analysis** (LBA) and dried blood layer analysis are techniques in which blood is observed under the microscope. Cells and blood layers can actually show a shiny grey-ish metallic outer surface if metals are present in the blood, and black specks can be seen at the outer edges of the blood layer under magnification.

- **Urine tests** - Surprisingly, a low urine mercury content may be more troubling than a higher level, since the low level is indicative of an inefficient excretory mechanism, i.e. the patient would be retaining mercury. Overall, urine tests without provocative chelation are relatively useless in determining body mercury [33]. A provocative chelation test uses chemicals such as DMPS [166-171] or DMSA to pull mercury and other metals and minerals out of the body and into the urine for testing. EDTA is not recommended for this purpose because it is likely to chelate out necessary minerals first, such as calcium, magnesium, manganese, zinc and others. The kidneys tend to hold mercury rather than releasing it in the urine. If there are other metals in the urine, this may be a sign of mercury in the body because metallothionein is occupied with detoxifying mercury.

- **Hair analysis** for mercury can be helpful, especially when compared with follow-up testing of new hair growth after removal of the amalgam. Not all people find hair analysis useful, however, since the procedure can destroy the mercury before it can be measured. In addition, mercury tends to be absorbed into the brain rather than into the hair.

- A **skin patch test** can indicate a high degree of sensitivity to mercury. Since the test involves additional exposure to mercury, it is not generally recommended.

- The **Jerome Mercury Vapor Analyzer** is used as previously described. A higher reading usually correlates to higher toxicity [53]. The body holds mercury so outgassing from fillings is one of the best indicators of mercury toxicity. The test is best performed both before and after chewing gum [166], which shows what happens when chewing, eating, or grinding the teeth.

Anyone who doubts or questions whether mercury is actually released from mercury amalgam fillings should be quickly convinced by readings from the Mercury Vapor Analyzer, which is specific for mercury testing and is often used for toxic spills and in mines. Test the air in the room, or the mouth of someone without metal fillings, and the reading is at or near zero. Test the mouth of a person with one or more metal fillings, and the reading is almost invariably more than the Environmental Protection Agency (EPA) would allow as being a safe *short* term exposure level. Whether or not mercury comes out of fillings - and from there is obviously inhaled with every breath - is not a matter to be decided by opinion, however vehement, when there is obvious and repeatable scientific proof.

- The **paraffin test** does not detect mercury directly, but picks up its "footprint" by looking at other indicators. This is analogous to seeing a broken window, ransacked drawers, and missing stereo and concluding that a burglar had been in your home, even if nobody saw the burglar.

- Many of the above tests are good for detecting other heavy or toxic metals. The presence of these, especially aluminum, is an indication that mercury has overwhelmed the detoxification pathways.

- Mercury may be detectable in the feces by **stool test** if it is present in the body, but the correlation has not been proven.

What can sheep tell us about mercury toxicity?

In a recent experiment done at the University of Calgary in Canada [172], sheep had amalgam fillings placed in their mouths. Sheep were chosen because their chewing and detoxification patterns resemble those of humans. The number and type of fillings and the way they were placed correlated as closely as possible with the way fillings are placed in the average person. After 29 days, tests were run on the sheep and their tissues to determine whether and where the mercury had migrated in the body. Keep in mind that fillings leach mercury into our bodies for far longer than 29 days.

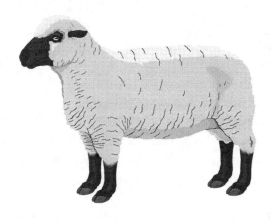

The results (tissue concentrations of mercury, Hg, in units of ng/g) are summarized in this chart and explained afterwards.

Tissue	ng Hg/g
Whole blood	9.0
Urine	4.7
Tooth bone	**318.2**
Gum mucosa	**323.7**
Stomach	**929.0**
Small intestine	28.0
Large intestine	63.1
Feces	**4489.3**
Kidney	**7438.0**
Liver	**772.1**
Spleen	48.3

Okay, so what does this chart mean?

Sheep without fillings were used as controls, and showed negligible amounts of mercury in their fluids and tissues. This means that the amounts of mercury indicated in the chart came only from the fillings. As an additional control, only mercury with radioactive tracers was picked up by the analytical instrumentation, ensuring that any small amount of regular non-radioactive mercury from the environment would not be reflected in these figures.

Highest amounts are shown in the kidneys, but comparatively little is found in the urine, which is where many doctors look. This means that the mercury concentrates in the kidneys and is not released into the urine; i.e. doesn't come out of you. Since the kidneys filter out all kinds of toxins for excretion as urine, the fact that mercury is concentrated there indicates that this detoxification pathway is blocked by the mercury and will not work as well as it should in removing other toxins. Since the kidney is involved in electrolyte balancing, blocking the kidney may cause electrolyte imbalance in the body, particularly of potassium, sodium, magnesium, and calcium.

Mercury is also found in the fetus and placenta (not shown on chart), indicating that, contrary to prior opinion, the fetus absorbs a substantial amount of this toxin before birth.

Large amounts of mercury are found in the feces, but little in the blood (another place where many doctors look), indicating that the fecal test would be a more accurate indicator of mercury exposure than a blood test.

Large amounts in the stomach indicate that mercury is indeed ingested from fillings during chewing.

Significant body burdens of mercury are also found by human autopsy [173-177].

Should fillings be removed?

If mercury is so universally toxic, then shouldn't everyone have their amalgam fillings removed and replaced? Not necessarily, although it is recommended for nearly everybody. Older fillings may be so low in mercury that their removal would bring only negligible improvement. For this reason mercury vapor testing is recommended.

Although there have been cases of dramatic and rapid reversals of debilitating symptoms, these cases are the exceptions. A more usual response is a slow but noticeable improvement, although most people who go to the trouble of replacing their amalgams are also making other positive lifestyle changes contributing to the improvement. Although any improvement is better than none, and some alleviation of symptoms usually occurs after replacement, the benefits should be weighed against the drawbacks:

- Even if the dentist is careful, the patient is exposed to more short-term mercury exposure during removal unless vitamin C chelation is done. The patient may feel worse before she/he feels better without chelation. Chelation involves the use of an intravenous metal binding agent to remove released mercury from the blood and body. The bound metal is then excreted.

- If a tooth is weak or has a very large filling, its structural integrity may be compromised by the procedure.

- Removal and replacement can be expensive, time-consuming, and, like all dental procedures, somewhat unpleasant.

- Allergic reactions to mercury, dental materials, anesthetics, and dental adhesives are possible.

For most people with the types of symptoms described in this book, however, the long-term benefits of replacement outweigh the short-term drawbacks. At the very least, the constant release of a known toxic metal into the body will be eliminated, which would certainly be to your benefit even if there is no immediate relief of symptoms. It comes down to the choice: tooth structure and temporary inconvenience versus your lifelong overall health.

The best policy is to visit a dentist who is aware of the dangers of dental mercury and knowledgeable about safe removal, and together you can make a decision based on your particular circumstances. It can be generally stated that no more amalgam should be placed in your mouth. If an amalgam filling needs to be replaced due to deterioration, have it replaced with one of the non-amalgam alternatives.

How can amalgam fillings be removed safely?

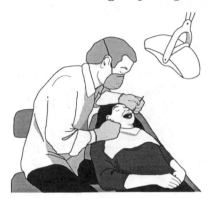

If you have decided to have all or most of your amalgam fillings replaced, it is important that the dentist you choose knows how to remove them safely. A dentist who simply drills out the old and puts in the new without treating the removed amalgam like the toxic material it is can do more harm than good. In fact, proceed with caution if the dentist places new mercury fillings at all in any patient, or recommends or does root canals. Such a dentist apparently does not understand the toxicity of mercury and other metals, or the dangers of electrical charges. Some recommendations for safe removal, and safe dental work in general, are:

- Use a rubber dental dam (latex sheet) in the mouth to keep from swallowing mercury particles.

- Use a high speed vacuum to remove drilled-out bits and mercury vapor.

- Use drapes so you don't carry mercury chips home on your clothes or absorb it through your exposed skin.

- Breathe oxygen or clean air through a nosepiece rather than mercury vapor-laden air from your mouth.

- Use a lighted magnifying instrument to see and remove every last bit of amalgam.

- Using a special blue light, the dentist should check teeth for cracks, which are common with mercury fillings. These cracks should then be repaired to stabilize tooth structure before crowns are needed.

- The dentist should protect him/herself with gloves and mask, otherwise this may be an indication that he/she does not take mercury toxicity seriously.

- Cut up the filling and remove it in sections rather than drilling it out, as drilling produces a fine mercury mist which can be inhaled or ingested.

- Use an air filtering system in the dental office.

- Have a biocompatibility test done for any replacement materials, adhesives, anesthetics, or other chemicals used. This can be a blood test or a muscle test.

What else is there to be concerned about other than mercury exposure?

Infection is a possibility when both you and the previous patient may have been bleeding. Bacteria, viruses, colds, hepatitis, and especially HIV (the so-called AIDS virus) are a possible danger if spread from one patient to another via unclean instruments. Such pathogens (disease organisms) can be spread through blood, saliva, and tissue (bone or gum).

Chemical exposure at the dental office is also a concern. It is a good idea to sniff the air during the first visit. Although nearly all dental offices have a characteristic smell, usually of formaldehyde and alcohol, a strong chemical smell is an indication that toxicity in general is not taken seriously. Also, if you are chemically sensitive, you could be putting yourself at risk by having your dental work done in an office filled with these toxins.

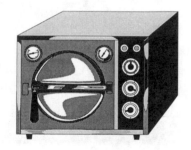

It is routine to wash and then autoclave instruments and dental drill bits by heating them in a special oven under pressure to kill any disease organisms. A wise precaution, and one rarely taken, is to also sterilize the handpieces of the drill. Handpieces are those parts of the dental drill which hold the drill bits and have gears and pulleys. They can easily become contaminated by blood, saliva, and tissue, and the quick alcohol wipe they are routinely given between patients is insufficient to kill pathogens.

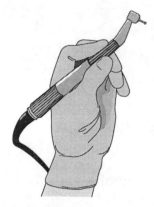

Ideally, handpieces should be removed after each patient and cleaned by ultrasound in a device called an ultrasonic cleaner or sonicator to remove any pieces of teeth or tissue. They should then be put into a special autoclave for sterilization. Each dental chair should have at least three handpieces: one in use, one in the autoclave, and one ready for the next patient.

Question your dentist to be sure he/she takes all of the above mentioned precautions.

Are you getting a charge out of your dental work?

Some nontoxic dentists, or medical clinics that work with such dentists, test the charge of each filled tooth with a special instrument, which is essentially an ammeter measuring in microamps. This records numbers such as +3, -13, etc., corresponding to the electrical charge. See the Battery Effect chapter for what this can mean. They then recommend removal and replacement in the following order: strongly negative, weakly negative, weakly positive, strongly positive. If positively charged fillings are removed first, they say, the patient's symptoms may even worsen. Other dentists feel the order of removal makes no difference. Since the evidence is inconclusive, it would be a good idea to have the fillings tested and removed in order of highest negative electrical charge first, since there is no reason not to do so and it may well be beneficial. Another way to remove fillings in order is to remove all fillings from one quadrant (quarter of the mouth) at a time, beginning with the quadrant which has the tooth with the most negative charge, then the quadrant with the next most negative charge and so on.

What is the cost for proper amalgam removal?

Dental work is rarely cheap, and a dentist who takes all or even most of the above precautions is likely to be even more expensive than most dentists, with good reason. A good dentist will have three sets of handpieces per chair rather than the usual single set; handpiece sets cost between $1000 (used) and $3000 (new). Washing, sonicating, and autoclaving handpieces after each patient is time consuming and expensive, but well worth it to the patient who does not contract AIDS or hepatitis after a dental visit.

Air and water filters are not cheap either. Testing for mercury vapor, electrical charges, and cracks in teeth requires special equipment which adds to the total cost. Masks, drapes, goggles, and rubber dental dams must be supplied and then cleaned or replaced for each patient. Biocompatibility testing can cost several hundred dollars.

The bottom line here is that you should be prepared to find that dentists who do the job according to the above guidelines will probably charge more than dentists who take only routine precautions. The difference in care, however, is well worth the extra cost. The quality of your life may depend on it.

What is the cost of improper amalgam removal?

Your health can be at risk when amalgam is removed improperly. Since your health is more valuable than money, this is a risk not worth taking.

What about mercury that gets into the body during removal?

For amalgam removal and replacement to have optimal results, adjunct therapy to detoxify mercury already in the body is recommended. Powdered charcoal tablets or capsules taken just before the procedure can help to soak up the mercury for excretion. An intravenous drip of vitamin C (ascorbic acid) during or immediately after the removal procedure binds with any mercury that escapes the precautions and gets into the body. This bound form is more easily excreted so the mercury doesn't enter the tissues to cause damage. Vitamin C is considered to be a mild chelating agent.

Won't the body get rid of the mercury after the amalgam fillings are removed?

Mercury is detoxified and excreted [178-182] through the following channels:

- *Liver [183]*
- *Kidney [83, 184-186]*
- *Sweat [80]*
- *Hair [187,188]*
- *Breath [12,189,190]*

However, it can take up to twenty years for the body to get rid of all of the mercury present in the tissues, if indeed it is possible to ever get rid of every last little bit, and assuming that no more mercury is entering the body from amalgam or other sources. It is therefore advisable to use chelation to help this process along.

Chelation therapy after removal of all fillings helps to bind mercury in tissues, where it is less accessible, and allows it to be excreted. DMSA, glutathione, DMPS, and EDTA are the most common chelating agents.

- DMSA   Takes metals out of the brain and central nervous system (CNS)

- Glutathione   Removes metals from blood

- DMPS   Removes metals from blood and tissue, more specific for mercury

- EDTA   Pulls out minerals more than metals, but opens up the detox pathways for the other chelators to work more effectively.

Although EDTA works best to remove mercury at a pH of 2.2, far more acid than the blood or tissues, EDTA is useful in opening up protein molecules so the other sulfur based chelators can work more effectively. These chelators, stronger than vitamin C, can only be used after all metal is out of the mouth. They are strong enough to pull metal out of the mouth and into the bloodstream and may do more harm than good under these conditions. You may then have the additive effect of mercury from two sources: that which is in the body already and that which is pulled from the teeth.

Since most chelating agents also remove desirable minerals such as sodium, potassium, magnesium, zinc, iron, copper, manganese, and calcium from the body, care must be taken to replace these during therapy, either orally or intravenously (IV). Homeopathic remedies can also be used to stimulate your body to dump the mercury [191].

Is there anything to worry about with chelation?
An important caution with any chelation therapy, including vitamin C: a plastic catheter is usually used for intravenous solutions, but a person with small veins may not be able to use a catheter and may require a smaller diameter needle. A stainless steel needle, safe to use for most applications, can be dangerous to use for chelation. The chelating solution, even vitamin C, can pull nickel out of the stainless steel needle and bring it into the body.

This is no trivial matter if the patient is allergic to nickel (sensitivity to cheap earrings is an indication). Potentially fatal anaphylactic shock is a possibility. Nickel brought into the body is toxic even if one is not allergic to it. Any acidic solution, not just chelating agents, can pull nickel out of a stainless steel needle.

Both authors have suffered severe allergic reactions to nickel during chelation, as have many patients. Another indication that you may be allergic to nickel, besides earring sensitivity, is vein collapse when a metal needle is introduced. A sign of vein collapse is a stoppage of the blood flow during blood collection for a blood test. Whole arm pain during most IVs is not usual and can also be a sign of nickel reactivity.

What else can help detoxify mercury?

There is some evidence that the "good" bacteria in the body can help in mercury detoxification. Acidophilus in capsules or yogurt will help replenish these good bacteria, since mercury acts as an antibiotic and, like other antibiotics, can kill some of the good bacteria. An even better idea is to first replace the colonizing bifidus bacteria and then take acidophilus. Bifidus establishes colonies on the intestinal wall, like condominiums the acidophilus workers live in.

If acidophilus is taken alone when mercury is present, the mercury will kill the acidophilus and the bacterial dieoff may cause you to feel sick. Human acidophilus is preferable to the more common cow (bovine) acidophilus, as it is a better match for our human system. In addition, people who are allergic to milk products or beef may also have an adverse reaction to cow acidophilus.

Good nutrition and other positive lifestyle choices, as detailed in this book and *Thriving In A Toxic World*, will enhance the benefits of amalgam replacement.

Once the mercury amalgam is removed, what material(s) should replace it?

The decision should be based on whether a filling or crown is needed, patient sensitivity to certain materials, aesthetics, and cost. The best alternatives are, in order of preference, indirect plastic composite or porcelain, direct composite, and gold or other noble metals platinum or palladium.

Comparison Summary of Dental Filling Materials				
Quality	**Mercury**	**Gold**	**Dir. Comp.**	**Indir. Comp.**
Toxicity	High	Medium	Low	Low
Battery Effect	High	High	None	None
Cost	Low	High	Medium	High
Longevity	Medium	High	Low	High
Appearance	Silver/black	Gold	Natural	Natural
Sensitivity / Pain	Medium	Medium	High	Low
Time Required for Procedure	Quick	Long	Medium	Long

Amalgam appears to have some benefits, such as relatively low cost for both the material and shorter procedure, and higher longevity than direct composite. However, it is unsuitable as a dental restoration material for a number of reasons:

- *Outgassing of mercury from the filling*
- *Toxicology [192-194], as well as discussed throughout this book.*
- *Poor in primary treatment of decay [195-197]*
- *Can cause periodontal (gum) problems [198,199]*
- *Poor for structural restoration [200-203]*
- *Expands and contracts with temperature changes and often cracks, often eventually needing a crown.*
- *Aesthetics - unattractive blackish color*

Plastic composite (sometimes called resin), desirable for a natural tooth-like appearance, is cheaper than porcelain. However, it has many drawbacks, including sensitivities to the materials used to make it. The procedure is more difficult and time-consuming than amalgam for the dentist to work with, and therefore more costly.

Composite can be placed using the direct method, in which the material is placed directly into the cleaned cavity and hardened using a special blue light. The indirect method is preferred for strength and longevity. In this procedure, a mold is first made of the cleaned cavity. From this mold, the filling is made and hardened in the laboratory and then cemented into place. Two appointments are needed, and a temporary filling is used between the appointments.

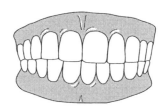

The indirect method is more time consuming and expensive, but the filling lasts longer and tooth sensitivity is less likely. Another approach which will work and may be cheaper is to place direct fillings, treating them as temporary. If or when the fillings loosen, replace them as needed using the indirect method. Alternatively, use the more expensive indirect fillings only on heavy biting surfaces such as the tops of molars.

Conquest and Herculite are two brand names of plastic composite. Conquest, especially, is unlikely to cause an adverse allergic patient reaction based on biocompatibility testing. Glass ionomer on a silver base to make it stronger is another type of composite. The silver, which can be toxic, should be completely enclosed by the ionomer or it may cause a reaction, either allergic or electrical (battery effect). Glass ionomer / resin mixed product would be a better alternative.

Porcelain is about as good as indirect composite. It is closest in appearance to natural teeth. The procedure, however, is longer and the cost higher than for other materials. Porcelain may be cast over mixed metals, but the metal should be completely enclosed by the porcelain and is unlikely to cause trouble unless some of the metal is exposed. Cheap porcelain crowns may have a visible metal band and should be avoided. Better quality porcelain crowns have porcelain right down to the gumline.

Gold is the material of choice for many dentists, although it has enough drawbacks to put it in third place as a desirable dental filling material. Pure gold is best, but may be too soft for high stress applications, as well as being expensive. Alloys of gold are cheaper and stronger, but alloys contain metals such as copper, nickel, or zinc to which the individual may be sensitive and, in combination, can cause an electric battery effect (discussed in the Battery Effect chapter). For the same reason, gold is not recommended if there are other metals in the mouth (braces, root canal posts, nickel crowns), or elsewhere in the body (bone pins, surgical staples). Gold is so conductive of electricity that it is used in the best stereo systems to conduct the electrical impulses which produce sound.

Another note on dental materials - if you have extractions done, you may get a temporary device or retainer sometimes called a flipper. This consists of a plastic tooth or teeth embedded in a clear or pink plastic base that fits over the gum. The pink base contains mercury or cadmium sulfate to produce the pink color, just as mercury produces a pink color in sunsets after volcanic eruptions. Request a clear base instead, which does not have mercury. A minor cosmetic problem with the clear base: the gums under the base could look black due to light refraction.

What kind of improvement is expected after removal?

Nobody can make any guarantees about the amount, type, or timing of improvement after amalgam removal. Some patients, especially those with a mercury sensitivity or electrical charges, report a dramatic and almost immediate (within one day) improvement. Some report an improvement so slow and slight that it was only noticed several months later upon looking back. Some report no improvement at all, or improvement in only some of their symptoms. This may be due in part to the fact that, although mercury is out of the mouth, it may take some time to get it out of the body. Removing the fillings is like turning off the faucet. Now you still have to drain the tub through chelation.

Many patients and both authors feel strongly enough about mercury toxicity that they have had their amalgam fillings removed and replaced. Most patients and both authors experienced noticeable improvement after removal.

What are some statistics for improvement?

A large study was done in December 1992 by the Foundation for Toxic Free Dentistry (FTFD) [14]. In this study, 762 patients who had their mercury fillings removed filled out a report detailing a wide variety of symptoms present before amalgam removal. The patients then evaluated whether each symptom improved after removal. These reports were originally submitted to the U.S. Food and Drug Administration (FDA) and a duplicate copy was then evaluated by the FTFD, removing a possible source of bias.

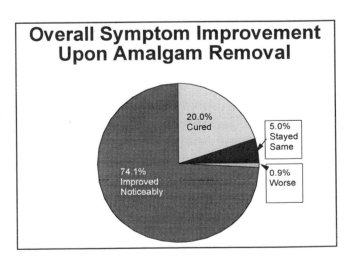

Overall Symptom Improvement Upon Amalgam Removal

- 20.0% Cured
- 5.0% Stayed Same
- 0.9% Worse
- 74.1% Improved Noticeably

Each symptom experienced by each patient was looked at separately. 3792 symptoms were reported by the 762 patients. Of these 3792 symptoms,

- *758, or 20%, were reported cured after amalgam removal*
- *2812, or 74%, improved noticeably*
- *188, or 5%, stayed the same six months after removal*
- *34, or 0.9%, reported a worsening of the symptom*

This improvement is convincing evidence of the toxicity of mercury fillings. It also provides cause for optimism for those who are considering amalgam removal.

What kinds of symptoms showed the most dramatic improvement?

Symptom	Initially reported by	Improved or cured
Depression	181, or 23.8% of total	All 181, or **100%**
Fatigue	325, or 42.7%	310, or **95%**
Allergies	221, or 29.0%	196, or **88.7%**
Headaches	233, or 30.6%	222, or **95%**
Memory loss	109, or 14.3%	102, or **93.5%**
Multiple sclerosis	42, or 5.5%	33, or **78.5%**

How can you increase your chances for improvement?
Some patients simply do not show improvement after amalgam removal. A study of what characteristics these patients might have in common [204] has led to some suggestions for increasing your chances of improvement following removal.

One of the main methods of mercury excretion is through the feces. Many people who do not improve following amalgam removal have fecal impactions in the intestines or diverticula, which are outpouchings in the intestinal lining that can hold waste matter. In both cases mercury is trapped and retained, then released slowly back into the bloodstream to cause the original symptoms rather than being eliminated.

With this in mind, it would be a good idea to eat a healthy diet high in fiber and enzymes for at least a week before amalgam removal - a good idea in any case. The eight day detoxification diet described in the Nutrition chapter in ***Thriving In A Toxic World*** is ideal for this purpose. Colonics after amalgam removal will also help to clear the bowel of mercury and other waste materials which may otherwise not be excreted. Metal crystals can sometimes be seen in the evacuation tube during a colonic.

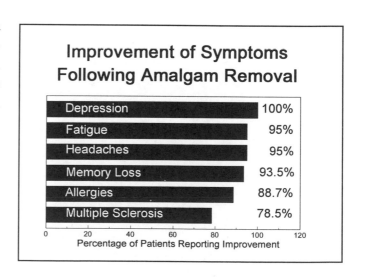

The other detoxification and excretion pathways should be kept as clear as possible so they can concentrate on ridding your body of mercury rather than dealing with other toxins. These pathways are:

- *Liver*   *uses glutathione*
- *Skin*   *by way of sweat*
- *Lungs*   *toxins breathed out*

To this end, reduce chemical and drug exposure even more scrupulously than usual for as long a period as possible before removal. Sulfur based amino acids such as glutathione will help detoxify mercury, but will also react with +2 valence minerals like iron, calcium, zinc, or copper.

Minerals should not be taken on days of glutathione detoxification to avoid competition with mercury removal, but take plenty of minerals before and after detoxification. The recommended glutathione dosage is one capsule (about 150 mg) per 25 pounds of body weight; a 125 pound person should therefore take five capsules.

Sugar, which becomes acid in the body and acts as a chelator, pulls out mercury from teeth and from storage sites in the body so it can cause symptoms. This is yet another reason to avoid sugar. All sweeteners are acid, and any sweet taste becomes acid in the mouth, so fruits and the artificial sweetener aspartame should also be avoided.

Patient Profile

One patient, a nurse married to a doctor, had symptoms since 1977, and was positively diagnosed with multiple sclerosis (MS) in 1992. Doctors told her that the disease would worsen over time, and the only treatment was steroids for symptomatic relief. The steroids made her ill and were discontinued. By January 1995, she had facial paralysis on one side, trigeminal neuralgia (severe facial pain), extreme fatigue, vision problems in one eye, numbness in one leg, couldn't keep her balance, pins-and-needles feeling in hands and feet, and urinary problems. She used a walker to get around, and used a wheelchair as needed to cover longer distances.

Kathy came to Comprehensive Health Center in March of 1995. Tests showed her level of mercury to be 81 - normal / optimal should be below 1, and 81 is higher than that of most dentists. She had her mercury fillings replaced with non-toxic dental composite material, and had chelation to remove the mercury from her body. She went on an eight-day detoxification diet and felt much better after three days, with the numbness and tingling subsiding. Other than this, however, the changes were at first slow. It is typical with MS that some days are better and some are worse, without any apparent pattern. Over several months she noticed that there were more good days, fewer bad days, she could walk farther, and no longer needed an afternoon nap. By June 1995 she was able to walk around EPCOT Center in Florida - and she was previously barely able to shop for a few groceries without leg pain.

Her MS tests used to be positive, and are now negative. No brain lesions show on the MRI test, and her spinal tap is negative.

What Can You Do?

1. If indicated by testing and symptomology, have your mercury amalgam fillings removed - safely, as per the guidelines in this chapter.

2. Follow the detoxification / chelation protocols outlined in the Metal Detoxification chapter.

3. Mercury acts as an antibiotic and kills the beneficial bacteria in the intestine, allowing yeast and other parasites to proliferate. Yeast and parasite testing and treatment (see Microorganism section) and supplementation with the beneficial bacteria acidophilus and bifidus (see Digestion chapter in *Thriving In A Toxic World*) would likely be indicated.

Summary

Mercury has been known to be poisonous for centuries. Most of the mercury we are exposed to comes from the amalgam fillings in our mouths, and this practice continues primarily for political and financial reasons. The best course of action is to have your amalgam fillings removed by a dentist who knows how to do so safely.

| References and Resources |

- The Burton Goldberg Group, "Biological Dentistry", pp. 80-96, *Alternative Medicine: The Definitive Guide*, Future Medicine Publishing, Puyallup WA, 1994

- Huggins, Hal, and Sharon Huggins, *It's All in Your Head*, Life Sciences Press, Colorado Springs CO, 1986.

- Manning, Betsy Russell (editor), *Candida: Silver (Mercury) Fillings and the Immune System*, Greensward Press, San Francisco CA, 1985.

- Stortebecker, Patrick, *Mercury Poisoning From Dental Amalgam - A Hazard to the Human Brain*, BioProbe Inc., Orlando FL, 1985.

- Taylor, Joyal, *The Complete Guide to Mercury Toxicity from Dental Fillings*, Scripps Publishing, San Diego CA, 1988.

- Ziff, Sam, *Silver Dental Fillings - The Toxic Time Bomb*, Aurora Press, Santa Fe NM, 1986.

- Ziff, Sam and Michael, *Infertility and Birth Defects*, BioProbe Inc., Orlando FL, 1987.

- Ziff, Sam and Michael, and Mats Hansen, *Mercury Detoxification*, BioProbe Inc., Orlando FL, 1990.

- Ziff, Sam and Michael, *Dental Mercury Detox*, BioProbe Inc., Orlando FL, 1993.

- Ziff, Sam and Michael, *Dentistry Without Mercury*, Bio-Probe Inc., Orlando FL, 1993.

- Ziff, Sam and Michael, *The Missing Link*, Bio-Probe Inc., Orlando FL, 1992. *Explores the relationship between mercury and heart disease.*

- **American Academy of Biological Dentistry**, P.O. Box 856, Carmel Valley CA 93924. Phone 408-659-5385. *Promotes nontoxic dentistry.*

- **International Academy of Oral Medicine and Toxicology**, P.O. Box 608531, Orlando FL 32860-8531. *Provides listing of non-toxic dentists.*

- **Foundation for Toxic-Free Dentistry**, P.O. Box 608010, Orlando FL 32860-8010. *Provides listing of non-toxic dentists; send self-addressed stamped envelope (52 cents) for information and referrals.*

- **Environmental Dental Association**, 9974 Scripps Ranch Blvd., Suite 36, San Diego CA 92131. Phone 800-388-8124 or 619-586-1208. *Referral service, books, and products relating to alternative dentistry. Call for free packet of information.*

- **DAMS** (Dental Amalgam Syndrome), 725-9 Tramway Lane Northeast, Albuquerque NM 87122. Phone 505-291-8239. *Support and study of those with mercury amalgam toxicity.*

NICKEL AND ROOT CANALS

You Need A Root Canal Like You Need A Hole In Your Head

Do you have root canals, or do you use cosmetics or eat margarine ? Do you have any of the following symptoms? There may be a connection between your symptoms and exposure to the toxic metal nickel.

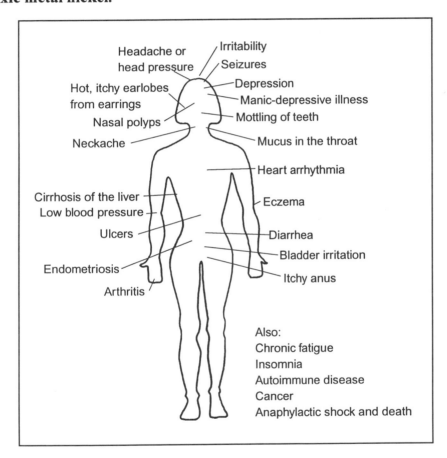

Thirteen things in this chapter that can change your health:

1. *Nickel is both the most allergenic and the most carcinogenic metal we are exposed to.*
2. *What are some symptoms of nickel allergy?*
3. *How do scientists use nickel to cause cancer in lab animals?*
4. *How are the immune system and other body systems affected by nickel?*
5. *What are some sources of nickel?*
6.-10. *Why are root canals so bad for you? - five major reasons*

11. Why and how are root canals done?

12. What can be done if you already have root canals?

13. What kind of improvement is possible from having root-canaled teeth re-moved?

What is one of the most harmful metals?

Nickel is one of the most common severe metal toxicities in humans in industrialized societies. Like mercury, the primary source of poisoning is right in your own mouth.

Trace amounts of nickel are needed to enable the enzyme system to run properly, but other than that nickel has no known use in the human body.

What kinds of harmful reactions can nickel cause?

Basic types of adverse nickel reactions in the body include:

- *Sensitivities/allergies*
- *Organonickel toxicity*
- *Carcinogenicity*
- *Immune system effects*
- *Other effects*

Is it possible to be allergic to a metal?

Nickel is the most potent allergen of all the trace elements, accounting for more contact dermatitis and other allergic reactions than all other metals combined.

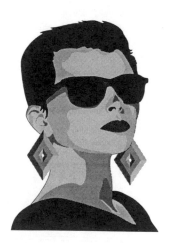

Up to 33% of women and 17% of men are allergic to nickel. A sign of nickel allergy is the development of hot, red, itchy earlobes soon after putting on inexpensive earrings. Inexpensive earring wires or posts are usually made of stainless steel, which contains nickel; this is also the case for cheap gold-colored earwires. Nickel is the component in inexpensive earrings that is most likely to cause problems. Expensive earrings are likely to be made of gold or silver, which rarely cause a reaction. Lack of a noticeable reaction, however, does not mean that one is not allergic.

The wearing of cheap earrings does more than just provide a visible means of identifying nickel allergy. They can actually cause nickel allergy by sensitizing the person to a metal they might not otherwise come in contact with. Men with pierced ears have thirty-three times the nickel sensitivity as men without pierced ears [1]. Women are even more likely to have nickel allergy because of earrings, jewelry, and nickel oxides in cosmetics which sometimes contact sensitive mucous membranes.

If you have all of the following there is a good chance that you have problems related to nickel allergy:

- *A reaction to earrings*
- *Root-canaled teeth, and*
- *Allergies and health problems, especially those discussed in this chapter*

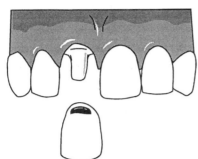

Nickel is commonly used in dental work to make crowns, and as components of orthodontic braces and root-canal posts. 12% of the stainless steel rod in a root canal post is nickel. Removable partial dentures have up to 30% nickel. About 80% of the dental community use nickel based alloys for porcelain fused to metal crowns [1]. In other words, 80% of all porcelain crowns have nickel in them.

Nickel does not pass government allergy test standards (ADA 41), but it is allowed to sneak in as stainless steel. If stainless steel can be compared to the Trojan horse, nickel is the soldiers inside that do the damage.

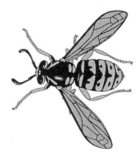

Nickel is toxic in itself, and much more so in someone who is allergic to it. Imagine being allergic to, say, poison ivy, or peanuts, or bee venom, and spending much of your life in constant contact with this substance. Life wouldn't be very pleasant, would it? Yet many people who are allergic to nickel have it in their mouths, and the result is a variety of symptoms ranging from inconvenient to life-threatening.

What kinds of symptoms can nickel allergy cause?

Most allergic symptoms from nickel in the mouth are systemic, not oral. These symptoms include:

- *Eczema or dermatitis on the eyelids, groin, elbows, and elsewhere*
- *Asthma from inhalation of the dust*
- *Autoimmune disease such as lupus or arthritis*
- *Headaches and neckaches*
- *Mucus in the throat* • *Nasal polyps*

Itchy anus, if pinworms, fungus, and food allergy have been ruled out as a cause, is often caused by nickel irritating the lining of the intestinal and anal mucosa as it is excreted. The itching and soreness is essentially the same reaction as sensitive individuals have on their earlobes from inexpensive earrings.

Nickel can cause an anaphylactic reaction, an acute (sudden) allergic reaction in which the body's systems are overwhelmed by a massive histamine reaction that can be fatal within minutes.

What happens when nickel combines with organic compounds?

An organic compound is one which contains carbon. When carbon monoxide is passed over finely divided (powdered) nickel, the organic

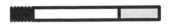

compound nickel carbonyl is formed. Nickel carbonyl is toxic and carcinogenic, especially to lung tissue. Conditions for its formation exist in motor vehicle exhaust where the gasoline contains nickel additives, and as pollutants from the incomplete burning of coal and petrochemicals. It is also found along with cadmium in cigarette smoke, and may in fact be partially responsible for the cancer that often results from smoking.

The carbon monoxide in cigarette smoke may further react with nickel in the smoker's mouth. Acute exposure to nickel carbonyl can cause symptoms that may be delayed for several hours after exposure. These symptoms include pulmonary (lung) and cerebral (brain) edema [2]. Nickel carbonyl is metabolized in the body back to Ni^{+2} (ionic form of nickel) and carbon monoxide, which is a potent asphyxiant, i.e. causes suffocation by stealing oxygen.

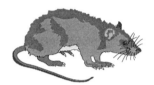

How do scientists cause cancer in lab animals?

The carcinogenicity, or cancer causing potential, of nickel is so well known that laboratory scientists who want to study cancer in animals will inject the animals with a nickel solution to reliably cause cancer.

In addition to the carcinogenic effects of organonickel compounds, nickel and nickel dust can themselves cause cancer. The RNA and DNA of the cell nucleus, where the blueprint for the making of new cells originates, are damaged by nickel. Lung and nasal cancers can develop when nickel dust is inhaled. Nickel dust is a known carcinogen with an incubation period of 25-30 years, similar to that of cigarettes [3].

Other nickel-caused cancers are intestinal cancer and oral cancer, which can result from nickel in the mouth. One patient, a nurse, got braces at age 26. A sharp end of the braces poked her repeatedly in the side of her mouth. A cancerous tumor developed at the site of irritation and quickly enlarged to the size of a melon. She was dead from cancer at age 28, only two years after she got the braces.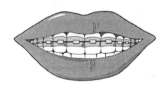

Good doctors learn more from patients than from any other source. Information learned from this nurse's condition was used to save the life of another patient in a similar situation.

A 20 year old male had a wire dental retainer made from nickel-containing stainless steel. For five years, he had ulcers, digestive problems, mucus in his throat, and recurrent lung infections. He took the wire out and dealt with fungus problems caused by the antibiotics the doctors had given him for the presumed lung infections. The health problems, caused initially by nickel allergy, cleared up.

This was not an isolated case. Another 20-year-old patient with a wire dental retainer was experiencing seizures of unknown cause. He was on Dilantin, an anticonvulsant medication. As soon as he had the retainer taken out and was chelated for metals, the seizures, throat mucus, low energy and attention problems cleared.

The temporomandibular joint (TMJ) where the upper and lower jaws meet can sometimes be out of alignment and cause problems such as facial pain. Artificial TMJ joints have been made of nickel-containing stainless steel. One company that made these joints has gone out of business from lawsuits. These lawsuits resulted when a large number of patients developed nickel-related complications. Some patients had their intestines removed due to inflammation, and others developed cancer. Other stainless steel artificial joints such as knees and hips are still being used.

Is the immune system also affected?
Nickel's effects on the immune system include decreased resistance to disease, decreased antibody formation, and decreased phagocytosis (the immune system's first line of defense) [2], all of which can result in infection and cancer. Nickel can cause or at least contribute to autoimmune disorders such as:

- *lupus*
- *arthritis*
- *ulcers*
- *endometriosis*
- *digestive system inflammations*

What else can nickel do?
Other symptoms caused by nickel and its compounds include [4]:

- Chronic fatigue, which usually has multiple causes

- Digestive system difficulties such as nausea, diarrhea, colitis, ulcers, and poor digestion

- Capillary damage and multiple hemorrhages, especially in the brain, lungs, and adrenals

- Mottling of teeth from nickel fluoride

- CNS stimulation leading to muscle tremors, tetany, and paralysis

- Malaise, dizziness, insomnia, irritability, muscle weakness

- Meningeal contraction from nickel irritation can cause headache and head pressure, low back and neck pain, and light sensitivity.

- Cirrhosis of the liver

- Low blood pressure, with accompanying dizziness on arising and lack of energy

- Nasal septum necrosis

- Nasal polyps from root canals in the top front teeth

- Bipolar disorder, also known as manic-depressive illness, can be caused by the nickel in dental braces.

- Both nickel and mercury suppress iron, copper, and cobalt (found in vitamin B12), leading to anemia.

- Nickel can block calcium channels in the heart, lowering magnesium levels and leading to heart arrhythmias.

- Seizures from electrical charges or allergy - one patient who was given a nickel dental retainer developed epileptic seizures within three weeks, which stopped when the retainer was removed.

- Depression

Where is nickel found, and how does it get into the body?

The primary sources of nickel are dental, dietary, and industrial. Dietary sources include [5]:

- *kelp*
- *tea*
- *herring*
- *legumes*
- *refined and processed food, especially those with hydrogenated fats and oils*

- *cabbage*
- *oysters*
- *buckwheat, oats*
- *unrefined grains and cereals*

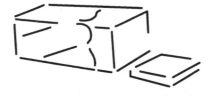

Nickel is used as a catalyst in the hydrogenation of vegetable oils (corn, peanut, cottonseed, margarine). Grains may be stone ground, in which case the label will proudly point this out. Otherwise stainless steel is used in grinding, and the nickel in the stainless steel may contaminate the ground grain.

Industrial and other sources include nickel plated alloys, fossil fuel emissions, batteries, stainless steel, nickel plating, some cosmetics, super-phosphate fertilizers, tobacco smoke, and "white gold" metal. Stainless steel cookware may transmit some nickel to foods, particularly acidic ones which can cause metal leaching. Frequent handling of coins, especially - not surprisingly - nickels, can cause sensitization to the metal.

Why are root canals so bad for you?

Root canals are a major source of nickel poisoning, but they are sources of other problems as well. The problems caused by root canals are due to:

- The presence of toxic and allergenic nickel in the stainless steel post

- The presence of a nonliving body part

- Infection due to stagnant infectious fluid in the tubules of the teeth

- Chemicals used to clean out and fill the tooth interior, including formaldehyde and mercury

- Electrical charges due to the battery effect, discussed in the Battery Effect chapter

Are teeth dead?

Teeth, contrary to the way many people think of them, are a living part of the body. They have a blood and nerve supply, take in nutrients, and pump calcium in and out as needed. The part of the tooth that is visible is a mineralized collagen shell which does not change much in appearance even years after the body dies.

Why are root canals done?

The living inner part of a tooth may die due to a hard blow that severs nerve and blood connections in the tooth with their source in the gums. A severe abscess (infection) can also kill the tooth. In a surprising number of cases, iatrogenic (treatment-caused) trauma from improperly done dental work can injure or kill the tooth.

The dying nerve supply in the tooth can cause severe pain. The dead or dying inner part of the tooth should be removed to keep the dying tissues from becoming food for bacteria and to keep the tooth from discoloring. Since the hard outer shell of the tooth is still functional for appearance, chewing, and proper space maintenance, it is left in place. This makes sense in theory, but read on.

How are root canals done?

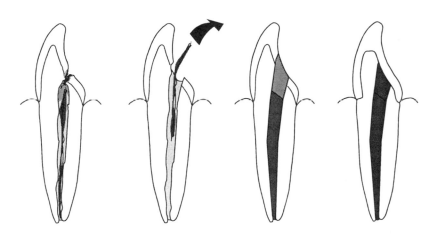

The dental specialist most likely to do root canals is called an endodontist. He or she drills a hole in the top of the dead or dying tooth and removes the dead material within, including pulp, blood supply, and nerves. The inside of the tooth is then cleaned with antiseptics and bleaching agents, all of which have potential for toxicity and allergic reactions. What you appear to have at this point is a clean, hollow ceramic-like tube.

Why don't you have a clean hollow tube?

What you actually have is a tooth that is full of microscopic dentin tubules, like little packets. If all the tubules in a front tooth were laid end to end they would reach for three miles. Although microscopic in size, their width is such that they can accommodate streptococcus bacteria eight abreast [6]. These tubules cannot be cleaned out by the standard root canal flushing procedure and become home to billions of multiplying bacteria and the infectious liquid they produce. The body cannot keep these bacteria under control any more since the blood supply is now missing, and bacteria and the biological toxins they produce can continue to leak out into the body for many years after the root canal procedure was done.

How harmful are these bacteria?

These bacteria are often the cause of chronic maladies and death suffered by people who do not suspect the root cause (pun intended). A dentist named Dr. Weston Price, who was in charge of the ADA toxicology department for years, demonstrated the connection between root canals and disease over sixty years ago. He observed that people with such ailments as kidney and heart disease, arthritis, and lupus often improved soon after their root-canaled teeth were extracted.

To further prove the connection, he implanted fragments of the removed teeth under the skin of rabbits, which are animals with an immune system similar to our own. The rabbits soon died of the exact disease, kidney or heart, that afflicted the human donor. These experiments were repeated and verified hundreds of times. It appears that different toxins are produced, each of which targets a specific organ or system. In similar experiments, 3 milligrams (mg) of material from root-canaled teeth caused death within one and a half minutes when injected into rabbits [7]. 3 mg of toxins can be found in the mouth of one person with root canals.

What happens after the tooth has been hollowed out?

Once the tooth has been hollowed out and the dentist wrongly assumes that it is clean and sterile, a stainless steel root canal post, which can be approximately 12% nickel, is inserted. This post is screwed into the bone for stability, and the tooth is then sealed. However, before inserting the post, the dentist will often put a drop of some type of antibiotic into the bottom of the tooth. Mercury used to be used for this purpose for its antibacterial properties; some dentists may still use mercury and if you have an older root canal there is a good chance that mercury was the antibiotic used. The bottom of the tooth is right next to the blood supply to the rest of the body, so it is not hard to figure out where the toxic mercury ends up - in the rest of the body. The combination of mercury and stainless steel also creates a miniature battery, which puts out damaging electrical charges (see Battery Effect chapter).

What is wrong with the logic of doing root canals?

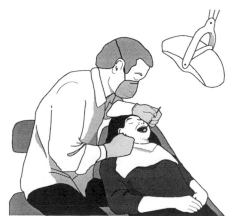

When a tooth has been killed, it is often better to extract it than to have a root canal done, although it appears on the surface that it would be better to "save" the tooth via a root canal. If your arm or toe were gangrenous and dead, with no blood or nerve supply and no hope of recovering life in the limb, any doctor would advocate amputating it and allowing the healthy remaining tissue to heal, so infection doesn't spread through your entire body. No doctor would suggest cleaning the arm to make it look lifelike, inserting a metal post to keep it from flopping, and leaving it attached, dead and nonfunctional, to the body. Yet this is what is done routinely to dead teeth. The body, instead of healing an extraction site and going on with life, must constantly cope with bacteria and toxins produced in the tooth.

The immune system is constantly stressed by what has become a foreign object that it is unable to consume or expel. This immune system stress can show up in later life as allergies, autoimmune disease, pain, or chronic fatigue.

Saving the external structure of a tooth is trivial compared to the importance of your overall health and well-being.

What if you already have root-canaled teeth?
It may be best to have them extracted if you have signs of nickel allergy such as sore earlobes from earrings, or other problems as described in this chapter which may be related to nickel. A doctor or clinic familiar with nickel toxicity may be the best place to get information to help you make the decision to extract the tooth or not. Be aware that a dentist, even if knowledgeable, may be prevented by law from discussing the health aspects of the procedure.

However, both nickel and bacteria may have penetrated into the bone surrounding the removed tooth. It is therefore important to use a slow speed dental burr to clean out this bone, which is often soft and mushy from infection. The removal of the bone by the burr also stirs up the bone cells and stimulates the formation of new bone growth to close up the hole left by the extraction. This procedure is painless with local anesthetic used for the extraction. The extraction site is then rinsed with a zinc and insulin mixture called PZI to facilitate healing. A prosthetic device such as a bridge or denture, sometimes called a flipper, is then worn to replace the extracted tooth.

What kind of improvement can occur?
There have been many cases of dramatic improvement of symptoms after extraction of root-canaled teeth. Some people report feeling better before even leaving the office, or within the same day. One patient stated that she felt as if a weight had been lifted off her shoulders almost immediately. Other people report a gradual improvement over the next few months. Still others do not notice a difference.

It is possible for a person to undergo what is called a healing crisis for about three days after extraction and to feel worse before getting better. The root canal may have been suppressing the immune system, and when the tooth comes out the immune system gains strength and goes after the pathogens. The ensuing fight, called a die-off or Herxheimer reaction, can cause unpleasant flu-like symptoms. These symptoms normally last a maximum of 72 hours and then the person should feel much better. If the symptoms last longer they can be due to nickel allergy or electrolyte (mineral) deficiency.

One patient had such a reaction. After researching information on root canals, she chose to have three root-canaled teeth removed in 1993. The damage leading to the root canals had been done in a car accident 23 years previously, and since the teeth were next to each other they were all removed at once. She felt sick within half an hour of the procedure and ran a fever for nine days afterward before improving in health. Fear not - this type of reaction is relatively rare, with a feeling of well-being more common following extraction. In this patient's case, the toxins that had been contributing to her health problems for years by leaking out slowly were released all at once. Her dramatic and rapid negative reaction was caused by toxins that were already present and were stirred up by the removal procedure. Recall that 3 mg of such toxins can kill a rabbit within minutes.

This unpleasant reaction might have been avoided if she had taken an intravenous solution such as vitamin C. The acidic solution acts as a safety net and would have helped to clean out the bacteria that were set loose.

One patient with an abscessed tooth had numb hands and feet. He had the tooth extracted, then had his mercury fillings removed, had chelation to remove the mercury from his body, and started getting better. Three other patients who had root-canaled teeth extracted reported that their problems -- low back pain (a runner in mid-30's), brain fog (environmentally ill patient in his 50's), and prostate problems (a man in his 40's) -- cleared after extraction.

What Can You Do?

If nickel is a problem for you, the solution is twofold:

- Remove the root canaled teeth or other sources of the metal.

- Chelate out the remaining nickel (and other metals) with DMPS (IV), which is preferred, or with DMSA (oral). DMPS chelation should not be done if there is any metal in the mouth, including mercury amalgam fillings. An exception is noble metals such as gold and platinum; chelation can be done with these in the mouth.

Summary

- Nickel is responsible for more allergic reactions than all other metals combined.

- Nickel is so toxic that it can cause a wide variety of symptoms, including deleterious effects on the immune system.

- Dental root canals are harmful for several reasons, including the nickel/ stainless steel post, the presence of bacteria that the body can no longer reach to eliminate, and the battery effect from dissimilar metals.

- Root canals can cause problems as diverse as heart disease, kidney disease, and autoimmune disorders.

- Root-canaled teeth should often be extracted, sacrificing the dead tooth in favor of your overall health.

References and Resources

- The Burton Goldberg Group, "Biological Dentistry", pp. 80-96, *Alternative Medicine: The Definitive Guide*, Future Medicine Publishing, Puyallup WA, 1994

- Meinig, George E., *Root Canal Cover-Up*, Bion Publishing, Ojai CA, 1994.

- Huggins, Hal, *Position Papers: Amalgam Issue, Root Canals, Cavitations*, Huggins Diagnostic Inc., Colorado Springs CO, 1991.

The following organizations promote the use of non-toxic dental materials, and may be able to provide information on the hazards of root canals as well as other dental materials.

- **American Academy of Biological Dentistry**, P.O. Box 856, Carmel Valley CA 93924, phone 408-659-5385.

- **Environmental Dental Association**, 9974 Scripps Ranch Blvd., Suite 36, San Diego CA 92131, phone 800-388-8124 or 619-586-1208.

- **Foundation for Toxic-Free Dentistry**, P.O. Box 608010, Orlando FL 32860-8010.

- **International Academy of Oral Medicine and Toxicology**, P.O. Box 608531, Orlando FL 32860-8531. *Provides listing of non-toxic dentists.*

OTHER METALS

Metals Belong In Cars, Not Bodies

Do you have any of the following symptoms? They could be due to toxic metals (other than mercury and nickel, covered in previous chapters).

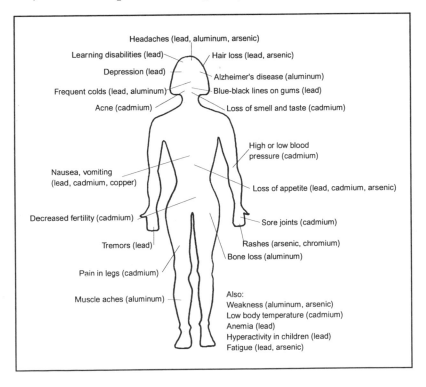

Headaches (lead, aluminum, arsenic)
Learning disabilities (lead)
Hair loss (lead, arsenic)
Depression (lead)
Frequent colds (lead, aluminum)
Alzheimer's disease (aluminum)
Blue-black lines on gums (lead)
Acne (cadmium)
Loss of smell and taste (cadmium)
High or low blood pressure (cadmium)
Nausea, vomiting (lead, cadmium, copper)
Loss of appetite (lead, cadmium, arsenic)
Decreased fertility (cadmium)
Sore joints (cadmium)
Tremors (lead)
Rashes (arsenic, chromium)
Bone loss (aluminum)
Pain in legs (cadmium)
Muscle aches (aluminum)

Also:
Weakness (aluminum, arsenic)
Low body temperature (cadmium)
Anemia (lead)
Hyperactivity in children (lead)
Fatigue (lead, arsenic)

In this chapter you can learn:

- *What other metals besides mercury and nickel are toxic, and how are they harmful?*

- *What are the symptoms of poisoning from these metals?*

- *Where are these toxic metals found?*

- *Are lead pencils really made of lead?*

- *Why does cigarette smoking make it harder to smell and taste?*

- *What is the link between aluminum and Alzheimer's disease, and how are mercury fillings involved?*

- *Why are deodorants not a good idea?*

What other metals besides mercury and nickel are toxic?

There are several metals which are both prevalent and toxic, and it is wise to avoid them whenever possible, although copper in ionic (charged) form rather than metallic form is needed in trace amounts for body function.

These metals include the following, discussed in this order:

- *lead*
- *arsenic*
- *cadmium*
- *copper*
- *aluminum*
- *platinum*

Lead

Get the lead out

Lead is a poison which targets cell protoplasm and the nervous system. Most of the body's lead, like the necessary mineral calcium, is deposited in bone and released in times of stress [1]. People may then think that stress caused their illness, when released lead or other toxins may be the culprit.

Where is lead found?

Lead exposure used to be much more prevalent than it is today. Major sources were, and to a certain extent still are:

- Paint chips containing lead, sometimes still found in older homes

- Leaded gasoline emissions - twenty years ago lead from motor vehicle exhausts came to two pounds per person per year [2].

- Old metal roll-up toothpaste tubes contained lead, one of only a few metals which bend that easily. If you are old enough to remember using these tubes, you may have taken in a measurable amount of lead from this source.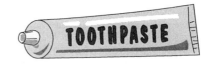

- Urban dirt, in which children played, was full of lead from motor vehicles and industrial processes.

- Acid foods leach lead out of glazed pottery, especially that made in most foreign countries. Lead was banned for use in glazes in this country around the late 1970s, about the same time it was banned in paints.

- The solder line in "tin" cans used to be lead.

- Moonshine liquor was made in old automobile radiators, which were soldered with lead.

- Lead pipes and soldered joints were found in old plumbing.

- Solder used for welding

One of the best known symptoms of lead poisoning is learning disabilities and mental retardation in children who usually ingest the metal by chewing on paint chips in older houses. Lead based paint, although banned since 1978, is still a major problem. A child can attain a level of 35 mcg/dl of lead by ingesting an amount equivalent in size to one sugar granule per day during childhood. Children with 25-30 mcg/dl are six times as likely to have reading and learning disabilities [3]. The Center for Disease Control (CDC) guidelines were 30 mcg/dl in the 1970s, 25 mcg/dl in 1985, and these guidelines may be lowered to 10-25 mcg/dl as more becomes known about the toxicity of smaller amounts. More attention is being paid to the effects of chronic exposure to lead and other toxins such as mercury. As effects become known, perceived safe levels of these metals become lower and lower.

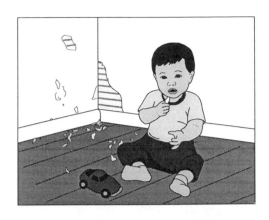

Lead damage is to a great extent irreversible, as chelation with DMSA can remove lead only from blood and not from the brain. DMSA is approved by the FDA for removing lead from the brains of children, a task for which it is not suited.

Today, paint, pottery glazes, cans, and most gasoline sold in the United States are free of lead, as public awareness and legislation has led to the development of substitutes which are perceived to be safer. However, contaminated paint and piping are still found in older houses, and leaded ceramics can be purchased in some foreign countries. Also, since lead excretion is very slow, you may be carrying lead around from earlier exposures, and this lead may still be causing you problems.

Many historians believe that a major contributor to the fall of Rome was poisoning by the lead in the plumbing.

Where else is lead found?
Present-day sources of lead include:
- *Cosmetics*
- *Bullets and buckshot*
- *Car and other batteries*
- *Certain calcium supplements such as bone meal and dolomite may be contaminated*
- *Caulking and plaster*

Rats inhale so much lead from discarded batteries burning in dumps that they get kidney tumors [1]. Lead that enters the air from burning and that enters the water table from discarded material in landfills is probably doing us similar harm.

Are lead pencils really lead pencils?

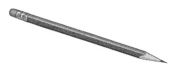 One place that lead is **not** found, contrary to popular belief, is in pencils, sometimes erroneously called lead pencils. Pencil leads used to actually contain lead, which was soft enough to make a mark on a surface. Graphite replaced lead long ago because it works more effectively, but the original name remains.

Today's pencils are not harmless, however. The graphite they contain is a form of carbon, and is a common allergen.

Newsprint ink contains both graphite and lead and is a common cause of allergy and toxicity from contact with hands and from inhalation. One patient's illness was traced to the ink in the books stored in the headboard of his bed.

What are the symptoms of lead exposure?
Lead accumulates in the body from slow exposure. Symptoms of lead poisoning include:

- CNS symptoms - seizures, learning disabilities, headaches, tremors, muscular weakness and pain, sight loss, dizziness, fatigue, malaise, nervousness, depression, disorientation, hyperactivity in children

- Nerve damage to hands and feet

- Frequent colds and other infections

- Gastrointestinal symptoms - nausea and vomiting, diarrhea or constipation, colic, abdominal rigidity and pain, loss of appetite and weight loss

- Cirrhosis of the liver

- Anemia, raised serum iron with lowered total iron-binding capacity; i.e. more iron in the blood but lowered ability to use it.

- Lead lines - blue-black line on gums; opaque lines on bone or material in gut visible on x-ray

- Lead can cross-fiber in bone, replacing calcium with resulting skeletal problems.

- Hair loss
- Thyroid dysfunction

- Birth defects
- Mental retardation

- Heart problems
- Kidney disease

The average lead body burden today in the United States is 240 mg (about 1/100 ounce) for an adult man, 120 times higher than in prehistoric times [4]. Our bodies were likely never meant to deal with the amount of lead (and other toxins) that we are exposed to today.

Why is lead more toxic if you have mercury amalgam fillings?

Mercury and lead are more harmful together than separately, since one amplifies the effects of the other. Both metals have a high molecular weight. Lead, mercury, and beneficial minerals such as calcium, iron, and zinc all have a +2 charge. They all fight for molecular sites in the body. Like two heavy bullies in the school yard instead of one, lead and mercury together are more likely to defeat or replace the lower weight necessary minerals.

In addition, two heavy metals instead of one are more likely to overwhelm the body's detoxification systems. For both of these reasons, people with mercury amalgam fillings are at greater risk of harm from lead exposure.

Cadmium

How is cadmium like mercury?

Cadmium is in the same group in the periodic table as mercury and zinc. Like mercury, cadmium blocks the usage of the essential mineral zinc in the body. Zinc is needed for the immune system, and lower zinc levels correlate to lowered immune function. Cadmium, having a +2 charge, also interferes with other +2 minerals such as iron (needed in blood) and calcium (needed in bones).

Where is cadmium found?

Cadmium is found in:

- *Paints*
- *Silver polish*
- *Metal plating*
- *Galvanized pipes*
- *Dental amalgam*
- *Cigarette smoke*

- *Photographic processes*
- *Fish from polluted water*
- *Batteries (nickel-cadmium)*
- *Zinc products and processes*
- *Particles from auto tires and brakes*
- *Incineration of rubber and plastic goods*

What happens when you are exposed to cadmium?

Cadmium tends to accumulate until the threshold of resistance is overcome, then strikes with apparent suddenness. One of the first symptoms of cadmium overexposure is high blood pressure. Cadmium can promote hypertension [5]. Those with high blood pressure have been shown to have blood cadmium levels 3-4 times higher than those with normal blood pressure [6]. With higher exposure, the kidneys and liver are damaged and the blood pressure then falls. This may be due to cadmium's effect on aldosterone, a hormone which affects blood pressure.

It has been found that patients with emphysema, a lung disease linked to smoking, have more cadmium in their kidneys and livers than do people without emphysema [1]. Since the kidneys and liver are the body's filters, it is not surprising that, when these filters are blocked with cadmium (or any other toxin), other toxic suppressors can more easily work their damage. The symptoms of cadmium poisoning are subtle and may not be noticed - the higher blood pressure puts strain on the heart, which can lead to an apparently sudden heart attack.

Other symptoms of cadmium poisoning include

- *Abdominal pain, anorexia, weight loss and vomiting*
- *Antibody suppression and immune dysfunction*
- *Sore joints, slow healing, acne, anemia*
- *Disrupted iron, copper and manganese metabolism*
- *Decreased fertility*
- *Sodium retention*
- *Lung disease*
- *Decreased body temperature*

Anorexia (loss of appetite) and weight loss may be a result of cadmium replacing zinc, the mineral responsible for taste and appetite. Decreased body temperature is a symptom of decreased thyroid func-

> **Zinc can help anorexia and leg pains.**

tion, which can result when cadmium blocks the copper that, along with iodine, promotes proper thyroid function. Decreased fertility may be a function of decreased progesterone and testosterone production. Sore joints can be caused by the suppression of potassium by cadmium. Cadmium lowers potassium by causing the kidneys to dump toxins. The kidneys will also dump electrolytes such as potassium directly.

Cadmium displaces zinc in the body, but the converse is also true. Zinc, taken orally, displaces cadmium and can stop and even reverse symptoms of cadmium poisoning. When cadmium causes leg arteries to narrow with resulting poor circulation and pain, zinc can reverse the spasms in the minor arteries and thus alleviate the symptoms.

Another example of the zinc-cadmium relationship is the symptom of anosmia, or lack of smell. Anosmia is attributed to zinc deficiency but could just as well be caused by an unbalanced excess of cadmium or mercury. Since cigarette smoke is a significant source of cadmium, it is not surprising that smokers lose their sense of taste and smell and their appetite. A person who quits smoking will usually get her or his taste back even without taking zinc supplements because more zinc in the body is now available for use, since the cadmium is no longer fighting for zinc's biochemical sites.

Aluminum

Does aluminum cause Alzheimer's disease?
Aluminum has been in the news due to its link with Alzheimer's disease. Alzheimer's disease afflicts an estimated 2.5 million Americans, and is characterized by ever-worsening senility and memory loss. High concentrations of aluminum have been found in the brains of Alzheimer's victims. Although the exact nature of the correlation is not known [7], it is very likely that the

high aluminum concentrations are themselves a result of mercury toxicity, as the body is less able to clear out the aluminum when the body's filters (liver and kidneys) are clogged with mercury. Since mercury inhibits the body's ability to clear out metals, aluminum builds up.

Aluminum also adversely affects the cytochrome P450 and metallothionein detoxification systems. The aluminum found in the brains of Alzheimer's victims may be the secondary cause of the disease, or may simply be another symptom of mercury toxicity and may not have a part in causing the disease. In animal experiments, aluminum given orally collects in brain nerve fibers and animals show memory loss and confusion [8].

In a study comparing aluminum levels in drinking water for 2344 patients with Alzheimer's disease or presenile dementia versus the water used by controls, it was found that the higher the aluminum in the water, the higher the correlation for Alzheimer's or dementia [9-11]. In a placebo controlled trial of desferroxamine, a chelator which removes aluminum from the body, it was found that the use of the chelator (i.e. less aluminum in the body) was correlated with a reduction in the decline in function in patients [12].

Aluminum is one of the metals used to make special effects in fireworks and sparklers. It causes sparks to form, in contrast to magnesium, which burns with a steady white light. Aluminum also makes sparks of a sort in the brain, causing intermittent function typical of Alzheimer's disease.

Strictly speaking, aluminum metal is relatively nontoxic. It is the soluble aluminum compounds which are readily formed from the metal that are powerful brain poisons.

Aluminum interferes with the electrical activity of the brain and contributes to slow learning as well as senile dementia and non-Alzheimer's memory loss.

Zinc supplementation has been shown to slow the accumulation of toxic aluminum in the brain [13,14].

What are other symptoms of aluminum toxicity?
Other symptoms include:

- *Bone loss*
- *Debilitation*
- *Headache*
- *Dryness of mucous membranes and skin*
- *Aversion to meat*
- *Susceptibility to colds*

Bone loss may be due to interference with calcium and magnesium. There is a possible correlation between aluminum and multiple sclerosis (MS). Aluminum lowers the amount of the phosphate group in the body, leading to muscle aches and weakness.

Where can aluminum be found?
Sources of aluminum include [15]:

- *Some baking powder*
- *The base for some dentures*
- *Many antacids (read labels)*
- *Some toothpaste*
- *Automotive exhaust*
- *Cake mixes*
- *Self-rising flour*
- *Sliced process cheese food*
- *Aluminum paints, including spray paints*
- *Sodium silicoaluminate (found in some salt)*
- *Antidiarrheal preparations such as Kaopectate*
- *Aluminum cookware (especially if used with acid foods)*
- *Antiperspirants and deodorants, both roll-on and spray*
- *Aluminum silicates in cat litter, shampoos, and cigarette smoke*
- *Aluminum-coated wax containers such as those for orange and pineapple juice*
- *Aluminum lauryl sulfate is a common ingredient in many commercial shampoos.*

- *Aluminum foil*
- *Acid rain*
- *Buffered aspirin*
- *Cigarette filters*
- *Aluminum cans*
- *Frozen dough*
- *Some douches*

How can aluminum exposure be reduced?

Spray deodorants are more hazardous than roll-on due to inhalant exposure of the spray (which also contains other toxins). Inhalation of aluminum from any source may be transported via the olfactory nerve in the nose to the brain, where it may cause nerve cell destruction and senility over time.

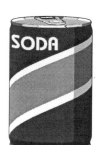

Some deodorants and antiperspirants, including those shaped like rock crystals, contain magnesium, which does the job and is far less hazardous. Keep in mind that body odor which is considered socially unacceptable is a sign of toxins being eliminated from the body Make sure you are drinking plenty of water to help your body eliminate toxins.

Most beverages in aluminum cans are not very healthy anyway (sodas, beer, fruit punch, etc.). It is better to drink these from glass bottles if you drink them at all.

In an experiment, water was heated in an aluminum coffeepot to determine whether aluminum leaches into the water. Tap water containing 22 mcg/liter of aluminum was heated to 88 degrees C (below boiling). After heating, the aluminum content increased to 1640 mcg/liter, a 75-fold increase [16], showing that aluminum does indeed leach into water or food from aluminum cookware. The recommended water limit of aluminum is 50 mcg/liter. Stainless steel cookware does not contain aluminum, but it contains nickel, and Teflon coated cookware contains toxic fluoride. Glass or ceramic cookware is least toxic and is recommended.

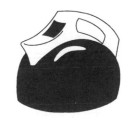

Buyer Beware! | Baking powder and salt from a health food store is less likely to contain aluminum than commercial brands, but read labels carefully. Look for any ingredient with -alum- in the name. Buyer beware: It was found that a particular brand of health food store salt was packaged in two nearly identical boxes, one with magnesium and one with aluminum.

As essential minerals go down, body concentration of aluminum tends to go up. This is yet another reason to keep your mineral level up. Keeping other toxic metals such as mercury, lead, or cadmium out of the body is another way of keeping the level of necessary minerals where it should be.

Arsenic

Arsenic and Old Lace
Ask someone to name some commonly known poisons, and arsenic will usually come to mind from murder mysteries, although it is not necessarily more toxic than other metals and is actually less toxic based on lethal dosage than mercury. Arsenate (the organic form) has a low toxicity, while arsenite (inorganic) is the highly toxic form.

Where is arsenic usually found, other than in murder mysteries?
Arsenic is most often found in:

- *Arsenical soap*
- *Seafood and kelp*
- *Wine*
- *Psoriasis and leukemia treatment*
- *Store-bought grains due to insecticide or rodenticide contamination*
- *Insecticides, herbicides, rat poison*
- *The manufacture of mirrors*
- *Some paints and dyes*

Meat, fish (especially shellfish), poultry and cows' milk are the foods which contain the greatest amount of arsenic [17].

The anti-protozoal drug metronidazole (trade name Flagyl) contains arsenic as one of its active ingredients. The bitter taste experienced by many Flagyl users is due to arsenic.

Arsenic poisoning mimics a number of other conditions, partially accounting for its popularity in murder mysteries. It is said that Napoleon had arsenic in his body according to hair analysis done after his death.

What are some of the symptoms of arsenic poisoning?
Symptoms of arsenic poisoning include:

- CNS effects - fatigue, dizziness, headache, weakness, confusion
- Gastrointestinal effects - anorexia, diarrhea, constipation, abdominal pain
- Body odor of garlic, probably due to interaction of arsenic with detoxifying sulfur-containing compounds in the body

- Thyroid dysfunction, iodine and folic acid deficiency, goiter

- Liver and kidney damage, jaundice

- Fluid and electrolyte loss

- Pigmentation (darkening) of skin, vitiligo (blotchy lighter areas of skin)

- Other - hair loss, edema, impaired healing, dermatitis, fever, skin cancer

Copper

Copper - mineral or poison?

Copper in small amounts is necessary for the body's proper functioning, but it is possible to get too much. Copper deficiency is more common than copper toxicity, since vomiting and diarrhea tend to clear an overdose of copper from the body, but chronic low level overexposure can occur. People with Wilson's disease tend to accumulate copper in the body, with resulting symptoms of toxicity. In this case copper is stored in the body rather than used, and symptoms of both overdose and deficiency may develop.

How can you get too much copper?

Sources of excess copper are

- *Copper plumbing*
- *Beer*
- *Copper cookware*
- *Copper releasing intrauterine devices (IUDs) used for birth control*

- *Sewage sludge*
- *Too-high doses of mineral supplements*
- *Gold fillings and crowns*

What are the symptoms of copper toxicity?

Symptoms of copper toxicity include

- *Nausea*
- *Mental disturbances, hyperactivity*
- *Toxemia of pregnancy, postpartum psychosis*
- *Liver problems (hepatosis)*
- *Myocardial infarction (heart attack)*

Copper, or foods that increase its availability such as citrus fruits, has been implicated in causing migraine headaches [18].

Some patients are so sensitive to copper that they can't even tolerate copper in nutritional supplements without becoming nauseated.

Platinum

Are catalytic converters a good thing?

Platinum has not been much of a health problem until recently. Why? Catalytic converters have been added to cars to enable them to run on unleaded gasoline. These catalytic converters have reduced the lead levels of the air, but have released large quantities of platinum into the atmosphere. One toxin has simply been substituted for another and added to gasoline toxins and carcinogens such as PCBs and benzene.

There has been a dramatic recent increase of alveolar lung cancer in states and countries where catalytic converters are required in cars. Some of the increased illness is directly attributable to the platinum. On inhalation platinum atoms may be energized to form free radicals. Toxic gases produced by the converter include hydrogen sulfide (rotten-egg smell), cyanide and cyanic acid and phosgene gas. Phosgene was a combat gas used in World War I [19].

Other Metals

What other metals can be toxic?

Barium is used as a contrast medium in X-rays and other radiographic methods to make certain organs and structures (usually the intestinal tract) stand out visually. Although danger is limited in the body due to its very low water solubility, it is extremely toxic.

Tin is right above lead on the periodic table, and so has many of the same toxic qualities as lead.

Beryllium is sometimes used in dental materials to improve the castability of metal alloy by lowering the melting temperature. Its use also reduces corrosion of the alloy. However, the fumes and dust of beryllium are hazardous. Acute exposure can cause pneumonitis (lung infection), granulomas (benign tumors) and interstitial fibrosis.

Chromium, like beryllium, is used in dental materials to improve corrosion resistance. Exposure to chromium can lead to a thirty- to forty-fold increase in the risk of lung and nasal carcinoma (cancer) 10-20 years after exposure. Dermatitis (skin rashes) can also be caused by chromium.

Summary

- There are a number of metals which are toxic. Their primary, but not only, toxic effect lies in their substitution in the body for necessary minerals.

- If there are metals in the body, certain blood tests (metal screen) and urine tests (provocative chelation) can bring this to the attention of your health practitioner.

- Chelation, discussed in the chapters on Metal Detoxification and Mercury, can help remove the metal from your body.

References and Resources

- The Burton Goldberg Group, "Cadmium Toxicity", pp. 896-7, *Alternative Medicine: The Definitive Guide*, Future Medicine Publishing Inc., Puyallup WA, 1994.

- Shroeder, Henry A., *The Poisons Around Us*, Indiana University Press, Bloomington IN, 1974.

- Shroeder, Henry A., *The Trace Elements and Man*, The Devin-Adair Co., Old Greenwich CT, 1973.

METAL DETOXIFICATION

Get The Lead Out!

Do you have any of the following health problems, or any of the problems listed on the first page of the Mercury, Nickel and Root Canals, or Other Metals chapters in this section? Your problems may be caused at least in part by metals, and metal detoxification, discussed in this chapter, may be of benefit.

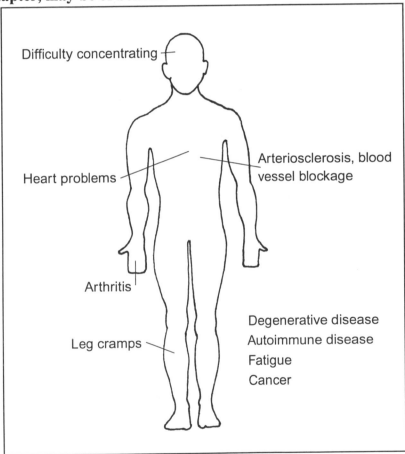

Things in this chapter that can change your health:

- *Toxic metals can adversely affect your health and even cause life-threatening conditions.*

- *Chelation is a way to remove these toxic metals from your body.*

How can you tell whether you have toxic metals in your body?

You or your doctor may suspect that you have metals in your body if you have symptoms of metal toxicity, if you work with metals, if you have metal dental work or if you have recently had mercury fillings or root-canaled teeth removed. In these cases a test for metals may be wise, followed by treatment if indicated by the testing. Sometimes the indications of metal toxicity are so strong that a test is considered to be unnecessary (however, you may want to document metal test results for insurance purposes)

There are tests which can determine the level and types of metal in your body. Tests for mercury and their pros and cons are discussed in the Mercury chapter. Tests for other metals include blood tests, although special tests are needed as metals are not typically screened for on a routine blood evaluation. Blood tests are not very accurate, as it is the amount of metal in the tissues, not in the blood, which is of greater concern. Tissue biopsy is a more accurate test, but it is invasive.

Urine tests are sometimes used, but they are often inaccurate because they measure only what is being excreted, not what is in the body. Provocative chelation is a more accurate type of urine test. A chelator, or metal-grabbing molecule such as EDTA, DMPS, glutathione, or even vitamin C is introduced into the body, usually intravenously (IV). The chelator binds with the metals in the blood and allows them to be excreted in the urine, which is then analyzed.

Hair analysis is a good test for metals other than mercury, which is volatile and is sometimes vaporized during preparation for the test. A small sample of hair is sent to a laboratory for metals testing. Another advantage of hair analysis is that it can reveal levels of necessary minerals in the body.

What if a toxic level of metal is found or strongly suspected?

If a person has a problem with metal toxicity, the treatment is twofold:

1. *Identify and eliminate continued exposure to the metal*
2. *Remove existing metal from the blood and body tissues*

Metal in the body will be slowly eliminated over a period of about 25 years if no more toxic metal is entering the system, even if nothing is done to speed up the process. However, the metal remaining in the body during the natural detoxification process is still doing its damage. It is therefore advantageous to intervene in order to help the body to eliminate the metal faster. The usual method is through chelation.

What is chelation?

Chelation is a term whose root means "claw" or "to bind". Most chelation is done by introducing an intravenous chelation solution into the veins. The chelator grabs hold of metal ions, forming a chemical compound which can more easily be excreted by the body. Excretion is done via urine, feces, and sweat. Some detoxification processes make use of a sauna to promote sweating for this purpose.

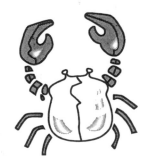

Why is chelation done?

Chelation helps to remove metals from the body tissues. These metals come from a number of sources including metal dental materials and mercury amalgam fillings. Metals can cause free radical damage in the body, and this damage can lead to:

- *Arteriosclerosis and atherosclerosis, blood vessel blockage*
- *Heart problems*
- *Cancer, autoimmune disease, arthritis, and other degenerative disease*
- *Fatigue and difficulty concentrating, particularly from mercury*
- *Leg cramps*

Arteriosclerosis and heart disease are the #1 killers in the U.S. Cancer is #2, with one third of Americans developing some form of cancer in their lifetime.

Not everyone needs chelation. The use, amount, and type of chelation should be determined by a knowledgeable practitioner after an evaluation of your health.

How can chelation reduce heart attack risk?

Chelation with EDTA and other chelators has been used to reduce calcium plaquing on the insides of arteries. This plaquing narrows the blood vessels, possibly leading to a heart attack in time if blood flow is sufficiently reduced. Chelation's action is believed to be twofold: it directly removes the excess of calcium from the arteries, and it removes heavy metals such as mercury from dental amalgam fillings, cadmium from cigarettes, and lead from gasoline, from the body. These metals set up conditions conducive to inflammation, causing calcium to be drawn to an area as a buffer. The calcium coats the inflamed areas in the blood vessels like a bandage, patching up one problem but creating another.

Metals can also change the blood pH (acidity), and calcium is taken from the bones to try to buffer the body fluids back to their normal pH. The end result of this is that the removal of calcium from the bones can lead to osteoporosis, so chelation can be beneficial in curtailing this process also.

Plaque in the arteries can also be related to structural or other problems, so it is important to identify and treat the basic problem and to use the correct chelator for the problem.

What are some chelators?

A naturally occurring chelator is **glutathione** (sometimes called GSH), which is produced by the body and is the first line of defense against mercury, cadmium, and other heavy metals. Ideally the metal exposure will be mild and short-term, in which case the glutathione will bind to the metal in a two-to-one ratio called a di-thiol bond. The word "thiol" refers to the sulfur in glutathione; the sulfur is the active ingredient. If there is more than one part metal to two parts available glutathione, they bind in a one-to-one ratio, or mono-thiol bond, which is itself harmful to the body. In other words, if there is more metal in the body than the body can deal with, both the metal and the body's attempt at detoxification can be toxic. Injected glutathione can boost the body's natural supply and increase the efficiency of the detoxification. Since glutathione can cross the blood-brain barrier, it can remove mercury and other toxic metals from the brain. The effective dosage is 1000 mg/day orally about once every five days. Antioxidants such as vitamin C in a 3:1 ratio with glutathione and vitamin E should be taken along with glutathione to prevent free radical damage from the mono-thiol binding.

Metallothionein is the second naturally occurring line of defense against metal poisoning. It is made in the liver and kidneys and is used in response to chronic, low dose exposure to +2 charge metals. Both glutathione and metallothionein make use of the thiol, or sulfhydryl, group, which is sulfur-hydrogen (-SH). This is the part of the molecule which grabs the metal ion. However, if nothing is done to remove the metal exposure and support the detoxification process, these and other natural systems become overwhelmed [1].

N-acetylcysteine (NAC), a nontoxic compound which is derived from the amino acid cysteine, is a nutritional precursor for the making of glutathione. Oral administration of 1200 mg/kg of NAC to mice increased liver glutathione levels 200-300% [2]. Increased glutathione levels will in turn reduce the metal levels in the body.

D-penicillamine and **dimercaptopropanol** (also called dimercaprol or British anti-Lewisite, or BAL) are thiol-containing compounds, not naturally found in the body, that have been widely used as heavy metal chelators. Their usefulness, however, is limited due to high toxicity.

2,3-dimercapto-1-propanesulfonate (**DMPS**), a water-soluble derivative of dimercaprol, is less toxic than dimercaprol due to higher water solubility and lower lipid (fat) solubility. Unlike some of the other chelators, it is effective when given orally [3] or as an intramuscular injection, although one of the most effective methods of administration is a ten minute IV push. Most chelators other than DMPS are most effective when administered as an intravenous drip.

Desferoxamine (trade name Desferal) is another chelator. A side effect is reduced blood pressure.

Chelation with desferoxamine has been shown to help diabetics with high levels of iron. In a study of 32 diabetics with high iron levels, 24, or two-thirds, were free of medication in 8-13 weeks [4].

Calcium or sodium ethylenediaminetetraacetic acid (**EDTA**) is one of the better-known chelators, but kidney problems (nephrosis) and reduced urine output can occur with its use [5].

DMSA (dimercaptosuccinic acid) is one of the best chelators for crossing the blood-brain barrier. It is given orally, about one 100 mg capsule per 25 pounds of body weight per day. It is an important adjunct to DMPS which doesn't cross the blood-brain barrier to pull mercury from the brain.

240

What should be done before chelation treatments start?

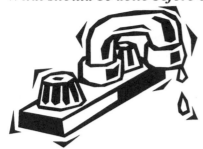

It is important to stop the source of the metals, such as removing mercury fillings, or chelation will have to be done indefinitely to remove the metals that have accumulated since the last chelation. In fact, some chelators can pull mercury out of the teeth and into the body as fast as they get rid of the mercury, like leaving the faucet on and the tub drain open at the same time. For this reason metal must be removed from the teeth before beginning chelation treatment.

A complete physical and blood test should be done to assess your overall condition and to provide a baseline by which your progress toward health can be measured.

How is chelation treatment administered?

Chelation treatment is usually administered intravenously (IV), although it can also be given orally or by intramuscular injection. However, oral chelators are not usually as effective as intravenous administration.

Each treatment lasts between ten minutes and three hours depending on the type of chelator used and the health problem being treated. The number of treatments is determined by your practitioner, with the severity of your metal-related health problems taken into consideration. The usual range is 3 (DMPS) to 20 (EDTA) treatments, with ten being about average. The number of treatments can go as high as about 40 in severe cases, but this is still safer and cheaper than bypass surgery.

What else should be done during chelation?

Zinc should be given during treatment with any chelating agent, preferably as zinc aspartate. Zinc by itself or in combination with chelators can be useful in detoxification, since it competes with heavy metals for sulfhydryl protein binding sites in the body. The more zinc (within reason) in the body, the more toxic metal is changed from a protein-bound state to a free state. Metal in the free state is more readily grabbed by the chelator. Because chelation causes losses of zinc and other divalent (+2) metals that are necessary to the body's function, mineral supplements should be taken to make up for this loss. Mineral IVs are effective in replacing minerals quickly.

More specifically, the following mineral supplements should be taken if the following symptoms are experienced during chelation:

- Magnesium   Constipation, heart palpitations, also potassium-deficiency symptoms, below (excess magnesium can cause diarrhea)

- Calcium   Fatigue, loose stools / diarrhea, bone and joint pain, lack of stamina (excess calcium can cause constipation)

- Potassium   Rapid / pounding heartbeat, water retention, kidney pain, cramps, tight / painful muscles, anxiety, difficulty sleeping

- Sodium (salt)   Fainting, low blood pressure, cold or numb hands and feet,
  (1 tsp / glass   heavy fatigue, nausea
  of water)

Calcium and potassium deficiency symptoms can also be brought on by diarrhea or excess urination, which can deplete the supplies of these minerals. Sodium deficiency symptoms can be brought on by sweating or vomiting, which can cause sodium loss.

The above minerals are important in balancing and keeping electrolytes balanced, which is important to keep in mind since chelation can cause minerals to be depleted.

How safe is chelation?

Chelation therapy has been used safely on more than five hundred thousand patients over the last forty years [6]. According to current drug safety standards, aspirin is about three and a half times more toxic than EDTA, one of the more common chelating agents [7].

What can I expect after treatment?

As with all therapies, individual progress can vary. Typically, the patient may feel a bit tired and weak immediately after the treatment due to mineral depletion, since chelators also grab onto and remove minerals. The appropriate mineral supplementation as indicated above or as recommended by your practitioner can prevent or alleviate these symptoms. Often the patient reports feeling noticeably better as soon as the day of or the day after the first treatment, with continuing improvement with successive treatments.

What kinds of results have been achieved with chelation?

Many people have benefited from chelation therapy. A number of patients with multiple sclerosis (MS) or Amyotrophic Lateral Sclerosis (ALS, or Lou Gehrig's disease) have improved. Not all patients will improve with chelation - the degree of improvement depends to a great extent on the degree to which mercury or other metals were a possible root cause of their health problems.

Ten patients in Canada with Alzheimer's disease were chelated to remove mercury and aluminum. Nine of them showed improvement. Chelation can often improve the condition by impeding further deterioration, but cannot reverse cellular damage.

One patient, an 80 year old man, had problems with impotence, low energy and brain fog. His wife suspected senility or early Alzheimer's disease. His problems improved markedly after 1 1/2 to 2 months of chelation therapy.

Many patients who had EDTA chelation therapy reported relief from angina pain, healing of gangrene, increased vigor, and improved memory, sight, hearing and sense of smell [8]. Nearly 90% of patients with peripheral vascular disease (blocked leg arteries) showed marked improvement after chelation therapy. Another study showed that all patients with peripheral vascular disease had significant improvement after only ten treatments of chelation therapy [9]. Fifty percent of cardiac arrhythmias were normalized [10]. Memory and concentration related to diminished circulation improved [11,12].

What types of nutrient support are recommended?
Home metal detoxification methods include a high fiber diet, apple pectin as apples or supplement, pumpkin seeds, beans, 8 glasses of water per day [13]. Also:

- Oral chelators can complement IV chelation. These include:
  - Glutathione complex
  - Vitamin C
  - DMSA and DMPS
  - ToxiCleanse (Metagenics), which contains apple pectin

- Supplements that support the body's detoxification systems include:
  - Life Solubles (Integris)
  - Sun Chlorella
  - Kyolic garlic
  - CoQ10
  - Bioflavonoids
  - ACES (Carlson Labs)
  - Mitochondrial Resuscitate (Metagenics)
  - Lymph Clear (Enzymatic Therapy)
  - Red Root tea
  - Ultra Clear Plus (Metagenics)

A recommended protocol uses glutathione before and after a liver/gallbladder flush to bind metals coming from the liver, followed the next day by a colonic. Dark metal crystals are sometimes even seen in the colonic viewing tube.

Sauna detoxification (see Chemical Toxicity chapter) is a method of eliminating fat stored chemicals. It is also useful in removing metals from the body, as metal salts eliminated through sweat and other channels. In addition, by removing chemicals, sauna can help free up detoxification pathways to more effectively deal with metals.

Summary

The three steps to getting the metal out of your body are:

1. Identify and eliminate the sources, such as mercury amalgam fillings and others.

2. IV, intramuscular or oral chelation to remove the metal in your body tissues.

3. Nutritional support, including mineral replacement, so your natural chelators can work optimally.

• The Burton Goldberg Group, "Chelation Therapy", pp. 126-133, and "Cadmium Toxicity", pp. 896-7, *Alternative Medicine: The Definitive Guide*, Future Medicine Publishing, Puyallup WA, 1994.

• Brecher, Harold and Arline, *40-Something Forever*, Healthsavers Press, NY, 1992. *Chelation and a healthy heart.*

• Cranton, Elmer, *Bypassing Bypass*, Hampton Roads, Troutdale VA, 1990. *The chelation methods discussed can enhance the benefits of bypass surgery and in many cases eliminate the need for the surgery.*

• Halstead, Bruce, *The Scientific Basis of EDTA Chelation Therapy*, Golden Quill Publishers Inc., Colton CA, 1979. *Scientific basis of chelation therapy; technically oriented rather than for the layperson.*

• Julian, James, *Chelation Extends Life*, Wellness Press, Hollywood CA, 1982. *This book discusses the prevention and treatment of arteriosclerosis.*

• Trowbridge, John P. and Morton Walker, *The Healing Powers of Chelation Therapy*, New Way of Life Inc., Stamford CT, 1992. *Focuses on IV chelation therapy; written for the layperson.*

• Walker, Morton, *The Chelation Way*, Avery Publishing Group Inc., Garden City Park NY, 1990. *A complete how-to book on chelation, including how to find and use over-the-counter chelating agents.*

• Walker, Morton and G. Gordon, *The Chelation Answer: How To Prevent Hardening of the Arteries and Rejuvenate Your Cardiovascular System*, M. Evans and Co. Inc., NY, 1982.

• Ziff, Sam and Michael, *Dental Mercury Detox*, Bio-Probe Inc., Orlando FL, 1993.

The following organizations present information on chelation therapy and in some cases can refer you to a qualified administrator of chelation in your area.

• **American Board of Chelation Therapy**, 70 West Huron Street, Chicago IL 60610. Phone (312) 266-7246. *Provides certification of physicians trained in chelation therapy, and can provide a list of these professionals.*

• **American College of Advancement in Medicine (ACAM)**, P.O. Box 3427, Laguna Hills CA 92654. Phone (714) 583-7666. *Establishes standards and certification in the field, and gives training and seminars. Provides worldwide directory of trained professionals.*

THE BATTERY EFFECT

Are You Getting A Charge Out Of Your Dental Work?

Do you have the following symptoms? Believe it or not: You could have a battery in your mouth!

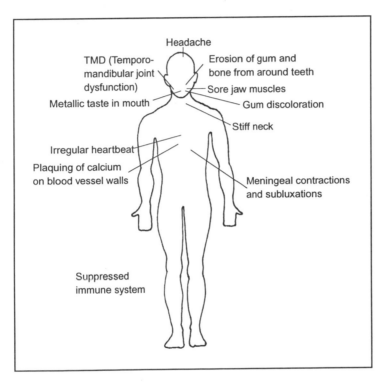

In this chapter you can learn:

- *Why do you sometimes get an odd tingling when you bite down on foil?*

- *How do metals in your mouth act like a battery, affecting the electrical systems of your body?*

- *What are some symptoms of the battery effect?*

- *What can be done about the battery effect?*

Have you ever chewed on foil?

If you have ever bitten down on a piece of aluminum foil (for example, a piece of foil wrapper stuck to your chewing gum or baked potato), what happened? If you are among the majority of people with amalgam fillings, you probably felt an unpleasant tingle in your mouth that gave you goose bumps, along with increased salivation and an odd metallic taste.

What caused that sensation?

What you felt was a small electric current, similar to that in a battery. When you have two different metals in a liquid with dissolved salts called an electrolyte - and saliva is such a liquid - then a reaction occurs to produce electricity. Metals have different potentials; that is, some metals will give up electrons more easily than others. In a situation like the one above, electrons will flow from the metal that gives up electrons more easily to the other one, in what is called an anode/cathode relationship. The flow of electrons, which are small parts of the metal atoms, is called electricity. All electricity, whether it is from a wall socket, a car battery, or two different metals in your body or mouth, is the same. It differs only in intensity.

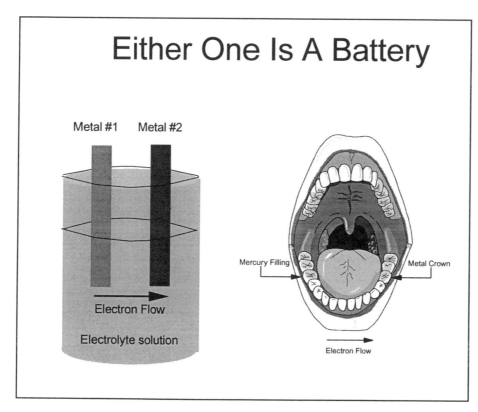

Either One Is A Battery

Metal #1   Metal #2

Electron Flow

Electrolyte solution

Mercury Filling   Metal Crown

Electron Flow

This battery effect is also called electrogalvanism. Toxic material from the fillings can erode from the current and leak out into the rest of the body, like the buildup on the terminals of a car battery [1].

The body electric

Many of the body's systems are electrical in nature. These include the heart's natural pacemaker, mineral transport systems, and primarily the nervous system, by which signals for proper action are sent from the brain to other parts of the body.

How is your body like a flashlight?

If you hooked a flashlight to household current, what do you think would happen? Since a flashlight is designed to work on a low direct current charge from a battery, the high alternating current from your household wiring would likely burn out the bulb filament immediately and damage the flashlight.

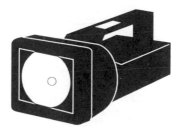

In the same manner, the electrical systems of the body are adversely affected by electricity other than that produced naturally by the body. Although the amount of electrical current generated by, say, biting on foil or the metals in your mouth is much less than that produced by a household electrical system, the body's electrical system is much more sensitive than a flashlight, so significant damage can still occur.

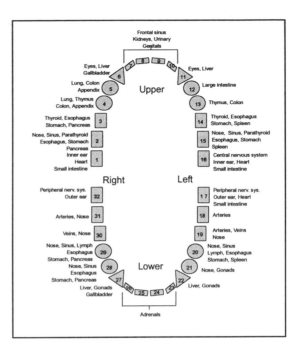

How is this relevant?

You may be thinking that this doesn't have anything to do with you. After all, how often do you chew on foil? Any two metals in the body can set up an electrical charge; that is, a miniature battery. If you have silver/mercury amalgam fillings in your mouth, along with a stainless steel post from a root canal, a gold or nickel crown, or metal braces, you have a battery that is putting out a weak electrical current 24 hours a day for many years. This can't help but produce a damaging effect. Particular areas of the body can be affected by currents in different teeth, as shown in this chart.

Electrical activity can cause corrosion of fillings and dental metals in addition to chemical corrosion. Corrosion can reduce the strength of the filling and increase the breakdown of the amalgam; the breakdown products end up absorbed and distributed throughout the body [2,3].

What if you no longer have metals in your mouth?

If metal is removed from the mouth, this does not mean that it has automatically been cleared out of the body, and metal in the body can still cause an electrical reaction. For example, if you have had your mercury amalgam fillings removed but still have your root canal posts in place, the nickel in the root canals can react with the mercury in your body to produce a battery effect.

This effect is much weaker and less destructive than if you still had mercury in your teeth, but it is still there. Gold salts taken for arthritis can also contribute to a battery effect.

What other metals can contribute to the battery effect?

Metal can be found elsewhere in the body, not just in the mouth, and all body fluids are conductive. Other sources of body metal include surgical staples, metal pins to hold together broken bones, metal earrings for pierced ears, artificial limbs and joints, spinal posts, and heart pacemakers.

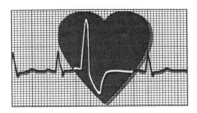

What are some symptoms of the battery effect?

The battery effect can cause premature ventricular contractions, or PVCs. These are felt as an irregular heartbeat that alternately appears to stop and then thump extra hard, causing an awareness of your heartbeat, shortness of breath, and sometimes chest pain. The body's own heart rhythm regulator is electrical in nature, so it is quite possible that many cases of PVCs are caused by metals in the body producing competing current. It is possible also that some artificial heart pacemakers would not be necessary if the root cause of the PVCs were sought and found. It seems strange to say that a person with a heart rhythm problem might be better off going to a dentist than to a cardiologist (heart doctor), but this may be worth considering.

Another example of the detrimental battery effect on the cardiovascular system involves the increase in the plaquing of calcium on the blood vessel walls. This process resembles the plating of metal using electric current.

Aberrant electrical currents in the body can also cause meningeal contractions, just as a wire carrying enough current to produce a small shock will cause the muscle to contract when touched to your skin. Meningeal contractions can result in spinal subluxations, or misalignments. These subluxations can cause a number of symptoms such as headache and stiff neck and back as detailed in the chapter on Structural Problems.

Local signs of the battery effect are erosion of gum tissue and bone from around the teeth, and mouth lesions and sores. The four top front teeth drain into the nasal area, and electrical charges in these teeth can cause nasal polyps with resultant difficulty breathing through your nose.

Systemic effects include a wide variety of nervous system and cardiovascular symptoms, which is not surprising considering the electrical nature of both of those systems. Spastic colon, accompanied by digestive difficulties, problems with elimination, and pain, can be caused by unwanted twinges of electricity causing the muscular walls of the colon to contract inappropriately. Depression of the immune system is not uncommon. Problems and symptoms can occur any way along the pathways in the tooth chart earlier in this chapter.

Electrical potentials in the mouth can reach 900 millivolts; 400 to 450 millivolts can cause a nerve cell to fire, a phenomenon which can register as pain or other disruption. Dental work can thus put out voltages more than sufficient to not only cause pain, but cause systems to dysfunction as well. Nerves act as transmission lines carrying electrical charges to other parts of the body, and it follows that pain and disruption related to dental metals can affect any part of the body. For example, electrically generated nerve impulses can travel to the hypothalamus and pituitary of the brain and affect these structures that control the autonomic nervous system and hormone-generating endocrine glands [2].

How long has medical science known about electrogalvanism?
Most doctors and dentists appear to be unaware of the existence and effects of electrogalvanism. However, the discovery of dentally caused electrical charges is nothing new. The phenomenon, and the adverse health effects, were reported as far back as 1878, nearly 120 years ago [4,5].

Much study on electrogalvanism was done, especially in Germany, in the early 1930s. Lippman (1930) reported 3 cases with both visible lesions and systemic symptoms, which improved greatly after metal removal. To verify his results, he then replaced the metals and the symptoms returned [6]. Ullman (1932) reported nine cases of similar problems, which abated after metal removal. Like Lippman, he replaced the metals for experimental purposes and the symptoms returned [7]. Freidlander (1932) reported 76 cases of symptoms from electrogalvanism [8]. Hyams (1933) studied orthodontic materials in 33 cases and recommended that materials be chosen that did not set up galvanic currents [9]. Macdonald (1934) reported 5 cases of galvanic burns which rapidly improved after metal removal [10]. Rattner (1935) reported a case of a patient experiencing prompt relief after the removal of two amalgam fillings [11].

Lain (1936, 1940) did a carefully tabulated study of over 1500 adults with dissimilar dental metals. He found that 69% had metallic taste, tingling or tongue sensations, 34% had electric shocks or tongue erosion, 28% had tongue patches, geographic tongue (fissures in the tongue), 6.2% had leukoplakia and other precancerous lesions. The more serious lesions such as ulcers and cancers in many cases did not appear for 10-25 years after the metals were placed in the mouth [12,13]. Solomon et al (1933) also noted the development of precancerous oral lesions linked to electrogalvanism [14]. Hyams (1933) was another researcher who described a number of symptoms attributed to dental metals [15]. The authors were able to verify the metal-symptom connection by ruling out other causes and noting the often dramatic alleviation of symptoms following metal removal or replacement.

More recently, Hal Huggins found that both low white blood cell counts and high counts (leukemia) were normalized following dental metal removal. Amalgams were removed in sequence from most negative to most positive [16].

Others have also discussed the relationship between dissimilar dental metals and a wide variety of symptoms [17].

Do you have gum discoloration?

If you have crowns, posts, a bridge, or a metal filling that is next to your gums, take a bright light and a mirror and look closely at the gum tissue that is next to the metal, and compare it to gum tissue elsewhere in the mouth. Is it pink and healthy? More likely it is reddened, purplish, or greyish, and has pulled back somewhat from the metal in the tooth. This is a sign of chronic tissue and cell damage that is severe enough to be visible. The fact that the discoloration can last for as long as the metal is in the mouth in spite of the fact that new gum tissue cells are constantly being formed is evidence that cell damage is continuously occurring. Gum problems and discoloration, not limited to areas next to metal, can also be due to periodontal problems or infection. A dental examination may be necessary to determine the cause of the gum problem.

How can stress worsen the symptoms of the battery effect?

Stress can cause tooth grinding at night, a condition known medically as bruxism. Bruxism can increase voltages from metal in the mouth. Morning fatigue or awakening with a metallic taste in your mouth or TMJ headache may be linked to tooth grinding for this reason. TMJ headache and sore jaw muscles can be caused by a misalignment of the temporomandibular joint (TMJ) in the jaw. A mouth guard such as that used in certain sports, worn at night, can help to alleviate the symptoms caused by tooth grinding and TMJ problems.

Is the amount and type of charge significant?

As discussed in the chapter on Mercury, teeth with metal of any kind can individually have an electrical charge. This can be measured with a voltmeter. High negative charges usually correspond to nerve related symptoms such as headache and depression. High positive charges can cause immunological symptoms such as increased susceptibility to infection, autoimmune diseases, and allergy. Gold in fillings facilitates the release of mercury from fillings, worsening symptoms of both mercury toxicity and electrical charges [18].

A "silver bullet" solution?

Mercury fillings should be removed in order of charge, with the highest negative ones taken out first. If your symptoms were caused by the battery effect, it is quite possible for them to be alleviated almost instantly after all metal is out of the mouth.

Mary, a patient in her mid 30s, became agoraphobic (afraid of leaving her home), developed chemical sensitivities, and had post-partum depression. It was so severe that institutionalization was necessary for a short time. She was found to have a high voltage in a tooth and had the tooth removed. She reported feeling her depression lift and her feeling of well-being return almost immediately. She stated that she "felt the weight of the world come off her shoulders."

Patient Profile

Lou, another patient in her 50s, had sudden and dramatic symptoms due to very high dental electrical charges, and an equally dramatic recovery after the problem was identified and corrected. In the early 1990s, she went to a dentist to have metal based porcelain crowns installed. Since neither she nor the dentist knew any better, the crowns were placed over mercury amalgam fillings. The instant he put in the last crown, on the upper left, she felt an immediate electric shock down her left arm. Within the next month her left arm curled up into a semi-paralyzed position, and the skin of her arm was so sensitive that the slightest touch was excruciating. She had the dental electrical charges test done, and the test showed charges, especially in the upper left crown, that were about the highest the tester had ever seen.

The upper left crown was removed, and the pain and paralysis in her arm was relieved considerably. Later she had her lower right crown removed, and right afterward she wrote out a check to the dentist for the work. She noticed immediately that her handwriting had changed - it was now like it had been when she was 25 years old. When she went home her husband noticed that her appearance had also changed - her face had relaxed visibly. The electrical charges had been contracting her facial muscles.

She has since made other changes in her diet and lifestyle, working with the same progressive clinic that pinpointed her dental crowns as the major part of her problems. The mild fibromyalgia (overall pain) that she had had, even before the placement of the crowns, is now gone, and she hasn't had a cold in years. She is now about 60 years old, but with her naturally blonde hair, nearly unlined face and alert mind she is regularly mistaken for a woman in her 40s.

References and Resources

- Huggins, Hal, and Sharon Huggins, *It's All in Your Head*, Life Sciences Press, Colorado Springs CO, 1986.

- Ziff, Sam, *Silver Dental Fillings - The Toxic Time Bomb*, Aurora Press, Santa Fe NM, 1986. Chapter 5, "Do We Really Have Electricity In Our Mouths?", pp. 65-70.

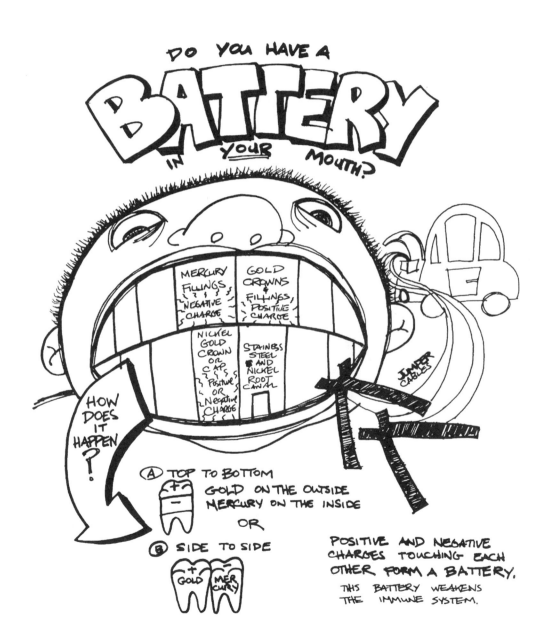

Primary Toxic Suppressors - Electromagnetic Radiation

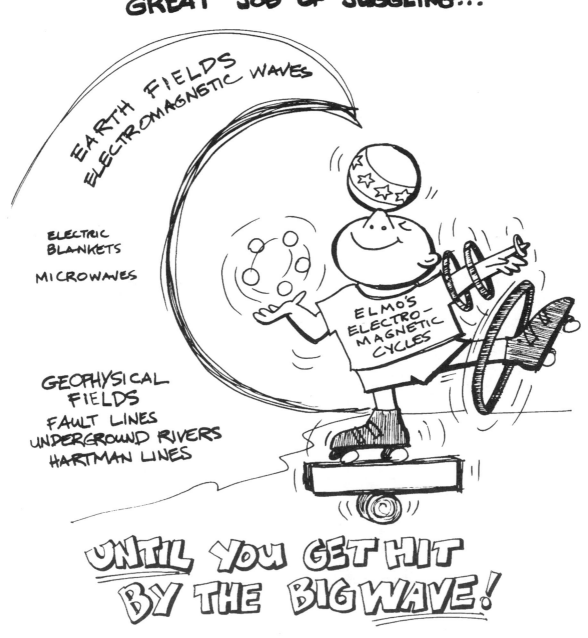

ELECTROMAGNETIC FIELDS AND RADIATION BASIC CONCEPTS

Are You Playing The Fields?

In this chapter you can learn:

- *What is radiation, and what kinds of radiation are there?*
- *How are electricity and magnetism involved in the animal world?*
- *How do homing pigeons find their way home?*
- *What types of natural radiation affect us?*
- *What are some sources of radiation?*
- *What is the link between radiation and cancer?*

What is radiation?

Radiation is energy, or more accurately a byproduct from an energy source which spills over into the surrounding environment. Although many people think of nuclear radiation or x-rays when they think of radiation, these are only two of many types.

This is the electromagnetic spectrum, which will be explained and referred to throughout this chapter and the next two chapters.

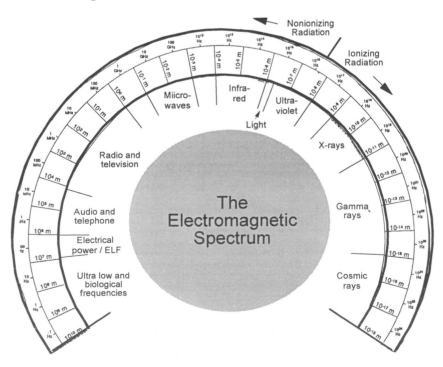

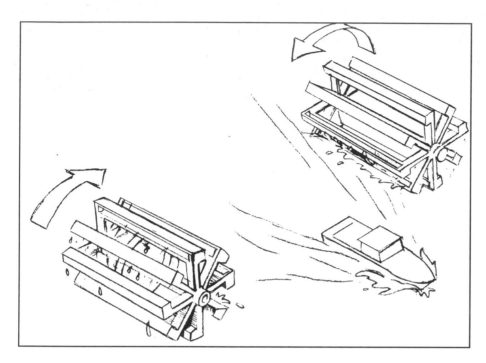

Just as a stone dropped into a bucket of water, creating ripples radiating from the path of the stone, radiation comes off its source like the wake of a boat going through the water. In a similar way, electromagnetic and other radiation emanates from many sources.

What types of radiation are there?

Some types of radiation, both natural and artificial, include:

- *ELF (Extremely Low Frequency) radiation*
- *Electromagnetic fields*
- *Radio waves*
- *Heat and infrared*
- *Ultraviolet (UV)*
- *Nuclear gamma rays*
- *Sound waves*
- *Microwaves*
- *Light and colors*
- *X-rays*
- *Cosmic rays*

These all have biological effects, some good and some bad, i.e. some are and some are not in harmony with the cells in our bodies. The beneficial effects, which, when deliberately applied, are called energy medicine, are discussed in the **Alternative Medicine** book referenced at the end of this chapter. The bad effects are discussed in this chapter and the next two chapters, along with ways to protect yourself from them.

What is an electromagnetic field?

When alternating electrical current (AC) flows through a wire, a magnetic field is set up around the wire.

Current is electron flow, and as it flows it puts out a magnetic field like a rock dropped into a pond puts out ripples perpendicular to it.

Stated in another way, if electron flow is like a boat plowing through water, electromagnetic

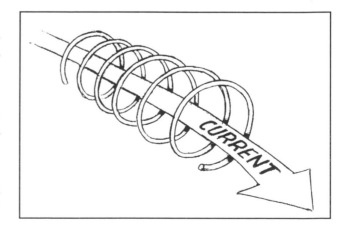

radiation is like the boat's wake.

If you are using an electrical appliance, the electrical current does not affect you directly, but the magnetic field produced by running the appliance can have a harmful biological effect. An electromagnetic field (EM field) is a combination of electrical and magnetic fields, and is one of many types of radiation.

Alternating current (AC) is more economical to generate and transmit long distances. This is the type of current used in this country and in most countries. It converts to direct current (DC) in some non-motor appliances such as stereos and televisions. Only AC, not DC, produces the harmful EM field. An electric shaver is AC, while a rechargeable shaver which is not plugged in at the time of use generates DC fields.

All mass, including ourselves, has fields, including gravitational and electromagnetic. These fields cause both attraction and repulsion, like north and south poles on a magnet.

What are some examples of electricity and magnetism in the animal world?

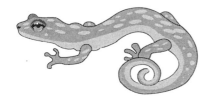

There are many examples of electrical or magnetic effects which are naturally occurring in the animal world. For example, a salamander can regenerate a limb or tail that has been amputated. Research has shown that the cut ends of nerve cells in the limb connect with the skin cells that form over the cut end of the limb. If this junction is prevented from forming, regeneration does not occur. A negative electrical current is then formed, which changes normal cells at the cut end to primitive, undiffcrentiated (not specific as to type) cells. These cells grow and then redifferentiate into skin, muscle, and bone. Without the natural electrical current, this process would not occur. A similar process is used in medicine when broken bones do not reunite when set. An applied weak electrical current can stimulate bone cell growth at the broken ends, with subsequent joining of the broken ends to mend the break [1].

Homing pigeons were studied to determine how they can return to a central reference point regardless of where they are released. It was discovered that their homing mechanism is magnetic, and it tunes into the earth's magnetic field to determine its location. The earth is a huge magnet, complete with a north and south pole just like the bar or horseshoe magnets that you played with in school. Pigeons which were temporarily visually impaired by contact lenses still found their way home. However, those pigeons to which a small magnet was attached became disoriented and could not find their way back. Our new grid missile guidance system used in the Gulf War used a technique similar to that of the pigeons.

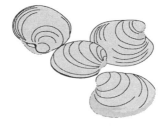

Some shellfish open and close their shells in response to high and low tides, which are caused by the magnetic (gravitational) pull of the moon in orbit around the earth. Shellfish in a salt water tank a mile from the coast still opened and closed their shells in rhythm to the tides, showing that the water's motion was not the signal they needed. In fact, when clams were flown from the East coast to the Chicago area, 1000 miles away, the clams changed their opening pattern to reflect when high or low tide would occur in Chicago if Chicago had been an oceanfront city.

Many other animal and plant experiments have shown that electricity, magnetism, sound, light, and other types of radiation have a profound effect on biological systems.

Why are animal effects significant to us?

Since we as human beings have biological and electrochemical systems, it is reasonable to assume that we too are similarly affected by radiation. It is also reasonable to assume that, since we can be very sensitive to different types of radiation, even in tiny naturally produced amounts, we would also be sensitive to the much larger amounts of artificially produced sources of radiation that we all come in contact with daily. More and more evidence is accumulating as proof that this is indeed the case. Furthermore, the changes produced in the body's cells from non-deliberate exposure to electromagnetic fields, x-rays, radio waves, and others are not what nature intended, and the effects are almost invariably harmful.

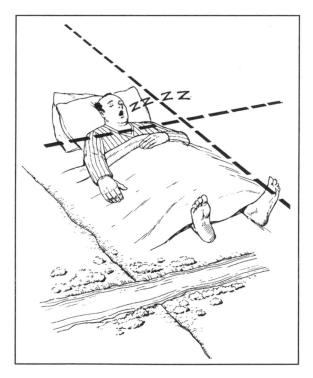

What other types of natural radiation affect us?

Regular lines of radiation, at right angles to each other like latitude and longitude lines, exist in the earth. These are called Hartman or Curry lines. These lines are about fifteen feet apart, ranging from about ten feet apart at the poles to about twenty feet apart at the equator. A node is the intersection of two of these perpendicular lines, and is the area of highest radiation. In some cases, cancer in a particular part of the body of a person can be traced back to a node located where that part of the person's body lies during sleep.

These fields along with underground rivers or earthquake fault lines are what a dowsing rod picks up.

Radon, a radioactive byproduct of uranium decay, is a gas which seeps up from the ground. The Environmental Protection Agency (EPA) estimates that radon may pose a serious threat to eight million U.S. homes as of 1987. The National Cancer Institute states that radon may be responsible for at least 30,000 lung cancer deaths each year [2,3], and is second only to tobacco as a lung cancer cause.

Parts of the United States which are most affected by radon include:

- *Parts of New York State*
- *Eastern Pennsylvania*
- *Northwest New Jersey*
- *Appalachian mountain area*
- *Parts of Montana, South Dakota, Colorado, and Florida*

Partial solutions, other than moving to a different area, include installing fans to circulate the air inside the home as well as venting it to the outside, and sealing any cracks in the basement floor. Tightly insulated homes tend to concentrate the radon gas inside the home.

Radon monitors for the home can be purchased by contacting local EPA or public health representatives.

What are some useful definitions?

Some definitions and explanations are helpful in understanding the different types of radiation and their effects. All energy, or radiation, occurs in the form of waves. The **frequency** refers to the number of times the wave peak occurs in a given period of time, usually one second. The **wavelength** is the length between wave peaks.

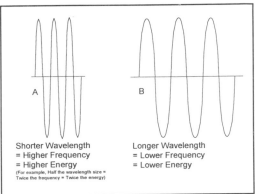

The shorter the wavelength, the higher the frequency, and vice versa. For example, a rubber band has a shorter wavelength (about two inches) than a jump rope (about four feet). The rubber band can vibrate, or move, much faster than the jump rope can. The higher the frequency, the more energy is being emitted, and the greater the potential for cell damage. In this picture, (A) has shorter wavelength and higher frequency, i.e. higher energy than (B).

Shorter Wavelength
= Higher Frequency
= Higher Energy
(For example, Half the wavelength size =
Twice the frequency = Twice the energy)

Longer Wavelength
= Lower Frequency
= Lower Energy

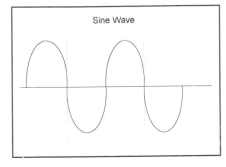

Sine Wave

Wavelengths are usually expressed in meters (m). A meter is about 39 inches, or just a bit longer than a yard. The longest wavelengths (such as those which power our appliances or are used for submarine communications) are thousands of miles between peaks, while the shortest are not much longer than the width of an atom. Frequencies are expressed in Hertz (Hz), or cycles per second. 10 Hertz means that 10 high-and-low cycles occur in one second.

One kilohertz   (kHz) =   one thousand hertz
One megahertz (mHz) =   one million hertz
One gigahertz (gHz) =   one billion hertz.

Numbers used for frequency and wavelength are expressed in what is called scientific notation, in which the numbers in superscript refer to the number of zeroes. For example, $10^2 = 100$, $10^5 = 100,000$, etc. A negative superscript refers to a fractional amount: $10^{-2} = 1/10^2 = 1/100$, etc. $10^0 = 1$. The picture on the first page, with wavelengths in meters (m) and frequencies in Hertz (Hz), is hopefully beginning to make sense.

What are the two major types of radiation?

The electromagnetic spectrum can be divided into two parts for purposes of health discussion - nonionizing and ionizing radiation. The higher, more powerful frequencies, located approximately above the visible light range, are **ionizing**, while the lower frequencies are **nonionizing**. Ionization is the electrical disruption of the atom or molecule, causing the ejection of electrons from the atom. The resulting atom or molecule is now electrically unbalanced, or charged, and is referred to as ionized. Ionized molecules are chemically very active and the resulting abnormal reactions are damaging to the body's cells. The DNA of the cells is damaged, potentially leading to cancer.

It has been known for some time that ionizing radiation such as x-rays and gamma rays are harmful to cells. Much evidence is mounting that nonionizing radiation such as electromagnetic radiation and microwaves can also cause cellular damage such as cancer.

ELF radiation, for **e**xtra (or **e**xtremely) **l**ow **f**requency, refers to radiation up to 1000 Hz. The 60 Hz radiation that powers our electrical appliances, long believed harmless unless one is holding a live wire, is now suspect in causing cellular and immune system damage due to magnetic radiation effects and the moving of the electrons in our bodies.

What are some sources of radiation?

Almost all frequencies of radiation are produced by both natural and artificial sources. Magnetic fields can come from the earth or the moon, or from electromagnets and electric currents. Microwaves come from space and from microwave ovens. X-rays come from space or from x-ray machines. Natural radiation is no less harmful than a similar artificially created field, but the body has learned to cope with and sometimes even use natural radiation. With natural sources, the body is usually exposed to far less radiation than the more powerful artificial sources.

Most radiation frequencies, regardless of source, are stressful to the body, and we are exposed to much more radiation daily than the body was designed to deal with. Radiation effects add up and accumulate over a period of time.

The U.S., with the possible exception of the remotest areas, is polluted with what can be considered to be electronic smog. Electromagnetic radiation is estimated to be 100 to 200 million times greater than natural nonionizing background radiation [4]. Since even natural radiation is proven to have an effect, it is highly unlikely that this level of radiation is harmless.

What is the link between EM radiation and cancer?

Of 35 international studies on electromagnetic radiation, 33 made a conclusive link with cancers. In a school in San Francisco, 22 cases of cancer were found in staff working in the front of the school, and no cancer was found in those who worked in the back. Large electrical transformers were located at the front of the school. Similar results have been found in Colorado, Sweden, and most recently in Manhattan Beach, California. In Sweden, the high power transmission lines are now buried in insulated piping with counterbalancing EM fields.

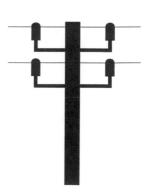

There was also found to be a 300% increase in brain tumors in children whose mothers used electric blankets during pregnancy [5]. This is why there are warnings on electric blanket instructions that the blankets should not be used by pregnant women. These warnings should apply to all of us.

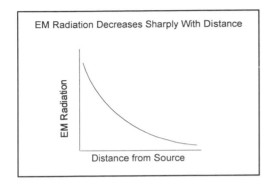

Danger from exposure falls off sharply with distance, explaining why there was such a difference in effect between those at the front and those at the back of the San Francisco school. EM exposure danger follows a logarithmic curve, and the greatest difference in harm is found at the closest distances to the source. There is a greater difference in exposure between being one to two feet from an electrical transformer versus being between 50 to 75 feet from it.

What is the link between muscle weakness and EM radiation, and why is this significant?
In one form of kinesiology testing, the test subject holds her/his arm out and the tester presses down on it while the subject resists. Certain toxic chemicals, foods to which one is allergic, and some types of radiation cause a dramatic, immediate, and temporary weakening of the arm muscle. This is indicative of the toxic weakening that is going on in the entire body. Russian scientists have done extensive research on this link between radiation and muscle weakness.

There is an energy field around the body which can be made visible in a technique called Kirlian photography. The body's energy fields can be changed adversely by the application of external electromagnetic fields. These changes are most likely due to the effects of electromagnetic radiation on the central nervous system.

It was found that many electrical or electronic devices can cause muscle weakness. These include:

- *Motors*
- *Transformers*
- *Fluorescent lights*
- *Battery powered and digital watches and clocks*
- *Electric blankets, waterbed heaters*
- *Video display terminals (TVs, computer screens, video games)*

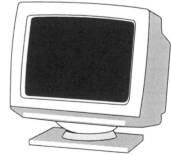

By implication, undesirable effects are occurring throughout the entire body.

A statistical correlation has been shown between the relative incidence of use of fetal monitors in hospitals and the hospital's rate of Cesarean birth. It is probable that the use of the monitor, in addition to other electronic equipment and fluorescent lights in the labor room, can weaken the uterus, a muscle whose strong contractions are necessary for a normal birth. One reason for a Cesarean section is a uterus which is unable to push sufficiently.

In another example of body weakness, an ionizing type smoke detector within 60 feet of the bed can diminish male and female sex drive. A 60 foot radius is nearly anywhere in an average size house, including the floors above and below. An ionizing smoke detector is not the same as a negative ion generator sometimes used for its beneficial health effects.

What are the lowest frequencies?
In following the electromagnetic spectrum from lowest to highest frequencies, we start with the biological frequencies, found in brain waves (from highest to lowest frequency: alpha, beta, theta, delta) and in the bodies of living things. These frequencies are intended by nature to be beneficial, and are utilized in energy medicine of various types such as homeopathy and acupuncture, which are discussed in the **Alternative Medicine** guide.

In the next chapter we will take a look at ELF, the next highest frequencies, and then review the remainder of the electromagnetic spectrum in the chapter entitled Other Frequencies. Ways to protect yourself from radiation exposure are discussed in both of these chapters.

References and Resources

- Becker, Robert O., *Cross Currents*, Jeremy P. Tarcher Inc., Los Angeles CA, 1990. *Discusses two trends - the rise in electropollution and the rise in electromedicine - the destructive and the healing potential of electromagnetic radiation.*

- Becker, Robert O. and Gary Selden, *The Body Electric: Electromagnetism and the Foundation of Life*, William Morrow and Co. Inc., NY, 1987.

- Becker, Robert O. and A.A. Marino, *Electromagnetism and Life*, State University of New York, Albany NY, 1982.

- The Burton Goldberg Group, James Strohecker (ed.), "Energy Medicine", pp. 192-204, *Alternative Medicine: The Definitive Guide*, Future Medicine Publishing Inc., Puyallup WA, 1994. *This chapter discusses ways that electromagnetic radiation can be used as a healing tool.*

- Davis, Albert and Walter Rawls, *Magnetism and Its Effects on the Living System*, Acres USA, Kansas City MO, 1993.

- Lee, Lita, *Radiation Protection Manual*, Grassroots Network, Redwood City CA, 1990, 3rd ed.

- Philpott, William, and Sharon Taplin, *Biomagnetic Handbook*, Enviro-Tech Products, Choctaw OK, 1990.

- Schechter, Steven R., *Fighting Radiation with Foods, Herbs, and Vitamins*, East West Health Books, Brookline MA, 1988. *Natural methods of strengthening the body's defenses against radiation of many types.*

- Smith, Cyril W. and Simon Best, *Electromagnetic Man: Health and Hazard in the Electrical Environment*, St. Martin's Press, NY, 1989.

Other resources:

BEMI Currents - Journal of the Bio-Electro-Magnetics Institute, 2490 West Moana Lane, Reno NV 89509-3936, phone (702) 827-9099. *BEMI Currents has articles pertaining to electromagnetics, and is also affiliated with the* **Bio-Electro-Magnetics Institute***, same address and phone, which was established to provide research and education in the field.*

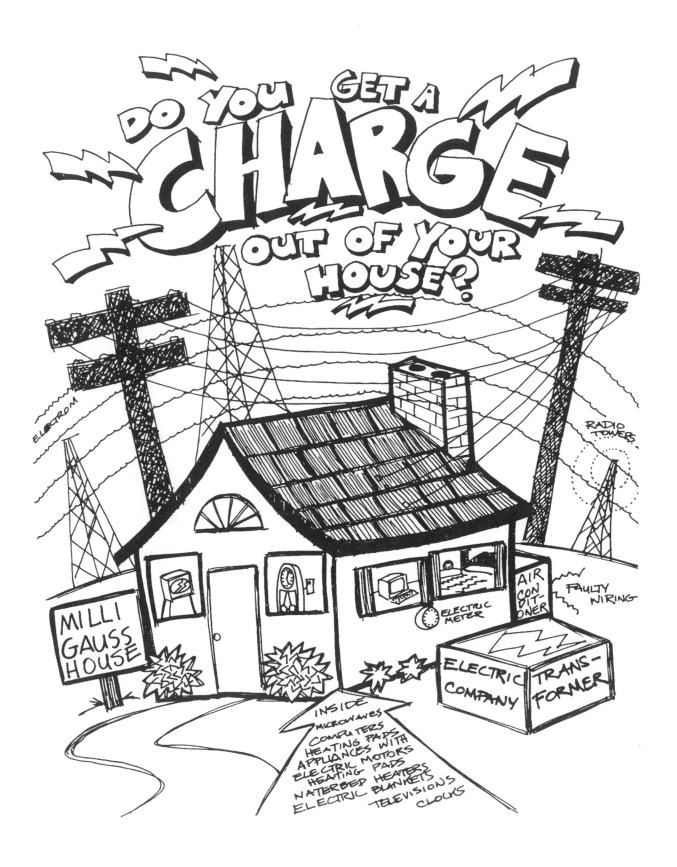

ELECTROMAGNETIC FIELDS AND RADIATION HOUSEHOLD CURRENT AND APPLIANCES

Are You Plugged In?

Do you have the following symptoms? Electromagnetic radiation from common household appliances may be involved.

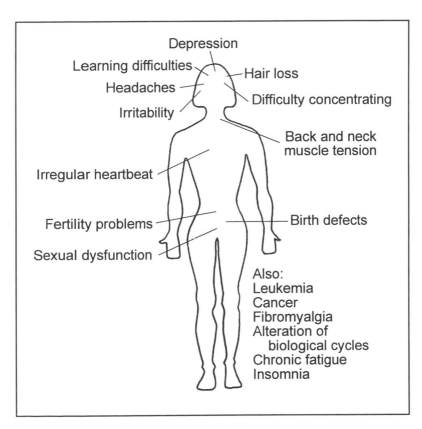

Things in this chapter that can change your life:

- *If your home or workplace is near high tension wires, you may be at greater risk of leukemia.*

- *Depression, learning difficulties, fertility problems, fatigue, and insomnia can be caused at least in part by exposure to electrical appliances.*

- *Some common household appliances such as electric blankets and clock radios can contribute to the development of cancer.*

You can also learn:

- *Why exposure to the electromagnetic fields coming from your household appliances can be hazardous.*

- *What exactly is electricity?*

- *What are motors, generators, and transformers and how are they relevant to your body?*

- *How does distance affect electromagnetic danger?*

- *What are some sources of harmful electromagnetic fields?*

What kind of radiation comes from our electrical sockets?

ELF (Extra Low Frequency) radiation, most notably the 60 Hz electrical currents in the United States (and 50 Hz in Europe) powers our electrical appliances. These frequencies and their attendant electromagnetic radiation have been shown to be harmful. Some people feel that 60 Hz is both a higher frequency and at greater disharmony with the body and is therefore more harmful than 50 Hz, but this has not been proven. Both are way out of phase with the body's many frequencies and systems, such as the heart which beats at 60 beats per minute.

What are the dangers of exposure to this frequency?

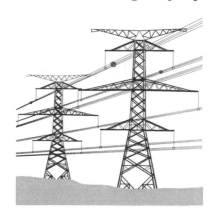

A recent study in Sweden has shown a four-fold increase in the incidence of leukemia among children who live near high-tension power lines. A number of U.S. studies have reported an increased risk of leukemia, lymphoma, and brain tumors among children living near power lines and workers exposed to EM fields on the job. Exposed adults had 1.7 times the normal risk of developing leukemia and three times the risk of chronic lymphocytic leukemia [1]. This increased cancer risk is due to cellular changes and stressing of the immune system. Animals exposed to EM fields have reduced melatonin, a cancer-fighting hormone which also controls sleep cycles.

Cancers from EM fields are more likely to be cancers of less dense tissue, such as leukemia and lymphomas. Cancers of dense tissue such as organs are less likely. This is why lawsuits against utility companies based on such effects as kidney cancer (which is more likely due to nickel, mercury, or benzene) have little chance of winning.

Other effects of exposure are:

- **CNS** effects - headaches, memory loss, learning and concentrating difficulties, depression and suicidal thoughts, irritability, behavioral abnormalities, Parkinson's disease, ALS, fibromyalgia, multiple sclerosis (MS)

- **Reproductive** effects - sexual dysfunction, miscarriages, birth defects

- **Cardiovascular** effects - irregular heartbeat

- **Other** effects - back and neck muscle tension, alteration of biological cycles, hair loss, chronic fatigue, insomnia and sleep disturbances

Effects on the heart and nervous system are not surprising, since both of these systems are electrical in nature and are susceptible to other types of electrical currents. Cell mutations from EM fields not only lead to cancerous changes but also to birth defects and resulting miscarriages.

One patient, an actress in her mid 30s, whose house was located in close proximity to high voltage lines experienced chronic low energy and was losing her hair. Her symptoms went away when she moved out of her house. In another example, a building had a cross-wired light, and employees who worked near it were chronically irritable and tired. Correcting the electrical problem corrected the health problems.

If you touch an exposed electrical wire, your muscles will contract instantly and painfully. Lesser electromagnetic exposure can also cause muscle and meningeal (brain and spinal cord covering) contraction to a lesser extent, and may be partially responsible for stiff neck and back and for some muscle cramps and aches. Touching an exposed wire will also cause the heart to try to go from its normal 60 beats (cycles) per minute to 60 cycles per second, and it fails. Lesser EM fields can cause lesser heart arrhythmias.

What exactly is electricity?

The 60-Hz frequency which powers our appliances is what we usually think of as electricity. The word "electricity" comes from the same root as the word "electron", no accident considering that electricity is electron flow. Electrons, discussed in the chapter on Basic Chemical Concepts, are the negatively charged particles on the outside of any atom, including the metal atoms which make up the inside of the cord that leads from your wall socket to your toaster. Electrons are interchangeable, and can be passed from one molecule to the next like a baton passed by runners in a relay race. This passage of electrons down a wire, atom by atom, is called electricity.

Some terms are useful in understanding electricity, which can be compared to water flowing through a hose.

- **Current** is the flow of electrons along the outside of a wire, similar to the way water flows through a garden hose. The ampere, or amp, is the measure of current flow. One amp represents the flow of 1.6×10^{17} electrons, or about one and a half times the huge number formed when 1 is followed by 17 zeroes. This is equivalent in concept to the amount of water in gallons which flows through a hose.

- **Resistance**, measured in units called ohms, is a measure of how hard it is to push the electrons through the wire, and is similar in effect to a constriction of part of the water hose or to the substitution of a small for a large hose.

- **Voltage** is equivalent to the force pushing the water through the hose. Voltage is the amps multiplied by the resistance in ohms. It takes more pressure (force) to push ten gallons of water per minute through a hose, and it takes more power to send a certain amount of current through a wire of high resistance.

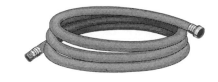

- **Wattage** is the amount of power at the exit end, and is calculated by multiplying the amps times the volts. In the garden hose analogy, this is equivalent to how much water comes out of the hose. It can be visualized by noting that either raising the water-pushing power or widening the hose (lowering the resistance) increases the amount of the water coming out the exit end.

To summarize:

Current	electron flow	measured in amps
Resistance	constriction	measured in ohms
Voltage	pushing force	measured in volts
Wattage	power out	measured in watts

Electricity is, in short, the flow of electrons along the outside of a wire. A magnetic field is produced by this flow; if electricity can be compared to a boat moving through the water, the magnetic field produced is analogous to the boat's wake. The magnetic field both causes and is caused by this flow of electrons much as a water wheel both moves water and is moved by water.

What is a kilowatt-hour?

Did you ever wonder about the phrase "kilowatt-hour" which may be on your electric bill? A kilowatt-hour is a measure of power (one kilowatt = 1000 watts) multiplied by the number of hours that the power was used. If you burn a 100 watt bulb for 10 hours (100 watts x 10 hours = 1000 watt-hours or one kilowatt-hour), this will cost you the going rate for one kilowatt-hour.

What are motors and generators, and what makes them work?

When electricity is moved through a wire, a magnetic field is created. When magnets are moved by an electric wire, the magnet moves the electrons down the wire. This is called a power generator.

If electricity is moved past a magnet, the electrons are alternately attracted and repelled. Electrons, which have a negative charge, are repelled by a negative charge and attracted by a positive charge. This is much like the two north sides of magnets being repelled by each other, while a north and a south side attract. An electron can thus be moved by pushing it with a negative charge or pulling it with a positive charge. In the generation of electricity, shoving the electrons forward is alternated with breaking the field, and this creates a vacuum that pulls the next electron into place. This is similar to the way a bullet is pulled by vacuum into a gun's chamber after the previous bullet has been fired.

This process spins an armature like water from a boat's wake can move a water wheel; this is a motor. The largest magnetic fields come from motors.

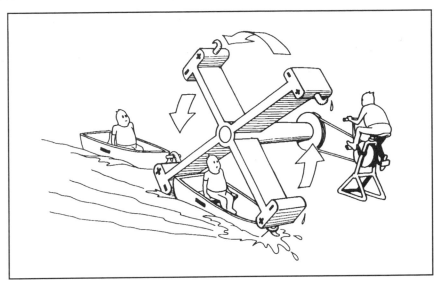

In this picture, the whole picture represents the generator, and the boats are the electrons. The movement of the electrons is the power.

What are transformers and why are they necessary?

When electric fields are moved next to each other, and different numbers of coils are wrapped around each side, you have a transformer. If you go from fewer to more coils (for example from 100 to 1000), a step-up transformer is created; the opposite situation creates a step-down transformer. Voltage decreases and current increases, or vice versa, in proportion to the difference in the number of coils.

When current is produced, it is produced as direct current (DC). It is then converted to alternating current (AC), which is cheaper to send. Very high voltages go longer distances like water in a high pressure hose. Our appliances are powered by much lower voltages, so a series of transformers is used to step down the voltage, in substations and then again at our homes. Transformers inside some appliances such as stereos step down the voltage still further.

How are our bodies like transformers?

There are billions of electrons in your body. If a magnetic field, generated by a motor or other electrical appliance, is near the body, then the electrons within the body will move just as they do in a wire. Our bodies in effect are like step-down transformers, and current within the body will increase accordingly. A cellular phone held near the head is a lot like a transformer.

The motion of electrons in the body in response to a magnetic field is not what is supposed to be happening in order for our bodies to function optimally. Another name for electrons which are moving in a way that is not orderly to the body is free radicals. As discussed in other contexts, free radicals can cause cell mutations, arterial problems, and cancers. The many studies which point to an increased incidence of soft tissue cancers in those exposed to strong electromagnetic fields makes sense in light of this understanding.

Every molecule in the brain and body of a person standing in a strong 60 Hz AC field also vibrates to and fro sixty times a second. This has been shown to alter normal activation of enzyme and cellular immune responses, leading to the chain of events causing cancer [2].

Did you know that a wire can be electrified without it touching the source of electricity?
The wires in a transformer are wrapped around a core which doesn't touch the nearby core with a different number of wires wrapped around it.

A wire with electrons moving through it puts out a field which can cause a lesser movement of electrons in a nearby wire - or in our bodies. This is called inductance, or an induced field. In other words, electricity (or more accurately electromagnetic fields) can essentially jump from a wire to another wire - or to you!

High voltage transmission lines necessarily put out high voltages, and therefore high electromagnetic fields. In the past, some farmers found a way to tap into these fields. They put coils under high voltage lines to get electricity by inductance. They were charged by the electric companies with theft of electricity. These same utility companies then deny in cancer lawsuits that EM fields radiate from their lines. If enough radiation leaks out to light a farm, it is certainly enough to affect your body.

Metal fences around substations must be grounded at intervals or they can become dangerously electrified by the induced current field.

EM fields can cause radio and phone static, burning out of light bulbs, and warping of a TV picture. Strong EM fields can distort the TV picture by interfering with the path of the electron beam that forms the picture.

Like a television picture tube, you have many billions of electrons in your body, and electromagneticfields nearby can set up a magnetic field in your body. The result is abnormal electron flow, which in turn can result in free radical damage. Free radical damage is that caused by uncontrolled and random electron flow, causing chain reactions throughout the body. This is one possible explanation for degenerative diseases such as arthritis, cancer, and heart disease.

What determines the hazard of EM fields?
Several factors determine the toxicity of EM fields:

- The frequency, with higher frequencies usually (but not always) more damaging.

- The amount of EM field emitted, measured in units called milliGauss (mG). Cellular changes are possible at a level as low as 1-2 mG. The amount can also be expressed as the power of the source. A more powerful radio station is one which can be heard louder and at a greater distance, and the more powerful station (or appliance) puts out more EM radiation.

- The distance from the source. The number of milliGauss one is exposed to decreases by the square of the distance. In other words, if you sit twice as far from the TV set as you used to, you are now exposed to only one-fourth the EM radiation. There is no absolute safe distance agreed on by the experts.

- The duration of exposure. An electric razor or hair dryer has a much higher mG reading than an electric blanket, but the blanket is more dangerous because it is used for a much longer period of time. For those living under high-tension wires, duration of exposure can be measured in years.

- Individual sensitivity, which is itself linked to the presence of other toxic burdens.

There are concepts called near field and far field. The far field leaves the antenna or source and does not return. The near field interacts with the far field and comes back to the source. The larger the transmission antenna, the longer are both the near field and the far field. The near field, which, as the name suggests, is much closer to the source than the far field, is more hazardous due to the numerous and more intense interactions.

What are some sources of EM fields?
Sources of EM fields include:

- Nearly all electrical appliances and motors, especially those which draw large amounts of current

- Office equipment such as fluorescent lights, copy machines, computer terminals and printers, telephones in frequent use

- Large numbers of overhead wires or transformers. Underground wires can also pose some risk, without a resident knowing where the wires are concentrated. Underground wires can be less hazardous if they are properly shielded by metal conduits. If not properly shielded, underground wires are more hazardous than overhead wires because they are nearer to your body.

- Waterbeds with electric heaters, electric blankets, heating pads. These can produce fields even when turned off if still plugged in, a phenomenon known as electrical potential. These heaters are most safely used to preheat the bed, and then unplugged before bedtime. Waterbed heaters advertised as EMF-free have recently become available.

- Household wiring behind a wall, especially next to the head of the bed or if improperly grounded. Be sure the bed is located as far as possible from the fuse or circuit breaker box.

- Electric clocks on the nightstand a foot or so from the head of someone sleeping can pose a significant risk over a period of years, as they are an AC motor.

- A transformer box on or near your property labeled "high voltage" or "property of electric company". These boxes are usually olive green and may emit a humming noise.

- Electric power meter

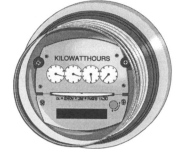

- Television sets and computer screens - since EM fields pass through walls, be aware of what is located on the other side of the TV wall (bed, baby crib). TV sets emit EM radiation even when they are not on as long as they are plugged in. The back and sides emit higher EM fields than the front, but the front emits higher free particle radiation.

- Electrical major appliances, such as electric heat, hot water, clothes dryer, air conditioner, oven, refrigerator. Appliances with motors are particularly hazardous. Motorized appliances are usually those in which something turns; for example, fan blades, electric razor, blender, vacuum cleaner.

How much electromagnetic radiation do these appliances emit?

Actual measurements taken with a Gauss meter (also called an EM field detector) on some common household appliances are shown here. The distance between the meter and the appliance is important, since there is a sharp drop-off with distance. To measure your own appliances, hold the meter at a distance representing your actual typical distance from the appliance.

The EM field is measured in milliGauss (mG), just as distance can be measured in miles. Keep in mind that as little as three mG for about forty hours a week for several years has been linked with an increased incidence of cancer.

Appliance	Distance	EMF, mG	Comments
Microwave oven	2 feet	10-50	fluctuates
Light bulb, on	2 inches	0.2	
Refrigerator	1 foot	4	
Television	2 feet	4	
Power meter	6 inches	over 50	wall opposite meter
Computer monitor	1.5 feet	5	working distance
Elec. outlet, unused	1 inch	0-9	results differed
Waterbed heater	on mattress	15-30	
Hair dryer	6 inches	6-15	
Digital clock, LED	3 inches	15	near head in bed
Phone, regular	by earpiece	0.8	
Fluorescent lights	2 feet	2	
Dimmer switch	3 inches	4-30	highest when dimmest
Electric blanket	as used	33	
Electric range	1 foot	40	

As noted above, an electric dimmer switch puts out more electromagnetic radiation (mG) when it is dimmer. This is an example of electrical potential.

How much difference does distance make?

Distance from the appliance makes a huge difference. For example, a hair dryer held six inches from the head produces about 10 mG, doubling if only an inch closer and dropping to about 5-6 mG if an inch further away. By comparison, recall that 2-3 mG can cause cellular changes. Other results with distance (microwave oven fluctuates about once per second due to magnetron) are:

	1 ft	2 ft	3 ft	4 ft	6 ft
Microwave		50-100	10-50	2-40	2-8
Television	9	4	1.5	0.7	0

This is shown here in graphic form:

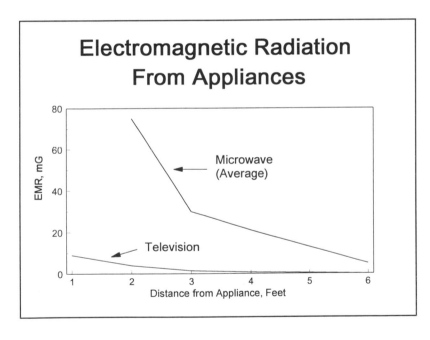

The television figures can be misleading. Televisions work by the firing of electrons directly at the screen by an electron gun. Many of these electrons pass through the screen toward the viewer. These are detectable by a Geiger counter.

Computer monitors work on the same principle, and are more hazardous because of the closer proximity involved.

Electron motion secondary to magnetic fields, rather than magnetic fields themselves, can cause free radical damage.

How can electricity be used for diagnostic purposes?

Electrical monitoring techniques allow the study of bodily organs and processes which generate electricity. These are the heart and the brain.

An electrocardiogram (EKG or ECG) shows whether the heart is contracting properly and, if not, it provides information for diagnosis of the problem. Electrical leads are temporarily attached to the chest with suction cups or tape, and

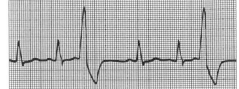

more leads are attached to the arm and/or leg as a ground. Electrical impulses show up on a monitor or graph paper as jagged lines that convey meaningful information to a trained person.

A type of portable electrocardiograph called a Holter monitor can be worn for 24 hours during normal activity to detect intermittent irregular heart rhythms. The patient presses a button on the monitor when symptoms are experienced. The electronic signals that are recorded from the button pressing will alert the interpreter who reads the result after the monitor is detached that these segments of the readout deserve particular attention. If arrhythmic episodes occur less often than once a day, a small portable device can be carried for as long as necessary and used to record heart rhythms only when symptoms are experienced. The readout can be transmitted by telephone, where the electrical signals and beeps are converted electronically to a recognizable EKG at the medical facility.

For your information, a cheaper and safer alternative to EKGs when irregular or fast heartbeat is suspected is to take the nutrient minerals magnesium (heart arrhythmia is a common symptom of deficiency) or potassium, whose lack can cause fast heartbeat. This may solve the problem without resorting to expensive testing.

The other type of electrical monitoring is the electroencephalogram (EEG). This records brain waves, and brain disorders from epilepsy to insomnia can be diagnosed and studied. Electrical leads are attached by suction or, where hair is present, by thin needles inserted just under the skin of the scalp.

Can such testing be harmful?
Although an electrical circuit is produced by the placing of the leads in a standard EKG, this is not known to be harmful, and the procedure is painless. The suction cups used in this procedure sometimes leave red imprints on the skin, but these disappear overnight.

Other than the insertion of the needles in the EEG, the procedure is painless, and like the EKG is considered to be relatively harmless.

What Can Be Done

There are many ways to minimize exposure to electrical fields:

- Replace your heated waterbed with a regular mattress, or unplug the waterbed heater and put a thick pad between the water mattress and the sheet. The waterbed can be left on during the day and unplugged (not just turned off) at night when it is used; it will retain the heat until morning. A timer between the outlet and the waterbed, set to go off at night and on in the morning, will serve the same purpose. If you replace the waterbed, a futon is even better than a regular mattress, as the coils in the box spring of the mattress can act as an antenna for radiation.

- Use a thick quilt, down comforter, or more blankets to replace your electric blanket.

- Use a battery operated or rechargeable electric razor instead of one attached to a power cord.

- Use an EM field detector (Gauss meter) to find areas of concentrated EM fields in your bedroom wall, and relocate your bed to a safer spot. Alternatively, sleep with your head away from the wall.

- A television generates EM fields even when not in use as a response to consumer demand for an instant-on or remote controlled picture. Unplug the set when not in use, or at least keep it over ten feet from your bed even if it's on the other side of the wall.

- Avoid using dimmer switches, especially those which do not click off.

- Electromagnetic shielding for your home or appliances is available. There are also certain types of transmitters that can smooth out EMFs in a building.

Summary

Nearly all household appliances, especially those with motors, produce damaging electromagnetic fields. The danger drops sharply as you put more distance between yourself and the appliance.

Other ways to protect yourself from electromagnetic fields and their effects are discussed at the end of the next chapter.

References and Resources

- Becker, Robert O., *Cross Currents*, Jeremy P. Tarcher Inc., Los Angeles CA, 1990.
- Brodeur, Paul, *The Great Power-Line Cover-Up*, Little, Brown, and Co., New York, 1993.

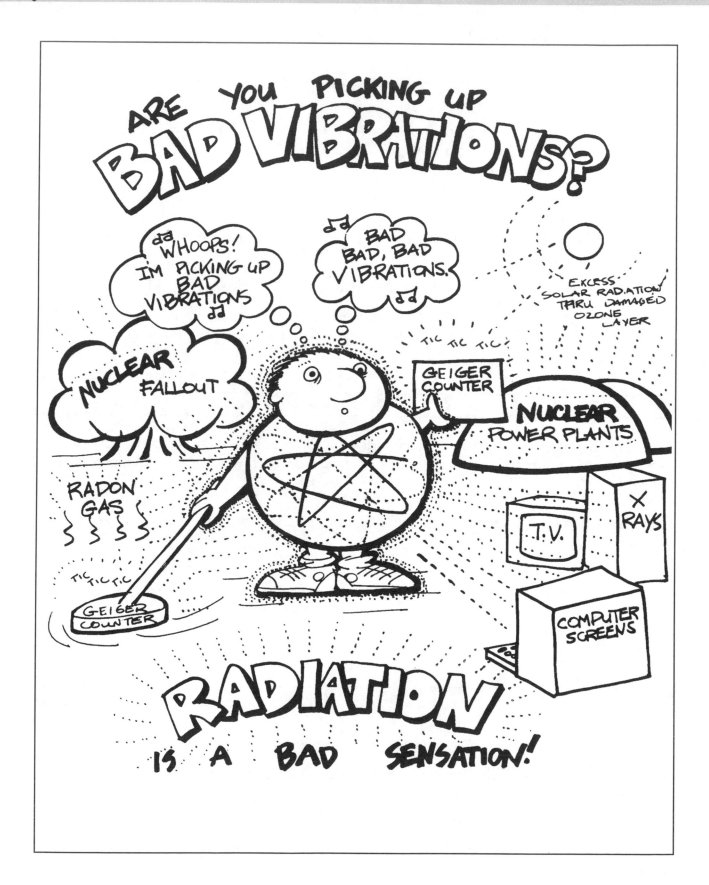

ELECTROMAGNETIC FIELDS AND RADIATION - OTHER FREQUENCIES

Bad Vibrations

Do you have any of the following symptoms? They have been linked to the types of electromagnetic radiation indicated (other than effects from electrical appliances).

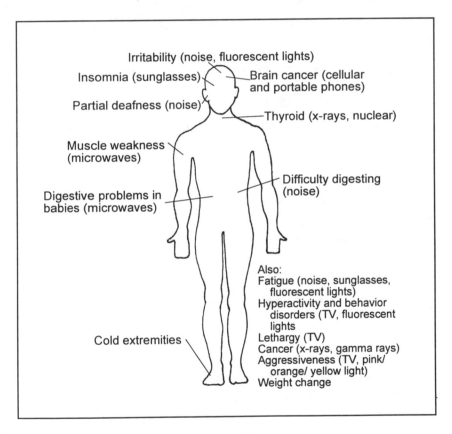

Irritability (noise, fluorescent lights)

Insomnia (sunglasses)

Brain cancer (cellular and portable phones)

Partial deafness (noise)

Thyroid (x-rays, nuclear)

Muscle weakness (microwaves)

Difficulty digesting (noise)

Digestive problems in babies (microwaves)

Also:
Fatigue (noise, sunglasses, fluorescent lights)
Hyperactivity and behavior disorders (TV, fluorescent lights
Lethargy (TV)
Cancer (x-rays, gamma rays)
Aggressiveness (TV, pink/ orange/ yellow light)
Weight change

Cold extremities

Fifteen things in this chapter that can change your life:

1. *Frequencies other than electromagnetic - sound, radio, microwave, infrared, light and color, ultraviolet, x-rays - can have harmful effects. You are probably exposed to many of these on a regular basis, whether or not you are aware of it.*

2. *Noise can be stressful, causing fatigue, irritability, and even difficulty digesting your food.*

3. *The Magnetic Resonance Imaging (MRI) diagnostic technique is probably not harmless.*

4. Television can be hazardous to your health, not just your mind.

5. Hyperactivity in children, reduced attention span, lowered test scores, and lethargy have been linked to too much TV.

6. Microwaves do more than cook food, and that's bad news.

7. Microwaving a baby's milk can make a baby sick.

8. Light can act like a nutrient in the body.

9. Different colors can affect our health for good or bad.

10. Sunglasses and colored contact lenses can lead to fatigue and insomnia.

11. The yellowish sodium lights that are in increasing use in our cities may actually be making crime worse.

12. Fluorescent lights, standard in our schools, have been linked to hyperactivity and behavior disorders.

13. Supermarket laser scanners and shoplifting detectors may be harmful.

14. Watch out for irradiated food.

15. There are ways to protect yourself from radiation exposure, even after the exposure.

The electromagnetic fields we are most commonly exposed to are those generated by 60 Hz household current and household appliances, as discussed in the previous chapter. However, there are other frequencies which have their hazards.

Sound

What frequencies can be heard?

The next highest frequencies above household current, about 1-10 kHz, are audio and telephone. These include all audible frequencies, which start at about 30 Hz, which is the lowest note that most people can still hear. The vibrations of the lowest bass guitar or piano strings are so slow as to be almost visible.

The inverse relationship between wavelength and frequency can be seen in stringed instruments. The shortest and smallest piano wires produce the highest frequencies, or highest sounds, and the longest and thickest wires produce the lowest notes or frequencies. Shortening the effective length of a guitar string by pressing on the string between the frets causes it to vibrate at a higher frequency and produce a higher note.

Lower frequencies travel farther than higher frequencies. This is true for sound waves and for all EM frequencies. To illustrate this, think back to the last time you heard a loud stereo that was some distance from you, such as from a neighbor's house, boom box, or nearby car. You hear the bass notes, which are the lowest frequency, much more than you hear middle range notes, and you can't hear the high notes at all.

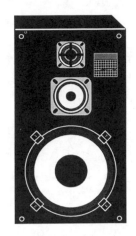

Bass frequencies are not directional, while treble (higher) frequencies are. One bass speaker is sufficient to produce good sound, while two treble and midrange speakers are necessary to produce good stereo.

How can sound waves be dangerous?
The danger of sound lies both in the potential for hearing damage and in the stress reaction it causes. The sounds we hear, such as stereos, traffic, jackhammers, and household appliances are more than the ears and the body were designed to deal with. Loud noise such as music at rock concerts or through portable radio headphones right next to your ears can, over time, paralyze the delicate sound receptor system inside the ears. The partial deafness that can result is usually irreversible.

A loud unexpected noise is usually greeted by a blast of adrenaline, as you jump and get ready to face possible danger. Loud, more or less continuous noise has the same effect, although at a lesser level. Noise is stressful because of the effect on the adrenals, and the noise levels we are exposed to keep us in the sympathetic fight-or-flight mode rather than in the parasympathetic restorative mode. The parasympathetic mode is the mode in which digestion takes place, so it follows that noise-induced or other stress can interfere with digestion and the accompanying assimilation of nutrients.

What is ultrasound and how is it used?
Ultrasound is at the high end of the sound wave part of the spectrum. If you go higher and higher on a musical scale until you can no longer hear the notes, this is the ultrasound range. Some animals such as dogs can hear notes that are a bit too high for us to hear.

Ultrasound imaging, or sonography, uses high frequency sound waves rather than ionizing radiation. A hand-held transducer is placed over the body area to be imaged, often with a slippery gel between skin and transducer to enhance conductivity. The transducer emits sound waves which penetrate the skin and bounce off tissues and organs to produce echoes which reveal the location and depth of internal structures. The principle is much the same as radar or sonar. The echoes are picked up by the transducer and are electronically converted to recognizable images on a computer screen. The images can also be recorded as a still picture or videotape.

Ultrasound is most often used on a pregnant woman to visualize the developing fetus to determine its position and development. The picture is sometimes clear enough to determine the baby's gender. Ultrasound is also used to analyze heart structure and function, for example to see whether the valves are closing properly. It can be used as well to see kidney and gallbladder function.

Is ultrasound harmless?

Ultrasound can be used nondiagnostically to clean dirt from jewelry, delicate electronic parts, and other items in liquid. It does so by causing high-speed vibrations in the liquid that vibrate dirt loose. Although the medical establishment says that ultrasound is harmless (remember that this is the same medical establishment that contends that mercury amalgam is harmless), ask yourself if you want this kind of energy vibrating through your body or that of your developing baby, even though the amount is less than that used for cleaning. The technique has not been around long enough to assess long-term effects.

On the plus side, it can provide valuable information, the procedure itself involves no discomfort, and it is cheaper than most other modern imaging techniques.

Radio Frequency

What are radio frequency waves and where are they found?

Radio and television waves are about 100 kHz to 100 mHz; these are called RF (radio frequency) waves. If you are able to receive radio and television signals, i.e. if you are anywhere other than very remote areas of the country, then these frequencies are filling the air. This is true whether or not you have receivers such as TV or radio. RF waves, not all of which are audible, include:

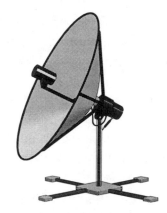

- *AM and FM radio waves of various frequencies*
- *All television channels*
- *CB radios*
- *Garage door openers*
- *TV remote controls*
- *Walkie-talkies*
- *Beepers and pagers*
- *Satellite dishes*
- *Cellular telephones*

Imagine what the air would look like if all of these waves were visible! Although they are not visible, they are passing through our bodies. Television gives off several frequencies, including 60 Hz from the electrical source, RF frequencies, sound wave frequencies, visible light frequencies, and possibly other frequencies as well. Sleeping with a nearby TV on is a significant source of EM exposure.

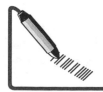

It is probable that we are exposed to radiation from shoplifting detectors in stores and libraries, from bar code readers at supermarket and department store checkouts, and from metal detectors in airports. The people who work with these sensors are exposed to much more of the radiation.

What is magnetic resonance imaging (MRI)?

Magnetic resonance imaging (MRI), which uses magnetic and radio frequency (RF) fields to view the interior of the body by bouncing magnetic frequencies off dense organs, is a valuable diagnostic technique which is probably not without risk. It is a procedure which utilizes a large high-strength magnet, radio frequency signals, and a computer to generate images of the inside of the body.

The patient is placed in the MRI scanner, which generates a magnetic field 30,000 times that of the Earth. This field surrounds the patient in order to do the scan. The technical details of the procedure would not be easily understood by the layperson, but essentially the atoms of the body align themselves with the strong magnetic field, which causes them to vibrate at a specific frequency. In so vibrating, they act as radio frequency receivers and transmitters. The scanner receives the radio signals and characterizes the body tissues based on the strength and duration of the signals. The computer reconstructs the information to produce an anatomic image.

MRI is used mostly to evaluate diseases of the brain and spine, and may eliminate the need for arteriography of the brain or myelography of the spinal column. It can also be used to study joints, and bone and soft tissue abnormalities [1].

Despite claims of its safety, MRI, like ultrasound, has not been around long enough to assess its long-term hazards. It has been demonstrated (see chapter on Electromagnetic Fields and Radiation - Basic Concepts) that even the Earth's far weaker magnetic field has an effect on living beings. It shall be left to the imagination what a magnetic field 30,000 times more powerful than this, which is capable of rearranging our atoms, can do.

On the other hand, lifesaving information can be obtained, and the test, which is very expensive, involves no discomfort other than apprehension. The potential risk should be weighed against the benefit in the use of MRI.

What are the dangers of television?

Television poses dangers - apart from the programming content - to those who watch it regularly.

Addiction can be said to be a maladaptive response to an environmental toxin, such as addiction to alcohol and other drugs. Millions of people appear to have an addiction to television. They flip channels idly, not even caring what is being shown as long as the TV set is on, often for hours at a time. A great many children are seemingly hooked on video games, which also use video display terminals similar to television. They can often play for hours, spending their money and then borrowing more to spend at the video arcade. This appears to be a genuine addiction not unlike alcohol addiction, and may be due in part to a physical maladaptive response to the radiation put out by the video display terminals. Attention span is adversely affected. Hyperactivity in children has been linked to television watching and video games.

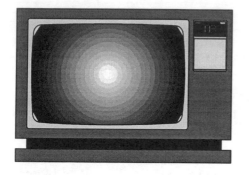

John Nash Ott, who has studied the effects of light and other radiation on living beings, did a study involving rats and television. He placed two cages of rats in front of operating television sets. The first set was shielded only with black paper, which blocked the visual image but not the radiation. The second set was shielded with a lead sheet, which blocked the radiation. The rats in the first cage became hyperactive and aggressive, and then increasingly lethargic with continued exposure. The rats in the second group behaved normally. Do the rats in the first group remind you of any children or adults you know?

In another study done by John Ott in a school for students with learning disabilities, it was found that many of the students lived in homes with an older or malfunctioning TV set. When the TV was repaired, replaced, or discarded, many of the learning disabilities improved or disappeared.

12th grade students who watched TV six or more hours a day scored 14% lower in standardized test scores than those who watched one hour or less per day [2].

Microwave Radiation

What do microwaves do besides cook food?

Microwaves are the next set of frequencies. Microwaves in a microwave oven cook food, i.e. produce permanent and killing cellular changes. A leaking gasket around the oven, more common in older ovens, can leak enough radiation to be harmful at close range. People with artificial implanted heart pacemakers are warned to keep their distance from microwave ovens in use, as enough microwave radiation can leak out to disturb the pacemaker's rhythm. It is likely that the cells of the heart's natural pacemaker, present in all of us, are also disturbed by microwave radiation. Microwaves also affect the way cells and the immune system communicate with each other.

There is some evidence that microwaving food can change its structure in a way that conventional cooking does not. Microwave ovens can cause muscle weakness in kinesiology testing at distances of six to sixty (!) feet from the oven. In an experiment [2], a hamburger with all the trimmings was cooked conventionally, and another identical hamburger was cooked in a microwave. The hamburgers were then eaten by test subjects. The microwaved burgers caused muscle weakness, while the conventionally cooked ones did not.

Microwaving a baby's formula or even mother's milk can chemically change the product. Milk heated this way can make a baby sick. The baby, whose stomach is not equipped to deal with the chemically changed (denatured) protein, may vomit and/or develop symptoms of malnutrition.

Radar guns, which employ microwaves, are used by police to determine vehicle speed and have been linked to cancer of the area of the body that the radar gun is held close to over an extended period of time, even when it is set between shootings or turned off. Testicular cancer in particular has been linked to the use of radar guns, as the gun is often held between the knees.

A look at the electromagnetic spectrum at the front of this section shows a wavelength of about a third of a meter, or about one foot, and a frequency of about 1000 megacycles, or one billion Hz. The first wavelength is 100 times as strong as the second. What this means is that if you are one wavelength, or one foot (near field), from a leaking microwave oven you are getting 100 times the microwave radiation that you would get if you stood two feet away (far field). This principle applies to other wavelengths as well, the distance vs. exposure related to the size of the particular wavelength.

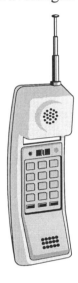

Cellular phones, relying on microwaves for transmission, are necessarily held next to the head, another potential source of cancer hazard. This was a source of concern even in the late 1980s, and will be of greater concern as cellular phone use increases. More than 10% of the American public now own cellular phones, and eight million new cellular phone customers were added in 1995 [3].

Portable cordless phones use lower voltages but are held closer to the person. It is unknown which of the two types of phones is more hazardous.

One patient developed and died of brain cancer. Soon after that, her husband, an engineer in his mid 40s, also developed brain cancer. They both had used car phones and portable house phones extensively.

Infrared Radiation

How is food kept warm in restaurants?
Infrared radiation, just below the threshold of visible light, is used for radiant heat. The reddish bulbs used to keep food warm in restaurants are infrared. Other infrared sources are flames, the sun, electric irons, steam radiators, hot pavements, and even our bodies [4]. Some saunas use infrared lights as a heat source.

Infrared film can be used to pinpoint tumors, veins, and skin problems because slight differences in temperature such as heat caused by tumor growth will show up. Infrared photography is also used to make aerial photographs to locate sources of water pollution and to provide other types of information not visible in a regular photograph. A light bulb, which radiates visible light, also radiates heat from the infrared part of the spectrum.

How can infrared radiation be used for diagnosis?
Thermography is a technique used to diagnose certain medical conditions. "Thermo", a word root found in the words thermometer, thermal, and Thermos, means heat. "Graphy" means writing, and thermography traces body heat patterns.

The technique makes use of the differences in temperature caused by certain conditions within the body. Many tumors are warmer than the surrounding tissue due to increased blood supply to the tumor site. Infections and other inflammatory processes are also hotter than their surroundings; an infection under the skin even feels hotter to the touch. On the other hand, a part of the body receiving decreased blood flow or that is underactive will often be cooler than normal.

Infrared film picks up the heat-producing infrared wavelengths of the spectrum in much the same way as regular camera film picks up the lights and colors of the visible part of the spectrum. Infrared film can be used for thermography, but usually an infrared detector is used, often linked to a computer which can enhance even slight temperature differences. A person who knows what a normal organ or tissue looks like with this technique can then spot abnormalities.

Conditions which can be diagnosed using thermography include:

- *Breast and other tumors*
- *Inflamed joints, bone infection*
- *Underactive or overactive ("cold" or "hot") thyroid gland nodes*
- *Decreased circulation in the hand or legs due to diabetes or cardiovascular problems*
- *A part of the liver or kidney that is not working properly*

Thermography, unlike most other imaging techniques, seems to be as safe as getting your picture taken. No harmful rays or wavelengths bombard the body, and nothing is injected or otherwise taken into the body.

Why are dark clothing colors hotter when worn outdoors?

Dark colors are dark because they absorb visible light wavelengths, and light colors such as white reflect light. Dark colors also absorb more of the non-visible infrared radiation than light colors. More infrared radiation is felt as more heat.

Light and Color

Which frequencies can we see?

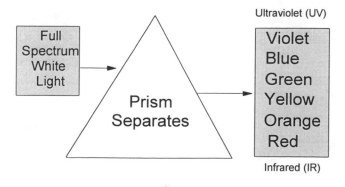

Visible light ranges from red (lowest energy, just past infrared) through orange, yellow, green, blue, to violet (highest energy, just below ultraviolet). This is the order in which colors are found in a rainbow. A prism breaks white light up into these colors in the same order. Red has a wavelength of about 700 nanometers (nm, or billionths of a meter; one meter is about three feet), while purple is about 400 nm. This distance, by comparison, is much smaller than a smoke particle. Visible light contains enough energy to stimulate cells in the retina. White light, as from the sun, light bulbs, or fluorescent tubes (especially full-spectrum fluorescent tubes), contains all light frequencies, although in slightly different proportions.

How do the wavelengths of light affect us?

Many biological responses, both good and bad, are due not just to light but to specific wavelengths within the light spectrum. If any of these wavelengths are missing in an artificial light source, or from being blocked by sunglasses or colored contact lenses, the biological receptor for that wavelength behaves as if it were completely dark. As an example, some bugs and moths are attracted to an ordinary incandescent light bulb, but appear not to see a yellow "bug light" because they lack the receptors for yellow.

Certain wavelengths (colors) of light can cure certain ailments, such as special lights for curing depression. It logically follows that lack or insufficiency of these wavelengths may cause the ailment in the first place. Light, in a sense, acts as a nutrient, and may not be all that different from vitamins or protein in the way the body needs and uses it.

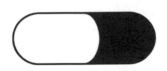

The so-called placebo effect of some drugs, in which non-active substances in colored capsules can produce relief, may be due in part to the color of the capsules themselves, if the capsule color corresponds to a color that one is deficient in.

Different minerals or metals have different frequencies, which cause different colors when used in fireworks or paints:

- *Copper*   *green-blue*
- *Cobalt*   *blue*
- *Sodium*   *yellow*
- *Strontium*   *red*
- *Magnesium*   *white*

The effect of minerals or metals may be in part related to their associated color.

How can sunglasses or colored lenses be harmful?

When light enters the eyes, it stimulates the pineal and pituitary glands which control the endocrine glandular system. Pink or amber (yellow-orange) tinted eyeglass lenses block the beneficial blue and ultraviolet (UV) wavelengths from entering the eyes, leading to endocrine deficiency due to understimulation of the pineal gland. The adrenals, thyroid, and thymus may then in turn be understimulated, leading to fatigue, insomnia, and poor quality sleep.

Some people who are blind wear very dark or opaque glasses to hide eye disfigurement. Although their sight is not affected by the glasses, it is possible that preventing light from stimulating the pineal gland may have an adverse effect on the rest of the body.

Bodies need clear day or night signals in order to function properly, as different body functions are activated at different times of the day. Jet lag is a common example of what happens when the day/night signals come at a different time than the body has come to expect. Many people get too little light during the day due to indoor jobs and the wearing of sunglasses when outside, and then get too much light at night. Such people often have depression and sleep problems due to the disruption of their day/night cycles.

Beneficial light wavelengths enter the body through the skin as well as the eyes. If this were not the case, there probably wouldn't be a healthy blind person around.

Is the effect of color on mood only psychological?

It has long been recognized that certain colors have psychological effects regardless of culture. Red is stimulating, blue is calming, etc. This may be due to biochemical effects of specific wavelengths on the cells and the endocrine glandular system. These biological effects should be considered before painting a room in which you will spend a large amount of time a strong color.

John Ott has done a number of studies on the pink/orange/yellow end of the spectrum [2]. He found in both animal and human experiments that the color pink, whether from wall paint or lights, causes muscle weakness and relaxation and reduces aggressiveness after short term exposure of about 15 minutes. Such muscle weakness is produced even in those who are color blind. However, a longer exposure of four or more hours actually increases aggressiveness.

Orange has a similar effect. Many cities have installed sodium crime lights, intended as a deterrent to crime by lighting up the city's dark corners. Sodium was chosen for economy. Ironically, the orange-yellow sodium lights may actually be increasing the crime rate by increasing aggressiveness.

Comment: Given that these wavelengths are relaxing for up to about 15 minutes, it is interesting that the pinks and oranges of sunset last for about this length of time.

How can fluorescent lights cause problems?

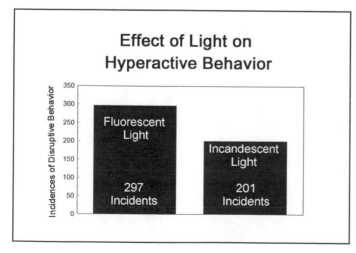

Incandescent light (ordinary light bulbs) emit light which is yellower than sunlight, and fluorescent tubes can be yellowish to bluish. Irritability and fatigue in an office environment has been linked to fluorescent light radiation. A study was done by John Ott [2] on emotionally disturbed and hyperactive students in a Santa Cruz, California, classroom. An observer counted 297 incidents of hyperactive or inappropriate behavior in a classroom lit with standard fluorescent bulbs. The following week incandescent lights were used instead, and hyperactive incidents were counted for the same time period as before. 201 incidents were reported, a 32% decrease; the only thing changed was the lighting. A number of teachers have noticed that turning off the fluorescent lights will calm an unruly class.

The ballast of a fluorescent light is a transformer. If you listen closely, a hum can be heard from the ballast when the light is on. Fluorescent lights can do damage in three ways:

- The transformer effect from the ballast

- The distorted color spectrum

- Fluorescent lights flash on and off sixty times a second. The flashing and flickering is sometimes visible in bulbs that are wearing out. The flashing, even when consciously imperceptible, fatigues the central nervous system.

Are all fluorescent lights created equal?

Anyone who has ever bought fluorescent light tubes at different stores has often found out the hard way that they can vary markedly in color, from orange-ish to bluish. These color differences may affect people in different ways. So-called full-spectrum fluorescent light bulbs are recommended, as these are closest to natural sunlight.

Fluorescent light bulbs at a small health clinic were changed to the full spectrum type, and there was a noticeable difference in the level of friction among staff working in a highly pressured environment. The constant pressure and demands in dealing with a patient load of sick and debilitated people tended to create levels of frustration and tension and a noticeable difference in lessening tensions and calmness in staff interaction was soon apparent.

What is a laser?

A laser is a light beam, highly focused at exactly one frequency, or wavelength. Lasers are in the light range of wavelengths, and can be any color. A red light bulb is a group of wavelengths of about 700 nm, and can include anything from about 650 to 725 nm. A red laser is just one frequency/wavelength, for example (but not necessarily) exactly 700 nm. This allows it to be highly focused.

How do you win a tug-of-war?

Another reason for the intense focus of lasers is the fact that all the waves of energy emitted are in phase, or are working together optimally. Think of a group of people engaged in a rug-or-war as an example of working in phase. A group of strong people all pulling on a rope in the same direction rather than in several directions at random. The people working in phase will cause the rope to move in the desired direction with the greatest efficiency. If people pulling on a rope expend their maximum energy at the same time, as in a pull-rest-pull-rest pattern, they are in phase both in direction and in time, and their effectiveness is increased still more. Lasers which are pulsed, with their waves synchronized, share this phenomenon.

Lasers can be "hot" or "cold". Hot lasers can burn tissue, and are increasingly used instead of scalpels in some types of surgery, as they can be aimed very precisely. Cold lasers are sometimes used in art, or as a supermarket price scanning device.

The difference between hot and cold lasers is the amount of power used to produce the desired effect, and whether the power is continuous (hot) or on-and-off many times a second (cold). Hot lasers can incinerate cells in a fraction of a second. Cold lasers do not produce any obvious damage in the short run, but it is logical and possible that longer exposure to the lower power lasers can cause damage cumulatively.

Supermarket checkout personnel who pass their hand over a cold laser beam many times a minute and stand next to the laser generating device for hours every day may be endangering their health. These devices have not been in use long enough to say for certain that they are safe long-term, and those who use them should be aware of the potential danger.

Lasers are used in meridian balancing instead of needles by some acupuncturists. It follows that careless exposure to lasers can cause imbalance.

Ultraviolet

What kinds of rays from the sun can burn us?

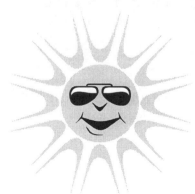

Ultraviolet (UV) light is just beyond the violet. Near UV (lower energy) is required for bodily function, while far UV (higher energy) is toxic. Blacklights are deep purple UV tubes which cause certain colors to glow brightly through the stimulation of the light on fluorescent paint. Blacklights emit enough energy to damage the eyes if stared at for long, even though the light isn't bright at all. UV rays from the sun can be responsible for sunburn and skin damage, including cancer, although small amounts of sunlight are necessary for the metabolism of vitamin D in the skin and for stimulating the pituitary gland.

Tanning lamps utilize UV radiation, but while they can tan you faster than the sun, they are also capable of causing more damage in a shorter period of time. Ultraviolet waves can kill microbes, so they are sometimes used for disinfectant purposes. However, an amount of energy sufficient to kill microbes, which are cells, is also sufficient to kill or at least damage the cells of our bodies.

What problems can be caused by sunglasses or contact lenses?

As discussed previously in this chapter, certain light wavelengths can be blocked by sunglasses or contact lenses, especially colored ones. In addition, UV light has its effect. The eye pupil muscle (the iris) contracts in response to UV light. In an experiment [2], test subjects wore a UV transmitting contact lens on one eye and a UV blocking lens on the other. There was no difference indoors, but the pupil in the eye with the UV transmitting lens contracted more than the other outdoors.

The pupil contraction is a normal response which keeps too much light and UV radiation from entering the eye. When this response is blocked, as by most contact lenses, especially colored ones, the pupils do not contract as much as they should and too much light, in an imbalance of frequencies, enters the eye. This causes squinting, eyestrain, and light sensitivity. The wearer of the lenses then feels the need for sunglasses, which makes the problem worse. Sunglasses, which are intended to reduce the amount of light reaching the eye, actually open the pupil and let more light in for the same reason as do contact lenses. Most contact lenses, glasses, sunglasses, windows, and car windshields block UV rays unless specified otherwise.

Ionizing radiation starts at the far UV range, just before x-rays.

X-Rays

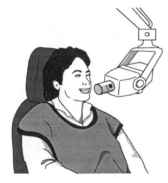

How are x-rays used?
X-rays are useful for taking pictures of bones, teeth, and to a lesser extent soft tissue. They are able to penetrate tissue and cells, and so can be quite dangerous. X-ray exposure is cumulative, so the fewer x-ray pictures taken, the better. CAT scans (Computerized Axial Tomography) take a visual slice from the body by bombarding a section of the body with x-rays from all directions, and so the x-ray exposure is considerable.

Ironically, x-ray technicians hide behind walls and lead shields while doing x-rays, and at the same time assure you that your x-ray exposure, which is much more direct and at closer range, is essentially harmless.

Wear a lead apron or shield when having x-rays done, especially over the neck and pelvis to protect the thyroid gland and reproductive organs. You may have to insist on this, as technicians, doctors and dentists may not want to bother with the shield and might try to convince you that you are worrying unnecessarily. Insist anyway.

Does this hazard mean that x-rays and CAT scans should never be used?
These can be valuable diagnostic tools, but there is danger involved. The risk should be weighed against the benefits. The danger of x-rays can be lessened by taking iodine (not the same as radioactive iodine), preferably in the safer form of liquid dulse, and the antioxidant nutrients vitamin A, vitamin C, and zinc.

X-rays are used in high doses to treat some medical conditions, most notably cancer, because they are well known to be potent cell killers. Ironically, x-rays themselves are quite carcinogenic due to free radical damage. A tumor that recurs years after x-ray treatment may well be the result of the treatment itself rather than part of the original cancer.

What are some of the imaging procedures using x-rays?
The film x-rays taken at the dentist or for diagnosing a broken arm are the most common x-ray procedures, but they are not the only ones. Others include:

- *Mammography*
- *CAT scans*
- *Fluoroscopy*
- *Angiography*

Film x-rays are one of the oldest imaging techniques. Interestingly, and perhaps not coincidentally, the doctor who discovered the technique died of cancer back when cancer was far less prevalent than it is today.

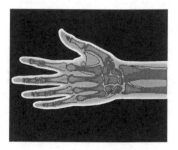

X-rays pass through body tissue and are absorbed to a greater or lesser degree by body tissues depending on their density. The x-rays pass through the body or body part and make an image on film.

Dense structures such as bone block, or absorb, x-rays the most, and show up on film as white areas. Air and fat block x-rays the least, and are darkest on the film.

The most common film x-rays are dental x-rays, chest x-rays for lung diseases, and diagnosis of broken bones. X-rays are also used for the abdomen, spine, sinuses, skull, and kidneys.

Mammography is an x-ray examination of the breast. It can detect tumors too small to be felt, especially if deep in the breast. The earlier any tumor is found, the higher the cure rate. There is some discomfort to the procedure; the breast is flattened top to bottom and then side to side between plastic plates for best visualization. Newer mammography machines, used only for this purpose and called "dedicated", emit lower doses of radiation than older machines.

Any amount of radiation is dangerous as described in the chapter on Electromagnetic Fields and Radiation - Basic Concepts, and the results are cumulative. It is an undisputed fact that x-rays are themselves carcinogenic (cancer causing). It is argued that the low dose of radiation provides less risk than benefit. Many women who undergo mammography have a family history, or genetic susceptibility, to breast cancer, and are at an age (over 40) when the disease most often starts. Is it possible that directly bombarding the breast of such a woman with x-rays in even a low dose triggers as many tumors as it detects?

It's sobering to consider that exposure to ionizing radiation, primarily medical and dental x-rays, might have a causative effect in possibly 75% of breast cancers. [5]

Fluoroscopy is an x-ray technique which provides a moving image over time. First developed in 1896, it uses a source of x-rays, a fluoroscopic screen, and more recently an image enhancer to intensify the image while requiring a lower dose of x-rays. It is used to view organs at work, including the heart, diaphragm movement, gastrointestinal function, and angiography. Those readers over the age of forty may remember fluoroscopes in shoe stores, where as children you may have watched your greenish foot bones wiggle in your new shoes. The advantage of fluoroscopy is in getting a dynamic picture of how part of the body works. The hazards are the same as for other x-ray techniques.

Angiography is the radiologic study of blood vessels. Arteriograms and venograms are studies of arteries and veins respectively. Since they are not normally visible to x-ray, a radiopaque iodine compound is injected for contrast. Angiograms can be still pictures or fluoroscopic (moving), or a series of still pictures which performs the function of fluoroscopy. Some abnormalities detected by angiography are:

- *Narrowing of blood vessels by arteriosclerosis*

- *Clogging of blood vessels which could lead to stroke or heart attacks if not treated*

- *A diffuse pool of blood, indicating internal bleeding*

- *A dense growth of blood vessels, indicating the presence and location of a tumor*

- *Diminished blood flow to an organ or extremity*

The angiographic technique involves inserting a long narrow catheter (tube) through a needle puncture in an artery, usually in the groin. The catheter is carefully threaded through the arterial system, guided by fluoroscopy, until it reaches the desired location. The contrast medium is then injected.

A relatively new angiographic technique is digital subtraction angiography, in which pictures of the area of interest are taken both before and after injection of the contrast medium. The first image is subtracted from the second by computer to provide an unobstructed picture of the blood vessels alone. Although more expensive than traditional angiography because of the equipment required, digital subtraction angiography requires less of the potentially hazardous contrast medium.

The contrast medium in either case diffuses through all of the blood vessels and is eventually eliminated. While flowing through the brain, it has been reported by many patients to cause headaches and optical disturbances such as bright flashes of light. Nearly all patients report some discomfort due to the contrast medium, such as a burning sensation.

Computerized axial tomography, or computerized tomography (CAT or CT scan) is a scanning technique which combines x-rays with computer technology. The patient is positioned on a narrow table that slides into the large tubelike scanner. The scanner emits a very narrow x-ray beam continuously as it rotates around the body, and the image is recorded by a detector opposite the x-ray source. The detector emits tiny flashes of light in proportion to the amount of x-radiation it receives, which itself is a function of tissue density. The computer collects these tiny light flashes as data points, and fashions an image that is the equivalent of an axial slice of the body, i.e. a slice perpendicular to the long axis of the body. CT scans can also be used to visualize the interior of an individual organ. Three-dimensional images can be generated using specialized computer software. The test is very expensive due to the complexity of the equipment, and is not without its hazards due to multiple x-ray exposure.

Are there hazards of x-ray procedures other than the x-rays themselves?

Contrast media are compounds which are radiopaque, or block x-rays. They are used to outline certain anatomic structures to distinguish them from nearby tissues of similar density. They have their dangers, some of which have been mentioned already.

Barium compounds form a chalklike liquid material which is swallowed or given as an enema to visualize the upper or lower gastrointestinal tract respectively. The barium is eventually excreted in the feces. Both still x-ray pictures and fluoroscopic (moving) pictures can be taken of the digestive tract using barium. It is well known that barium is extremely toxic, but its use is defended on the grounds that barium salts are insoluble in water and therefore will not be absorbed into and react with body tissues. A chemist knows that everything is soluble if only to a very limited degree, even metal in water. It follows that barium will in fact enter the bloodstream and react, and even if the amount involved is very tiny it is inadvisable to have something this toxic in the body. As with all of these diagnostic procedures that have potential for harm, the benefit may still outweigh the risk. It is important to know the risk to help make this determination.

Iodine-containing compounds are also radiopaque. They can be:

- *Injected into arteries and veins (angiography) to detect abnormalities*
- *Injected into the spinal cord to study it and the spinal nerves*
- *Used to study the shape and function of the kidneys*
- *Used to enhance images of CAT scans*

Iodine is one of a chemical group called the halogens, which also include chlorine, fluorine, and bromine. Although chlorine and iodine are needed by the body in very small amounts, all halogenated compounds are toxic to a greater or lesser extent.

Gamma Rays

What are the highest frequencies?

Gamma rays come from space and thermonuclear explosions. Cosmic rays come from space. These powerful ionizing frequencies are largely shielded by our atmosphere. However, airplane flight crew members and frequent fliers are at higher cancer risk from cosmic radiation than is the general public. 220 people out of 1000 will die, statistically, from any kind of cancer. After

20 years of flying, flight crews and frequent fliers will add 10 (230 per 1000) and 5 (225 per 1000) more cancer deaths per 1000 respectively [6].

This increase in death rate, however, could also be due in part to the closed-in cabin and accumulative, detrimental effects of breathing stale air (see Air Pollution chapter).

The free particles of such high frequency ionizing radiation are detectable using a Geiger counter. Each individual click heard is a free particle hitting a detector.

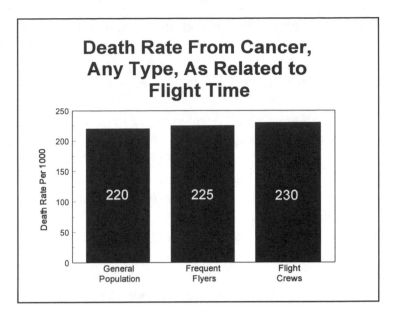

How can gamma rays be used diagnostically?

Nuclear medicine uses radionuclides, which are radioactive compounds that emit gamma (or sometimes beta) rays. The method of ingestion - swallowing, inhalation, or injection - and the type of compound used allow the radionuclide to collect temporarily in the part(s) of the body to be studied. A camera sensitive to gamma radiation is suspended above the patient who is lying on the examining table, and it records the distribution of the radionuclide within the body. This image is called a scintigram.

A heart scan is used to evaluate cardiac function, and a bone scan can detect cancer or infection. Although bone and heart scans are most common, scintigrams are also used to evaluate the lungs, liver, gallbladder, kidney, thyroid gland, and brain.

As mentioned, gamma rays are among the highest electromagnetic frequencies, higher even than x-rays. Would you want such a radioactive compound to be deliberately placed into your body?

Positron emission tomography (PET) is used to study the metabolic activity inside an organ. It has been shown to be useful in the study of brain disorders such as epilepsy and Alzheimer's disease. Single-photon emission computed tomography (SPECT) is used to obtain visual thin slices of organs such as the heart, brain, and liver in greater detail than with scintigrams [1].

Food Irradiation

Is food irradiation dangerous?

Irradiation of food has been in the news, and has been the cause of some controversy. Proponents say that irradiating food kills bacteria, molds, and parasites, which is true. It allows foods that otherwise need refrigeration or freezing to be kept on the shelf, including juice and milk in individual serving boxes, and even whole entrees and dinners. It increases shelf life for many types of foods, including fresh fruits, vegetables, meats, herbs and spices. This translates into greater corporate profits, since there is less spoiled, unsaleable food. Proponents also give the assurance that irradiation leaves no residue on the food, nor does it make the food radioactive.

However, there is another side to the story. The frequencies involved are, of necessity, sufficient to kill and mutate cells (bacteria and parasites are cells, as are once-live foods such as vegetables and meat), and it is not known what taking these damaged cells and the resulting enzyme-free dead food into our bodies will do over time. Experiments have shown that irradiated foods produce tumors and kidney abnormalities in test animals, and therefore potentially in humans. Long term human toxicity studies have not been done, and cancer can take decades to develop. In addition, the new irradiating plants that are being built are adding radiation to the environment, which will affect all of us, including those who avoid irradiated food.

The radiation of food exposes the foods to radiation doses from 100,000 to 6,000,000 times that of a chest x-ray. Food irradiation can cause fats in food to turn rancid, which affects not just taste, but health (see Oils and Fats chapter in *Thriving In A Toxic World*). Irradiation can also be responsible for the destruction of lifegiving enzymes. As of 1993, several food companies including HJ Heinz, Quaker Oats, Ralston Purina, McDonald's and Campbell's refuse to use irradiated foods. Also as of 1993, Maine, New York and New Jersey prohibit the sale of irradiated food. 37 radiation facilities use nuclear waste to sterilize medical equipment, tampons and sanitary napkins [7].

Food irradiation kills enzymes, coenzymes, and nutrients, making the food harder to digest and less nutritious. Nutrient losses have been linked to food irradiation, especially the loss of vitamins A, B, E and K. It also causes brown discoloration of raw meat and softening of fruit [8].

Does it make sense that mutated enzyme-free dead food can be expected to feed and nourish a healthy body?

Many European countries do not irradiate food. They appear to be watching us, the guinea pigs, to find out the long term effects of irradiation before they will permit it.

Does irradiation prevent food poisoning - or contribute to it?
Salmonella is a type of bacteria which causes food poisoning characterized by gastrointestinal distress. It rarely causes complications or death. However, the botulinus bacterium releases potent toxins which cause botulism, a type of food poisoning which can cause nerve damage and can be fatal. Both types of bacteria grow and multiply in food which is improperly stored. Salmonella causes a foul odor, while botulinus is odorless. Irradiation kills salmonella but not botulinus. Spoiled nonirradiated food will therefore have an odor which will keep the consumer from eating it and possibly ingesting the deadly botulinus. Irradiating food, by killing only the salmonella, may keep nature's warning signal from operating, with serious consequences. Leave these two together - breaking up can be hard on you.

How can you recognize irradiated foods?

Proposed legislation to inform the consumer that food is irradiated has been fought by the food industry, who claim that the word "irradiated" might create panic and an irrational fear that this food would glow in the dark. As a compromise measure, a symbol called a radura is placed on some, but not all, irradiated food, without explanation. This cute little stylized flower in a circle is deliberately misleading and evokes images of health, nature, and the environment.

Existing Radura

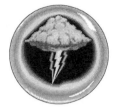
Proposed Radura

Cigarette commercials often use the same tactic, using symbols such as the Marlboro man. Very few people are aware of what the radura means. A picture of a nuclear mushroom cloud or a lightning bolt might be more appropriate and convey more information.

If you want to avoid irradiated food, look for the radura on food products, avoid single serving beverages in flat boxes with straws (usually sold in three-packs), avoid on-shelf (non-frozen) boxed entrees and dinners, and shop at health food stores. These precautions will minimize, but not eliminate, exposure to irradiated foods.

The radura is not found on foods sold in some states such as California because irradiated food is prohibited in these states at the time of this book writing.

Solutions that could save your life

What can be done about the hazards of electromagnetic and radiation pollution?

There are four approaches, and all four should be utilized for best effect:

- *Get involved on a community level.*

- *Avoid as much future radiation exposure as possible.*

- *Use foods, herbs, and nutrients such as iodine, vitamins A and C, and zinc to detoxify your body.*

- *Build up your immune system.*

Get involved. Educate your neighbors and organize against electrical wire grids in your neighborhood, lobby for consumer information on irradiated foods and electrical appliances, push for better shielding of computer terminals and microwave ovens, make the higher-ups at your workplace aware of office safety, and choose not to use unsafe products (vote with your dollars). Research and inform people in positions of political and other power of radiation dangers.

Avoid exposure to radiation whenever possible. Now that you are aware of the dangers - and there are many books and articles to increase your awareness - you can make informed risk-versus-benefit decisions. Some suggestions:

- Use an EM field detector (Gauss meter) to find areas of concentrated EM fields in your bedroom wall, and relocate your bed to a safer spot. Alternatively, sleep with your head away from the wall.

- A television generates EM fields even when not in use as a response to consumer demand for an instant-on or remote controlled picture. Unplug the set when not in use, or at least keep it over ten feet from your bed even if it's on the other side of the wall.

- Avoid irradiated foods when possible.

- Avoid unnecessary x-rays. Obtain copies of previous x-rays when changing dentists or doctors so the new doctor won't need to make a new set.

- Electromagnetic shielding for your home or appliances is available. There are also certain types of transmitters that can smooth out EMFs in a building.

- Avoid car phones, portable phones, and radar.

- Natural earth radiation, found in nodes, is not harmless. Cats like these nodes; if your cat likes to sleep on your bed, especially near where you put your head, consider changing the bed location or sleeping position.

What You Can Do

What can you do if you have already been exposed to radiation of any type?
The foods, minerals, and vitamins which detoxify the body are essentially those that build up the immune system, as detailed in the Supporters section in ***Thriving In A Toxic World***. Books on the subject of healing the body specifically from radiation exposure are available [9]. Other immune system building methods, described throughout this book and especially the in Supporters section in ***Thriving In A Toxic World***, will help the body resist cellular changes caused by electromagnetic radiation. Some of these methods, foods and substances include:

- *Calcium*

- *Vitamins A and E*

- *Zinc, copper*

- *Antioxidants to counteract free radical damage*

- *Bioflavonoids - rutin, grape seed extract, quercetin, pycnogenol*

- *Iodine, preferably in a natural form such as Liqui-Dulse, helps protect the thyroid gland, a particular target of radiation.*

- *Sea vegetables such as arame, wakame, hijiki and kombu are a good natural source of iodine and other nutrients.*

- *Bee pollen and propolis*

- *Garlic (such as Kyolic brand) and onion are good sources of the detoxifying mineral sulfur.*

- *Chlorophyll, Sun Chlorella*

- *Oils, especially olive and fish liver oils*

Summary

Protecting yourself against electromagnetic radiation of any type is a three-step procedure:

- Become aware, through self-education and the use of an EM field detector, where the radiation sources are in your home and your life.

- Avoid sources of radiation whenever possible.

- Build up your immune system through proper nutrition, avoidance of other toxins, and taking antioxidants.

References and Resources

General

- The Burton Goldberg Group, ***Alternative Medicine: The Definitive Guide***, Future Medicine Publishing, Puyallup WA, 1994. *The following chapters discuss therapies related to electromagnetic frequencies:*

"Energy Medicine"	pp. 192-204
"Light Therapy"	pp. 319-329
"Sound Therapy"	pp. 439-449

- Schechter, Steven R., ***Fighting Radiation with Foods, Herbs, and Vitamins***, East West Health Books, Brookline MA, 1988.

Sound

- Black, D., ***Healing With Sound***, Tapestry Press, Springville UT, 1991.

- Glass, L. and MC Mackey, ***From Clocks to Chaos - The Rhythms of Life***, Princeton University Press, Princeton NJ, 1988. *Sound Therapy.*

Light

- Ott, John Nash, ***Light, Radiation, and You***, The Devin-Adair Co., Old Greenwich CT, 1982.

- Freeman, Ira M., ***Light and Radiation***, Random House, NY, 1968.

X-Rays

- Gofman, John W., ***Preventing Breast Cancer: The Story of a Major, Proven, Preventable Cause of the Disease***, Committee for Nuclear Responsibility, San Francisco CA, 1995. *Discusses the connection between x-rays and breast cancer.*

Food Irradiation

- Webb, Tony, Tom Lang and Kathleen Tucker, ***Food Irradiation:Who Wants It?***, Thorsons Publishers Inc., Rochester VT, 1987.

- Millichap, J. Gordon, ***Environmental Poisons In Our Food***, PNB Publishers, Chicago IL, 1993. *Covers many types of environmental toxins in food, including discussion of the dangers of food irradiation.*

- **Consumers United for Food Safety**, P.O. Box 22928, Seattle WA 98122, phone 206-747-2659. *Information on food irradiation.*

Primary Toxic Suppressors

-

Structural Problems

STRUCTURAL MISALIGNMENTS

Balancing The Unbalanced Body

Do you have any of the following symptoms? They may be caused by a structural problem.

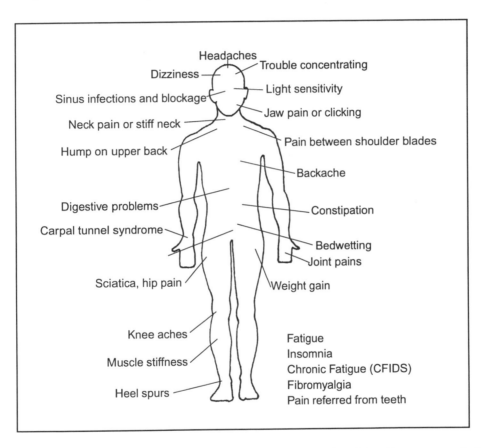

Do any of the following apply to you? If so, information in this chapter and the next one can have a powerful impact on your health.

- *Were you or your children delivered by forceps? Forceps injuries can cause spinal misalignments and resulting symptoms which can be mistaken for a birth defect.*

- *Did you ever have a concussion, whiplash, traumatic fall, sports injury, orthodontic braces, dental crowns, or a blow to the face?*

- *Did you know that allergy, toxicity, or infection can cause spinal defects and vice versa?*

- *Have you recently given birth, or are you planning to do so in the future? Learn why it is important to have a spinal and pelvic adjustment within a few months of having a baby.*

- *Do you carry a heavy purse over one shoulder, or a wallet in your hip pocket?*

- *Do you have impotence or other sexual problems? A correctable misalignment in the lower back may be the cause.*

- *Do you know why many women gain weight after a Cesarean birth?*

- *Do you go to a chiropractor but only get temporary relief? An understanding and appropriate treatment of secondary structural problems, discussed in this chapter, can lead to permanent and lasting relief.*

- *Did you know that chiropractors and osteopaths specialize, and you may be going to the wrong type for your particular problem?*

- *Do you have a dental bridge spanning your two top front teeth? You may be setting the stage for autoimmune disorders as well as head, neck and low back problems.*

- *Do you have any symptoms at all? They just might be caused, at least in part, by a structural problem. Some of these problems include:*

Headaches	*Fatigue*	*Digestive problems*
Light sensitivity	*Brain fog*	*Depression*
Problems with the knee, foot, shoulder, elbow, wrist, neck, low back		

- *Did you know that there is a lot more to structural problems and their associated symptoms than just spinal misalignments:*

Cranial	*Whiplash*	*Hips*
Dentures	*Dental bridges*	*Meningeal contractions*
TMJ and TMD	*Forceps delivery*	*Unbalanced feet*

  These can cause:

Allergy	*Toxicity*	*Emotional problems*
Digestive problems	*Infection*	*Meningeal contractions*

- *Structural problems are a component of the symptom or problem in over 80% of people's chronic health issues.*

How can problems with your spine lead to all these diverse symptoms?

There are many types of structural defects or problems possible in the body, either inborn or acquired. These include malformed organs, damaged heart valves, muscle and skin injuries, and spinal problems. The focus of this chapter is on musculoskeletal injuries and anomalies, especially spinal subluxations, or misalignments (vertebrae out of place). These subluxations can affect every organ and system in the body, depending on their location. They can cause back or neck pain, not surprisingly, but they can also be responsible for ailments as diverse as headaches, vision problems, digestive difficulties, and even faulty immune system function. This diversity is because nerves, blood, and fluids go from the spine area to all parts of the body.

These nerves also go from the parts of the body back to the spine to complete a feedback loop. This is like a stereo system which has both input and output cables between the amplifier and the tape deck.

Why is the anatomy of the spine significant?
To understand what spinal subluxations are and how they can affect the entire body, it is first necessary to have an understanding of the anatomy of the spine. It is particularly important to see the relationship between the vertebrae and the spinal nerves.

What is the spine made of?
The spinal column is a S-shaped flexible column of bones that extends down the back from the base of the skull to the hips. These bones are called vertebrae (singular: vertebra), which are named from the Latin word vertere, meaning "to turn". The vertebrae are held together by ligaments, which are connective tissue. This connective tissue is like plastic (less flexible) rather than rubber. A system of muscles attaches to the vertebrae, and these muscles together with the flexible ligaments allow the spine to rotate, flex, and bend in all directions, up to a point.

The spinal cord pushes through an opening between each of the vertebrae. The spinal cord, which originates in the brain and hangs downward, carries all of the messages from the brain and is necessary for life. Nerve impulses regulate every organ's function, and these impulses are carried down the spinal cord, through the spinal nerves, and to the organs and muscles. Sensations such as pain, touch, and heat are carried in the reverse direction to the brain.

The meningeal system is the covering of the brain and spinal cord. This can cause your muscles to tighten down as a counterbalancing or stabilizing agent in response to toxins, infection, or allergens, and cause the spine to go out of alignment. The converse is also true.

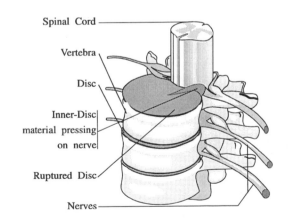

The delicate spinal cord is surrounded on all sides by vertebral bone for protection. The 31 pairs of spinal nerves branch off of the spinal cord and pass through vertebral notches called foramina (singular: foramen).

What are the different types of vertebrae?
The spine, which is normally about 24 to 28 inches long in an adult, contains four curves (two S-curves) to optimize load bearing and shock absorption. The 33 vertebrae which make up the spine are, from top to bottom:

- Seven **cervical** vertebrae in the neck, which curve forward. The top one, which supports the head, is called the atlas, named after the Titan in Greek mythology who supported the world on his shoulders. The cervical vertebrae are abbreviated C-1 (the Atlas) and C-2 (the Axis, so named because of its turning capability) through C-7. The Axis is the pivot for the Atlas. These vertebrae are sometimes called 1C to 7C.

- Twelve medium sized **thoracic** vertebrae, which curve backward, running from the shoulder area to mid-back. This is the area that supports the ribs. These vertebrae are designated T-1 (uppermost) to T-12.

- Five **lumbar** vertebrae. These are the largest and heaviest vertebrae, and they support the weight of the upper body. They are located in the area of the waist, curve towards the front of the body, and are designated L-1 to L-5.

- Five **sacral** vertebrae, which curve backward. These are separate in childhood, but fuse by adulthood to form the sacrum.

Atlas
Axis
Cervical spine
Thoracic spine
Lumbar spine
Sacrum
Coccyx

- Four (sometimes five) tiny bones are fused together to form the **coccyx**. The coccyx (usually pronounced cock-six) is also called the tailbone, as it is located where animals have tails.

Some books say there are 24 vertebrae rather than 33. They are counting only the non-fused vertebrae so those sources are equally correct.

How is the spinal cord like a telephone line?

The spinal cord carries information from the brain to the organs and muscles via the spinal nerves. The spinal cord can be compared to the main telephone line running down a street. The spinal nerves, like a series circuit, are then comparable to the phone lines leading to individual houses. If the main line is cut or badly damaged, all houses beyond that point do not receive their messages. Similarly, if the spinal cord is severed, everything controlled by regions below the break will not work, nor will the brain sense the messages from these areas. If individual phone lines are damaged, pinched, twisted, or short-circuited, communications to the house will be garbled by static. In the same way, pinched or damaged spinal nerves will not communicate at full capacity with the organ or body part that they lead to.

The picture at right shows the nerves from the brain and spinal cord going out towards the rest of the body.

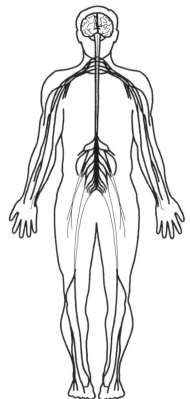

What are subluxations?

Subluxations are caused by vertebrae being out of alignment. The misaligned vertebra indirectly pinches one or more spinal nerves, like a water hose which is pinched and thus delivers less water. Anything served by that nerve will function less than optimally as a result.

The classic view of subluxation has been the idea that the subluxed vertebra pinches the nerve directly. Anatomically this is incorrect, or at least incomplete. The subluxed bone compresses the intervertebral foramen (IVF), which in turn compresses the spinal nerve, artery, and vein which are surrounded by fatty tissue and run through the IVF.

How do subluxations damage organs and muscles?

Sustained compression of the nerve will cause the nerve to first hyperfunction, then hypofunction, and finally not function at all. For example, if the nerve leads to a muscle, the muscle may first go into spasm (hyperfunction), then become weak (hypofunction), and may finally go into a state of flaccid paralysis (no function) if untreated. In another example, if the nerve leads to the skin, the first stage may be skin hypersensitivity or itching, then progressive numbness may follow.

After treatment, itching and pain may return temporarily. This is a sign of improvement.

What is the connection between nerves, muscles, and organs?

Nerves weave over and under muscles on their way to organs. Muscles can contract due to non-nerve-related causes such as calcium deficiency or overexercise. This contraction can affect nerves which in turn affect the associated organs.

Referred pain is another example of the interrelatedness of nerves, muscles, and organs. Let's say the gallbladder is infested with parasites. The T5 spinal nerve leading from the spine between the shoulder blades to the gallbladder is affected, and the impulse can "jump the tracks" to adjacent nerves serving muscles and other organs. The nerve-muscle-organ connection can also explain why some women have low back pain during their periods when the back muscles are nowhere near the uterus.

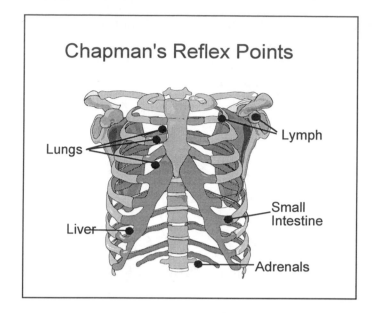

Chapman's Reflex Points

Pressure on certain body points (nerves and muscles), applied with a finger, can affect particular organs. The application of this technique is Chapman's reflexes, taken from osteopathy. If you know what to do, you can treat yourself using these points. Chapman's reflexes can also be used to help with diagnosis - the technique can point to a liver problem, kidney problem, etc. A few representative Chapman's Reflex points are pictured.

Which spinal nerves serve which parts of the body?

It is known which spinal nerves serve which parts of the body based on human and animal dissections and on observation of people whose nerves have been cut due to accident or trauma. The following list shows some of the areas controlled by the nerves from each vertebra and some of the effects that can be caused by a subluxation in that area. It should be noted, however, that the human body is more complex than is indicated by this list, and few of the conditions listed are totally under the control of one nerve.

Blood vessels are also compressed by subluxations, and these compressions also have deleterious effects on the rest of the body.

The Chinese have recently shown us galvanic or surface feedback energy systems (like a lie detector) which can change blood, pain, and function by putting small needles in junction boxes called trigger points. This is additional evidence that small changes in nerves can cause major changes in the body.

Vertebra	Areas	Effects
C-1	Head, pituitary gland, brain, ear, sympathetic nervous system	Headaches, fatigue, dizziness, high blood pressure
C-2	Eyes, sinuses, tongue	Sinus problems, allergies, eye problems
C-3	Teeth, facial nerves	Neuralgia, acne, eczema
C-4	Nose, mouth	Hay fever
C-5	Vocal cords, neck glands	Laryngitis, throat problems
C-6	Neck muscles, shoulders	Stiff neck, croup
C-7	Thyroid gland, shoulder bursae, elbows, wrists	Bursitis, thyroid conditions Carpal tunnel syndrome

T-1	Arms, hands, esophagus	Asthma, cough, difficult breathing, pain in arms and wrists
T-2	Heart, coronary arteries	Heart and chest conditions
T-3	Lungs, chest	Bronchitis, influenza, congestion, pneumonia
T-4	Gallbladder	Gallbladder problems, jaundice, shingles
T-5	Liver, solar plexus, gallbladder	Liver conditions, fevers, blood anemia, poor circulation, arthritis, low blood pressure
T-6	Stomach	Indigestion, stomach problems
T-7	Pancreas, duodenum	Ulcers, gastritis
T-8	Spleen, diaphragm	Hiccups, lowered resistance
T-9	Adrenals	Allergies, hives
T-10	Kidneys	Kidney trouble, chronic tiredness, arteriosclerosis
T-11	Kidneys, ureters	Skin conditions, eczema, boils
T-12	Small intestine, lymph	Rheumatism, gas pains
L-1	Large intestine	Constipation, diarrhea, hernias, colitis
L-2	Appendix, upper leg, abdomen	Cramps, difficult breathing, varicose veins
L-3	Sex organs, bladder, knees	Bladder problems, menstrual problems, impotence, knee pains, bedwetting
L-4	Prostate gland, lower back muscles	Sciatica, backaches, urination problems
L-5	Lower legs, feet, ankles	Poor leg circulation, weak ankles, leg cramps
Sacrum	Hip bones, buttocks	Sacroiliac conditions, spinal curvatures
Coccyx	Rectum, anus	Hemorrhoids

Subluxations in these areas can cause the indicated problems in the body, but the converse is also true. Problems in the certain organs or systems can send signals through the spinal nerves and cause subluxations of the associated vertebrae. For example, gallbladder problems caused by parasites, mercury, sludge, or gallstones can lead to subluxation in the T4-T5 area. This misalignment can result in pain between the shoulder blades, tight trapezius muscles, neckaches, and headaches. Problems with the tailbone can lead to constipation, and conversely constipation from non-structural causes can affect the tailbone.

Are there other nerves involved besides the spinal nerves?
Both cranial and spinal nerves are involved in the body's function. Autonomic nerves (those which control non-voluntary or automatic activities such as heartbeat and digestion) are divided

into two categories by function: sympathetic (fight-or-flight) and parasympathetic (repair, restore, digest). The nerves are also divided into two categories by structure: cranial (skull) and spinal. Most sympathetic and a few parasympathetic nerves are found in the spinal region. Cranial nerves are about a 50-50 split between sympathetic and parasympathetic.

It is necessary to have both sympathetic and parasympathetic responses in good working order to have proper bodily function. By way of analogy, both the plumbing and electrical systems serve your dishwasher. If one of these two doesn't function, it doesn't matter whether the other does. The dishwasher still won't work. Similarly, the vagus nerve, for example, exits the skull and travels down the front of the neck. It is the parasympathetic nerve which controls digestion. The sympathetic nerve which affects digestion is the spinal nerve from the T6 vertebra. Both are needed for digestion. For this reason, both spinal adjustment and the lesser-known cranial adjustment (discussed later in this chapter) may be needed to restore proper function.

How do subluxations occur?

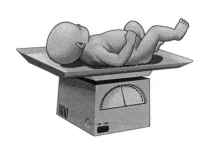

Subluxations are acquired in a number of ways. They may be present before birth, perhaps due to a less than optimal position in the uterus. Subluxations often occur during birth, such as a torsion (twisting) injury or partial dislocation of the infant's neck, pelvic, and hip bones. Birth subluxations are especially common when forceps are used, and forceps injuries may be mistaken for a congenital defect. Immediately after birth, the newborn's body, curled up for nine months, may be abruptly straightened by the doctor. The baby's cry at this time may not be entirely a reflex to stimulate the lungs, but may instead be a cry of pain from having the vertebrae moved suddenly and unnaturally. In addition, delivery room nurses usually pull the baby full length within an hour of birth to get its length measurement for the delivery record.

The stress of childbirth can cause misalignment of the mother's pelvic and pubic bones, with resulting pain and an uneven walking gait. This can be easily corrected if the adjustment is done within a month or so after the birth.

Babies and children fall, roll, slide, and stumble while learning to walk and while playing, and may sustain injuries that leave no lasting effects. However, minor misalignments caused by these mishaps can cause problems later on.

Are subluxations always a primary injury?

Subluxations can be either primary or secondary. In primary, or acute, cases the problem is directly caused by an external event such as whiplash, a concussion, or a heavy purse worn habitually over one shoulder. Primary subluxations are usually fully correctable with chiropractic or other spinal manipulation if they are caught early.

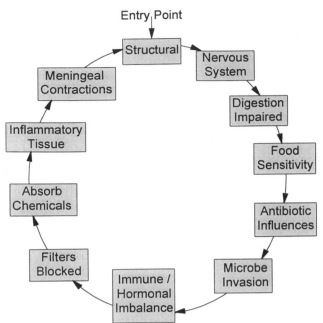

Entry Point
Structural
Nervous System
Meningeal Contractions
Digestion Impaired
Inflammatory Tissue
Food Sensitivity
Absorb Chemicals
Antibiotic Influences
Filters Blocked
Microbe Invasion
Immune / Hormonal Imbalance

Secondary subluxation can be caused by meningeal or muscle contraction which in turn can be caused by toxins, allergy, stress, parasites, fungus, or dental work. Repeated treatment will not correct the subluxation or its attendant symptoms, at least not for very long, until and unless the underlying cause is also dealt with.

It is possible for secondary subluxations to clear up once the causes of the subluxation have been dealt with, although this does not always happen. One patient had an x-ray of her neck done by a chiropractor, and the x-ray showed a cervical spine that was ruler straight, a condition sometimes called "military spine", rather than with its normal curve. She was treated for multiple chronic problems, including exposure to chemicals. An x-ray of her neck taken after treatment, and about six years after the first x-ray, showed a cervical spine with a nearly normal curve The meningeal contractions from the chemicals and toxins relaxed after treatment, allowing the spine to assume its normal contour.

Military spine is normally compensated for by an outward curve lower in the back. People with such a curve are sometimes diagnosed as having ankylosing spondylitis, a condition related to arthritis. Classical medical thought is that it has no known cause and therefore no cure. Before giving up, check whiplash injury, TMJ, unbalanced bite, cranial sinus problems, allergy and microorganisms.

Normal Neck and "Military Spine"

7 pounds   7 pounds   10 pounds   4 pounds

Normal   "Military Spine"

Concept from Lowell Ward, D.C.of Long Beach, CA. Used with permission.

What is a slipped disk?

Small pads of cartilage called disks are located 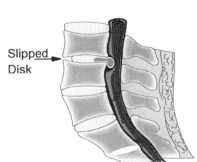 between each of the vertebrae for a total of 23 disks. These form a cushion against shocks and aid in the flexibility of the spine. Spinal misalignments due to injury, improper muscle tension, meningeal contraction, wear and tear over the years, or improper lifting can cause the disk to bulge, move, or herniate (squeeze out of its proper location). This is commonly known as a "slipped disk".

Slipped Disk

A slipped, or subluxed, disk, if untreated or treated improperly, can progress to more serious problems. The usual progression is **subluxed → bulged → deteriorated → herniated → fused.** With a collapsed or fused disk, the cushioning liquid is gone from the disk. Once a disk is fused, the damage is usually considered to be impossible to repair.

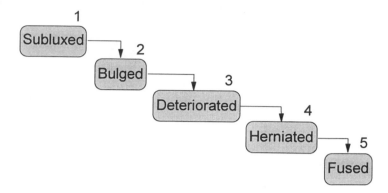

The Five Steps of Spinal Disk Damage

A surgical procedure called a laminectomy is sometimes used to alleviate the pain. This procedure, which fuses the disks in some cases, makes the adjacent disks overcompensate. Then these disks get worn out by having to do more than their share of the work, and the disk problem spreads.

What is whiplash?

Older children and adults can also fall or be involved in sports or auto accidents. Whiplash injuries are best known as the result of rear end auto collisions, which causes the neck to rapidly snap backwards and then forwards. Like the cracking of a whip, the greatest impact is at the point where the whip, or neck, abruptly changes direction.

Think of your neck with its delicate curve, and your head perched on top like a fourteen pound weight. The inertial, or gravitational forces of an accident makes the head more like a 100-pound ball. This 100-pound ball snaps backwards and then forwards in a car accident. Imagine the potential damage to your neck! If the head is forward, the spine curves outward to compensate, creating the well known "dowager's hump" over time if uncorrected. What you have is a weight equivalent to a fourteen pound ball - the actual weight of your head. If you have six pounds of unbalanced weight more out in front than intended, the body tries to compensates for this additional burden by bowing forward.

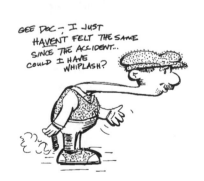

Try lifting a six-pound weight to get a feel for how heavy this is. Then picture a six-pound shot-put in your mouth, which is in effect what is happening when the head is more forward in front of the body. Is it any wonder that your shoulders and low back ache? They are having to bear the strain and tension from trying to keep you balanced, with this six pound weight pulling in the opposite direction.

How else can whiplash occur?

In addition to being struck by a car from behind, whiplash-type injuries can also result from auto accidents involving forward motion, in which the person's head is stopped abruptly by the steering wheel, dashboard, or windshield, again causing the head to be snapped back. Another effect of this is a compressed front facial bone which can lock up the cranial bones and affect the sinuses, meninges, and back.

Other causes of whiplash can be:

- *Forceps deliveries and other birth injuries*
- *Poor head position over a long term*
- *Some amusement park rides*
- *Horseback riding accidents*
- *Sudden quick movements*
- *Sports injuries*
- *Falls*

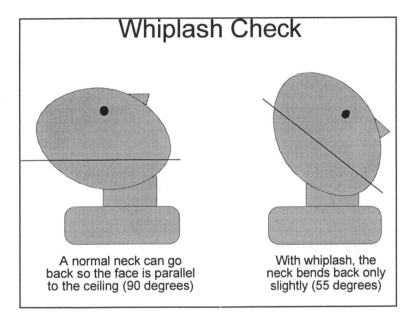

Whiplash Check

A normal neck can go back so the face is parallel to the ceiling (90 degrees)

With whiplash, the neck bends back only slightly (55 degrees)

How can you tell if you have had a whiplash injury?
Try tilting your head back as far as it will go. Your face should be parallel with the ceiling. If you can't tilt it back that far, you probably have a whiplash-type injury that may be affecting your health. Another indication - when standing erect, have someone observe you from the side. Your ear should be directly over the center of your shoulder. If it is forward, this may be an indication of whiplash or other structural imbalance.

How can whiplash change your life?
If you have had whiplash and haven't had it treated correctly, chances are other parts of your body aren't working properly. A whiplash injury can cause your entire spine to be out of alignment, with resulting compromised organ function. In addition, if you have had a whiplash injury, your jaw is also whiplashed and is probably out of alignment. The importance of this is discussed in the next chapter.

> **Most chronically ill patients have whiplash and/or jaw misalignment**

Since the nerves, muscles, and organs are interrelated, whiplash can adversely affect the cranial nerves which go down the front of the neck, such as the vagus nerve which controls digestion. Digestive difficulties such as poor nutrient absorption can result from whiplash for this reason.

The C2 axis vertebra, sometimes along with C3 and C4, is usually pushed back in a whiplash accident, producing a "military spine" effect. This pushes the head forward. When the head goes forward after a whiplash injury, the jaw goes forward, the teeth don't mesh properly, and the sutures of the head are not aligned. Cerebrospinal fluid is then not pumped effectively. The importance of the teeth and head sutures is discussed later in this chapter.

Jim, a 40-plus-year-old truck driver, had had a whiplash problem for years. After having a whiplash adjustment and bite balancing (described in the next chapter), as well as removal of mercury and treatment for parasites, he experienced relief of his low back pain, digestive difficulties, depression, headaches and low energy.

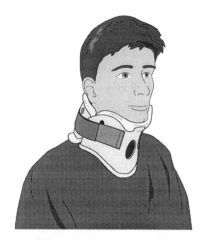

How is whiplash often mistreated?

The cervical collar (a bulky neck collar that restricts neck movement) often applied by paramedic technicians only keeps the injury from moving, thus keeping short term pain from worsening, but does nothing to correct it. The collar makes the muscles more comfortable, but this is like applying a cast to a broken arm without setting the bone. Ideally, having a chiropractors on staff in emergency rooms to correct whiplash injuries before they worsen, and a dentist to correct TMJ displacement (discussed in the next chapter) would be advisable in dealing with the displacement and misalignment that usually occurs as a result of whiplash injury.

Most doctors and many chiropractors don't know how to properly treat a whiplash injury. When chiropractors adjust the neck after a whiplash injury, they often only do a side-to-side adjustment. In fact, they sometimes erroneously push the head forward, causing whiplash in an attempt to open the occiput (back and base of head). It is necessary to also adjust the neck forward to back to position the C2, 3 and 4 vertebras forward where they belong, and the dowager's compensating hump back in place.

How can sports injuries cause subluxations?

Sports injuries, especially those involving body contact such as football tackles, can cause spinal injuries. Many cases of injury cause pain or dizziness, and require a cervical collar and/or painkillers or muscle relaxants. Other injuries are so minor as to go unnoticed. As an example, this can happen during some of the wilder amusement park rides or by hitting a bad pothole in the road while traveling at high speed. The resulting subluxations can cause problems to surface anywhere from one month to years later, and can even last a lifetime if untreated.

How can structural abnormalities set up a vicious cycle?

Structural abnormalities can cause impingement of a nerve, but the reverse is often true. In many cases the misalignment and irritated nerve(s) perpetuate each other in a vicious cycle. The muscles are also involved, as irritation can cause them to contract defensively to compensate and can further lock in and worsen the misalignment.

This vicious cycle can cause a progressive worsening of the situation. For example, a torsion injury to young child's pelvis may make one leg functionally shorter than the other due to the way the leg sits in the hip socket, even though the leg bones are the same length. However, during the child's growth period, the unbalanced shifting of weight while standing and walking can cause one leg to grow more slowly, since growth is mediated partially by nerve impulses; in time one leg is actually shorter than the other. Furthermore, since the feet, legs, and pelvis are the foundations for the structure of the spine, such an imbalance can cause weakening of the spine, with later scoliosis (spinal curvature), disk degeneration, and even arthritis. Scoliosis is often a compensation for meningeal mediated contraction.

If a man habitually carries a wallet in his hip pocket on the same side, or has chronic constipation, the same kinds of unbalanced shifting of weight can occur. This, in essence, shifts his hips like a chiropractic wedge, but in the wrong direction.

If you have the type of pinched nerve that causes pain, for example in the neck, then the nearby muscles and meninges will cause the muscles to contract to protect the injured area. Your neck may tilt visibly to one side and you will most likely want to limit your range of motion. If the situation were to persist for some time, the unbalanced muscle contraction and restricted movement would sooner or later pull the upper spine out of alignment. One might think that this would not happen in real life, as the pain would cause you to run to the nearest chiropractor, osteopath or physician for relief before permanent damage could be done. However, some pinched nerves do not produce immediate excruciating pain and the damage can continue unnoticed.

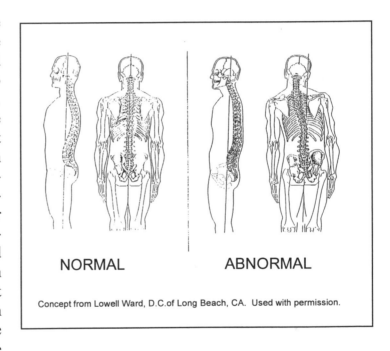

NORMAL   ABNORMAL

Concept from Lowell Ward, D.C. of Long Beach, CA. Used with permission.

What can happen if the nerve irritation is minor?

If a nerve is irritated to a lesser degree, below the threshold of pain, the same type of damage can occur. Because the nerve irritation is less, you are unlikely to seek out a doctor for nerve irritation you are not aware of, so the chronic damage can be greater over time. Several different types of stresses can cause this kind of nerve irritation, which can in turn lead to subluxations, leading to irritation of other nerves, leading to dysfunction within the body.

Have you ever watched a toddler walk?

In this culture, a toddler's legs usually emerge from either side of a large, bulky diaper. This causes the toddler to walk with the legs spread far apart. However, most toddlers, once past the diaper stage, start walking with their legs closer together. So it is possible that some damage may be done to the relatively soft and rapidly growing bones and joints as the baby is forced to walk, sit, lie down and live 24 hours a day with her/his legs in this unnatural stance. But the effects of this damage may not show up for decades.

In some societies and in other cultures, especially in the past, people who habitually carried heavy loads learned to walk side-to-side to stabilize the load, rather than front-to-back like Westerners. This may lead to some of the same conditions faced by those who wore bulky diapers as toddlers.

What types of nerve irritants are there?

The primary types of nerve irritants are physical, chemical, emotional, and electrical. Physical irritants are the most obvious. There may or may not be pain at the time of injury, and if there is pain treatment may not relieve the subluxation. For example, whiplash injury shock may be treated by wearing a cervical collar until the soft tissue injury heals and the pain is gone, but the spine may still be painlessly out of alignment. Muscle compensation and meningeal contraction may follow, worsening the problem.

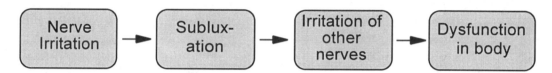

What can cause physical nerve irritation?

Physical irritation may be the result of a single event or an accumulation of years of spinal abuse. Trauma or injuries leading to physical irritation include:

- *Poor posture*
- *Shoveling snow*
- *Falling down*
- *Slipping on the ice*
- *Physically demanding work, such as athletics or dancing*
- *Automobile accidents*
- *Falling off a bicycle or swing*
- *Lifting repeatedly or lifting heavy objects*
- *Misstepping on the stairs*

The meningeal system will mediate muscle contractions to stabilize the body if the head is habitually held out in front of the body.

What about chemical irritation?

Physical irritation seems fairly obvious. Chemical irritation is much less obvious. Environmental toxins, cigarette smoke, allergic reactions, parasitic or microbial infections, and drugs can cause nerve irritation initiating the chain of events including meningeal mediated contraction which culminates in bodily dysfunction.

How long has the medical profession known about chemical irritation of nerves?

D. D. Palmer, who started the science of chiropractic in its modern form a century ago back in 1895, wrote:

"The poison, acting on certain nerves, irritates their structure. They in turn contract muscles which draw vertebrae out of alignment, thereby impinging upon nerves which go and affect certain portions of the body."

Since then dozens of medical studies have substantiated Palmer's claim. However, meningeal contractions are the missing ingredient that completes the picture.

Is something getting on your nerves?
Emotional irritation can cause the same cascade of events. The connection between nerves and emotions has been known at some level for a long time; consider the following metaphorically emotional expressions:

- *"You're getting on my nerves"*
- *"I'm a nervous wreck"*
- *"After a day like this, my nerves are shot"*
- *"I'm about to have a nervous breakdown"*
- *"I've earned this nervous breakdown and I'm going to have it!*

There are many ways your state of mind can make you ill, and this is one of them. Tension, anger, worry, fear, and hate can themselves cause nerve irritation, meningeal mediated contraction, and muscle tension. It should be mentioned here that a lot of emotion attributed to nerves is actually a function of the adrenal glands and their output of adrenaline (epinephrine), or of adrenal exhaustion.

In addition, postures characteristic of these emotions can contract or stretch certain muscles which, over time, can cause misalignment. An angry person might have tension in the neck and other muscles, a clenched jaw, squinted eyes, and a head jutted forward - a typical fight position. A depressed person tends to slouch, droop, and lower the head.

Dr. Wilhelm Reich, who studied the mind-body connection, found that people with shame, fear, or anxiety over sex tend to retract the pelvic area. A teenage girl, self-conscious about her developing breasts, may begin a lifelong habit of slouching over and rounding her shoulders. All of these emotion-induced postures can, over time, change the curvature of the spine.

Because a tense person often tenses the neck muscles, and because the vagus nerve which controls digestion comes from the skull and runs through the neck, neck muscle tension can affect this nerve and interfere with digestion.

What about electrical irritation?
You may have heard of those early biological experiments in which frogs' legs, not attached to the frog, can be stimulated to jerk and twitch by the application of an electric current. Our bodies are subjected to electrical currents on a daily basis, from electromagnetic fields caused by the running of electrical appliances and from electrical currents generated in the mouth by dissimilar

metals, as previous discussed in the chapters on Electromagnetic Radiation and The Battery Effect.

What happens after a misalignment occurs?

Once a misalignment has occurred, other changes can take place within a relatively short time. Misaligned vertebrae and joints develop adhesions and contractures, and ligaments and muscles often conform themselves to the misalignment.

What are some of the effects of misalignment?

Misalignment can cause a wide variety of symptoms and malfunctions, which includes things you might expect, such as back pain. But misalignments can also cause some pretty surprising ailments. Such ailments fall into two categories - musculoskeletal and organic (or visceral).

Headache can have a number of causes, only some of which are structural. Problems with the cranial sutures can also cause headaches. The location of the headache can give some indication as to the cause:

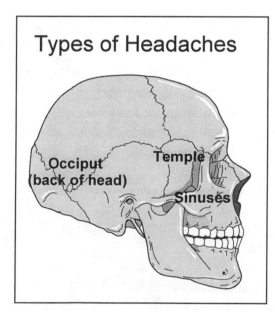

Types of Headaches

- Tight in back (occiput), front, or top - misaligned vertebrae reduce blood flow to head and can cause meningeal mediated contractions. Misaligned jaw, popularly called TMJ and discussed later in this chapter, can also cause occipital headache. (O/M)

- Temple to temple - vascular (blood vessel dilation or constriction), sometimes caused by allergy (V)

- Sinus area - allergy or sinus infection. (S)

Each of these three types of headache can have a number of causes. These lead to the occipital/meningeal (O/M), vascular (V), or sinus (S) headache type as indicated.

- A misaligned vertebra can compress an artery, reducing blood flow to the brain. Osteopathic or chiropractic work can help correct this. (O/M)

- Liver or gallbladder blockage (O/M), which also can cause tight trapezius muscles and an ache midway between the shoulder blades.

- Emotional upset can cause the muscles in the head and neck to contract, resulting in reduced blood flow and then a tension headache. (O/M, V)

- Microorganisms and their toxic byproducts (O/M, S)

- A displaced bony segment in the neck can apply direct pressure to a nerve, resulting in a neck muscle spasm (stiff neck) and then headache. (O/M)

- Toxins and allergies (S, V, O/M)

- Poor posture, either the result of laziness or a lower spinal misalignment, can also cause spasms of the head and neck muscles. (O/M)

Major Misalignments - Disk problems and backache - Misalignment can cause disks to slip out of normal position and cause pain. The converse is also true, as slipped disks can cause misalignment. Muscle spasm anywhere in the neck or back can be caused by impingement on a nerve. According to chiropractic theory, the disks between vertebrae absorb essential nutrients from tissue fluids, lymph, and blood capillaries which surround them. A subluxation can cause disk "starvation" and eventual deterioration. Disk starvation can come from insufficient blood or spinal fluid flow and/or nerve electricity.

Whiplash is an acute neuromuscular injury caused by a sudden back and forth jolt to the neck, like snapping a whip or a wet towel. The head snaps back and then rapidly snaps forward. Ligaments and muscles are torn, vertebrae move, nerves are pinched, disks are compressed, and inflammation (noninfectious) can develop around the nerve root. The jaw can also be displaced. These injuries can cause headaches, dizziness, neuralgia (nerve pain), blurred vision, and loss of normal neck motion. Long-term damage such as disk degeneration and bone spurs can follow if the whiplash injury is not adequately treated, i.e. **adjusted forward and back and not just side to side**.

Joint pains include bursitis, tennis elbow, carpal tunnel syndrome, hip pain, housemaid's knee, long bone pain, and others. Most of these, which involve the shoulder, knee, or wrist, are long bone pain of a sort because they involve the ends of a long bone. Bursitis, on the other hand, is an inflammation of the bursa, a fluid-filled sac that cushions adjacent joint tissues. Joint pain often results from overuse or misuse of the joint, or not enough weight-bearing exercise, but can also occur when subluxations cause muscle spasm which inhibits the normal motion of the joint. This can be detected by lying flat on your back and having someone observe whether one foot is further from vertical than the other, as in the adjacent picture.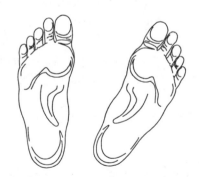

If the inguinal ligament in the groin is out, this can affect the ileocecal valve of the digestive system and vice-versa. The ileocecal valve prevents toxins in the colon from backing up into the intestines and being absorbed into the rest of the body.

Calcium can be taken from the long bones and muscles if there is inflammation elsewhere in the body, such as the arteries. If you have any of these joint pains, this may be the cause. It may be a good idea to have your arteries checked and take antioxidants for protection. Allergy, toxins, and waste byproducts of microorganisms can have the same effect on calcium as does inflammation.

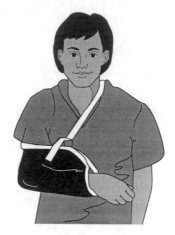

Carpal tunnel syndrome is an inflammation of the nerves caused by irritation by the bones of the wrist, from repetitive actions such as prolonged typing or working at a calculator or cash register. It can also be caused by nerve, vascular or muscle irritation, lesions or scar tissue, or a misalignment of the vertebrae C-7 and T-1, as well as problems in the shoulder or elbow, or in the bones themselves. Either a deficiency or a severe excess of vitamin B6 can also contribute to the ailment, as vitamin B6 supports the nerves. If there is a deficiency, vitamin B6 should be taken for at least six weeks before improvement is noticed. Omega-3 oils and choline can be useful in treatment.

Carpal tunnel syndrome can also be caused by a reaction to Yellow Dye No. 5 or tartrazine, a food additive. Other nutritional recommendations include the B vitamin complex, folic acid, magnesium, and essential fatty acids [1].

Tarsal tunnel syndrome involves the analogous, or similar, structure of the feet. If all else fails a wrist or foot adjustment can be done, although the problem is usually not in the wrist or foot but in the spine.

Scoliosis is an abnormal sideways curvature of the spine. It is estimated to affect about twenty percent of children to some degree. It usually shows up in adolescence, and more often in girls than in boys. Scoliosis tends to worsen if untreated. It can be caused by a muscle spasm. The spasm causes misalignment, which worsens the spasm in a vicious cycle. The worse the misalignment, the worse the spasm. The meningeal system may also be involved.

The spine is designed to curve front to back. If it straightens out, it has to bend somewhere else instead to compensate. This can be scoliosis.

Poor posture and scoliosis are also both cause and effect of each other. A misaligned jaw can lead to scoliosis as the body turns to compensate. This is discussed in the next chapter.

A biofeedback device has been developed which sounds an alarm if the wearer slouches. This has proven effective in treating scoliosis (side to side curvature) and kyphosis (front to back curvature) [2].

To detect scoliosis in your child, have her/him stand as straight as possible and check for the following, which may or may not be signs of scoliosis:

- *One pants leg, or one side of a skirt hem, that is shorter than the other even with a change of garment*
- *The head tilts consistently to one side*

- *One shoulder higher than the other*
- *One hip higher than the other*
- *Shoes show uneven wear*
- *Leaning to one side*

Try this - Other ways to detect spinal abnormalities in a child or adult include seeing whether the head turns or moves from side to side or shoulder to shoulder more easily in one direction than the other. A problem with shoulder-to-shoulder motion points to a problem with the C1 vertebra (the atlas), while side-to-side difficulty is more likely a C2 (axis) problem).

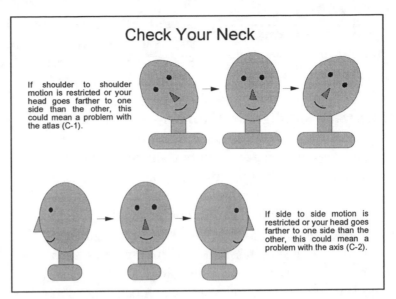

Check Your Neck

If shoulder to shoulder motion is restricted or your head goes farther to one side than the other, this could mean a problem with the atlas (C-1).

If side to side motion is restricted or your head goes farther to one side than the other, this could mean a problem with the axis (C-2).

Thyroid problems - The thyroid gland in the neck is served by nerves and blood vessels that come from the nearby cervical spine, so it is not surprising that a cervical subluxation can affect thyroid / parathyroid / adrenal function. A patient suffered a whiplash injury in an automobile accident. She wore a cervical collar for a while, and in time the pain and obvious whiplash symptoms went away. After the accident, the patient started gaining weight rapidly even after reducing her food intake. She was sluggish, dry skinned, and puffy-faced. She saw several doctors who put her on diets, gave her drugs, and suggested she go for counseling. Chiropractic treatment was able to successfully find and treat the cause - an underactive thyroid gland caused by the whiplash injury. TMJ problems can also adversely affect thyroid function.

> **88% of people with neck subluxations have thyroid dysfunction.**

The *Journal of the American Osteopathic Association* [cited in source 3] reports that 88 percent of subjects with cervical lesions, or subluxations, also suffered from thyroid dysfunction, as compared with a 34 percent incidence of thyroid dysfunction in control subjects with no cervical lesions. Check this before taking, and becoming dependent on, thyroid medication.

Referred pain is pain that is perceived by the brain as coming from a site other than its true origin. Subluxation or spinal curvature resulting in nerve interference can produce radiating pain that appears to come from the heart, gastrointestinal tract, gallbladder, or elsewhere. This is diagnosed as being the case when spinal manipulation provides immediate relief, hopefully before more invasive treatment is performed for the apparent but incorrect cause. Tightness and pain between the shoulder blades (the trapezius muscles), neck and head pressure, and sunlight sensitivity along with apparent gallbladder problems point to a root cause that is possibly centered in the spinal area and not in the gallbladder.

The converse is also true, as problems with the organs can cause pain to radiate back along the spinal nerves and cause back pain in the area served by those nerves.

> **Sexual difficulties can result from lower back problems.**

Sexual difficulties, especially male impotence, can be caused by subluxations in the lower back (the spinal vertebrae S2, S3, and S4). The resulting nerve and fluid impingement can affect the sexual organs.

Intestinal and digestive problems such as colitis, constipation, and intestinal cramps can be caused when an out-of-place vertebra impinges on the nerves servicing the intestine and digestive organs.

Meningeal mediated contractions can be caused by misalignments, and can lead to neck pain and headache. On the other hand, health problems such as chemical toxicity or psychological stress can cause meningeal contractions, which can then pull the spine out of alignment. The importance of the meningeal system is discussed in the chapter on Body Systems in *Thriving In A Toxic World*.

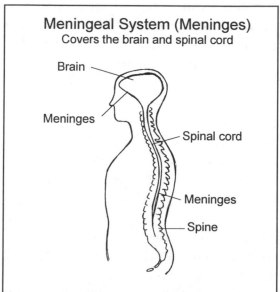

How does one prevent subluxations?

There are a number of ways to minimize misalignment and the resulting nerve impingement, or to keep it from worsening:

- Observe children for signs of scoliosis, as described earlier in this chapter.

- Have regular chiropractic and/or osteopathic checkups, and have your children checked as well.

- Watch your posture when sitting or standing. Look in a mirror or ask a friend for feedback.

- Lift properly, letting your legs rather than your back move the weight upwards.

- Replace shoes or shoe heels as necessary. Minor misalignments can result in uneven wear of shoes, and the uneven shoe support can then exaggerate the misalignment.

- Keep your weight within normal range, as extra weight will push on and worsen any misalignment.

- Have a structural checkup and adjustment after having a baby or after a car accident.

- Have proper dental balancing by using muscle testing after a whiplash injury or after orthodontia or the installation of crowns. If certain muscles are weak, this can tell which associated teeth are out of alignment and need adjustment.

- Do not develop the habit of carrying heavy purses or cases with one arm, especially the same arm regularly over a period of years.

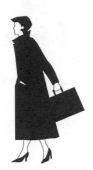

- A wallet worn in the back pocket in the same position for years can press on the hip joint and rotate the hips, increasing apparent leg length. This can cause eventual hip abnormalities and knee and hip degeneration because a disproportionate amount of weight is on one knee and hip.

- Be aware of things that appear to be non-structural but can have an effect on subluxations: meningeal contractions, allergy, toxins, microorganisms, hypoglycemia, and electrolyte imbalance, among others.

- Adjusting and balancing the feet is very important to get your center of gravity back where it belongs.

Are there any ways to self test for misalignments?

In addition to using a mirror or a friend to check for asymmetries as discussed above, there are a few other tests.

- Bend the head from side to side as if trying to touch the ear to the shoulder. If one side moves less easily, not as far, or with more pain than the other, the very important C-1 (atlas) or C-2 (axis) vertebrae may be out of alignment. Check whether it is the top of the head (C-1) or the shoulders and low neck (C-7), as shown in the picture a few pages back.

- Turn the head from side to side. If the head moves in one direction more easily than the other, the axis (C-2, top of neck), or C-7 (bottom of neck) or T-1 may be out.

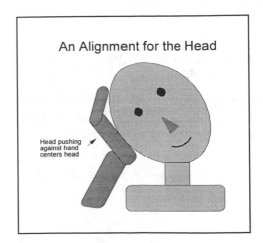

An Alignment for the Head

Head pushing against hand centers head

An alignment for the head, which can be done yourself but is best done by a professional, involves having someone hold your head as you push against their hand toward the easy side. Relax, and then push further until you feel balanced side to side. Then you can turn your head to the difficult side against pressure and release at the end.

What are the different types of structural treatment?

There are many types of structural treatments available. Some of the different treatments for structural problems, listed here and in some cases discussed immediately following, include [3,4,5]:

- *Spinal manipulation*   - *Chiropractic, osteopathy*

- *Soft tissue work*   - *Rolfing, Hellerwork, Feldenkrais, massage therapy, orthobionomy*

- *Energy balancing*   - *Acupuncture, acupressure, Jin Shen Jyutsu, energy work*

- *Emotional work*   - *Stressology, NET (Neuro-emotional therapy), NAET (allergy treatment)*

- *Cranial work*   - *Cranial-sacral therapy, nasal or sinus specific (balloons), resultant force vector (RFV) analysis, bite balancing*

- *Other*   - *Applied kinesiology, physical therapy, NAET (allergy treatment), Tai Chi*

This is only a partial listing of the many possible types of treatment.

What is chiropractic?

Chiropractic seeks to relieve the symptoms caused by subluxations of vertebrae and the resulting nerve impingement. This is done by manipulating the misaligned vertebrae to the full range of motion end point, then just a bit further and back into place, whereby a force applied to the spine in the same direction that is restricted allows the body's inherent recuperative powers to realign the appropriate spinal section.

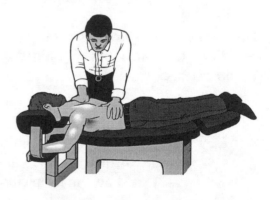

Chiropractors do not claim to cure disease or even diagnose it. Rather, what they do is remove structural and nerve barriers to the body's own healing systems. Chiropractic's belief is that a structurally sound body, freed from nerve interference, can fight disease more effectively than one with nerve blockage. Medical literature is full of enough anecdotal evidence of remission of disease through chiropractic to bear out this theory.

Pasteur said: "The body's environment determines everything."

Louis Pasteur, considered to be the father of the germ theory of disease, realized late in life that "the terrain is everything". Terrain, in this case refers to the body's physical (and emotional) environment. By his statement, Pasteur realized that, although germs (bacteria, viruses, microorganisms) have the capability to cause disease, the overall health of the body determines whether they will actually do so. This realization correlates with the chiropractic idea that a sound body that is free of blockages can better fight disease.

A Doctor of Chiropractic (DC) undergoes four years of intensive training and testing, a program as rigorous as that of a Medical Doctor (MD). They take about the same number of class hours of instruction, with the chiropractic curriculum focusing more on body structure and the medical curriculum focusing more on drugs and surgery.

Are all chiropractors created equal?
There are differences in theory and technique among chiropractors, and some chiropractors specialize in a particular type of treatment.

Some chiropractors, referred to as "straights", believe that spinal adjustment is all that is necessary. Others, sometimes called "mixers", feel that spinal adjustment is best combined with adjunctive therapy such as nutritional supplementation, detoxification, massage, and/or ultrasound. Chiropractic manipulation alone may be sufficient if the problem is an acute primary one, such as sports injury or whiplash.

Different chiropractors focus on different areas of the spinal column:

- One theory has it that all structural problems originate in the atlas and axis. Adjust these and the rest of the spine will fall into line. This is called the Palmer method.

- Other chiropractors focus on adjusting the hips to affect the rest of the spinal column.

- Some focus on cranial-sacral manipulation, others focus on TMJ problems.

- Some focus on the feet, using shoe inserts called orthotics to readjust the spine.

> **If about six weeks of chiropractic treatment does not bring relief, you may need to look elsewhere.**

If about six weeks of treatment does not fix your problem, the chiropractor may be a good one but his/her specialty may be unsuited to the totality of your particular problem. Alternatively, it is possible that the apparent chiropractic problem may be secondary to other causes, for which additional treatment may be needed. Chiropractic can give temporary relief if the structural problem is secondary or tied to the meningeal system, but in this case the chiropractic treatment can be considered to be symptom-suppressing rather than addressing the root cause.

How is osteopathy different from chiropractic?
Osteopathy is outwardly similar to chiropractic in that both disciplines believe structural anomalies, especially of the spine, can lead to poor health. Both seek to move misaligned bones to their normal position to restore normal body function. The difference lies in their primary focus. Chiropractic focuses on nerve interference, while osteopathy is concerned with proper circulation of

fluids, including blood, lymph, and spinal fluid. Recall that an artery and vein flow through the intervertebral foramen (IVF) leading from the vertebrae along with the nerve.

A practitioner of osteopathy is called a Doctor of Osteopathy (D.O.). A D.O., like a chiropractor, has as much training as a Medical Doctor (MD), but unlike a chiropractor the D.O. is licensed to perform certain types of surgery, give intravenous medications, and prescribe drugs. In some ways a D.O. can combine the best of both the chiropractor and the medical doctor

What are some of the other structural treatments?

Acupressure, known as Shiatsu in Japan, involves the use of fingertip pressure to activate certain pressure points along the body's twelve meridians, or pathways, as compared with acupuncture, which uses needles rather than fingers during the treatment. Acupressure has been used successfully to treat chronic back pain, hypertension, headache, and ulcers, among other ailments.

Acupressure's basic premise is that a blocked flow of energy within the body causes impaired function of body systems. The treatments seek to restore proper energy flow and balance to the body, so it can more effectively heal itself.

An example of the importance of meridians lies in the fact that many women tend to gain weight after a Cesarean birth. This can be partially attributed to the fact that meridians (energy pathways) as well as lymph channels have been cut, affecting the body's ability to stay in balance.

Applied kinesiology helps to locate and correct imbalances in the body's energy system through the muscles that relate to the body's twelve major organs. Applied kinesiology can also determine whether the imbalance is structural, nutritional, or psychological.

The tester puts pressure on the patient's arm or leg, which the patient attempts to resist. Lack of strong resistance indicates a weakness in the muscles or pathways to the related organ. Firm pressure is applied to the appropriate acupuncture point, which stimulates the weakened area. The muscle is then retested. Kinesiology testing is sometimes used to evaluate the effectiveness of chiropractic and other treatments. Kinesiology can be applied to either the whole body or to isolated muscle groups. The accuracy of kinesiology testing can vary by the skill and bias of the operator.

Physical therapy, also called physiotherapy, is often conducted under medical supervision. While chiropractic's goal is to remove nerve interference so that the body can function optimally, physical therapists or the associated MDs decide what the body needs and administer the appropriate treatment.

The objectives of physical therapy are to increase the range of motion of joints, for example in an accident victim or a person with cerebral palsy. It also aims to correct postural deviations and to decrease muscle spasm.

Techniques of physical therapy include:

- *Passive exercises to stimulate muscles and prevent atrophy*
- *Massage*
- *Heat*
- *Ultrasound*
- *Hydrotherapy*
- *Range of motion exercises*
- *Cold compresses*
- *Electrotherapy*
- *Drugs (pain killers, muscle relaxants)*

Physical therapy rarely deals with any underlying structural issues. It just makes you adapt to and feel more comfortable with your imbalance.

Jin Shen Jyutsu connects the painful points to the point of blockage of energy, like connecting the dots or using jumper cables. This opens up the surface energy pathways and allows the muscles to relax.

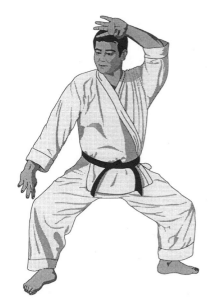

Tai Chi is a series of slow, deliberate movements, going from gross to fine motor skills. This recruits the muscle spindle bundle fibers which are not always used otherwise. Tai Chi appears to the casual observer to be like a precise, slow-motion dance. A complete set of Tai Chi exercises works every muscle group in the body.

Tai Chi can also be called slow movement exercises. An example of these is the following: Turn your head as far as possible toward the left shoulder. Very slowly, to the count of 16, rotate your head toward the right shoulder. Alternatively, raise or shrug the shoulders up very slowly and then let them back down slowly. Unless you are experienced in this type of exercise, chances are you will feel a jerkiness in the movement, as if it were being accomplished stepwise.

After you do the exercise for a while, the motion gets smoother as muscle spindle bundle fibers are recruited. The jerkiness you feel is how your whole body moves, and this throws the whole body out of balance. Muscle fibers are like bridge suspension cables. If the cables are weak or too few, the bridge sags. If the muscle fibers are weak or too few, the body structure will not hold together properly. Slow movement exercises which involve each part of the body in turn will optimize this part of your structure.

The **counterstrain technique** makes use of the principle of opposing movement. This gets the message to the brain that the muscle is too short, and the brain will then relax it. If, for example, you want to be able to lift your knee higher, first lift your knee as high as it will go. Have another person support your knee at this height, and use your leg muscles to try to press your knee downward. This is the opposite direction to where you want it to go ultimately. Relax, then see how high you can now lift your leg. It will often be much higher than before. Repeat this exercise several times. Surprisingly, the counterstrain technique will work more effectively than trying to force the muscle to go where you want it to, as for example trying to stretch your leg to lift it higher.

The **compression technique** utilizes the principle that if you want to lengthen a muscle, first shorten it. This works like Chinese handcuffs, which slip over the fingers and tighten if you pull them but relax if you push. If you have tight trapezius muscles on the side of your neck, have someone else push your shoulder towards your neck. This gets the message to the brain that the muscle is too short. The brain will then allow it to relax and lengthen.

Rolfing, developed by Ida P. Rolf, is also called Structural Integration. It is based on the idea that bodily and mental function is improved when the segments of the body (head, torso, pelvis, legs, feet) are in proper alignment. In many cases poor posture causes the other parts of the body to shift to compensate. After years of this, the fibrous fascial tissues covering the muscles holds the structures in this compensated position, restricting movement of muscles and joints and causing pain, reducing mental clarity and causing stress. In Rolfing, the body's fascial tissues are manually manipulated and stretched, using elbows, forearms and even knuckles sliding on ligaments, tendons and muscle. The process can be painful. The result is freer, more balanced movements and the relief of associated symptoms. Rolfing has also been found to help many arthritis sufferers [6-8].

Hellerwork is a spinoff of Rolfing, and is a series of related soft tissue manipulations. Soft tissue work helps release the musculature from chronic or acute spasm (contraction). Since muscle contraction can affect the nerves and the organs that they serve, release from muscle spasm can help restore normal nerve and organ function.

Trager work, developed in 1927 by Milton Trager, MD, is an approach to movement reeducation that uses a gentle rhythmical touch combined with movement exercises. By making a link between pleasurable feelings and certain motions, his work can help trigger tissue changes that can lead to increased flexibility, range of motion, and relaxation. Trager work has helped people with severe neuromuscular disturbances such as polio, multiple sclerosis and muscular dystrophy, and has helped professional athletes increase their efficiency of movement and stamina [9].

The **Alexander technique** involves retraining the person to stand, sit and move in a way that restores natural balance and responsiveness during movement. This has benefits as diverse as improving body image, helping actors and singers improve their performance, and relieving chronic pain [10,11].

Stressology, done by Dr. Lowell Ward in Long Beach, California among others, explores the possible emotional and psychological causes of subluxations by looking at meningeal system patterns. NET (Neuro-Emotional Therapy), developed by Dr. Scott Walker of Encinitas, California, also makes use of the relationship between emotions, meningeal mediated contractions, and subluxations.

How can you recruit or reprogram your mind to optimize movement?

Feldenkrais, a technique named after its originator Moshe Feldenkrais, focuses on changing the movement of the body by re-educating the mind. When a baby first learns to roll over, crawl, or walk, it learns a set of separate movements which become the action of, for example, walking. These movements are wired into the brain and are called upon when it is necessary to walk somewhere. Sloppy or inefficient habits often form over time, and by adulthood walking, or any other motion, is not done optimally. Inefficient ways of moving can lead to stiffness, limited range of motion, unnecessary bodily tension, poor or limited sports performance, and lowered stamina.

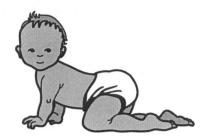

The principle behind Feldenkrais lies in the fact that our muscles do not function except as directed by the nervous system. When you learn a particular move, as for example a tennis serve, your brain learns a complex pattern of neural firings which it then uses to direct your arm. If you want to improve your tennis serve, according to Feldenkrais, it is necessary to repattern the mind, not simply practice serving tennis balls. You programmed, or wired, yourself in the first place, whether the action is walking or a complex gymnastics move. It follows that you can rewire yourself at any time once you know how to do so.

Repatterning (reprogramming) the mind is somewhat like following a map: you can't get where you're going unless you know where you are. To this end, it is first necessary to be aware of the many steps involved in even a simple action like moving your arm. Only then can you repattern each aspect of the motion. The mind can be used to repattern muscle movement, but the converse is also true: more mental flexibility is often the result of changing the way you move. Learning to change rigid, habitual patterns of movement can enhance your ability to learn other types of information.

Changing pathways in your nervous system does not take much time if it is done correctly. Only the mind, not the muscles, needs to be changed. In fact, it is possible to go through each step of a Feldenkrais exercise in your mind only to achieve retraining. Changing your purpose is an element of your retraining. For example, when you practice your tennis serve, you hit the ball back to the other person. However, in an actual game the goal is to hit the ball to where the other person *isn't*.

There are two basic Feldenkrais techniques. One is Awareness Through Movement (ATM), described in a book by the same name by Moshe Feldenkrais. ATM consists of verbally directed movement sequences, usually presented to groups of people. The other technique is Functional Integration (FI), which is an intensive, hands-on, one-on-one technique for repatterning that is done by a practitioner.

Are all structural problems below the neck?

Problems with the cranium (skull), the jaw, and the teeth can have major and surprising health effects. These are discussed in the next chapter.

Summary

Structural problems, or subluxations, can occur in many ways even when you are unaware of them. These injuries can compress nerves or fluid channels and compromise the function of the associated organ or part of the body. Structural problems can be primary, or secondary to toxins and allergies. Chiropractic, osteopathic and other structural specialties may be able to rebalance the spinal structure, restoring balance and health.

References and Resources

Structural, General

- The Burton Goldberg Group, *Alternative Medicine: The Definitive Guide*, "Chiropractic", pp. 134-142, "Osteopathy", pp. 405-411, "Carpal Tunnel Syndrome", pp. 898-900, Future Medicine Publishing, Puyallup WA, 1994.

Headache

- Ingram, Cass, *Who Needs Headaches?*, Literary Visions Publishing, Cedar Rapids IA, 1991.

- Lipton, Richard, Lawrence Newman and Helene MacLean, *Migraine: Beating The Odds*, Addison Wesley, Reading MA, 1992.

- Saper, Joel, and Kenneth Magee, *Freedom From Headaches*, Fireside Books, NY, 1981.

Chiropractic

- Altman, Nathaniel, *Everybody's Guide to Chiropractic Health Care*, Jeremy P. Tarcher Inc., Los Angeles CA, 1990.

- Coplan-Griffiths, Michael, *Dynamic Chiropractic Today*, Harper Collins, San Francisco CA, 1991.

- Langone, John, *Chiropractors: A Consumer's Guide*, Addison-Wesley Publishing Co., Reading MA, 1982.

- Martin, Raquel, *Today's Health Alternative*, America West Publishers, Tehachapi CA, 1992.

- Palmer, Daniel David, ***The Chiropractor's Adjuster***, Palmer College Press, Davenport IA, 1992. *Written by one of the fathers of chiropractic medicine.*

- Tousley, Dick, ***The Chiropractic Handbook for Patients***, White Dove Publishing Co., Kansas City MO, 1983.

- Wilk, Chester, ***Chiropractic Speaks Out***, Wilk Publishing Co., Chicago IL, 1975.

- **American Chiropractic Association**, 1701 Clarendon Blvd., Arlington VA 22209, phone (703) 276-8800. *Major source for chiropractic information.*

Osteopathy

- Chaitow, Leon, ***Osteopathic Self-Treatment***, Thorsons, San Francisco CA, 1990.

- Chaitow, Leon, ***Osteopathy: A Complete Health Care System***, Thorsons, London England, 1982.

- Fryett, HH, ***Principles of Osteopathic Technique***, American Academy of Osteopathy, Carmel CA, 1970.

- Northup, George, ***Osteopathic Medicine: An American Reformation***, American Osteopathic Association, Chicago IL, 1987.

- Still, Andrew Taylor, ***Philosophy of Osteopathy***, American Academy of Osteopathy, Colorado Springs CO, 1975.

Feldenkrais

- Feldenkrais, Moshe, ***Awareness Through Movement: Health Exercises for Personal Growth***, Harper and Row, NY, 1972.

- Feldenkrais, Moshe and M. Kimmey, ***The Potent Self: A Guide to Spontaneity***, Harper and Row, San Francisco CA, 1992.

- **Feldenkrais Guild**, P.O. Box 489, Albany OR 97321, phone (503) 926-0981.

Rolfing

- Rolf, Ida P., ***Rolfing: The Integration of Human Structures***, Harper and Row, NY, 1977.

- **International Rolf Institute**, P.O. Box 1868, Boulder CO 80306, phone (303) 449-5903.

Alexander Technique

- Barlow, Wilfred, ***The Alexander Technique***, Alfred A. Knopf, NY, 1991. *Reduce mental stress and muscle tension through balance, posture and movement.*

- Gray, John, ***The Alexander Technique***, St. Martin's Press, NY, 1991.

- Jones, Frank P., ***Body Awareness in Action***, Schocken Books, NY, 1976. *Alexander Technique.*

Massage

- Lidell, Lucinda, *The Book of Massage*, Fireside, NY, 1984. *Includes Shiatsu, reflexology and others.*

- Thomas, Sara, *Massage for Common Ailments*, Fireside, NY, 1989. *How to alleviate every-day health problems through Shiatsu and other massage techniques.*

- **American Massage Therapy Association**, 820 Davis Street, Suite 100, Evanston IL 60201, phone (312) 761-2682.

Bodywork

- Murphy, Michael, *The Future of the Body*, Jeremy P. Tarcher Inc., Los Angeles CA, 1992. *Bodywork.*

- **The Body of Knowledge / Hellerwork**, 406 Berry Street, Mt. Shasta CA 96067, phone (916) 926-2500. *Information, referral directory, training and certification.*

- **Trager Institute**, 33 Millwood, Mill Valley CA 94941, phone (415) 388-2688. *Information, referral directory, training and certification.*

Practitioners

The following practitioners are recommended for the structural work mentioned in this chapter, although these types of work are done at Comprehensive Health Centers, 4403 Manchester Avenue, Suite 107, Encinitas CA 92024, phone (619) 632-9042.

- Dr. Lowell Ward is the developer of Stressology. He is located in Long Beach, CA.

- Dr. Dean Howell, N.D. does cranial work and nasal specific therapy. He is located in Everett, WA.

- Dr. Suzanne Fuselier, D.C. can be reached at Comprehensive Health Centers, 4403 Manchester Avenue, Suite 107, Encinitas CA 92024, phone (619) 632-9042.

- Dr. David Olinger, D.C. can be reached at Comprehensive Health Centers, 4403 Manchester Avenue, Suite 107, Encinitas CA 92024, phone (619) 632-9042.

STRUCTURAL MISALIGNMENTS - HEAD AND BITE

Getting Your Head On Straight

If you have any of the symptoms listed at the beginning of the previous chapter, they may be caused by a structural problem involving the head, neck, jaw, or teeth.

Do any of the following apply to you? If so, information in this chapter can have a powerful impact on your health.

- *Did you ever have orthodontic braces, dental crowns, or a blow to the face?*

- *Do you have a dental bridge spanning your two top front teeth? You may be setting the stage for restrictive structural disorders such as head, neck and low back problems.*

- *Did you know that there is a lot more to the root causes of structural problems and their associated symptoms than just spinal misalignments:*
Cranial sutures	Whiplash	Dentures
Dental bridges	TMJ/TMD	Unbalanced bite
Atlas/Axis	Feet unbalanced	True differing leg length

Cranial Therapy

Does all structural therapy involve only the spine?

Cranial therapy was first introduced by a osteopath in the 1940s. Its goal is to remove obstructions to the flow of cerebrospinal fluid (CSF), which flows at about 6-12 cycles per minute and nourishes the nerves and promotes nerve transmission throughout the body. CSF flows along the wall of the skull and along the spinal cord. Its flow can be affected by abnormal pressure that can occur if the bony plates of the skull are misaligned. The cranial bones move every time you breathe or chew and help the flow of CSF. Insufficient chewing, as 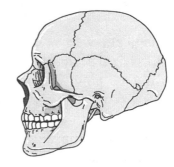 with meals gulped in a hurry or a processed food diet, can reduce the CSF flow. High teeth, unbalanced bite, TMJ or sinus bone collapse can greatly affect this.

Teeth should, by chewing, set up vectors that flex and move the cranial bones to pump spinal fluid. Any injury such as a jammed cheekbone from an accident can block the free movement of the cranial bones and hinder spinal fluid flow.

The cranial nerves are equal in importance to the spinal nerves in promoting or hindering organ and muscle function.

Such misalignments can occur due to injury, hits to the face, concussion, whiplash, stress, spinal misalignments, congenital deformity, and birth trauma (especially forceps delivery) that did not fully correct itself. The practitioner gently aligns the bones by pressing and moving the bones of the skull and at the base of the skull, and to a lesser extent the bones of the face. The palate inside the mouth can also be adjusted. Cranial therapy is especially useful for disorders of the eyes, ears, nose, and sinuses, and for sleep disorders.

Craniosacral work has been useful in the treatment of childhood autism and in reducing self-abusive behaviors such as head-banging, possibly by relieving chronic head pain [1].

Have you ever considered having a balloon blown up inside your face?
Nasal specific therapy is a specialized form of cranial therapy. A misalignment of the bony plates of the skull is rather like wearing a tight shoe every day. You may or may not notice the discomfort, but you will certainly feel the relief when the tight shoe is replaced with a comfortable one.

Nasal specific therapy, as well as other forms of cranial therapy, realigns the bones of the skull so they fit together as they were meant to, and the relief can be at least as great as that of removing a tight pair of shoes. Cerebrospinal fluid and blood can now flow properly to the brain and to other parts of the body.

Although cranial bones (skull plates) can be adjusted to a certain extent from the outside, Dr. Dean Howell of Washington uses the more effective nasal specific technique. In this technique, small balloons are inserted into the sinus cavity and quickly inflated; then the air is released inside the nasal cavities. This moves the bones of the skull from the inside. Dr. Howell compares it to banging out the dents in a car from the inside.

This treatment may sound a bit bizarre. It may be startling and may even bring up memories of the original accident, if any, that caused the cranial or facial misalignment. The sensation is one of intense pressure that only lasts about a second. It has been described as similar to what one feels when water gets into the sinus cavity during swimming or diving into water.

Many times immediate relief follows the procedure, even after the first treatment. The average course of therapy involves about 6-8 treatments. Dr. Howell and his mentor, Dr. J.R. Stober of Portland, Oregon, have done over 125,000 such adjustments between them with minimal ill effects [2].

Do you have a bridge across your front teeth?
A dental bridge across the two top front teeth can restrict the movement of the cranial sutures. This adversely affects the cerebrospinal fluid pump and can also restrict movement all the way down to locked hips.

In a dramatic example, one patient had an autoimmune disease which partially fused his spine and hips and made certain movements such as bending over difficult. After his dentist informed him of similar cases in which separating the two front teeth by cutting through the bridge produced striking improvement, he decided to have his dentist to do this procedure for him. He almost immediately felt as if something had released, and he was able to bend over more easily starting that day. Later, when the dentist installed an upper bite guard which blocked these same front teeth both the pain and the locking in the hips returned that same night. Removal of the bite guard again cleared the symptoms.

A more permanent solution involved the installation of a front bridge with a plunger between the two top front teeth that allows suture movement. This specialized bridge with plunger was developed by Dr. Smith, DDS of Pennsylvania, and is now available. However, at this time, it is available by only one lab.

How do you know whether you need cranial therapy?
There are a number of indications that you have a skull misalignment or compression [2]:

- A head that is pointed, flattened on top or in the back, lumpy, or other than perfectly round.

- Asymmetry of the face. Hold a piece of paper down the middle of your face and look in the mirror or enlist the help of a friend. If the two sides don't match, this could be a sign of cranial deformity or accidental damage.

- Another test for asymmetry involves laying a finger on top of each cheekbone with your fingers pointing toward your nose. Look in the mirror to see whether the fingers are lined up at equal heights.

- One eye is larger, lower, at a different slant, or more deeply set than the other.

- Your sinuses are chronically clogged.

- A feeling of pressure behind the eyes or a tight feeling at the base of the skull.

- Soreness or numbness near the skull sutures.

What kinds of ailments can be relieved by this therapy?
A partial list of treatable ailments includes:

- *Brain fog*
- *Backache*
- *Seizures*
- *Insomnia*
- *Fatigue*

- *Sinus infections and blockage*
- *Mental retardation*
- *Neck and back pain*
- *Head and face pain*
- *Emotional trauma*

Adjustments should go from major to minor:

1. First the head should be adjusted and positioned over the neck and shoulders.
2. Adjustments should be made to the sinus area, cranium, and skull sutures.
3. The jaw and temporomandibular joint (TMJ) should be aligned.
4. Last, the teeth are dealt with in the form of a bite adjustment.

All of these are discussed in this chapter. The head position dictates the jaw position, and the jaw should be in its proper place before the bite is adjusted.

TMD/TMJ Syndrome

A Flaw in the Jaw?

The jaw is a singular marvel in the human body. It is the only part of the body strong enough to crush ice, something that even the grip of a strong person can't accomplish. However, the same

> **The jaw is quite a miracle of engineering!**

jaw can perform such delicate movements as separating the sinews of celery. No other part of the body has this range of both control and power.

Temporomandibular joint syndrome (TMJ), less commonly but more correctly called TMJ dysfunction (TMD), is a misalignment of the upper jaw (skull) and lower jaw. It is estimated that at least ten million, and as many as seventy million, Americans have TMD, with more women than men affected. TMD is significant in that a large number of people are inconvenienced or disabled by the disorder, and in the fact that TMD can mimic other ailments. Pain, if present, can be quite severe and debilitating, and can occur elsewhere in the body, not just in the jaw. TMD can cause or contribute to:

- *Headache*
- *Neck and low back pain*
- *Fibromyalgia*
- *Nerve and blood flow ailments*
- *Muscle stiffness*
- *Chronic Fatigue Syndrome (CFIDS)*
- *Almost any recurrent structural ailment*

For this reason it can be mistaken for other disorders.

The initials TMJ refer to the joint itself, but the term TMJ is also commonly (if not quite correctly) used to refer to the syndrome or symptoms caused by misalignment.

The temporomandibular joint is a ball and socket-type hinge. It can be considered to be either singular or plural, as there is one bone with two hinges. They are the only bilateral (two sided) joints in the body. The ball (condyle) glides over the disk into which it fits. The temporomandibular joints contain over 50% of the neural receptors of the body.

Temporomandibular Joint

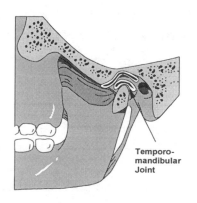

Temporo-
mandibular
Joint

The problem arises when, for any of a number of reasons, the ball and socket do not come together properly when the mouth is opened and closed. The result is a vicious cycle of nerve irritation, muscle spasm, and a worsening of the misalignment. The nerve irritation and muscle imbalance may eventually affect other parts of the body.

The joint may not pop out of place but if the teeth don't meet properly, or the jaw is turned slightly, this can set up the potential for problems elsewhere in the body.

The teeth, jaw, and cranium are related. When you chew, the sutures of the skull move as they are supposed to unless the jaw is out of alignment. In addition, the jaw joint is close to C-1 (the atlas) and a misaligned joint can adversely move or affect the atlas.

How important is TMJ to the rest of the body?
About 40% to 57% of the nerves leave the cranium through the temporomandibular joint. Misaligned TMJ can cause a restriction of any of these nerves and thus create health problems in the areas of the body served by these nerves. This accounts for the wide variety of apparently unrelated symptoms throughout the body.

The temporomandibular joint is also the primary intersection for the circulation of blood to and from the brain. Four bioelectromagnetic circuits pass through the TMJ area - the small intestine, gallbladder, stomach, and endocrine glandular system [3].

If the jaw is turned, the body can turn in the opposite direction to compensate. This twisting can lead to scoliosis (spinal curvature). Scoliosis with this cause can often be corrected by adjusting the jaw.

What are some of the causes of TMJ dysfunction?
There are many causes of TMJ/TMD syndrome. These include:

- An abscess can raise up a tooth so the bite is off.

- Teeth clenching or grinding (also called bruxism or bruxing). This may take place at night when you are not aware of it. Although bruxing may lead to TMD, the converse is more likely to be true as TMD can cause the bite to be unbalanced, and the teeth may be constantly trying to find a place to fit and land.

- A bad bite, in which teeth do not fit together properly. This can be due to loss of teeth, high crowns, or to whiplash.

- Poorly done dental work - high crowns or fillings hit improperly, while low crowns or fillings do not offer enough support.

- Bruxism may cause even more difficulty due to generated electrical currents if the teeth that are ground together have dissimilar metals in them, such as a mercury filling and a nickel crown. (See the chapter on the Battery Effect).

- Electricity from dissimilar metals in the mouth can cause TMD by causing the surrounding muscles to contract. This contraction can occur even without bruxism, or can be the cause of bruxism.

- Orthodontia done for cosmetic reasons can cause a bad bite by shifting teeth from the correct functional position to one that is more aesthetically pleasing but less functional. This is one of the most common causes of TMD.

- Regular gum chewing, ice chewing, or nail biting

- Poorly fitting dentures that don't come together properly or don't hit opposing teeth properly in four places top and bottom.

- Emotional stress which can lead to tightening of the jaw

- An injury to the jaw

- Deformed jaw joints

- Whiplash injury

- Cervical dysfunction - If the neck is out of alignment, the head will tilt to one side, but the jaw tends to be pulled straight down like a plumb bob. Over time, the jaw will not be symmetrical with respect to the rest of the face. The point of asymmetry in this case is the temporomandibular joint.

- Allergy, especially allergy to nickel which is found in root canal posts and orthodontic appliances, or to the metals copper or beryllium. Infection from root canal posts is another possible cause.

- Degenerative disease such as arthritis

If you have or do any of these, you may have TMJ dysfunction (TMD) without realizing it. Treatment could change your health for the better.

Both the incidence and severity of TMD has worsened over the years. This may be due in part to developmental abnormalities of the upper and/or lower jaw linked to the increased intake of processed foods, especially sugar and white flour [4], along with problems created by whiplash.

How can TMJ syndrome be diagnosed?
Since the problem is located near the teeth, TMJ is often first diagnosed by a dentist. In fact, the problem is often first noticed during a dental visit when, after holding her/his mouth open for an extended period of time, the dental patient notices discomfort or a popping feeling on finally closing the mouth. If TMJ is suspected, diagnosis can be confirmed by a doctor (MD, chiropractor, or osteopath) or dentist listening to the moving jaw with a stethoscope for telltale pops, clicks, and crackles, or by x-ray or other imaging techniques.

Four self-tests for TMJ dysfunction

- A self diagnostic test for TMJ is to put the little fingers in the ears and open and close the jaw. If you can feel a ball-type hinge joint move against your fingers in one or both ears, you may have TMJ syndrome.

- Open and close the mouth without using the finger technique and be aware of any pops, clicks, pain, or a feeling that the jaw is not closing smoothly. Repeated testing may be necessary as the symptoms may not show up or may not be the same every time.

- See if you can put three fingers, held vertically, in your mouth. If not, you may have TMD.

- Look for asymmetry in the opening and closing of the jaw by looking in a mirror or having a friend observe. A misaligned jaw may close at a slant, pop into position suddenly, or make an L shape or S shape as it closes.

What are some of the symptoms of TMD?

Symptoms of TMD include:

- A popping feeling or sound on opening the mouth wide or closing it

- Clicks and crackles while chewing

- Pain in the jaw joint in front of the ear

- Headaches, sometimes severe, and sometimes accompanied by nausea, blurred vision, or dizziness

- Earaches or ringing in the ears

- Pain in the teeth, which can be mistaken for abscesses or other tooth problems

- Facial muscles that cramp or go into spasm; facial pain

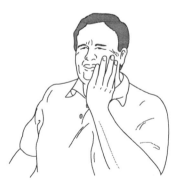

- Difficulty opening the mouth, especially wide or for a long time, or closing the mouth comfortably.

- Neck, shoulder, or back stiffness or pain, or whole body pain

- Brain fog from reduced blood flow to the brain

- Sunlight sensitivity

- Asymmetry in the opening or closing of the jaw - look in a mirror or have a friend observe

- Asymmetry in facial features

TMD and its symptoms can be present on one or both sides of the face. Some symptoms, such as joint pain, clicking, and popping, are practically diagnostic of TMD. Other symptoms take some real detective work, as they can be mistaken for sinusitis, back disk problems, ear infections, tooth abscesses, tumors, and other ailments.

How can you obtain relief from TMD?
Relief can be obtained by doing any of the following:

- Avoid hard or chewy foods .

- Avoid opening the mouth wide or for a long time

- Do stress reduction exercises such as alternately flexing and relaxing, or bio-feedback treatment.

- Use a bite guard to prevent tooth grinding.

- Jaw relaxation exercises

- Tai chi type exercise

- Avoid caffeine.

- Take bioflavonoids, especially pycnogenol or quercetin, and fish oils.

- Have a chiropractor or osteopath adjust the jaw, cranium, or do soft tissue work.

- Build up the teeth to balance the bite.

- Mild analgesics (pain relievers) such as aspirin or acetaminophen (Tylenol) can be used if other measures fail and the discomfort is severe.

- If malocclusion of the teeth is a cause, i.e. if the bite is off, this can be corrected by a dentist, especially one trained in vector work, which is discussed in the next paragraphs.

- Cold laser therapy and acupuncture have been useful in treating TMD [5].

These measures, other than correcting the bite, only relieve the symptoms of TMD. It is far more beneficial to the entire body to treat the cause of the TMJ dysfunction.

Bite Balancing

Beyond TMD: Is every tooth surface important to your health?
The relationship between the teeth and the rest of the body is demonstrated dramatically by work done by Daniel R. Gole, DDS, in Hastings, Michigan, and others. Dr. Gole uses the Resultant Force Vector technique (RFV) [6], in which very minor painless adjustments are made to the

teeth in order to make major changes in the body. Although few people in this country have heard of this technique, it is in fairly wide use in Europe, and over 2000 people are familiar with it and practice it with varying degrees of competence in the U.S.

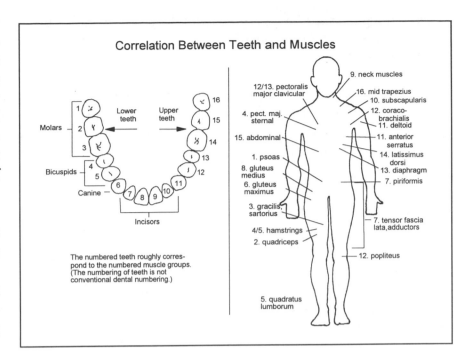

What is the relationship between the teeth and the muscles?
Each tooth or part of a tooth correlates with a compensating or counterbalancing muscle or muscle group.

This has been demonstrated empirically by noting that adjusting a certain tooth will cause certain muscles to unlock and relax reliably and predictably in thousands of patients. There is also a correlation between the pathways connecting teeth and muscle groups, according to pathway charts in use in Chinese medicine for the past 3000 years.

What can a piece of paper tell you about your bite?

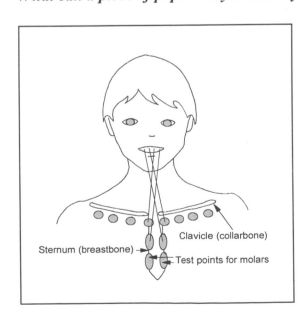

Press on spots just below the collarbone, starting close to the center of the body and working away from the center, and see if the spots are tender to the touch. Then press on spots going down the sternum, or breastbone, again checking for soreness. This test can point to tooth problems depending on the location of the pain. The closer the pain in the collarbone is to the front of the body, the closer the problematic tooth is to the front of the mouth, on the opposite side as the pain. As you go down the sternum, the location of the problem tooth is again shown by the location of the tender spot; the farther down the sternum, the farther back in the mouth the tooth is. The tenderness or soreness when pressed correlates to a high spot on the tooth on the opposite side.

Once you have figured out approximately which tooth or teeth may be high, put a folded piece of ordinary paper between the teeth on the opposite side, which is the same side as the clavicle or sternum pain. This raises the bite so it more closely matches the high spot on the opposite tooth, thus evening out the bite. Swallow with the paper in place - this clears what is called the gamma loop - and press the previously sore spot. If it is much less tender to touch now, the problem could be your bite.

The relationship between the pain and the high tooth spot, and pain relief with its temporary correction, shows the relationship between the teeth and the rest of the body. The soreness to touch is indicative of imbalance in the body, and the temporary correction with the paper approximates the permanent improvement when the high tooth is adjusted, as described in the next few paragraphs.

How is the tooth/body relationship utilized?

The practitioner "reads" muscle groups by noting areas of tenseness, knots, pain, and heightened pain response to pressure. S/he also notes how the person walks, any asymmetry in the body, range of motion, how the head moves, how the jaw moves up and down, rotation and flexion in limbs, and any stiffness or tenseness in any part of the body. Both individual muscles and total patterns or groups of muscles are significant. A chart such as the one on this page, with areas of tenderness, weakness or stiffness marked, makes patterns easier to spot.

Evaluation of muscles is done in several positions, including standing and lying down because this ties to the structure. This evaluation is more accurate than the "dental eye" and the use of articulating paper to show the high spots, usually the only gauges of bite problems. The "dental eye" has been shown to be wrong in demonstrations nearly 100% of the time.

Each tooth should ideally land in four spots on the opposing tooth. Many of us have only one or two such contact points per tooth. If the teeth do not meet properly, the jaw is constantly circling like a helicopter looking for a place to land. This instability is felt throughout the body.

The practitioner, guided by the anomalous muscle patterns and using a bite strip to confirm observations, makes very tiny adjustments to the teeth with a drill. The amount removed with the drill is as little as 1/1000 of an inch (less than the width of a hair), and dental material (fillings, crowns) is adjusted when possible rather than the natural tooth surface.

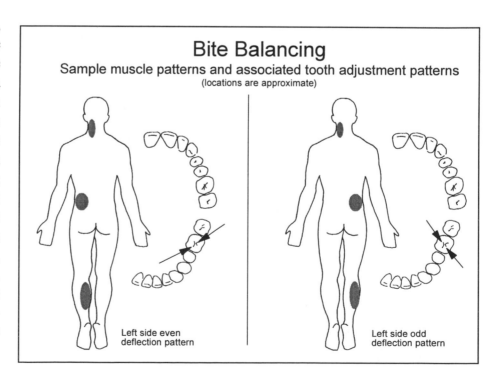

Bite Balancing
Sample muscle patterns and associated tooth adjustment patterns
(locations are approximate)

Left side even deflection pattern

Left side odd deflection pattern

The angle of the cut on the tooth is very important. This is dictated by the pattern of muscle weakness or tenderness - on the same side of the body (even) or on opposite sides of the body (odd). There are other types of patterns as well.

When this is done properly, both the patient and the practitioner can often feel entire muscle groups relax instantly.

How does this relationship affect the rest of the body?

Tense muscles can pull the spine, neck, and hips out of alignment, causing the many adverse effects discussed in the previous chapter. If your spine is out of alignment, muscles may then stiffen to compensate, worsening the problem in a vicious cycle. The stiffness so characteristic of many older people is often a result of such a cycle, and the RFV technique may prevent or alleviate this stiffness.

> Unbalanced Bite = Unbalanced Body

This misalignment may be partially or wholly responsible for Parkinson's disease, arthritis (especially ankylosing spondylitis), fibromyalgia, and nerve and muscle disorders such as multiple sclerosis (MS) and ALS (Lou Gehrig's Disease).

Movement of the jaw stimulates the fifth cranial nerve to the central nervous system (CNS). Nerve impulses from the CNS then affect every system in the body. In other words, if the bite is off, the jaw may not move properly, and body systems may then be adversely affected. However, when the bite is adjusted, jaw movement is smooth and relaxed, and through the jaw's action on the CNS, body function no longer has to compensate and is normalized to an extent.

The jaw is like a gyroscope or a plumb bob. If it is uncertain the body compensates by being tight, like the way a person who is dizzy might tighten the body when walking down the stairs. When the jaw/gyroscope is certain, or the plumb is level, the body is loose, as it should be.

What are some other implications of this technique?

As noted, an adjustment to the tooth as fine as 1/1000 of an inch can have noticeable results. Much larger adjustments are made to the bite without considering the effect on the rest of the body during cosmetic orthodontia (braces). The natural bite can be inadvertently improved or worsened by orthodontia, with resulting improvement in body function or, more often, the appearance of puzzling or even debilitating symptoms. High fillings or poorly fitting crowns or dentures can also adversely affect the person's entire body for the same reason.

Who is the most important doctor you have?

The dentist is the most important doctor most of us have. A caring dentist has the potential to solve more problems, but an uncaring or uninformed dentist can cause more problems than almost any other practitioner.

> A dentist can have more influence on health than almost any other practitioner.

What other treatment exists for TMJ?

Surgery is a remedy of last resort, and should be considered only if milder measures do not help, there is considerable damage to or deformity of the jaw joint, and symptoms are very debilitating. Stainless steel jaw joints, containing the carcinogenic and allergenic metal nickel, have been used. These are not recommended.

A patient who had these metal joints surgically implanted developed numerous severe health problems, including a cut facial nerve resulting in partial facial paralysis, a jaw that wouldn't open properly, and nickel allergy. She developed colon problems so severe that a part of her colon was removed, and she required a hysterectomy due also to complications from the surgery. She then became allergic to many substances. She finally died from the complications.

A fairly severe TMJ problem can develop into arthritis or an arthritis-like condition if untreated [3,6,7]. Fibromyalgia or multiple sclerosis (MS) can also result.

Getting your head on straight

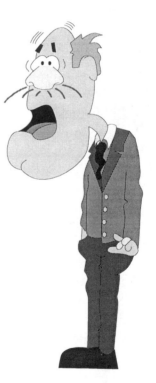

Many people carry their heads forward rather than in proper balance on top of their spines. This is especially visible on many older people. If a person stands up straight and is viewed from the side, the ear should be directly over the shoulder. One cause of the head-forward position is a jaw that is too far back, and the person thrusts their whole head forward to compensate and to keep their airway open. The unbalanced weight of a 14-pound head can throw the whole spine out, with a wide range of resulting problems and symptoms as discussed in these two chapters.

A head forward C2-4 adjustment and a "dowager's hump" adjustment, along with bite balancing, can allow a head that used to be too far forward to stay in place.

Dr. Joseph Lytle, DDS, uses a technique involving a splint to pull the jaw open and forward, which allows the head to go back where it belongs. The throat opens up and the person stands taller rather than bending forward. After this treatment, one 80 year old woman was able to stand straight up after being osteoporotic and bent over.

Summary

The mouth, jaw, teeth and head can have an amazing influence on the rest of the body. Most people, including many dentists, think of the teeth as being essentially separate from the body. However, they are so important to total body health that four chapters in this book are devoted wholly or partially to the influence of the teeth: this chapter, Mercury, Nickel and Root Canals, and The Battery Effect.

When correcting the head, go from major to minor, as in this building analogy:

- Get your head on straight   Whiplash, C1-C7   Plumb the house
- Don't get your nose out of joint   Nasal specific   Fix the door jamb
- Quit your jawing and do something   TMJ   Adjust hinges
- Provide a secure landing spot for your teeth   Bite balancing   Plane door

---

References and Resources

- The Burton Goldberg Group, *Alternative Medicine: The Definitive Guide*, "Craniosacral Therapy", pp. 149-155, Future Medicine Publishing, Puyallup WA, 1994.

- Upledger, John E., *Your Inner Physician and You: Cranio-Sacral Therapy and Soma-toEmotional Release*, North Atlantic Books, Berkeley CA, 1992. *For the lay reader.*

- **MyoData TMJ and Stress Center**, P.O. Box 803394, Dallas TX 75380, phone 1-800- 533-5131. *Has a catalog of TMD-related materials, books and services.*

Practitioners

- Dr. Joseph Lytle is the developer of the jaw splint. He is located in...

- Dr. Joe Smith is the developer of the split front-tooth bridge. He is located in Philadelphia, PA.

- Dr. Daniel R. Gole, D.D.S. does pioneering bite balancing work. He is located in Hastings, MI.

- Dr. Dean Howell, N.D. does cranial work and nasal specific therapy as described in the previous chapter. He is located in Everett, WA.

- Dr. Suzanne Fuselier, D.C. can be reached at Comprehensive Health Centers, 4403 Manchester Avenue, Suite 107, Encinitas CA 92024, phone (619) 632-9042.

- Dr. David Olinger, D.C. can be reached at Comprehensive Health Centers, 4403 Manchester Avenue, Suite 107, Encinitas CA 92024, phone (619) 632-9042.

Most of the above methods are incorporated into Comprehensive Health Centers, consisting of Integrated Healing Medical Center and Coastal Dental. Together they combine Medical, Dental, Chiropractic and Natural Therapeutics. They are located at 4403 Manchester Avenue, Suite 107, Encinitas, CA 92024, phone 619-632-9042.

Secondary Toxic Suppressors

-

Microorganisms

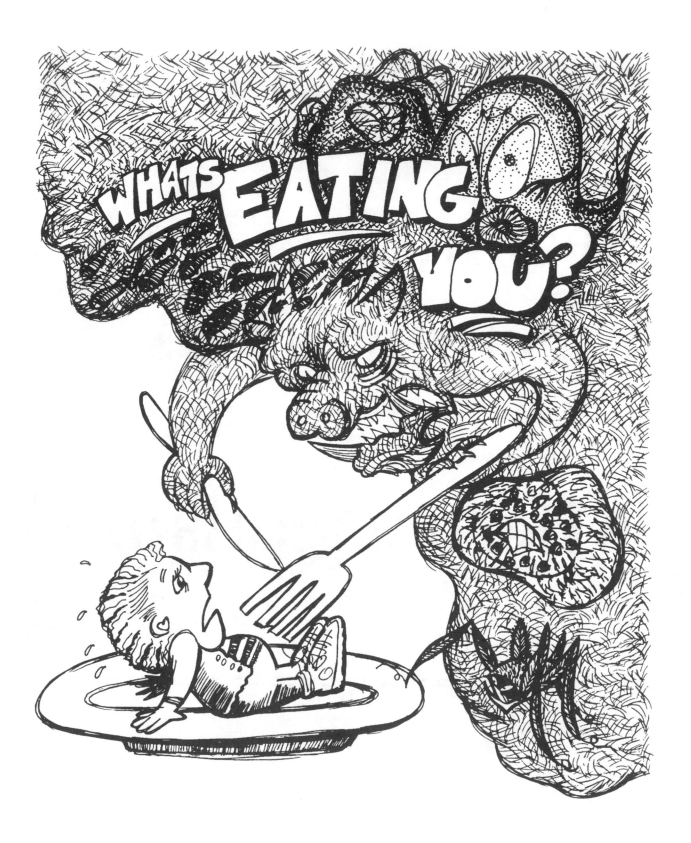

MICROORGANISMS - AN OVERVIEW

What's Eating You?

Do you have the following symptoms? You may have microorganisms, also known as parasites, and they might be adversely affecting your health.

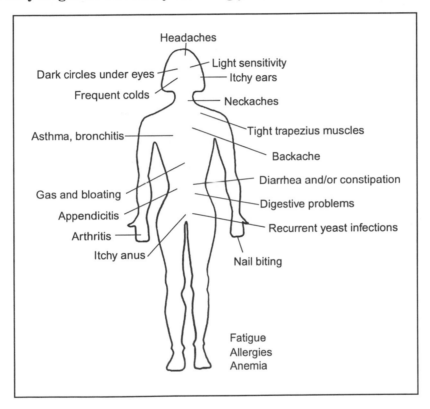

Fifteen things in this chapter that can change your health:

1. Parasite infestation, which involves more than the creepy-crawly things that most people envision, can have a powerful negative impact on your health.

*2. As many as 50% of the U.S. population has some kind of parasite. There's a 50% chance this means **you**. Almost anyone can have parasites regardless of personal habits.*

3. Parasites will infect or infest a body which is already weakened by primary toxic suppressors such as amalgam fillings. Parasites don't invade a healthy body.

4. Doctors don't usually look for parasites. This means that a parasite-caused illness will probably not be detected and treated.

5. *Parasites are not limited to tropical areas.*

6-11. *Parasites are a common cause of*

> *Allergies*   *Fatigue*
> *Nailbiting*   *Dark circles under the eyes*
> *Recurrent yeast infections*
> *Frequent colds and infections*

12. *Some cases of acne may be caused by anal-to-face parasite transmission.*

13. *Do you know exactly why infection makes you feel sick?*

14. *You may have had parasites since childhood, and some genetic predisposition to parasites may be passed on. Parasites rarely go away by themselves.*

15. *Why most labs can't find parasites. Both testing and treatment for parasites may need to be done more than once to be effective.*

Okay, now we've got your attention. What is a parasite?
A parasite is one form of a microorganism. However, not all microbes are parasites. A parasite is a living organism that stays alive through dependence on the body of an animal, called the host. This dependence is often to the detriment of the host. Humans can be hosts to a wide variety of parasites which can be transferred to them by animals or other humans, either directly or through such means as contaminated produce or water.

Parasites are everywhere. Once infected, they can stay within your body for decades. Parasites causing today's symptoms may have entered your body in childhood. They will rarely, if ever, go away by themselves.

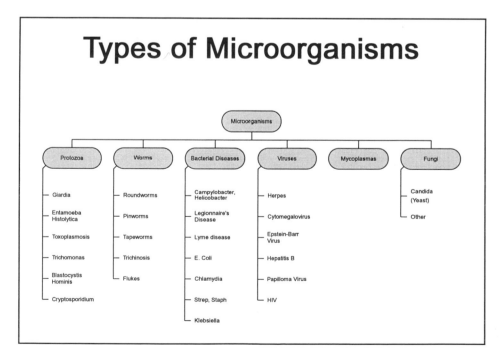

Parasites include bacteria and viruses as well as the creepy-crawly things that many people may envision.

What sets the stage for parasites to take up residence in your body?
Parasites are considered secondary toxic suppressors because they will rarely infect, or infest, a body which is not already

weakened by the primary toxic suppressors discussed in previous book sections. The primary suppressors set up the conditions in which parasites flourish. Once a person is infested, parasites will further depress the immune system and cause systemic problems (the type of problem depends on the type of parasite) as do the primary suppressors.

Parasites can be both the cause and effect of weakness and illness. To say that parasites make you sick is like saying that maggots and buzzards, which are also opportunistic organisms, cause an animal's death. The obvious question here is: which came first?

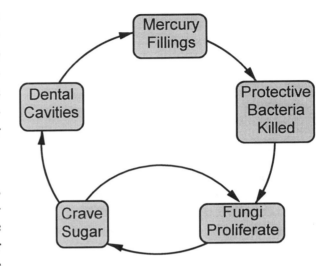

A vicious cycle of primary and secondary toxic suppressors can be set up. For example, beneficial bifidus bacteria in the gut which help keep parasites under control can be destroyed by mercury from amalgam tooth fillings, antibiotic drugs, and chlorine in the water supply. Whatever kills the beneficial bacteria opens the door for the parasites.

Fungi such as yeast can then grow out of control, causing craving for sweets which feed the fungus. You then eat sugar, which ferments in the body, providing an environment favorable for many parasites. Sugar will also contribute to the development of dental cavities, leading to the placement of amalgam fillings, which contain mercury which is toxic to the friendly bifidus bacteria. The lack of these bacteria allow parasites to flourish. It's a vicious cycle.

Another common example of this kind of a vicious cycle is where parasites lead to allergies, which lower the hydrochloric acid (HCl) in the stomach. Since HCl kills parasites, a deficiency of HCl allows parasites to flourish.

To treat parasites effectively, first change the environment in which they best live and thrive.

Why doesn't everyone who is exposed to parasites get sick?
If a number of people are in the same room with someone who has a cold, some people will catch the cold but most won't. What makes the difference?

Those who catch the cold are those whose bodies and immune systems are already weakened by some of the primary toxic suppressors already discussed. Similarly, not everyone who is exposed to the HIV virus will develop AIDS. The contributing toxic suppressors, covered in more detail in the chapter on HIV and AIDS, include drugs (not only IV drugs), semen (an immune suppressor), and various parasites.

The condition of the host is more important than the organism.

> **The condition of the host is more important than the organism.**

Who, me?

You may be thinking that a chapter on parasites doesn't apply to you. After all,

- *You've never been to Africa.*

- *You don't go backpacking or drink from mountain streams.*

- *You wash your hands.*

- *You can't possibly have something crawly and socially unacceptable inside **your** body.*

> **You couldn't possibly have something crawly and socially unacceptable inside your body, could you?**

Unfortunately, you may have one or more types of parasites, especially considering the symptoms that may have led you to read this book. Estimates vary, but it should be safe to say that 15-50% of the population has at least one type of parasite in their bodies, defining parasite as something living that doesn't belong in your body and lives off of you.

Why don't doctors suspect parasites more often?

There is a common misconception that parasites are tropical diseases, and the tropics sounds like some place far away. Actually, tropics and subtropics are defined as areas where the ground doesn't freeze in winter. Much of the southern third of the United States falls into that category, including much of California, Florida, and Texas.

Widespread and comparatively easy travel has contributed to the spread of parasites. Visitors to Mexico, South America, Africa, and other tropical areas bring these unwelcome hitchhikers back to all parts of the country. A parasite does not need a visa to cross the border. Food handlers and vegetable pickers from these countries carry parasites with them to the U.S.

Doctors often do not suspect parasites because they don't see this as a tropical area. Also, symptoms such as fatigue and asthma may seem far removed from, say, worm infestation, which may indeed be causing the symptoms.

What are the major types of parasites?

Types of parasites include:

- **Amoebic protozoa** such as entamoeba histolytica can cause a very serious infestation.

- **Flagellate protozoa** such as giardia are less harmful than amoebic protozoa but in large numbers can interfere with food absorption and fat metabolism.

- **Worms** such as pinworm or roundworm.

- **Bacteria** such as streptococcus, which can cause strep throat, and helicobacter pylori.

- **Viruses** such as flu virus, HIV, herpes, Epstein-Barr virus, and cytomegalovirus.

- **Mycoplasmas**, which are very tiny organisms.

- **Fungi** such as yeast, which are plants.

These parasites range in size from single celled protozoa, to viruses which are even smaller, to roundworms several feet long. All of these parasites are discussed in greater detail in this book section.

Why doesn't the immune system eliminate parasites?

If our immune systems are so vigilant, why don't they recognize the parasites as outside invaders and eliminate them?

Parasites, which have coexisted over time within their hosts, have developed the ability to evade the immune response by a variety of mechanisms [1]:

- Antigenic variation - this is the best-known evasive tactic. A parasite such as the trypanosome can go through a genetically programmed series of mutations and so stay one step ahead of the immune system.

- Molecular mimicry - Some parasites make antigens that resemble those of the host to take advantage of the immune system's safeguards against autoimmunity - like "wolves in sheep's clothing".

- Parasites may avoid stimulating the immune response by colonizing in sites not well serviced by the immune system, like criminals congregating in spots which are not well patrolled by police.

- They may interfere with the immune system's normal control processes by redirecting the immune system into nonproductive channels.

Parasites are not totally exempt from immune system effects, however, or they would multiply out of control and eventually kill the host. The parasites and the immune system often appear to achieve a balance where the parasite population stays relatively constant over the years.

Strengthening the immune system would tip the balance in the host's (your) favor. On the other hand, the presence of parasites can weaken the immune system or cause "leaky gut" which can lead to allergies, which are a natural immune system response to undigested non-self protein. Eliminating the parasites would strengthen the immune system and improve your general health.

Do parasites cause symptoms other than tummyaches and "trots"?

Parasites can cause both acute and chronic symptoms, depending on the type of parasite and individual sensitivity. Acute (short term) symptoms are unmistakable, such as stomach pains and explosive diarrhea, or deadly malarial fevers. If untreated or mistreated, acute infection or infestation can become chronic.

A single episode of parasitic infestation such as food poisoning can increase intestinal permeability, i.e. "leaky gut" syndrome, which sets the stage for food allergies [2].

Chronic (long term) symptoms, on the other hand, can be so subtle that they cannot be traced back to a particular infection. You've felt this way for so long you don't even remember when it started. Some symptoms are specific enough, especially in combination, that an alert doctor can make a diagnosis of parasite infestation. Other symptoms, such as fatigue, although they are very real and debilitating to you, are vague enough that they could be attributable to almost anything.

What are some indications that you may have a parasite infestation?

While some symptoms are specific to a particular type of parasite, there are some general symptoms which, especially in combination, can be due to parasite infestation. For example, weight problems and gland problems (thyroid, gonads, adrenals) can have chronic parasitic infection as their source. Other general symptoms include: [3]

- *Fatigue*
- *Arthritis*
- *Low-grade fever*
- *Chronic anemia*
- *Light sensitivity*
- *Nail biting*
- *Stiffness and pain*
- *Widespread allergies*
- *Autoimmune disease*
- *Itchy ears or anus*
- *Dark under-eye circles*
- *Headaches, neck and back aches*
- *Diarrhea or constipation, constant or alternating*
- *Elevated eosinophils (white blood cells)*
- *Chronic viral infections, frequent colds*
- *Irritable bowel symptoms (gas, intestinal pain, bloating)*

Cycle of Parasite Reinfestation

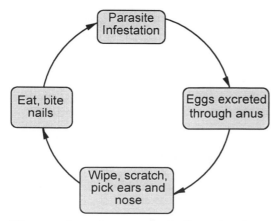

Nailbiting and nose picking may be caused by parasites, which use these routes to reinfest your body.

The desire to bite the nails is a craving which may be puzzling because it provides no real pleasure and resists efforts to stop by using willpower or self-condemnation. Many people, even those who have bitten their nails for decades, find that they lose the desire to bite their nails after being treated for parasites.

> **You may be able to stop biting your nails easily!**

How serious is parasite infestation?

Although chronic parasite infestation can cause symptoms that are vague and elusive, the infestation can be quite serious rather than simply inconvenient. Many protozoa can penetrate vital organs such as the brain, lungs, and liver. The most prevalent parasite worldwide is the roundworm, which can grow so large that it can block the human intestine or fill the appendix and cause it to burst. Amebiasis is one of the most deadly parasites, and can cause death if untreated. One parasite, the schistosomiasis worm, kills more people worldwide than all forms of cancer put together. If you have reason to suspect parasitic infection, you can't afford **not** to be diagnosed and treated.

Why exactly does infection or infestation cause you to feel so absolutely debilitated?

Let's say you have an acute infection, such as the flu. You are tired and weak and achy, you are both cold and feverish, and you just want to sleep. Food is unappetizing, your sex drive has dropped to zero, and you can't even think straight. Have you ever wondered how a bunch of germs that have temporarily gotten out of hand can cause these particular symptoms?

> **Ever wonder why you feel sick when you're sick?**

Every one of these symptoms - the fatigue, fever, aches, and loss of appetite and sex drive - happens for a reason, with the ultimate goal of triumphing over the invaders. A complex series of immune system responses brings all this about.

When an invader such as a bacterium or virus enters the body, the immune system sounds the alarm, a scavenger (attack and cleanup) cell called a macrophage cell grabs the bug and presents it to the T cells, which confirm that the invader is non-self and should be dealt with. The macrophage sets off a chain of events, in which a substance called interleukin acts as messenger, that leads to killer T cells attacking the intruders.

Interleukin also has another job, that of temperature regulation. A higher body temperature both helps the immune system to work faster and puts pathogens at a disadvantage, since many of them multiply more slowly at higher temperatures. The hypothalamus, which functions as a thermostat, is normally set at about 98.6 degrees Fahrenheit; if the body temperature goes below that, you shiver and feel chilly. When the hypothalamus gets the message that higher temperatures are needed, the thermostat setting is moved up, you run a fever, and 98.6 now feels chilly. You shiver and pile on the blankets. Taking aspirin or a similar medication will lower the fever, reduce the body aches, and make you feel better in the short term, but will thwart one of the immune system's ways to make you feel better in the long run.

When the body senses danger, whether from a car bearing down on you as you cross the intersection or from a large number of invading bacteria or parasites, a chain of events is set into motion which signal the adrenal glands to prepare you for an emergency, the sympathetic fight-or-flight response. Energy is diverted to the muscles where it would be needed, and at the same time is diverted from activities which are not useful or would be distracting at the time. For this reason, appetite, digestion, reproductive processes, and sex drive are suppressed. When you are sick, you aren't much interested in food, and sex is probably the furthest thing from your mind. You find it difficult to concentrate on anything but the danger, so you can focus on only the simplest reading material or TV shows. After the sympathetic fight-or-flight response is depleted, the parasympathetic repair-and-restore response kicks in, making you feel fatigued but doing more good in the long run.

Since the body senses danger, all of your senses are on full alert. Your sensitivity threshold to pain and other stimuli is lowered, so your body will react to things it would normally ignore. Your joints ache, your skin is unpleasantly sensitive, light hurts your eyes, music is too loud. You are emotionally hypersensitive, or irritable, as well.

It takes a lot of energy to mobilize the immune system, fight off the invaders, and stay on full alert. Since much of your body's energy is being used in this way, it isn't surprising that you feel tired and listless and want to sleep a lot. The tiredness is also nature's way of making you conserve energy for the internal battle [4].

What does this have to do with chronic parasitic infection or infestation?

This explains what goes on when you have the flu and feel awful for a week, but what does this have to do with chronic parasitic infection? The difference between the two is like the difference between an enemy invasion and rapid counterattack as compared with a long drawn-out war in which a great deal of energy is expended over the years in simply trying to keep the front line from moving in the enemy's favor. In both cases, however, there is fighting, and the need for constant vigilance.

In chronic infection or infestation, as with the flu, the immune system is mobilizing and fighting, the adrenal glands are on alert, and your energy is diverted towards the battle and away from nonessential functions. The difference is that in chronic infections this process goes on for years, although at a lower level than with the flu. You end up with a milder but much longer lasting set of flu-like symptoms, and for much the same reason.

Your internal thermostat is out of whack, so you may run a low-grade fever and probably feel chilly. Energy is diverted from activity which is nonessential in an emergency, so your appetite may be low, your sex drive may be low to nonexistent, and you may have trouble getting or staying pregnant. Your digestion is off, both for this reason and because many parasites that live in the gut cause digestive problems of their own. You can't concentrate or stay focused on what you are doing.

Your sensitivity threshold is lowered, explaining in part the joint aches and other pains, sensitivity to light and noise, and general irritability. Your fatigue, dragginess, and desire to sleep make sense now, since so much of your energy is going towards fighting a battle that your body, at best, is only able to keep from getting worse.

All of these symptoms caused by immune system response are in addition to symptoms caused by toxicity from the waste byproducts of the parasites themselves. The battle can last from the time the parasite enters the body until treatment or death, which could be a period of many years, during which time you may be becoming progressively more debilitated.

How do parasites enter the body?

Whether or not you have parasites, it is important to know how they enter the body and how this entry can be prevented.

Water - Parasites, especially giardia and roundworm, can be ingested from contaminated water, whether from a pristine-looking mountain stream or from the tap. Even if you don't drink water, if you use it to wash fruits and vegetables which you then eat raw, you can still be infected. Use filters or bottled water that has been tested.

Drinking water is a major source of parasites. A study of surface water sources in Kansas showed that 86% of them were contaminated with giardia and/or cryptosporidium [5].

Pets - Animals harbor parasites that can be transmitted to humans. Wash your hands after petting an animal, changing your cat's litterbox, or cleaning up after your dog. Keep your pets wormed and vaccinated. Cats and dogs looking for a bathroom and your children are all attracted to the sandbox or the grass in the park, and this is a common way for children to become infected. Allow your children to play only in your own sandbox, and keep it covered when not in use. Pets, especially dogs, use their tongues to practice personal hygiene and then lick people, potentially transmitting any diseases the pet may have.

Meat - Some parasites, such as trichinosis and toxoplasmosis, can be transmitted through raw or incompletely cooked meat and fish if the animal was infected before butchering, or if the butcher carried the infection from another animal. It is best to give up steak tartare and sushi, and to cook all meat, especially pork, thoroughly. The e. coli bacteria in meat caused fatal infections in customers at Jack in the Box restaurant in 1993.

Produce - Fruit pickers, often from tropical areas, pick fruits and vegetables in the field. Sanitary facilities may be deficient or nonexistent, and farms may lack even a sink and soap for use by the workers. An infected worker can therefore transmit parasites to the produce being picked. The produce is often not washed before selling, especially from roadside stands. Produce should always be washed thoroughly before eating, especially if it can't be peeled. A few drops of food grade hydrogen peroxide (preferred) or chlorine bleach in a dishpan full of wash water has a microbe-killing effect.

Sex -. Disease can also be spread through any sexual practices in which body fluids from one partner come in contact with a membrane surface (vagina, mouth) of another. Contact with fecal material can spread disease. Scrupulous hygiene is important.

Babies and young children - Day-care centers are notorious for parasite epidemics, such as giardia and pinworms, since there are a lot of baby diapers and hand-to-mouth contact in that age group. The bugs, which may come originally from a child's pets, can survive for quite a while on toys and faucets, thereby infecting parents and caretakers. Swimming pools used by toddlers not yet toilet trained are another source of risk [6]. Since it is rarely possible or desirable to isolate your child from contact with others, wash your hands and your child's hands frequently, and keep an eye on your child's stools. Some parasites such as pinworms are visible in the stool.

Restaurants - One of the unknowns you face when eating in a restaurant or at a salad bar is the personal hygiene habits of the workers. One food preparer who doesn't wash after wiping can infect an awful lot of people. To be safe, limit restaurant eating and make your own salads at home with vegetables you have washed yourself. If you eat out, eat only cooked foods. Foods containing a lot of garlic or cayenne have a protective effect against worms. Ideally, food handlers should be tested for parasites.

Insects - Many parasitic diseases can be transmitted by fleas, houseflies, mosquitoes, and ticks. These insects are said to be disease vectors. Lyme disease is transmitted by a particular type of tiny tick, the deer tick. Minimize insect contact by avoiding woods and tall grassy areas, especially at dawn or dusk, and wearing long sleeves and pants. Check yourself for ticks after being in wooded areas, and check your pets for fleas and ticks.

Soil - Animal parasites can enter the soil through fecal and other contact. Wear gloves when gardening and/or scrub your hands and nails afterward. It is not uncommon for young children to eat dirt, and they may become infected in this way.

What are other ways to protect against parasites?
Preventive measures other than avoiding the above sources include:

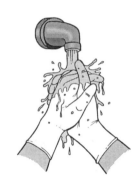

- **Washing** your hands regularly, especially after using the toilet, petting animals, gardening or changing diapers.

- **Hi-Tech Hygiene** makes an iodine-based hand and face wash; iodine kills parasites.

- **Resistance** - Keep your immune system in good shape. Avoid sugar and mucus-producers such as dairy products, as parasites don't favor clean intestines.

- **Stool testing** done on a regular basis, perhaps once a year.

How can you be tested for parasites?
Stool samples are often used for testing. In some cases, such as pinworms, the small wiggling white worms can be seen by the untrained eye. Stool samples are usually examined microscopically by a professional for the parasites themselves or for their eggs. Purged stool testing is believed to be more accurate than examination of solid stool [3]. Rectal swab tests, repeated three times, are also good for detecting parasites.

A word of warning - most parasites don't do the same thing throughout their life cycles. They will lay eggs, or enter the bowel, only at certain times in their lives. Therefore, a negative stool test does not mean that you are free of parasites. If you have a negative test, and parasites are still suspected, repeat the test at least once at a later date or do a different type of test for confirmation, since the parasites may have been in an undetectable part of their life cycle during the first testing.

String - A method to detect upper gastrointestinal parasites involves swallowing a capsule attached to a string, one end of which is left outside the mouth. The string is withdrawn through the mouth after a few hours and examined microscopically [6].

Endoscopy - This is an invasive procedure in which intestinal tissue is extracted by way of the mouth. It is a very accurate test for some parasites, but they can usually be detected using less drastic measures [6]. Duodenal intubation and biopsy are other invasive procedures which are effective but drastic [7].

Tape applied to and then removed from the unwashed anus upon awakening will pick up pinworm eggs, which can be detected microscopically on the tape.

ELISA testing - This is a noninvasive laboratory test, using polyclonal rabbit antiserum, which can diagnose giardia and possibly other parasites [7].

IgG and IgM antibody testing can be done for giardia and entamoeba histolytica [3].

Kinesiology, or muscle testing, is sometimes used to detect parasites.

For all tests, it is important to realize that a positive result means that you have parasites, but a negative result does not mean that you don't have parasites. If you test negative but still believe you are infested, repeat the test, try a different test, or treat for parasites even though the test results are negative.

Proper diagnosis is over 90% of the battle against parasites.

> **Proper diagnosis is over 90% of the battle against parasites.**

What Can You Do?

What are some treatments for parasites?
There are several treatment options. These are discussed only briefly here and in the following chapters, as this book is not intended to prescribe treatment. Your doctor or health practitioner will do the appropriate prescribing after testing, diagnosis, and assessment of the severity of the problem. However, a few treatment protocols are listed in the appropriate chapters **for physician/practitioner use only**.

Allopathic drugs, such as vermifuges for worms or Metronidazole for amoebic infection, can be used. These may or may not do the job, but have the potential for serious side effects. Metronidazole (trade name Flagyl) contains the poison arsenic. Fasigyn (Tenidazol from Pfizer Pharmaceuticals) is more effective and less toxic than Flagyl, although it is only available in Mexico, Canada, and Europe, but not the U.S.

Botanicals and natural remedies work with the body in partnership against the parasites. They are much less likely than allopathic drugs to cause side effects. Biocidin and AP Mag are both herbal antiparasitic preparations. Black walnut, cayenne, garlic, artemisia annua and wormwood are also useful.

Immune system strengthening through a variety of methods as discussed throughout this book. This may be sufficient to empower the immune system to fight off the parasites without outside help. The parasite population can at least be reduced in this way, and there are no side effects except beneficial ones. However, immune system boosting will probably be insufficient to eliminate the problem entirely, and drugs or botanicals will be needed to complete or start the job.

Liver/gallbladder flush gets parasites out of the gallbladder, although the flush is also good for gallstones and to optimize liver and gallbladder function in general. A knowledgeable practitioner can give you a liver/gallbladder flush protocol and monitor your progress.

Citrus seed extracts such as Citricidal or Nutricidal brand grapefruit seed extract are active against viruses, protozoa, bacteria and yeast. It may be necessary to take it for up to several months, which is possible because it is nontoxic and rarely allergenic. Artemisia annua, artemisia absinthium (wormwood) and cloves are also recommended. Wormwood can be toxic, however, if taken by itself and is therefore recommended in combination with other herbs [8].

Parasites are plural
Once the stage is set for a parasite infestation, other parasites often follow or co-exist. For example, blastocystis hominis is normally found with either entamoeba histolytica or giardia, which tend to be found together, as are giardia and roundworm. A more complete solution to the parasite problem involves treating the "go-withs" as well as the diagnosed parasite.

Fungus often follows parasite infestation and may also follow parasite treatment, as the treatment may kill the protective bacteria which keep the fungus/yeast under control. It is therefore wise to treat for yeast/fungus after treating parasites.

Remember, prevention is better than treatment!

References and Resources

- The Burton Goldberg Group, *Alternative Medicine: The Definitive Guide*, Future Medicine Publishing, Puyallup WA, 1994. *The following chapters are relevant to Parasites:*

  "Parasitic Infections", pp. 782-9
  "Infections", p. 937

- Leventhal, R. and R.F. Cheadle, *Medical Parasitology: A Self-Instructional Text*, F.A. Davis Company, Philadelphia PA, 3rd ed., 1989.

AMOEBAS AND PROTOZOA

What's Bugging You?

Do you have any of the following symptoms? You may have a protozoal or amoebic infestation.

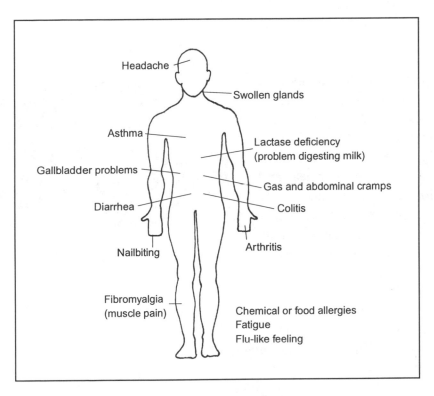

Twelve things in this chapter that can change your health :

1. Giardia is the most common human parasite in the U.S., and it can be very disabling.

2. Giardia is a major cause of asthma. Treating for the parasite in these cases often brings partial or full relief from the asthma.

3. Rheumatoid arthritis has been linked to giardial infestation.

4. Biting your nails, picking your nose, or even rubbing your eyes can keep the parasite infestation going.

5. The water from your household faucet can be transmitting a parasitic disease.

6. Intolerance to milk products can be an indication of giardial infestation.

7. Many people with gallbladder problems can avoid needless surgery by being treated for giardia, which may be causing their symptoms.

8. Treatment for protozoa should be given more than once to be effective.

9. Entamoeba histolytica, a protozoal disease, can be deadly.

10. Chronic fatigue and multiple chemical or food allergies can be related to protozoal infestation.

11. A parasite hazardous to pregnant women can be transmitted by a house cat.

12. What is the most common protozoal gynecological disease, and what can be done about it?

What are protozoa?

Protozoa are single-celled animals that are slightly larger than bacteria. "Protozoa" is the plural form; the singular form is "protozoan". Most protozoa are found in the digestive tract, particularly the bowel, causing diarrhea and general ill health in the short run. Some protozoa start out in the intestines but, if untreated, can migrate to vital organs such as the lungs, brain, and liver, causing chronic problems.

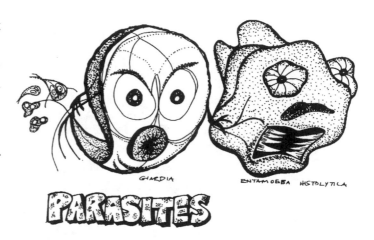

Many protozoa secrete a resistant covering and go into a cocoon-like resting stage called a cyst. They can thus survive for long periods of time in water or on faucets or toys before infecting the next person or animal. The cyst is the infectious form. The trophozoite, or active form, causes the symptoms. Trophozoite and cyst are like chicken and egg respectively.

Protozoa that are most likely to cause problems are giardia lamblia and entamoeba histolytica.

Giardia

What is the most common parasite?

Giardia lamblia, which is also called giardia intestinalis, is the most common parasite found in humans in the United States. The disease caused by the parasite, giardiasis, is not fatal but can be very disabling.

Giardia is a one-celled, flattened organism with an adhesive disk on its front surface, with which it attaches itself to a cell in the host's intestinal wall.

How does giardial infection occur?

Giardia is passed through fecal-oral contamination, as cysts found in the human or animal host's fecal matter are ingested by another person or animal. This is accomplished through:

- Drinking water contaminated by animal feces from mountain streams or even household faucets. Because of fecal contamination of streams, giardiasis has been called beaver fever.

- Engaging in sexual practices involving anal and/or oral contact.

- Changing diapers without washing hands.

- Eating food that has been handled by the un-washed hands of an infected person.

- Cleaning up after infected pets.

- Children crawling on carpets or yards where in-fected animals have been, then putting their fin-gers in their own or the pets' mouths.

- Reinfecting yourself by wiping, picking your ears or nose, and biting your nails, licking your fingers, or rubbing your eyes.

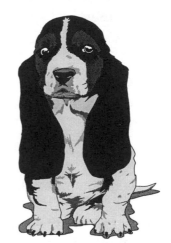

- 21-44% of children in U.S. day care centers are estimated to have giardial in-fections [1]. A study in Toronto, Canada showed an infection rate of 19% for the children and 14% for the staff from dientameba and giardia [2]. 38% of children in pediatric and dental clinics were found to be infected [3].

Sanitation is the key to preventing the transmission of this highly infectious parasite.

How does giardia gain a foothold in the body?

After the cyst is swallowed, it travels through the stomach and lodges in the duodenum, jejunum, and upper ileum of humans, i.e. the upper small bowel in the digestive tract. The adhesive disk of the trophozoite fits over an epithelial cell, and in a severe infection the free surface of nearly every cell can be covered with a parasite [4].

Since the gastrointestinal tract has a surface area the size of a football field [5], this represents a huge number of protozoa that can potentially be present in the body. Giardia may or may not spread beyond the digestive tract, including to the gallbladder and bile duct where they can inter-fere with oil absorption. Whether or not the infestation is limited to the gastrointestinal tract, such a huge number of invading organisms has the ability to affect the rest of the body in various ways.

Hypochlorhydria, an insufficiency of hydrochloric acid in the stomach, predisposes one to infec-tion, as the HCl, a first line of defense, "cooks" the parasites before they can infest the rest of the body. A deficiency of gamma globulin, an immune system component which fights infection and infestation, also allows parasites to gain a foothold [6].

What are the early symptoms of giardial infestation?

The incubation period is about one to three weeks after exposure to the parasite. After this incubation period, during which the protozoa are multiplying and getting themselves established, initial symptoms may - or may not - develop. These include [7]:

- *Watery, foul-smelling diarrhea*
- *Nausea*
- *Anorexia (appetite suppression) and weight loss*
- *Dehydration*
- *Gas and abdominal cramps*
- *Chills and low-grade fever*
- *Headache*
- *Malaise (flu-like feeling)*

These initial symptoms can last for a few days to several months.

What are the chronic symptoms of giardial infection?

If the giardial infection is not treated - and lack of treatment is common since these early symptoms can disappear on their own or may not even be present - the infection becomes well-established and can last a lifetime. A large and diverse number of symptoms have been linked to chronic giardial infestation:

- Chronic fatigue, lack of motivation, constant need to nap [8]. In one study, 218 patients complaining of chronic fatigue were tested for giardia; 61 (28%) of them were infected. Over two-thirds of these were relieved of their fatigue when the protozoal infection was cured [9]. Depression is also linked to chronic fatigue and to giardia.

- Immune system effects, especially a reduction in the production of immunoglobulin A. These effects include multiple allergies, autoimmune diseases, and decreased disease resistance. Immune system effects can be especially damaging if a patient is already immunocompromised, as with AIDS.

- Mucus in the throat and stool.

- Foul smelling stools.

- The gallbladder can be blocked by giardia, causing malabsorption of oils and resultant chemical sensitivity. Symptoms of this include brain fog, light sensitivity, stiff neck and back, pain between the shoulder blades, and headache.

- Giardia can get into the lungs, and is a major cause of asthma. Clearing the giardia can clear up the

> **Giardia, along with roundworm, is a major cause of asthma.**

asthma.

- Rheumatoid arthritis, made worse by exposure to solvents or to certain dietary components.

- Multiple gastrointestinal complaints, such as abdominal pain and diarrhea. Giardial infection has been mistaken for irritable bowel syndrome and duodenal ulcers. In a study done by Leo Galland, 197 patients with chronic intestinal problems were tested for giardia; almost half were infected, and 31 of them had previously been misdiagnosed as having irritable bowel syndrome [10].

- Lactase deficiency may develop, since, in the case of prolonged infection [6], normal intestinal flora are stripped away by the parasites. Lactase is the enzyme needed to digest milk sugar, and a deficiency will lead to diarrhea and abdominal distress after consuming milk products.

- The gallbladder may become infected, which can cause jaundice and colic [4].

- Pain, including myalgia (muscle aches) and headaches. A number of patients had headaches from giardia, and these cleared up when the giardia was treated.

- Flu-like feelings.

Gallbladder surgery is commonly done in the U.S. for relief of gallbladder pain. It is, in fact, the nation's second most common surgery, with 35% of the population losing their gallbladders to the knife. (The most common type of surgery is removal of wisdom teeth.) About half of these patients do not get appreciable relief from the surgery. Giardia can block the gallbladder or the common bile duct, causing gallbladder pain which is mistakenly treated by removing the gallbladder. It is simpler and healthier to test for and eliminate giardial infestation than to remove this useful fat-digesting organ.

> **Gallbladder problems? Check for parasites - you may be able to avoid surgery.**

What kind of testing is done for giardia?
Testing for giardia is often not done because symptoms are often attributed to some other cause, or may not be present. Testing methods include:

- Microscopic examination of bowel movements, preferably on multiple specimens (at least three), for cysts or trophozoites. However, in about 25% of people with giardiasis, stool specimens do not reveal the organism [6]. Purged bowel testing is considered to be more accurate.

- Examination of bowel mucus or duodenal juice.

- The string test, described in the chapter on Parasites.

- Blood testing for IgG and IgM antibodies to giardia.

- Rectal swab testing.

Negative results do not mean that the parasite is not there. They may be in a stage of their life cycle that does not show up on the test. Retest after a week or so. If you test negative for giardia but have symptoms of infestation, it may be worthwhile to treat for giardia anyway based on symptomatology.

How are treatments for giardia given?

Whether allopathic or botanical treatments are used, it is important to treat the parasite in cycles to kill the newly hatched parasites, as medication is ineffective against the egg or cyst form. This is also true for parasites other than giardia.

Treatment for giardia should be given on days 1-3, days 13-15, and days 21-23 to catch the parasites at optimal times in their cycle. If treatment is given only once, as with antibiotics, you simply move from acute short term illness to chronic long term illness when the eggs (cysts) hatch.

Roundworm and giardia are usually found together. It is best to treat for both of them at the same time.

For practitioners only

The following treatment protocol is to be prescribed by a health care practitioner after appropriate testing and diagnosis. Since giardia and roundworm are often found together, it is generally best to treat for roundworm first (see protocol in Worms chapter), then giardia, using the following protocol:

> For giardia: Flagyl (Metronidazole) can be used. Alternatively, Fasigyn (Tinidazole) can be used. Fasigyn has fewer side effects but is available only in Mexico, not in the U.S.
>
> > Day 1 - 2 tablets (500 mg tablets) at bedtime with Kavli or Wasa crackers
> > Day 2 - 1 tablet 3 times a day with food
> > Day 3 - 1 tablet 3 times a day with food
> >
> > Days 14 - 16   Same as days 1-3, then stop for 13 days
> >
> > Days 29 - 31   Same as days 1-3
>
> Also advised - Use Hi-Tech Hygiene Hand Wash Kit after each bowel movement to avoid reinfection, as well as 5 droppers of Hi-Tech iodine / Facial dip in a bath every five days.

What are some allopathic treatments for giardia?

There are four allopathic drugs used to treat giardia. These drugs, their trade names, and recommended dosages [11] are listed here and elsewhere in these chapters to provide information to your doctor. Since most allopathic drugs have side effects, it is best not to attempt self-medication with them.

- *Metronidazole*   *(Flagyl)*   *500 mg tid, 3 days*
- *Tinidazole*   *(Fasigyn)*   *500 mg tid, 3 days*

- *Quinacrine HCl*   *(Atabrine)*   *100 mg tid, 21 days straight*
- *Furazolidone*   *(Furoxone)*   *100 mg qid, 7 days x 2*
- *Tetracycline*

In case you have ever wondered about these medical abbreviations, bid is twice a day, tid is three times a day, and qid is four times a day. These letters are abbreviations from the Latin.

These drugs are most likely to be effective (up to 90%) on very recent infections, those contracted within three to six months. If taken for an older infection, symptoms will improve for about a month and then will often return [12]. Cure rates, derived from an analysis of 11 published studies, are [13]:

- *Metronidazole*   *(Flagyl)*   *46-95%*
- *Tinidazole*   *(Fasigyn)*   *88-100%*
- *Quinacrine*   *(Atabrine)*   *60-100%*
- *Furazolidone*   *(Furoxone)*   *58-95%*

Cure rates can go even higher if two of these drugs are used.

Another study is more pessimistic; the cure rate from a single course of treatment is less than 5% due to the fact that the protozoa are much more resistant than in the past [8]. At least three treatments may be necessary in order to kill both cysts and trophozoites as they enter different parts of their life cycle.

These allopathic drugs, especially metronidazole, can cause a number of unpleasant side effects, including nausea and gastrointestinal upset and cramps, metallic or bitter taste, or psychotic symptoms, as well as possible carcinogenic changes after long-term use [13]. Some of these effects of metronidazole, especially the bitter taste, are due to its active ingredient, the heavy metal poison arsenic.

What are some natural treatments for giardia?

A group of botanical agents has been shown to be effective in infections that have persisted for more than six months; these agents include artemisia annua and gossipol [12]. Another botanical preparation combines 22 herbs and claims success in treating 83 of 105 patients. It can also be used prophylactically by travelers [8]. An iodine hand and face wash such as that made by Hi-Tech Hygiene can help control reinfestation, as iodine kills the organisms.

Entamoeba Histolytica

What is the most deadly parasitic disease?

Entamoeba histolytica is the protozoan responsible for amebiasis. This is the most deadly of the parasites; unlike giardia, it can cause death if untreated. About 400 million people are infected worldwide, of whom 100 million suffer acute or chronic effects. The prevalence of infection in the United States and Canada is about 5%, and can be up to 40% in tropical areas [1]. There are several strains of entamoeba histolytica which vary in their virulence.

As with giardia, entamoeba is passed from one person or animal to another by fecal-oral contact. Fecal-oral contact includes poor hygiene between toilet use and eating, and certain sexual practices.

The life cycle of entamoeba is a bit more complex than that of giardia. It involves the passage through five stages, of which the cyst (infective) and trophozoite (damage causing) forms are most important.

How do entamoeba histolytica do their damage?
Unlike the other amoebas which infect humans, E. histolytica secrete enzymes which hydrolyze (digest) host intestinal tissues. They can then penetrate the epithelium (top intestinal layer) and move deeper. The resulting intestinal lesion usually develops initially in the cecum, appendix, or upper colon and then spreads the length of the colon. Ulceration and necrosis (death) of these tissues can result, accompanied by stabbing pains. A high percentage of deaths results from perforated colons with concomitant peritonitis (intestinal infection). Older lesions can be assisted by bacteria and cause further damage, including penetration into the muscle layers. Trophozoites can then be carried by blood and lymph to other sites throughout the body to form secondary lesions.

Secondary lesions can be found on nearly every organ, although the liver is most commonly affected (about 5% of all cases), with resulting liver function abnormalities and jaundice. Hepatic (liver) and pulmonary (lung) lesions can also result from infection [4].

What are the symptoms of E. histolytica infestation?
Acute amebic dysentery is most often contracted from contaminated water. Sudden and severe symptoms occur after an incubation period of 8-10 days. These include headache, fever, diarrhea, vomiting, and severe abdominal cramps. Death can occur from peritonitis due to gut perforation, or from cardiac failure and exhaustion.

More commonly the disease develops slowly, with intermittent diarrhea, cramps, vomiting, and general malaise. Symptoms of chronic infection can mimic other diseases, and include:

- Symptoms usually attributed to ulcerative colitis, spastic colon, or irritable bowel syndrome, such as frequent, loose, mucus-filled bowel movements and abdominal pain.

- Fibromyalgia, or progressive muscle pain or wasting that can leave the patient bedridden [5].

- Multiple chemical or food allergies

- Chronic fatigue

- Candida (yeast) related complex

- Diarrhea can cause dehydration and depletion of electrolytes, especially potassium and calcium.

- Constipation

What kind of testing is done for E. histolytica?

Testing is similar to testing for giardia. Allopathic drugs used in treatment of amebiasis include metronidazole, paromycin (trade name Humatin), iodoquinol, and tetracycline, as well as combinations of drug therapies that depend on the severity and location of the disease [detailed in source 11].

Artemisia annua is a recommended botanical treatment [5,12]. AP Mag (distributed by Inter-Plexus, Inc.), which contains magnesium malate in an herbal base of Bael fruit, chinaberries, bitter melon, basil leaves, longpepper, and hydrastis root, is also effective. Black walnut and wormwood can be useful, but these are static (keep the problem from worsening) rather than cidal (parasite-killing).

For practitioners only

The following treatment protocol for chronic amoeba histolytica (entamoeba histolytica), e. coli, e. nana, and blastocystis hominis is to be prescribed by a health care practitioner after appropriate testing and diagnosis. Rule out positive helicobacter prior to treatment. If positive for helicobacter, add Bismogel as directed on bottle for first 14 days of treatment.

Protocol:

1. Tetracycline: 500 mg. 4 times a day for 7 days, then 500 mg. 3 times a day for 14 days. Total tetracycline needed: 80 capsules/tablets. Minimum one hour away from food or any other substances. No dairy products through course of treatment and reduce fat intake to no more than 15% of total diet. Follow strict candida diet, including 10 mg. biotin per day. Tetracycline can cause sensitivity to the sun (may sunburn more easily).

2. Flagyl (Metronidazole) or Fasigyn: 500 mg. 3 times a day for 21 days. Total Flagyl or Fasigyn needed: 63 capsules/tablets. Take with food.

   (Fasigyn (Tinidazol) is available in Mexico, Canada, and Europe, but is not available in the U.S.A. If available, Fasigyn is preferable to Flagyl because it is both more effective and less toxic, with fewer side effects.)

   Wait at least one hour after medications, then take 1 tsp. Ultrabifidus or Ultra-dophilus (acidophilus), recommended to minimize chances of yeast infection.

3. AP Mag: 2 before each meal. Alternatively, an herbal mix called Paragone can be used - ten days of Paragone I, then ten days of Paragone II, then repeat for a total of 40 days.

4. Mycopril 680: 2 before each meal.

Every four days, put five droppers of Hi-Tech Hygiene iodine into a bathtub of water. Get the solution into your nose and mucous membranes, and open and close your eyes underwater. **Do not do this if allergic to iodine.**

Monitor blood chemistry / liver enzymes 7 to 12 days into program.

Toxoplasmosis

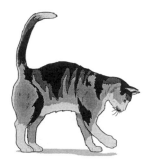

What parasite can be transmitted by cats?
Toxoplasmosis is caused by a parasite called toxoplasma gondii, which is most commonly transmitted to humans from cat feces via handling infected litterbox material or soil or the cats themselves. The central nervous system and brain, blood, and lymph nodes can be affected, causing confusion, headaches, dizziness, swollen glands, and malaise.

Cysts can remain inactive in the body for years, causing no symptoms during this period. The greatest danger in toxoplasmosis occurs when a pregnant woman contracts the disease. A wide variety of birth defects are possible depending on when during gestation the disease was contracted. Testing for the antibody specific to toxoplasma gondii is easy and accurate [4]. The medications pyrimethamine (25 mg/day) and sulfonamides (2-6 g/day), both for 3-4 weeks, are widely used in combination.

Trichomonas

What is the most common protozoal gynecological disease?
Trichomonas, one of the most common protozoan parasites in the United States, is best known as a gynecological disease. Trichomonas vaginalis, a protozoan, lives in the vagina and urethra of women and in the prostate, seminal vesicles, and urethra of men. It is generally a sexually transmitted disease, although infants can contract it during birth if the mother is infected. It is occasionally present in young children, suggesting that the infection can be spread by way of washcloths, towels, and clothing. Testing has shown that the organism can remain alive in damp cloth for as long as 24 hours [1].

The acidity of the normal vagina (pH 4 to 4.5) discourages infection. However, once established, T. vaginalis itself causes a shift towards alkalinity (pH 5 to 6), which is more favorable for the organism's continued growth. Female symptoms are tissue inflammation and a whitish to greenish vaginal discharge with a characteristic unpleasant odor which may worsen after menstruation. Symptoms may become chronic, lasting for years unless treated. Men are rarely symptomatic, but can develop prostatitis and eventually prostate cancer.

The protozoa are identified directly from vaginal smears or cultures. Metronidazole is the drug most often used for treatment, taken for 5-10 days.

Reduce intake of refined carbohydrates, especially sugar [14]. High dosages of zinc can help clear up trichomonas, even in cases which are not responsive to other therapies such as metronidazole [15]. It is also useful to douche once or twice a day with a solution of calendula, goldenseal and echinacea [14].

Blastocystis Hominis

What are some of the controversies regarding B. hominis?
Blastocystis hominis was first classified as a yeast (plant), but in 1967 it was reclassified as a protozoan (animal) and considered to be a pathogen, or disease-producing organism.

B. hominis lives in the digestive tract and has been implicated in cases of acute and chronic diarrhea and gastroenteritis, although there is some disagreement that the presence of both B. hominis and gastrointestinal symptoms is proof of a cause and effect relationship. When B. hominis or cryptosporidium are present, other organisms such as E. histolytica, giardia, or roundworms are often also present. These other organisms may be wholly or partially responsible for symptoms attributed to B. hominis.

It was once believed that blastocystis hominis, giardia, and cryptosporidium (another protozoan discussed in this chapter) were harmless. It is now known that they are harmful to humans.

What other diseases and symptoms are associated with B. hominis?
Colitis, a chronic gastrointestinal disease, has also been linked to B. hominis. In two studies, patients with colitis, diarrhea, and abdominal cramps have been found to have B. hominis in their digestive tracts. Treatment with metronidazole both eliminated the protozoa and alleviated the symptoms [16, 17].

The organism is present in small quantities in up to one-fifth of hospitalized patients, but is associated with diarrhea only in heavily infested patients. Other typical symptoms are [18]:

- *Osteoarthritis - B. hominis has actually been found in affected joints such as kneecaps*
- *Abdominal pain and gas*
- *Nausea and vomiting*
- *Low-grade fever and chills*
- *General malaise*

How is B. hominis detected and treated?
B. hominis is detected using purged bowel methods. In addition to metronidazole (1-2 grams per day in divided doses), diodoquine or non-chlorinated quinolines can be used for drug treatment. Botanicals are less effective with B. hominis than with other amoebas. Support nutrients coenzyme Q10, copper lysinate, and glutathione will boost their effectiveness [9].

Cryptosporidium

What protozoal disease causes many deaths in AIDS patients?
Cryptosporidium is considered to be an opportunistic parasite of humans, especially those who are immunodeficient. Although self-limiting in immunocompetent patients, it is an important contributing factor in the deaths of some AIDS patients [19].

After ingestion of the cysts, the organisms invade epithelial cells in the intestine. New oocysts, the infectious form, are passed as early as five days after infection. The primary symptom is profuse, watery diarrhea that can last for several months [4]. Cryptosporidium infections of the gallbladder and respiratory epithelium have also been reported [20].

Transmission from animals to humans can occur, but human to human transmission is far more common. Testing involves the detection of the oocysts in feces using stain. There is no established effective drug treatment for cryptosporidium [11]. A botanical treatment protocol similar to that for E. histolytica is recommended [12].

Are there other amoebic diseases to be concerned about?
There are a number of other amoebic diseases that can cause chronic problems, although to a lesser extent than giardia or amebiasis. Methods of transmission and testing are similar.

References and Resources

- The Burton Goldberg Group, *Alternative Medicine: The Definitive Guide*, Future Medicine Publishing, Puyallup WA, 1994. *The following chapter is relevant to Amoebic and Protozoal Infections:*
    "Trichomonas", p. 832

- Schmidt, Gerald D, and Larry S. Roberts, *Foundations of Parasitology*, Times Mirror/Mosby College Publishing, St. Louis MO, 3rd ed., 1985.

- Beaver, Paul Chester, *Animal Agents and Vectors of Human Disease*, Lea and Febinger, Philadelphia PA, 5th ed. 1985.

WORMS

The Worms Crawl In, The Worms Crawl Out...

Do you have the following symptoms? Worms may be one of your problems.

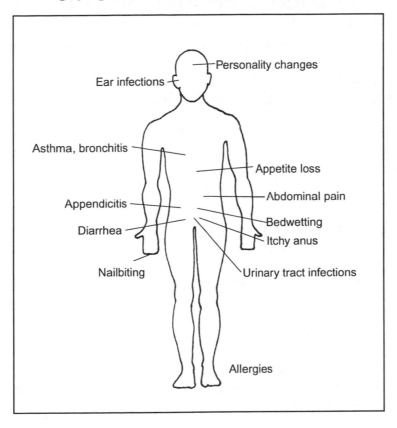

Personality changes
Ear infections
Asthma, bronchitis
Appetite loss
Abdominal pain
Appendicitis
Bedwetting
Diarrhea
Itchy anus
Nailbiting
Urinary tract infections
Allergies

Six things in this chapter that can change your health:

1-4. Asthma, nailbiting, ear infections, and bedwetting can be caused by worms.
5. Malnutrition can result from worm infestation even with a good diet.
6. Appendicitis can be caused by roundworm; surgery is not always necessary.

What symptoms can be caused by worms?
Worms, also called helminths, can cause a wide variety of symptoms, including [1]:

- *Diarrhea*
- *Nailbiting*
- *Bedwetting*
- *Asthma and bronchitis (very common)*
- *Anorexia (appetite loss)*
- *Immune deficiencies*

- *Allergic symptoms*
- *Abdominal pains*
- *Personality changes*
- *Urinary tract infections*

Many species of worms migrate through different organs as part of their life cycle, compounding the damage they can cause.

How are worms transmitted?

Worm eggs are passed in the feces of humans and animals. The eggs can survive for years in the soil and will still be capable of causing infestation. Hygiene, especially careful and frequent washing of the hands and nails, is the best preventive measure. Hi-Tech Hygiene hand and face wash is recommended to kill parasites on hands and under nails. It is possible to reinfest oneself by transferring eggs from the anus to the mouth as a result of poor hygiene.

What are the most common types of worms?

The most common types of worms in the United States are:

- *Pinworms*
- *Roundworms*
- *Threadworms*
- *Whipworms*
- *Tapeworms*
- *Hookworms*
- *Trichinosis*
- *Flukes*

Some of these are discussed throughout this chapter.

Roundworm

What type of worm is most prevalent worldwide?

Roundworms (ascaris) are the most prevalent worm infestation worldwide. They infest approximately 1.25 billion people worldwide and are perhaps the most powerful cause of allergies and hypersensitivity [1]. They infect about 25% of the world population and cause up to one million cases of disease annually [2].

Roundworms enter the body through the feet when walking in contaminated water or soil, or by ingestion from eating contaminated raw food or playing with an infected animal. Roundworms are the largest of the nematodes, and can grow up to 18 inches long and can lay up to 200,000 eggs per day.

What problems can be caused by roundworms?

Roundworms can cause a number of symptoms not generally associated with worms:

- Ascaris consume much of the liquid contents of the intestine. In moderate to heavy infestations, malnutrition can develop and become severe even with an otherwise adequate diet.

- Allergic responses to metabolites produced by the worms include rashes, asthma, and insomnia. Abdominal pains and nausea are not uncommon.

- Clusters of worms can knot up sufficiently to block the intestine. Penetration of the intestine or appendix can occur, with fatal peritonitis (abdominal infection) rapidly resulting. Some cases of appendicitis are caused by roundworms in the appendix. Medication to kill the roundworm can relieve the appendicitis totally, so surgery is sometimes not necessary.

> **Appendicitis can be caused by roundworm, and surgery may not be necessary.**

- A 17 year old female with anorexia was able to eat again and gain weight after being treated for roundworm and candida. This changed how she felt after meals - no more sick, bloated feeling.

- Roundworms can wander into the pancreatic and bile ducts, the esophagus, the trachea, or even the Eustachian tubes of the ears and the middle ears, causing extensive damage [3]. Persistent or recurring childhood ear infections may be due in part to roundworm infestation.

- Roundworms often inhabit the upper respiratory area, and are responsible for many cases of asthma and bronchitis. One patient, a 15 year old tennis player with asthma, was cleared for roundworm and candida. His asthma went away and he could play tennis again. A 12 year old with asthma and attention deficit disorder (ADD) was cleared of his symptoms in the same way.

What type of testing is used to detect roundworm?
Testing is usually done by identifying the characteristically shaped eggs in the feces. So many eggs are laid per day that one or two fecal smears are usually sufficient to verify the worms' presence.

What are some treatments for roundworm?
Treatments mentioned here are intended to be used by doctors, not for self treatment. Some drugs are cidals (kill worms), while others are statics (keep the infestation from getting worse). Drugs effective against roundworm, and their recommended dosages [4] include:

- *Piperazine citrate*   *75 mg/kg daily for 2 days*
- *Pyrantel pamoate (Antiminth)*   *11 mg/kg, single dose*
- *Mebendazole*   *100 mg bid for 3 days*

Another recommended protocol [1] is to give pyrantel pamoate (10 mg/kg at night) first to paralyze the worms so they don't migrate from the gastrointestinal tract to cause further damage. This protocol is also recommended for pinworms and some hookworms. Normal bowel activity should then dislodge the immobilized worms. Repeat in 10 days to catch those worms that were still eggs during the first treatment. Scrupulous hygiene such as careful handwashing immediately after bowel movements is necessary during the treatment period to prevent reinfection.

Paragone I and II (Integris) are less toxic than most allopathic medicines. It is often recommended that they be tried first, along with Replenz to replenish the beneficial bacteria.

If further treatment is needed, try mebendazole (Vermox), 100 mg, repeated in 14 days. If the worms are still resistant, 25 mg/kg of thiabendazole is recommended. Vermox is also effective [5], especially if taken several times, three days at a time, 2-3 weeks apart. Vermox is expensive if purchased in the United States (about $90 for three treatments), but it is available from Mexico for less than $9 or about one tenth the price. Botanicals such as Paratox 11 and the herb blue vervain are also available.

For practitioners only

The following treatment protocol is to be prescribed by a health care practitioner after appropriate testing and diagnosis. Since giardia and roundworm are often found together, it is generally best to treat for roundworm first, then giardia (see protocol in Amoebas and Protozoa chapter), using the following protocol for roundworm:

> 1. Chew one tablet of Vermox twice a day on an empty stomach (upon rising and before evening meal) before any nutrient intake for 3 days. Discontinue for 14 days.
>
> 2. Then chew one tablet twice a day for 3 days as above. Discontinue for 21 days.
>
> 3. Then chew one tablet twice a day for 3 days as above.
>
> Do not take the Vermox along with any other protocol, anti-amoebic drug, herbs, black walnut, Par Qing, Flagyl, Fasigyn, Atabrine, Quinacrine, or Yodoxin, etc.

Pinworm

What is the most common worm in the United States?

Pinworm is the most common worm infestation in the United States. As many as 50% of children have this worm infection at some time. Transmission is fecal to oral, with worm eggs in the feces taken into the mouth by unwashed hands or from contaminated food. The worms are easily visible on the surface of the feces as 1/4- to 1/2-inch white, moving, threadlike worms. They migrate to the anus at night to lay their eggs in a sticky chemical that causes intense anal itching. Since children tend to scratch where it itches and then to suck their fingers, bite their nails, and pick their noses, they keep the infestation going. The infestation can persist for years if untreated.

How easy is it to test for pinworm?

Testing is simple and accurate. The worms can be identified visually in the stool, as can the eggs with the aid of a microscope. A piece of tape applied to the unwashed anus upon awakening will pick up eggs and even whole worms.

What are the treatments for pinworm?

Effective medications are the same as for roundworm, with some variation in dosage [4]. With each of these drugs, repeat dosage after 2 weeks.

- *Mebendazole*   *100 mg single dose*
- *Pyrantel pamoate*   *11 mg/kg single dose*
- *Piperazine citrate*   *65 mg/kg daily for 7 days*
- *Pyrvinium pamoate*   *5 mg/kg single dose*

Again, Paragone I and II are less toxic, and should be tried first.

Tapeworms

What are tapeworms?

About 700 million people worldwide are infected with tapeworm [1]. Tapeworms are spread via the fecal to oral route, and from eating undercooked meat.

There are several types of tapeworms which can infest humans. They are generally flat, long, and segmented. Segments are sometimes passed through the feces. While they primarily infest the intestines, some species or their cysts can infiltrate almost any part of the body.

Tapeworms are more complex than roundworms in nutritional requirements from their host. The broad tapeworm of humans, diphyllobothrium latum, absorbs so much vitamin B12 from the intestine that the host can develop pernicious anemia [6], a disease associated with a vitamin B12 deficiency.

What is the testing and treatment for tapeworm?

Testing is done by checking the stool for eggs and segments. The drug of choice for treatment is niclosamide [1,3]. Point of interest: the head must be killed or the tapeworm will be able to regenerate.

Trichinosis

Why is it dangerous to eat undercooked pork?

Trichinosis is caused by the trichinella worm, which is most commonly transmitted to humans by eating undercooked pork and sausage. Trichinosis is capable of causing death if undiagnosed or untreated. Guanidine, a liver toxin, is also found in pigs and pork.

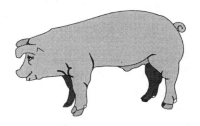

What are the symptoms of trichinosis?

The disease typically goes through three stages:

1. Low-grade vague symptoms appear 12-48 hours after ingesting contaminated meat.

2. The female worms then penetrate the intestinal epithelium (lining), depositing waste products which lead to the proliferation of enteric (intestinal) bacteria. 5 to 7 days after the initial symptoms, acute symptoms of food poisoning occur, such as vomiting, pain, and diarrhea.

3. After ten days, the juvenile worms infiltrate muscle tissue. Symptoms are varied and vague, and include muscular pain and heart damage. If untreated, death can result from heart failure, respiratory complications, toxemia, or kidney malfunction [3].

What type of testing and treatment is available for trichinosis?

The most accurate, although drastic, diagnostic method is muscle biopsy. Unfortunately, trichinosis is rarely tested for due to the vagueness of the symptoms and the specificity of the test.

Drug treatment for trichinosis is mebendazole (200-400 mg tid for 4 days, then 400-500 mg tid for 10 days) or pyrantel pamoate (10 mg/kg daily for 4 days) [4]. Corticosteroids can be taken if absolutely necessary for pain (20-40 mg prednisone daily, reduced as symptoms decrease).

Flukes

What is another common type of worm?

Flukes are among the most common and abundant of parasitic worms, and inhabit the bodies of all types of vertebrates, including humans. They belong to a class of parasites called digenetic trematodes. Flukes vary considerably in size, shape, and part of the body that is preferentially infested; i.e. where they develop into adults and deposit their eggs.

What types of flukes are there?

There are, for example:

- *Liver flukes*   (fasciola hepatica, clonorchis sinensis)
- *Intestinal flukes*   (fasciolopsis buski)
- *Blood flukes*   (schistosomes)
- *Lung flukes*   (paragonimus westermani)

Sheep liver flukes are indigenous to the United States and affect the liver and biliary tract in humans. If a person is heavily infested, these liver flukes can cause sharp, hard to diagnose pain in the area of the liver. Most flukes are flattened and oval in shape, and nearly all of them have a powerful oral sucker with which to cling to body tissues.

How can one become infested with flukes?

The life cycle of flukes is quite complex, involving as many as six different body forms and several different environments, including water and the body of a snail. A single snail can release

169 million worms in a month. In short, the egg leaves the host in feces, enters the water, and goes through several forms and changes. The encysted organisms enter the body of a human, either through the skin (blood flukes) or by being swallowed. The cysts mature into flukes in the human host, and then lay eggs to start another cycle.

Flukes are therefore contracted by swimming or wading in infested water. Blood flukes are most likely to enter the body via the skin between the toes, and other flukes can be swallowed with the water either directly or indirectly.

What are some symptoms of fluke infestation?

The pathologic changes in the human body are due to the eggs trapped in the tissues. A single fluke can deposit eggs in a given area for up to 20 years. The eggs set up an inflammatory reaction in the mucous membrane, resulting in wartlike thickenings. Fluke eggs are then excreted in feces, urine, or, in the case of lung flukes, sputum. The period of time between initial infection and the appearance of eggs in the stool is 6-10 weeks.

Schistosomes (blood flukes) are often parasitized in turn by salmonella bacteria. Salmonella's best known effect is food poisoning (salmonellosis), with its attendant gastrointestinal symptoms. However, the bacteria can also cause:

- *arthritis*
- *abscesses*
- *pneumonia*
- *meningitis*
- *endocarditis*

Salmonella infections can be deadly, and chronic salmonellosis often accompanies schistosomiasis (fluke infestation) [7].

What is the treatment for flukes?

Treatment for flukes includes praziquantel (25 mg/kg for 1 day), and bithional (alternate days for nearly a month) [4].

Summary

Worms are more common than many people realize, and they can be found in even the cleanest and most affluent people. Worms can cause a number of symptoms such as asthma, ear infections, appendicitis, gallbladder problems, nailbiting, and bedwetting. It is wise to test and treat for worms before undergoing more drastic treatments for these conditions.

References and Resources

- The Burton Goldberg Group, ***Alternative Medicine: The Definitive Guide***, Future Medicine Publishing, Puyallup WA, 1994. *The following chapters are relevant to Worms:*
  "Worms", p. 993
  "Childhood Parasites - Pinworms", p. 609

- Schmidt, Gerald D, and Larry S. Roberts, ***Foundations of Parasitology***, Times Mirror / Mosby College Publishing, St. Louis MO, 3rd ed., 1985. *Technical text.*

- Beaver, Paul Chester, ***Animal Agents and Vectors of Human Disease***, Lea and Febinger, Philadelphia PA, 5th ed. 1985. *Technical text.*

- Smith, Alice Lorraine, ***Principles of Microbiology***, C.V. Mosby Co., St. Louis MO, 9th ed., 1981. *Technical text.*

BACTERIA

More Than Just Bad Guys

Do you have the following symptoms? You may have a bacterial infection.

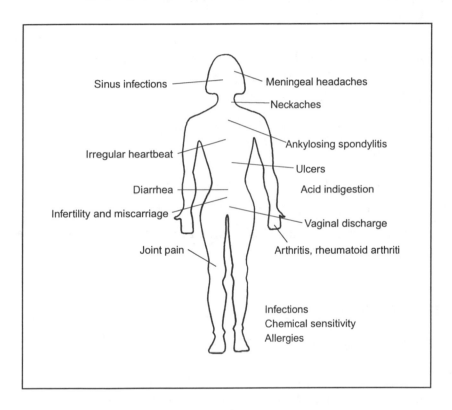

Eight things in this chapter that can affect your health:

1. Over 99% of all bacteria in the body are beneficial, and less than 1% are disease-producing. Antibiotics thus kill about 100 times more beneficial bacteria than bad ones.

2. How do bacteria cause disease?

3. Disease-producing bacteria are found in up to 90% of chickens.

4. Did you know that bacteria are the cause of most ulcers?

5. Why doesn't everyone exposed to bacteria get infected, and what can you do to increase your odds of being one who isn't?

6. What is the cause of the "tourist trots" and how can you protect yourself?

7. *What is the most widespread sexually transmitted disease?*

8. *Antibiotics are losing the battle against bacteria - you can't count on them for protection to the extent that you could in the past.*

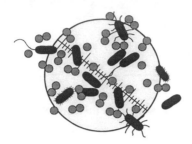

What are bacteria?

Bacteria are one-celled animals. Bacteria can be:

- *Endogenous, or naturally occurring within the body*
- *Exogenous, or introduced from outside the body*

A controversial theory is that bacteria exhibit pleomorphism, characterized by having different forms during different parts of their life cycle. This is not unheard of in the animal world; for example, tadpole / frog or caterpillar / pupa / moth. The different forms of one type of bacteria may be mistaken for different bacteria.

Are all bacteria bad?

Endogenous bacteria can be

- Protective (good) bacteria, which interact with the host for mutual benefit. They are called protectors or symbionts.

- Freeloaders, also called commensals, which live off the host but cause neither good nor harm.

- Pathogens, or disease causers.

Over 99% of all bacteria in the body are the beneficial type.

Bacteria can, then, be good, bad, or indifferent. Over 99% of all bacteria in the body are the beneficial type.

A pathogen, whether from within the body or from the environment, may not cause trouble if the protective bacteria are present in sufficient numbers to keep the pathogens in control. Antibiotics, whether prescribed or taken inadvertently as with antibiotic-fed meat or chlorinated water (chlorine has antibiotic action), will kill off some of the protective bacteria and disturb the body's healthy balance. Mercury from amalgam fillings also has an undesirable antibiotic action. Toxic burdens and immune system deficiencies can also give pathogens the upper hand.

Bacteria and fungi live in and create an alkaline environment. This is why acidifying urine is recommended in fighting bladder and kidney infections.

How do bacteria enter the body?

Bacteria enter the body in a number of different ways:

- **Skin** - many bacteria enter through broken skin, and a few can enter through intact skin. From there, they can be transported throughout the body via the circulatory system, or penetrate to deeper skin layers to cause a localized infection. Broken skin can occur not only through cuts and abrasions, but through skin eroded by skin rashes, burns, skin broken by hangnails, or through receding gums. Some bacteria are injected into the skin by insects such as mosquitoes.

- **Respiratory** - bacteria (and viruses) which enter the air via coughing and sneezing can be inhaled, and are then transported throughout the body by the bloodstream.

- **Alimentary tract** - bacteria on food or in water or beverages can be swallowed.

- **Genitourinary system** - sexually transmitted diseases.

- **Placenta** - most bacteria do not cross the placental barrier like chemicals and metals, but a few may. An infant can also pick up bacteria, both good and bad, from its mother's vaginal canal during delivery.

How do bacteria cause disease?

Most disease symptoms are the result of biochemical changes. These come from toxic secretions of bacteria which can interfere with metabolic processes or destroy body tissues. Bacteria can also incapacitate the immune system to a certain extent, thus ensuring their own continued survival. This explains how many bacterial infections can become chronic, and how one infection can follow another once the immune system is weakened.

Bacteria can be aerobic or anaerobic, which means oxygen-loving or oxygen-hating respectively. Keeping the blood well-oxygenated, as with deep breathing or aerobic exercise, will discourage the growth of anaerobic bacteria.

Campylobacter and Helicobacter

What types of bacteria are found in most chickens?

Campylobacter and helicobacter are spiral-shaped bacteria which are found in the intestinal tract and oral cavities of humans and animals. Campylobacter fetus can cause gastroenteritis, a diarrhea that can last for several days. An underlying condition such as alcoholism or cardiovascular disease may predispose to infection [1]. It is usually contracted through contaminated food or water. Campylobacter has been found to be present in most (up to 90%) chickens sold in supermarkets. The USDA does not require testing for this bacteria [2].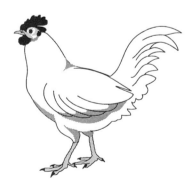

Acute food poisoning symptoms include vomiting, chills, and abdominal pain. Long-term symptoms include arthritis, pericarditis (inflammation of the heart lining), and neurological disorders. The disease can be fatal to the very young, the old, and those with weakened immune systems.

What is the cause of most ulcers?

Helicobacter pylori may cause up to 80% of stomach ulcers and nearly all duodenal ulcers. The bacterium is thought to burrow through and digest the layer of mucus that protects the stomach and duodenum from gastric acid. Only 5-25% of ulcer patients treated with antibiotics had a relapse the following year, as compared with a 75-90% relapse rate in those treated only with ulcer drugs [3]. A three-week course of treatment with tetracycline and metronidazole is recommended for infected ulcer patients [4], although these drugs have their side effects. Another study [5] blames campylobacter pyloridis for duodenal ulcers, and recommends a bismuth compound in combination with an antibacterial drug as treatment.

> **Helicobacter pylori causes most stomach and duodenal ulcers. Eliminate the bacteria, eliminate the ulcer.**

One of our patients, a man from Australia came to the clinic with ulcers which he was treating unsuccessfully with antacids. H. pylori treatment was instituted, as well as eliminating dental metals (mercury in amalgam fillings acts like an antibiotic and kills beneficial bacteria which keep infectious organisms under control), cleared his associated candida, and implanted the beneficial bacteria acidophilus and bifidus. This regimen cleared up the ulcer cause and therefore the ulcer symptoms.

The connection between H. pylori and ulcers was known by doctors in 1982 [6], and by veterinary medicine well before that [7], but this connection has only recently (1995) been made widely known.

Helicobacter pylori is also implicated in stomach cancer; chronic inflammation caused by the bacterium may add to other risk factors. There is evidence that people infected with H. pylori are three to six times as likely as non-infected individuals to develop stomach cancer over a 20-year period [8].

H. pylori may be responsible for some chemical sensitivities and allergic reactions, including hives, sinus infections, and even potentially fatal anaphylactic shock. These symptoms can be traced to an allergy to the bacterium [9].

Gallbladder problems are sometimes linked to h. pylori, as well as to giardia and roundworm. One patient, a 40 year old woman, had her gallbladder removed but still had pain, which went away when she was treated for helicobacter. (The unanswered question: Was the surgery unnecessary?)

Type O blood groups seem to be more susceptible than others to H. pylori infection [10].

Allergic symptoms such as hives, sinusitis and exercise-induced anaphylaxis may be caused by h. pylori [11]. The probable mechanism of action is a suppression of hydrochloric acid by the bacteria, leading to poor protein digestion and the development or worsening of food allergies [12].

Campylobacter and helicobacter are detected using a sensitive indirect hemagglutination test; the organisms are readily recovered in blood culture [1]. Recently (1996) a saliva test for helicobacter has been made available.

For practitioners only

The following treatment protocol for helicobacter pylori is to be prescribed by a health care practitioner after appropriate testing and diagnosis. Other protocols are available for resistant cases. This protocol has a reported 90% cure rate. Monitor blood chemistry / liver enzymes 7 to 12 days into program.

1. Take Bismogel for the first 14 days. Take 1 Tbsp. immediately before dose of Flagyl/Fasigyn and tetracycline to coat the stomach and allow the antibiotic to treat the bacteria.

2. Tetracycline: 500 mg. 3 times a day for 21 days. Eat food 15 minutes after taking dose. No dairy products through course of treatment and reduce fat intake to no more than 15% of total diet. Follow strict candida diet, including 10 mg. biotin per day. Tetracycline can cause sensitivity to the sun (may sunburn more easily). The antibiotic Biaxin can be taken instead if one is allergic to Tetracycline.

3. Flagyl (Metronidazole) or Fasigyn (Tinidazole): 500 mg. 3 times a day for 21 days. Eat food 15 minutes after taking dose.

   Fasigyn (Tinidazol) is available in Mexico, Canada, and Europe, but is not available in the U.S.A. If available, Fasigyn is preferable to Flagyl because it is both more effective and less toxic (fewer side effects).

   Wait at least two hours after medications, then take 1 tsp. Ultrabifidus or Ultradophilus (acidophilus), This is recommended to minimize chances of yeast infection.

4. Mycopril 680 or antifungal drug three times a day with food.

5. Zantac 150 mg: 1 capsule at bedtime to prevent release of stomach acid for 14 days. Prilosec can be taken instead.

Legionnaire's disease

Do you remember Legionnaire's disease?

Legionnaire's disease (Legionella), recognized and named in July 1976, made major news headlines at that time as an outbreak of respiratory illness in Philadelphia. 221 people got sick and 34 died of it.

Legionnaire's disease and its milder cousin Pontiac fever are caused by the aerobic bacterium Legionella pneumophilia. Legionnaire's disease causes acute flu-like symptoms after an incubation period of 2-10 days, followed by pneumonia. Legionella species are responsible for about 15% of community acquired pneumonia cases and 40% of hospital acquired cases. Abdominal pain, gastrointestinal symptoms, cough, or shortness of breath may be present. Liver and kidney complications can appear later. Although the primary target is the lung, other body systems are usually involved. Lung abscesses may form. 1-7% of those exposed become ill. The mortality rate is 15-25%, and is especially high in those with depressed immune systems.

Epidemics of Legionella are associated with aerosols from contaminated condensers, ice machines, and shower heads [13,14].

It is postulated that the organism is present in soil, and enters the air and is breathed in when the soil is disturbed. The outbreak in 1976 was thought to be spread through the air conditioning system. Legionella is rarely infectious on a person to person basis.

Diagnosis is done by various methods, such as blood or sputum culture, or direct immunofluorescence. Antibodies appear three weeks after onset, and these can be detected by an indirect fluorescent antibody test [1].

Why didn't everyone exposed get Legionnaire's disease and die?
The condition of the host is more important than the microorganism. Only those people whose immune systems have been weakened by the primary toxic suppressors discussed in the previous book section are likely to get Legionnaire's disease or any other parasite-caused disease. The immune systems of the others are strong enough to fight off the invaders.

Lyme disease

What is the most prevalent bacterial illness in the U.S.?
Lyme disease, first discovered and named in Lyme, Connecticut in 1975, is second only to AIDS as the most prevalent parasitic disease in the United States. It is caused by a spiral-shaped bacteria called Borrelia burgdorferi. The vector is the deer tick, Ixodes dammini (or Ixodes pacificus in California), a tiny black tick not much larger than a pinhead.

Most cases are concentrated along the northeastern coast, the upper midwest, and the Pacific northwest. 21,000 cases have been reported in 43 states since the Center for Disease Control began tracking the disease's incidence in 1982. The peak incidence period is in the summer.

What are the symptoms of Lyme disease?
Disease symptoms show up in at least two stages. The tick will inject the spirochetes (bacteria) 24 hours to 4 days after biting, which allows plenty of time to locate and remove it. Once infected, the first sign is a small red bump where the person was bitten, followed shortly by a ring-like or bull's-eye rash (called erythema migrans) around the bite site, which is two or more inches

in diameter. There may also be flu-like symptoms. These symptoms disappear within a few days. The disease is easily treated with antibiotics at this stage; the ringlike rash is characteristic enough to be diagnostic.

If untreated, there may be no symptoms for years, and then serious symptoms, difficult to treat, set in. There are a wide variety of symptoms, affecting nearly every organ system, and diagnosis is difficult unless the patient remembers the tick bite and bull's-eye rash. These symptoms, which can be chronic and disabling, include:

- *Arthritis, one of the most common effects*
- *Nervous system disorders, memory loss*
- *Psychological disorders, dementia*
- *Multiple sclerosis-like symptoms*
- *Heart rhythm abnormalities, heart damage*
- *Fatigue*
- *Joint pain and swelling, especially the knees*
- *Miscarriage and birth defects*
- *Jaw pain, facial paralysis*

E. coli

What is the cause of the "tourist trots"?
Escherichia coli (E. coli) is the organism most frequently associated with diarrhea in travelers to less-developed countries; it can account for 30-70% of cases of the "tourist trots". Both E. coli and klebsiella are short, rod-shaped (also called coliform) bacteria with similar characteristics.

E. coli is normally found in the digestive tract and does not cause trouble unless

- *The intestinal wall becomes diseased*
- *Host resistance is lowered*
- *Virulence of the organism is increased*

Under one or more of these conditions, coliforms can pass to the abdominal cavity or enter the bloodstream. At this point, their virulence, or disease-causing strength, is considerably enhanced.

What other problems can these bacteria cause?
Coliform bacteria can then cause such diseases as

- *Pyelonephritis*   *a kidney infection*
- *Cystitis*   *urinary tract infection*
- *Cholecystitis*   *gall bladder infection*
- *Abscesses*   *local infections, usually of the skin*

- *Peritonitis*   *infection of the peritoneum, or abdominal lining*
- *Meningitis*   *infection of the meninges of the brain*

The suffix "-itis" means inflammation or infection.

E. coli is the most common cause of urinary tract infections and the kidney infection pyelonephritis. The coliforms play a part in the formation of gallstones. They can team up with other bacteria such as streptococci and staphylococci to produce septicemia (bacterial poisoning). The bacterium Klebsiella pneumoniae can cause pneumonia, especially in chronic alcoholics [1].

3-5% of patients admitted to hospitals for any reason develop an infection while hospitalized. The most common infectious agents are the gram-negative (do not react to a particular microscopic stain) enteric bacilli as a group, which includes E. coli and klebsiella.

Chlamydia

What is the most widespread sexually transmitted disease?
Chlamydia is now the most widespread sexually transmitted disease. It is caused by a bacterium, chlamydia trachomatis. Three million to ten million people contract the disease every year [15]. Chlamydia is responsible for infertility in more than 20,000 American women annually [16], and is responsible for the rise in ectopic (tubal) pregnancies.

About seventy percent of infected women experience no symptoms at all [17]. Men may or may not experience symptoms. Chlamydia is then diagnosed when the woman is unable to conceive.

What are the symptoms of chlamydial infection?
Symptoms of infection include:

- *Vaginal discharge - copious cloudy, sticky discharge with little or no odor, rarely accompanied by itching.*

- *Lower abdominal pain in women*

- *Painful urination*

- *Bleeding between periods*

- *A dripping discharge from the penis, similar to that of gonorrhea*

Chlamydia begins as an infection of the cervix, and from there may spread to the uterus and fallopian tubes.

What are some complications of untreated chlamydia?
If chlamydia is not diagnosed and treated, it can cause a number of complications:

- *Infertility in women*

- *Sterility in men*
- *Ectopic (tubal) pregnancies*
- *Miscarriages*
- *Nongonococcal urethritis (inflammation of the urinary tract) in men*
- *Conjunctivitis, an eye inflammation, in newborns born to infected mothers*
- *Endometritis, a uterine infection*

- *Pelvic inflammatory disease (PID) - a painful infection which can lead to scarring of the fallopian tubes and subsequent sterility. Chlamydia is responsible for one third to one half of all cases of PID [18]*

How is chlamydia spread?
Chlamydia is spread via sexual contact. There are three million new chlamydia cases per year. As with nearly all sexually transmitted diseases, barrier methods such as a condom or (less effective) a diaphragm can provide some protection. Nonoxynol-9, a spermicide, has been shown to inhibit chlamydia in experiments with mouse cells. Several studies show that oral contraceptive users have two to three times the incidence of chlamydia than non-users, probably because oral contraceptives sometimes cause changes in the cervix that allow bacteria to enter more easily [15].

What testing and treatment are available for chlamydia?
Tests for chlamydia exist that either detect a characteristic enzyme or permit microscopic examination of cells grown in culture. To examine the cells, a bit of the cervical discharge is obtained during a gynecologic exam. Unfortunately, testing is not done routinely, since the test is neither simple nor inexpensive and the disease is not life-threatening. Testing is generally only done when the disease is suspected, and this may be the case only after permanent damage has been done.

Once diagnosed, treatment is fairly simple, especially if diagnosed in the early stages. A ten-day course of an antibiotic such as doxycycline or tetracycline will kill the bacteria. Unfortunately, scarring caused by advanced cases is not known to be reversible.

Other Bacteria

What else can bacteria do?
Bacteria such as klebsiella, proteus, pseudomonas and citrobacter may contribute to various autoimmune diseases, including [19-21]:

- *Diabetes*
- *Lupus*
- *Arthritis*
- *Ankyklosing spondylitis*
- *Thyroid disease*
- *Meningitis*
- *Ulcerative colitis*

Bacteria may contribute to autoimmune diseases

Two patients with klebsiella, one in the colon and the other in the prostate, had ankylosing-type symptoms such as back stiffening.

Antibiotics

Aren't bacterial infections a thing of the past because of antibiotics?
The use of antibiotics, which kill certain bacteria, was once heralded as the potential end to infectious disease. Many bacterial diseases such as diphtheria, syphilis, and bacterial pneumonia used to kill a large number of people but are not considered to be a cause for concern today. Antibiotics, sanitation, and refrigeration are the primary reasons for the dramatic drop in fatal bacterial diseases.

Unfortunately, bacteria have a survival mechanism known as mutation. Not all bacteria of a certain type are exactly the same; some have mutated, or changed, to be resistant to antibiotics. The antibiotic will kill most of the bacteria, but the mutated survivors will multiply, passing on their resistance to their descendants. A new infection starts that is resistant to the same antibiotic that worked before.

Medical science's answer to this is to come up with newer and stronger antibiotics, maintaining a slight lead over the speed of bacterial mutation. But science is running out of new ammunition, and the bacteria now seem to be catching up and even winning. Diseases such as tuberculosis and gonorrhea, once thought to be nearly conquered, are once again taking lives. Our overuse and inappropriate use of antibiotics over the years has contributed greatly to our present situation, as bacteria were forced to mutate to survive to a greater extent than they would naturally. Farm animals receive 30 times more antibiotics than people do directly [22], although people end up eating the antibiotic-containing meat and milk.

Antibiotic-resistant bacteria have become an increasing problem since the early 1980s. In addition to the misprescribing and overprescribing of antibiotics for colds and ear infections, the prophylactic use of antibiotics in hospitals and the routine use of antibiotics in meat-producing animals have been blamed. The number of infections in hospitals, called nosocomial infections, is rising. Many European countries such as Sweden have stopped or sharply reduced the use of antibiotics in the raising of food animals to try to prevent the further decline in usefulness of these drugs. A particular strain of penicillin-resistant gonorrhea has caused the number of affected individuals to double between 1983 and 1984 to almost 7000 cases in the U.S. and Canada - one can only guess the number of people afflicted now, over a decade later [23].

In 1941, only 40,000 units of penicillin a day for four days was effective against pneumococcus, and infectious bacteria which can cause fatal infections. Today, 24 million units of penicillin are often not sufficient [24].

Children with recurring ear infections which are treated with antibiotics repeatedly can develop fungal ear infections. These ear infections are often misdiagnosed as being bacterial and treated with more antibiotics in a vicious cycle [25].

Some bacterial diseases and the antibiotics which no longer work against them include [22]:

Microbe	Diseases caused	Ineffective antibiotics
Enterococcus	*surgical infections*	*erythromycin, cephalosporins, penicillin, tetracycline*
H. influenzae	*meningitis, ear infections*	*penicillin, chloramphenicol, tetracycline*
M. tuberculosis	*tuberculosis*	*rifampin, aminoglycosides*
N. gonorrhoeae	*gonorrhea*	*penicillin, tetracycline*
Strep. pneumoniae	*pneumonia*	*cephalosporins, erythromycin, penicillin, tetracycline*

Since antibiotics can no longer be counted on to protect you fully from bacterial infection, and their effectiveness is waning rapidly, it is of even greater importance to keep your immune system in top condition so you can fight infection the way your body was intended to.

References and Resources

- The Burton Goldberg Group, *Alternative Medicine: The Definitive Guide*, Future Medicine Publishing, Puyallup WA, 1994. *The following chapters are relevant to Bacterial Infections:*
  "Sexually Transmitted Diseases" -
         Chlamydia (pp. 828-830)
         Gonorrhea (p. 830)
         Syphilis (p. 831)
  "Tuberculosis", p. 983

- Lappe, Marc, *When Antibiotics Fail*, North Atlantic Books, Berkeley CA, 1986.

- Schmidt, Michael A., Lendon H. Smith and Keith W. Sehnert, *Beyond Antibiotics: Healthier Options For Families*, North Atlantic Books, Berkeley CA, 1992.

- Smith, Alice Lorraine, *Principles of Microbiology*, C.V. Mosby Co., St. Louis MO, 9th ed., 1981.

VIRUSES

A Ghost Of A Chance

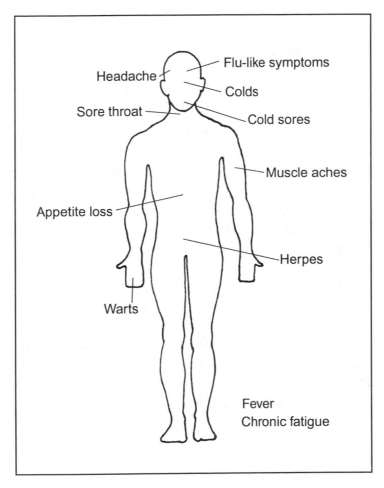

Do you have the following symptoms? You may have a viral infection.

Nine things in this chapter that can change your health:

    1. How can viruses cause damage?

    2. Can you catch a viral infection more than once?

    3. Why do we catch colds repeatedly?

    4. What treatments are useful against viral diseases?

5. *A virus with which most of the population is infected may be a trigger for atherosclerosis (hardening of the arteries).*

6. *People with genital herpes are twice as susceptible to HIV (AIDS) infection.*

7. *Did you know that a virus may be involved in diabetes?*

8. *What are some of the contributors to Chronic Fatigue Syndrome?*

9. *What is the correlation between an affluent lifestyle and Epstein-Barr Virus / Chronic Fatigue Syndrome?*

What are viruses, and how are they like airline hijackers?

To understand viruses, it is first necessary to understand the basic structure and function of a cell, whether a body cell or a bacterium. A cell is a self-contained unit which can:

- *take in nourishment*
- *excrete wastes*
- *produce energy*
- *reproduce itself*

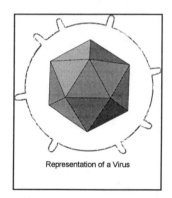

Representation of a Virus

In order to reproduce, the cell uses the information encoded in its genetic material, DNA and RNA, to make copies of itself with the same characteristics as the original cell. The DNA does not in itself cause reproduction; it is instead used as a blueprint for the "building crew" inside the cell to follow.

A virus is essentially a packet of genetic information surrounded by a protein covering. All viruses have an inner covering, called a capsid, to protect the genetic material; some viruses also have an outer covering made up of proteins, complex sugars, and fat. Viruses cannot perform any cellular functions by themselves, and so must hijack cells to carry out their intended purpose: replicating themselves. A virus can take over a cell like the invasion by an alien entity takes over a hapless victim in a science fiction movie.

Are viruses alive?

Viruses, by themselves, are not considered to be alive by most criteria. They more closely resemble molecules or crystals than they resemble cells. While bacteria are amorphous, or blob-shaped, many viruses have geometrical many-sided structures that fit together with mathematical precision. Viruses are barely larger than the largest macromolecules. If an average bacterium were blown up to the size of this paragraph, the average virus, in contrast, would be about the size of the period at the end of this sentence [1].

Other approximate relative sizes are:

- *Mycoplasma*   *golf ball*
- *Parasite*   *jacuzzi tub*
- *Sperm*   *jacuzzi tub*
- *Roundworm*   *swimming pool*

What are the basic types of viruses?

There are many types of viruses that infect humans. These are very specific in the types of cells they attach to, and will not affect other cells, tissues, or organs. For example, the mumps virus has a precise affinity for the human respiratory epithelium (lining of lungs and trachea). Because of this specificity, it is rare for viruses to affect more than one animal or plant species, although there are exceptions such as rabies. Viruses that infect bacterial cells are called bacteriophages. An example of a bacteriophage would be the T4 phage which infects the E. coli bacteria in the stomach.

What is the life cycle of a virus?

The viral life cycle consists of several stages. The amount of time required to complete this life cycle varies greatly depending on virus type.

1. **Attachment/adsorption/penetration** - When the virus finds a cell whose surface molecules correspond to its own, it fuses to these molecules in a process called adsorption. It may fuse with the cell's surface membrane and release its contents into the cell, or, if lacking an outer envelope, the virus may burrow through the cell membrane and enter the cell itself. Bacteriophages usually inject their genetic material into the appropriate spot on a bacterium like a bee injects venom into the skin.

2. **Eclipse** - After the virus penetrates the cell wall, its coat is removed by intracellular chemicals. During this eclipse period the virus cannot be detected by laboratory methods or recovered in infectious form. As a distinct virus, it has, in effect, ceased to exist.

3. **Maturation and replication** - There are thousands of proteins in a cell, and the manufacture of each of these is directed by a gene, a tiny part of the DNA. Viruses also have genes that direct protein synthesis, but lack the metabolic functions and chemicals to actually make the proteins, so they must use the raw materials and "factory workers" provided by the cell. The genetic material of the virus enters the nucleus of the cell and inserts its DNA into the DNA of the cell. The cell, thus commandeered, is then directed to make new viral particles. After replication, these new viral particles acquire protein coats to protect them between release from the cell and entry into new cells.

4. **Release** - The new mature viruses are released by the cell, at which point they each find new cells to infect [1, 2].

How do viruses enter the body?

Viruses enter the body through the same routes as bacteria - respiratory, ingestion, etc. Because of their specificity, viruses must enter the body in a particular way in order to cause infection. Inhaled stomach viruses (normally swallowed), cold viruses in contact with a cut in the skin (normally inhaled), or swallowed AIDS (HIV) viruses (normally transmitted through body fluids) are less likely to cause damage than if they entered the body by their preferred route. The susceptibility of the person to infection depends primarily on the state of the immune system, the presence of bacteria, and also upon the age of the host/victim, with the youngest and oldest being more susceptible.

How is viral infection prevented?

Prevention involves blocking the spread of infection by washing hands, covering sneezes, and carefully disposing of used tissues in the case of rhinoviruses (cold viruses), or by practicing abstinence or monogamy to help prevent the spread of the HIV or herpes viruses.

Using an iodine-based hand and face wash such as Hi-Tech Hygiene can help prevent the spread of infection, as iodine has a viricidal (virus-killing) effect like chlorine.

What types of viral infection are there?

There are several types of viral infections:

- **Acute** - When viruses cause an immediate set of symptoms with a short incubation period and a distinct onset and are then eliminated, the infection is said to be acute. An example is a cold or the flu.

- **Chronic** - A persistent infection such as infant cytomegalovirus causes low-grade symptoms and lingers on. The presence of these viruses can cause constant and fruitless attacks by the immune system, leading to autoimmune disorders. Viruses are, however, not the only cause of such disorders.

- **Latent** - Some viruses can enter a latent stage that can last for years or even decades. Viruses in this state cannot be detected, either by scientific methods or by the immune system. When the viruses enter, or re-enter, the active stage, infectious symptoms can come on suddenly and appear acute. An example of a latent virus is the herpes varicella virus, which causes childhood chickenpox. The virus lays latent in nerve cells, and can reappear decades later as a case of shingles. The virus is now called herpes zoster, and very painful poxlike vesicles erupt on the surface of the skin, primarily that of the trunk, where viruses in the nerve cells erupt through the nearby skin. Another example is the genital herpes virus, which can cause a painful, disabling first herpes attack years after infection.

- **Slow** - Viruses can slowly build up to the point of causing symptoms that come on and worsen gradually, as in the case of AIDS.

Many viruses such as herpes remain in the body for a lifetime. At best they are controlled, but not eliminated, by the immune system.

How can viruses cause damage?
Viruses cause their damage in several ways.

- They can cause destruction of the cell or its function, as for example polio's attack on the nerve cells, producing permanent paralysis. Damage is confined to the part of the body actually infected.

- They can, through stimulation of the immune system to attack, cause a local inflammatory response, although this rarely happens to any large extent.

- As previously mentioned, viruses can stimulate an autoimmune attack.

- They can cause hyperplasia, or a buildup of cells, as in skin or genital warts (papilloma). Warts can spread to nearby areas on the skin or mucous membranes, but don't travel freely through the body.

- They can cause DNA mutations which lead to uncontrolled cell growth, or cancer. Viruses probably do not act alone to cause cancer, but rather interact with other stressors when the immune system is suppressed.

- They can weaken the immune system so that other, more dangerous viruses and bacteria can gain a foothold and do their damage. Examples are encephalitis (brain infection) or meningitis following measles or viral or bacterial pneumonia following a cold.

Can you catch a viral infection more than once?
Since each virus has a specific shape, the immune system will attack it, usually successfully, once the immune system recognizes the invader and produces antibodies against it. This explains several things:

- Most viral infections are self-limiting - they run their course and are then eliminated.

- This immune system recognition also explains why vaccination works, although vaccination has its drawbacks, as discussed in the chapter on Treatment-Caused Trauma in *Thriving In A Toxic World*. A dead or weakened form of the virus is injected into the body, and the immune system mounts a defense and is forever after ready to attack immediately if live viruses later enter the body. The live viruses are killed before they have time to multiply to damage-causing numbers and to penetrate the body's cells.

- Similarly, once a person has had a particular viral disease, such as chickenpox, mumps, or measles, she/he cannot be reinfected at a later date because the immune system is primed to attack the invader if it ever again enters the body.

If this is the case, then why do so many of us catch colds, which are caused by viruses, repeatedly?

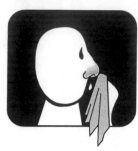

About half of all viruses which affect humans, including different types of adenoviruses, coronaviruses, and coxsackie viruses, attack upper respiratory and nasal membranes to produce the familiar symptoms of a cold. The cold symptoms produced by one virus are nearly indistinguishable from those produced by another. The symptoms vary from person to person depending on the individual's weak spots (throat, lungs, sinuses). After infection, the person is then immune, but only to that particular virus, one out of many. For the same reason, although a vaccine could theoretically be made against a particular cold virus, such a vaccine would not be very useful when hundreds of other viruses which cause cold symptoms would not be affected by the vaccine.

Are there effective treatments for viral diseases?

There is no true allopathic treatment for most viral diseases, if what is meant by treatment is a drug or agent that will selectively kill viruses in the body. Viruses are either nonliving crystalline matter or an indistinguishable part of an otherwise normal cell, depending on the stage of their life cycle, so it is unlikely that a virus-killer will be developed in the near future.

Antibiotics are useless against viruses and can cause harm of their own, but they are sometimes misprescribed for a viral infection through ignorance because the patient pressures the doctor to do something (however useless), or as a preventive measure against the bacterial infections that sometimes follow viral infections.

"Treatments" for viruses are therefore of three types:

- One type aims for symptom suppression, such as antihistamines, cold capsules, fever reducers, or cough drops. These suppress the immune system's effectiveness.

- The second type treats the opportunistic infections such as bacterial infection that may occur once the virus has weakened the immune system.

- The most effective measures for both prevention and cure are any ways in which immune system function is enhanced. Stronger and more numerous antibodies will then mount an attack on the viruses.

Some substances which support the immune system in fighting viruses include:

- Philmarten (phyllanthus amarus)

- Copper and the amino acid lysine which form copper lysinate

- Cyclic AMP (adenosine monophosphate)

- Gamma globulin

- Oxygenation methods such as hydrogen peroxide, ozone, or Dioxychlor (chlorine dioxide)

- Hyperthermia, in which the blood is heated outside the body and reinfused

- Rife and other frequency generators

- Germanium and Coenzyme Q10

- Antioxidants such as vitamins A, E, and C; bioflavonoids like pycnogenol, grape seed, quercetin, rutin; selenium. These control free radical damage and inflammation

- Transfer factor, also called complement, which tells the immune system what to attack. It programs the immune system to work normally.

- Alpha interferon

- Personalized vaccination, in which a vaccine is made from viral material from your own body.

- Colloidal silver

- Garlic is shown to protect against viruses and to enhance the production of antibodies. It should be eaten raw or as an extract, as it loses much of its medicinal value when cooked [4].

Moderate exercise increases resistance to viral and other infections. It supports immune system function and works the lymph glands. Even 45 minutes a day of walking has been shown to significantly reduce the number of respiratory infections in those who previously got them frequently [5].

What is a protocol for colds and flu?
If you feel a cold or flu coming on, it is a good idea to take any or all of the following supplements for maximum immune support. Dosages given are suggested amounts only. Check with your doctor for the dosages that are optimal for you. The injections must be prescribed by a physician.

- Garlic - Liquid Kyolic — 1/2 tsp. three times a day in water with meals

- Vitamin A (Nutri-Sorb A by Interplexus) — 2 drops (10,000 IU) three times a day tongue for 5 days

- SSKI (Super-saturated potassium iodide) — 10 drops three times a day in water for up to 10 days. Do not use if sensitive to iodine. Do not combine with colloidal silver.

- Vitamin C — 1000 mg 3 times a day in morning

- Calcium / Magnesium 2:1 — 2 in evening on empty stomach

(1000 mg / 500 mg)

- Gamma Globulin   (2cc) / c-AMP (1 cc) injection

- Colloidal Silver, Gold, Copper

- Vitamin B12   (2 cc) / Folic Acid (1 cc) injection once a week

- Copper and Lysine (Copper lysinate)

- Pro-Bioplex Intensive Care   Follow label directions
  (for gastrointestinal support)

- Immuplex Lozenges (Tyler)

What are some indicators of viral infection?

A comprehensive blood test can show a number of indicators that viral disease is present, although they are not diagnostic in themselves. The more of these that show up in the blood, the greater the likelihood that viruses have gone out of control.

- *Low uric acid*
- *High bilirubin*
- *High albumin / globulin (A/G) ratio, above 2.0*
- *High lymphocytes, white cells that fight viral infection*
- *High monocytes, another white blood cell type*
- *Lowered total white blood cell count*

If you have lowered immune system function from toxic immune suppressors such as chemicals or metals, or low levels of protective bacteria, copper, lysine, and gamma globulin, you are susceptible to viral infection. The environment is more important than the presence of the virus in determining whether viral infection will develop.

Stress greatly increases the likelihood of getting a cold or viral infection [6,7]. A study of people with strep bacteria in their throats showed that only 1/5 of those with low stress levels got sick, compared with 1/2 of those with high stress levels [8].

How are viruses classified?

Viruses are classified based on size and shape, presence or absence of an outer envelope, and pathological changes caused by the virus, among other criteria. Animal viruses can be broken down into 16 major groups in this manner. The viruses that are most likely to cause chronic problems in humans are several types of herpes viruses (varicella-zoster, herpes simplex I and II, Epstein-Barr, and cytomegalovirus), hepatitis B, and the HIV virus believed by some to be responsible for AIDS.

Herpes

What are the two types of herpes?

Herpes simplex I is said to cause "cold sores" and other mouth lesions, while Herpes simplex II causes genital sores. Since these lesions can be transferred from one site to the other via the hands or through oral-genital contact the distinction between I and II is not a clearly defined one, although type II is considered to be the more dangerous form.

What are the symptoms of Herpes simplex I?

Herpes simplex I affects 20% to 40% of the population in the United States. Primary infections include [3]:

- Cold sores and fever blisters on the lips and in the mouth. These are sometimes confused with canker sores, which are not virus caused and are not contagious.

- Infections of the oropharynx (throat area), such as pharyngitis, tonsillitis, and gingivostomatitis

- Keratitis, an eye inflammation

What are the symptoms of Herpes simplex II?

An estimated 30 million Americans have been infected with the Herpes simplex II virus, including nearly 20% of the sexually active adults in New York [9]. Genital herpes typically causes a severe initial outbreak of symptoms, followed by less-severe outbreaks. Between outbreaks, the virus is latent in nerve cells at the site of infection. The initial outbreak is quite unmistakable: visible, extremely painful genital blisters erupt, sometimes accompanied by general groin pain or swollen glands. The person may have flu-like symptoms, and a feeling of depression is not uncommon. Subsequent attacks are usually much milder, consisting of blisters that are less painful than the initial eruption, and an absence of most of the other symptoms.

Genital herpes outbreaks may be frequent, seldom, or may not recur after the initial outbreak. The virus remains in the body for life, however. Stress and the consequent immune system depression usually precipitates an outbreak. Many patients experience recurrences when emotionally stressed, when recovering from a cold, or around the time of menstruation. Herpes is considered to be infectious only when the blisters are present and are shedding virus particles. There have been cases in which herpes appeared to have been transmitted during an asymptomatic period, but this can often be explained by the fact that a woman can have blisters on the relatively insensitive and non-visible upper (inner) part of her vagina, or on her cervix, and be unaware of them.

Herpes can be passed from an infected mother to her baby during vaginal delivery. In one study, 10 of 56 pregnant, asymptomatic women passed the virus to their babies; one baby died and four others developed encephalitis [10].

What are some treatments for herpes?

Acyclovir (Zovirax) is often given to treat the initial outbreak, although it is not recommended for continued use or for subsequent outbreaks. Acyclovir, however, will not eliminate the virus. L-lysine, an amino acid, may have potential in inhibiting the growth of the herpes virus. An experimental group that received one gram of l-lysine daily had a reduced number of herpes lesion outbreaks [11]. Copper lysinate helps to boost the immune system, as copper is depleted by fighting infection. Arginine, found in nuts, acts against lysine and should be restricted.

Glycyrrhizic acid, the active constituent of the licorice plant, inactivates HSV-1 (herpes simplex virus) infected cell cultures [12]. Also recommended are lysine cream on the blisters and lysine taken orally, and vitamin B complex, zinc, vitamin C, thymus extract, acidophilus and vitamin E [13].

Essential oils are often effective against the herpes simplex virus due to their strong antiviral properties. Apply the oil to the lesion, or to the area of outbreak before the lesion appears. The lesions typically dry up and disappear within a few days. Oils recommended are lemon and geranium combined, eucalyptus radiata and bergamot combined, true rose oil or true melissa oil [14].

Stress reduction is one of the best things one can do to prevent herpes outbreaks [15].

Preventive measures include using condoms, preferably with the spermicide nonoxynol-9, and avoiding sex during outbreaks. It is important to understand that condoms will only reduce the risk by an unknown amount, not eliminate it.

What are some of the problems associated with herpes?

There are a number of chronic or recurring problems associated with herpes infections besides the blisters and discomfort themselves.

- People with genital herpes are twice as susceptible to HIV (AIDS) infection as people without the virus [16].

- Herpes infection can disarm key components of the immune system, explaining why the herpes virus persists for life in an infected person. The virus may also prevent other pathogens from being destroyed by the immune system [17].

- Herpes simplex I may cause atherosclerosis, a hardening of the arteries that may lead to heart attacks and strokes. It is hypothesized that herpes-infected cells become clogged with cholesterol buildup [18].

- Herpes encephalitis is caused when the virus migrates to the brain, where the immune system attacks it, but does not distinguish between healthy brain cells and the virus. Herpes encephalitis is rare but frequently deadly; there are only 1000 to 2000 cases in the United States annually [19].

- Since the virus can migrate to the brain, it can cause mood and behavior changes, such as manic depression [1].

- Women with genital herpes (and genital warts) have a higher risk of developing cancer of the cervix.

Cytomegalovirus

With which virus is most of the population infected?

Cytomegalovirus (CMV) is also a herpes virus, with which most of the adult population is latently infected. It can cause a syndrome similar to mononucleosis, and can also be involved in hepatitis. These are normally self-limiting diseases, and active CMV infection is rare in those with normal immunity, but these diseases can be threatening to immunocompromised patients. CMV is one of the leading serious infections of pregnancy, causing miscarriage, prematurity, fetal malformations, and fetal death. Even moderate prenatal infection can show up years later as intellectual impairment or subtle behavioral and learning problems [1].

What problems can be caused by cytomegalovirus?

Chronic effects of CMV include:

- CMV can destroy the cells of the pancreas and limit their ability to produce insulin, and so has been implicated in playing a triggering role in diabetes [1].

- Kaposi's sarcoma, an otherwise rare skin cancer that often afflicts AIDS patients, is thought to be actually caused by CMV [20]. CMV may be a cofactor that promotes infection by HIV (the so-called AIDS virus) [21].

- Like herpes simplex, CMV may be a trigger for atherosclerosis by causing the accumulation of cholesterol in human arterial cells [22].

- CMV encephalitis can affect the nerves and brain and can cause paralysis, loss of speech, and seizures; the disease can be fatal [23].

- CMV retinitis is a progressive retinal infection that can cause blindness. It is believed to afflict up to 20% of AIDS patients. Ganciclovir and Foscarnet are drugs used in treatment [24].

- CMV can also cause blindness by directly attacking the optic nerve.

Mononucleosis

What is mononucleosis?

Mononucleosis (sometimes called mono for short) is an acute infectious viral disease which causes sore throat, enlarged and tender lymph nodes and spleen, mild fever, and fatigue. EBV is found in the throat and saliva and is spread primarily via mouth to mouth contact; for this reason mononucleosis has been called the "kissing disease". It usually attacks children and young adults up to age 30, with peak incidence among those who are college age.

What are the symptoms of mononucleosis?

The incubation period of the virus can be as little as four days to as much as five weeks [2]. After several days to a week of flu-like symptoms, mononucleosis often causes several more weeks of fatigue which worsens after exertion. The immune system is adversely affected by mononucleosis, leading to opportunistic infections. One patient who contracted a severe case of mononucleosis at age 16 developed chronic, antibiotic-resistant ear infections starting about one month after the acute viral infection was past. These infections persisted for about six months.

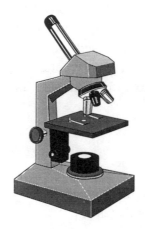

What are the cell changes of mononucleosis and how can they help in diagnosis?

A feature of infectious mononucleosis is the way the virus causes an increase in the number of white blood cells and a change in the appearance and behavior of a particular type of white blood cell, lymphocytes. Infected lymphocytes reproduce rapidly in somewhat mutated form, in a similar manner to cells that have undergone cancerous changes. There is also a characteristic change in the appearance of the lymphocyte. Observation of suitably stained lymphocytes is one method of diagnosis. (Staining causes certain cellular features to stand out under the microscope.)

Another method detects heterophil antibodies, which develop in 50-80% of patients with active clinical infection. A third method for diagnosis is an immunofluorescent test for antibodies to the EBV capsid antigen [2].

Is there any treatment for mononucleosis?

As with most viral diseases, there is no known external agent which will kill the mononucleosis virus directly. Treatment measures often employed are:

- Medication to alleviate some of the symptoms. Such medication is useless against the virus and can be harmful, as for example by suppressing the immune system.

- Antibiotics, which are useless against viruses but can treat or ward off opportunistic bacterial infection. They are useless if no pathogenic bacteria are causing a secondary infection, and can be harmful for the reasons discussed in the chapter on Drugs.

- Bed rest and time, helped by steam and hot baths.

- Measures as discussed in this book to boost immune system function.

- Cyclic AMP, gamma globulin, intravenous viral transfer factor, interferon.

- Liver extract, enzymatic therapy, silymarin (milk thistle), lipogen, protein powder, antioxidants, glutathione, and copper lysinate

Epstein-Barr Virus

What is the link between the Epstein-Barr virus, mononucleosis, and chronic fatigue syndrome?

Epstein-Barr virus (EBV) is best known as the virus that causes mononucleosis. It is also believed by many to cause or to be a cofactor in chronic fatigue syndrome. Its presence is also implicated in the development of several cancers.

Nearly everyone has EBV in their system, but whether symptoms develop and what type of symptoms they are depends on a variety of factors, such as immune system strength and age at the time of infection.

What is chronic fatigue syndrome?

Chronic fatigue syndrome (CFS) also goes by several other names:

- *Chronic Epstein-Barr virus syndrome (CEBV)*
- *Chronic fatigue immune deficiency syndrome (CFIDS, or CFS)*
- *The "Yuppie flu"*

Although it has been reported in all age groups, chronic fatigue syndrome is most prevalent in the 20-40 age range. Women sufferers outnumber men two to one, and 95% of the victims are Caucasian [25]. Chronic Fatigue Syndrome, which is discussed in the chapter on Diseases of the 21st Century in *Thriving In A Toxic World*, has been linked to the Epstein-Barr virus (EBV) in the past. EBV titers are often elevated in CFS patients, leading to the belief that there was a cause-effect relationship - that the elevated EBV levels were the cause of chronic fatigue. Since then it has been shown that elevated EBV levels can be found in non-CFS patients, while many CFS patients nave normal EBV levels.

Although some doctors still believe the cause-effect relationship, many others believe that EBV is not involved in CFS. The most likely theory is that the many toxic suppressors described in this book cause both the chronic fatigue symptoms and the EBV infection through immune suppression.

What other problems are linked to the Epstein-Barr virus?

A surge of EBV in the blood can aggravate a preexisting chronic condition, such as arthritis. Ankylosing spondylitis, a form of arthritis characterized by a hardening of the ligaments and tendons that bind the vertebrae together, is also believed to be brought on by EBV [26] or klebsiella bacteria.

Cancers believed related to EBV include [2, 20]:

- *Hodgkins' lymphoma*
- *Burkitt's lymphoma, which affects the jaw and abdomen*
- *Nasopharyngeal carcinoma, most common in Asia*
- *Leukemia*

EBV can be shielded in the body from the immune system and thus perpetuated as a consequence of chronic parasitic infection [27].

How is EBV detected and treated?
Detection of Epstein-Barr virus is similar to detecting mononucleosis. However, chronic fatigue syndrome is diagnosed by looking at the subjective list of symptoms and their duration.

Although symptom-relieving medication may be of some palliative use, measures used to boost the immune system will do the most good. An experimental treatment involves the use of Lauricidin (also called monolaurin or viricidin), alone or in combination with the food antioxidants BHA and BHT [28], which is not recommended here due to the toxicity of BHA and BHT, which contains the solvent toluene. Acyclovir and interferon are sometimes used prophylactically in high-risk individuals [3]. Homeopathic treatments include Echinacea angustifolia, 15 drops 3 times a day. Other measures such as those discussed earlier in the chapter for viruses in general can also be employed.

Hepatitis B

What is hepatitis B?
Hepatitis refers to inflammation of the liver (hepat- refers to the liver, -itis means inflammation). Several agents, viral and otherwise, can cause hepatitis. One of the most important of these is the hepatitis B virus. Hepatitis B is the ninth leading cause of death worldwide [29]. This deadly disease is at least 15 times more common than AIDS, with more than 300,000 cases reported in the United States in 1988 [30]. 5-10% of those infected become carriers.

How is hepatitis B spread?
Hepatitis B is spread through blood and body fluids. As little as 0.000025 ml (about 1/100,000 of a drop) of contaminated blood can transmit the disease [2]. The most common routes of transmission are contaminated needles (hepatitis B is often found among intravenous drug users), and through some sexual practices, especially anal sex. Health care workers are frequently exposed to the virus. A vaccine exists for hepatitis B, but most people at high risk have not been immunized.

What are the symptoms of hepatitis B?
The incubation period is 30 to 180 days. The virus can be found three months before symptoms occur, but one can be an asymptomatic carrier for up to five years. Although the virus can infect people of all ages, infection is most common at ages 15-24 [2]. The onset of the disease is slow and insidious, as compared with the acute onset of hepatitis A.

404

Early symptoms of hepatitis B infection resemble those of the flu:

- *Fever*
- *Achiness*
- *Fatigue*
- *Loss of appetite*
- *Bitter taste*
- *Nausea*
- *Rashes*

The hepatitis B virus targets liver cells, and swelling and tenderness of the liver and spleen, jaundice (yellow skin and eyes), and darkened urine can result [31]. An intolerance to food, alcohol, and medications may develop, as the liver, primarily involved in detoxification, is unable to function fully. Most people recover in two to twelve weeks, although some do not recover fully and these symptoms become chronic.

How is hepatitis B detected and treated?
Diagnostic methods include radioimmunoassay, reverse passive hemagglutination, and others [2]. Hepatitis B passed by blood transfusion used to be common, but screening of donated blood is now routine.

Treatment usually involves letting the disease run its course, as allopathic medication will tax the liver and often do more harm than good. A preparation of the plant Phyllanthus amarus, used for over 2000 years to treat jaundice in India and elsewhere, has been shown to be effective in treating 59% of patients [32]. Liquid liver and silymarin (milk thistle) are also recommended.

Genital Warts

What are genital warts?
Genital warts, also called condyloma or condylomata, are caused by the human papilloma virus (HPV). HPV causes two types of warts - visible, slightly raised painless lesions, and microscopic growths called flat warts. Both types of warts are found on or around a woman's vagina and cervix, on the anus, and on the head and shaft of the penis. They are not always visible.

Genital warts are twice as prevalent as the more highly publicized genital herpes. An estimated ten to twelve million people were infected with HPV as of 1988, with 300,000 to 500,000 new cases per year [33]. This means that about 14 million people are infected as of 1994. Unlike herpes, genital warts are painless and may not even be noticed, so they are not taken nearly as seriously as they should be.

What is a major danger of genital warts?
A number of research studies have linked HPV to an increased incidence of cervical cancer in women. The male reproductive tract may also be affected. About thirty percent of HPV warts

will progress to dysplasia, a stage of precancerous cell changes, within five years of infection [34].

How is the virus spread?
The virus is highly contagious, and is spread by sexual contact. Barrier methods such as the condom and to a lesser extent the diaphragm may help to prevent the spread of infection. However, as with other sexually transmitted diseases, abstinence or mutual monogamy with a non-infected partner are the best preventive measures. As with herpes, the lesions are treatable but the virus stays in the body for a lifetime, so prevention is of prime importance.

How are genital warts treated?

- HPV infection can be treated with a drug called podophyllin [35]

- The warts can be removed with conventional or laser surgery or with cryotherapy (freezing off the warts). They can also be burned off with acid. However, one study indicates that removing the flat warts by laser surgery doubles the risk of precancerous changes in cervical cells as compared with women who received no treatment [36].

- The immune system component alpha interferon, given by injection, is also useful in treatment.

- A treatment for genital warts is an ointment of vitamin A and the herbs thuja and lomatium. These herbs can also be taken orally, or thuja can be taken as a homeopathic. These herbs have both antiviral and immune supportive properties, and have been shown to inhibit HPV [37].

Summary

Viruses can cause a number of diseases and symptoms. There is no treatment at present which directly attacks the virus, although there is much that can be done to boost your immune system and thus reduce viral infections, including:

- *Gamma globulin, c-AMP*
- *Eliminate toxins*
- *Fungus-control diet*
- *Clear whiplash, balance the bite*
- *Support biochemistry (nutrition)*

References and Resources

Viruses, General

- The Burton Goldberg Group, *Alternative Medicine: The Definitive Guide*, Future Medicine Publishing, Puyallup WA, 1994. *The following chapters are relevant to Viral Infections:*

  "Chronic Fatigue Syndrome", pp. 616-624
  "Colds and Flus", pp. 632-9
  "Sexually Transmitted Diseases - Herpes", p. 831
  "Sexually Transmitted Diseases - Genital Warts", p. 832
  "Cold Sores", pp. 905-6
  "Hepatitis", p. 929
  "Mononucleosis", p. 948
  "Shingles", p. 971-2
  "Viral Infection", pp. 988-9
  "Warts", pp. 991-2

- Fettner, Ann Giudici, *Viruses: Agents of Change*, McGraw-Hill Publishing Co., New York, 1990.

- Smith, Alice Lorraine, *Principles of Microbiology*, C.V. Mosby Co., St. Louis MO, 9th ed., 1981.

- Alexander, Dale, *The Common Cold and Common Sense*, Fireside Books, New York, 1981.

- **Herpes Resource Center**, P.O. Box 13827, Research Triangle Park NC 27709, phone 919-361-8488.

Chronic Fatigue Syndrome

- Stoff, Jesse A. and Charles R. Pellegrino, *Chronic Fatigue Syndrome: The Hidden Epidemic*, Random House, New York, 1988.

- Rosenbaum, Michael and Murray Susser, *Solving the Puzzle of Chronic Fatigue Syndrome*, Life Sciences Press, Tacoma WA, 1992.

- Collinge, William, *Recovering From Chronic Fatigue Syndrome*, The Body Press / Perigree Books, NY, 1993.

- Crook, William, *Chronic Fatigue Syndrome and the Yeast Connection*, Professional Books, Jackson TN, 1992.

- Feide, Karyn, *Hope and Help for Chronic Fatigue Syndrome*, Fireside Books, NY, 1990.

- **CFIDS Association, Inc.**, P.O. Box 220398, Charlotte NC 28222-0398, phone 800-442-3437 or 900-988-2343. *This is the largest nonprofit organization dedicated to funding research and giving out information on Chronic Fatigue and Immune Dysfunction Syndrome (CFIDS).*

AIDS AND HIV

Don't Just Sit There - Do Something

Do you have many of the following symptoms? An HIV test may be in order.

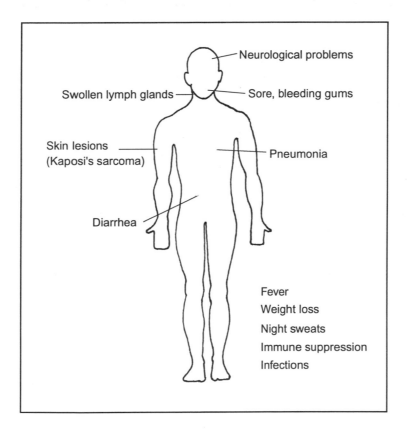

Neurological problems

Swollen lymph glands

Sore, bleeding gums

Skin lesions
(Kaposi's sarcoma)

Pneumonia

Diarrhea

Fever
Weight loss
Night sweats
Immune suppression
Infections

Eleven things in this chapter that can affect your health or even save your life:

*1. AIDS causes immune suppression, but AIDS is itself probably partially **caused** by immune suppression.*

2. Is AIDS actually caused by the HIV virus? - several viewpoints

3. Fungus along with HIV is more likely to cause AIDS than HIV alone.

4. If you have a diagnosis of HIV-positive, this is not necessarily a death sentence!

5. How can AIDS disrupt an entire immune system with so many different parts and backup systems?

6. How is AIDS transmitted?

7. Drugs other than IV drugs can contribute to AIDS.

8. Semen itself has properties which contribute to the spread of disease.

9. -10. Do condoms actually prevent infection? How can you protect yourself?

11. What are some immune-supporting treatments for AIDS?

What is AIDS?

AIDS is an acronym for **A**cquired **I**mmune **D**eficiency **S**yndrome. It is acquired as opposed to being genetic. Immune deficiency is the hallmark of the disease, allowing infections and cancers which would normally be controlled by the immune system to take hold. A syndrome is a collection of characteristic symptoms.

AIDS is one of the most feared diseases in the world now, as it is considered by most people (but not all) to be 100% fatal.

How many people are infected with HIV?

It is generally believed that HIV is the virus responsible for AIDS, but there is much evidence to the contrary, as discussed in this chapter.

The Centers for Disease Control estimated that between 1 and 1.5 million Americans were infected with HIV as of the end of 1991 [1]. This breaks down by gender to about 89% men and 11% women; 48% of infected women were intravenous drug users, and 36% of women contracted the infection through heterosexual contact. It is seventeen times more likely that an infected man will pass the virus to a woman than vice versa [2].

Statistics show that 0.4% of the U.S. population is HIV-antibody positive as of 1994; this is the same percentage that was positive ten years previously in 1984 [3,4].

The Global AIDS Policy coalition estimates that the number of people infected with HIV world wide is 19.5 million as of the end of 1992, up from 7 million at the end of 1987 [5]. More than three million people have already developed full-blown AIDS, and most of these have already died. Responsible estimates of cases of HIV infection by the year 2000 range from 40 million to 110 million. To put this into perspective, 110 million is about 2% of the world's present population.

New infections occur at the rate of one every 15 seconds [3]. Most of these are due to heterosexual contact, contrary to popular belief.

What is the historical background of AIDS research?

In 1953 it was shown that laboratory animals could be induced to develop cancer when infected with retroviruses. This was the first link made between viruses and cancer. In 1978 Robert Gallo of the National Institute of Health and National Cancer Institute showed that the virus-cancer connection was applicable to humans. HTLV, or human T-cell leukemia virus (leukemia is a type of cancer), attacks the T lymphocytes of the immune system and is a cause of adult T-cell leukemia (ATL).

Symptoms of ATL include enlarged lymph nodes, malignant circulating white blood cells, and skin lesions. Death can occur within six months of diagnosis [6]. HTLV-1, which is similar to but significantly different than HTLV, is associated with hairy-cell leukemia. HTLV-1 is thought to cause leukemia in only 1% of infected people, but a latency period (time between infection and symptoms) of up to thirty years makes it difficult to predict the future outcome for those infected [7]. So far these discoveries are coming to sound more and more like AIDS symptoms.

Gallo proposed that the virus, once in the body, did not need to spread from one cell to the next. The virus causes a genetic cell mutation, and this neoplastic (mutated) cell produces descendants that are cancer cells. Treatment lies in the prevention of transmission, which occurs through blood and bodily fluids. The Red Cross began screening blood donations for HTLV-1 in 1984.

HTLV-1 is also believed to be involved in the development of multiple sclerosis [8] and some forms of rheumatoid arthritis [9].

HTLV is transmitted through blood transfusions (prior to 1988), infected needles, sexual contact, and breastfeeding. 50% of intravenous (IV) drug users in New Orleans and 12% in New Jersey were found to be infected [10], although a link between infection and IV drug use is not necessarily cause / effect.

How does this research relate to HIV and AIDS?
The immune system disorder now known as Acquired Immune Deficiency Syndrome (AIDS) first showed up as a handful of isolated cases in 1979. By 1981, researchers were beginning to see a pattern primarily among intravenous drug users, male homosexuals, and Haitians. In 1983, several unrelated researchers discovered HTLV-infected white blood cells in up to 25% of patients with AIDS, which was their first clue that the disease may be caused by a virus, although, again, a link is not necessarily the same as cause and effect. The human immunodeficiency virus (HIV) is closely related to HTLV-1 and HTLV-2, although HTLV causes unrestrained cell growth, as in leukemia, while HIV kills cells.

Is AIDS caused by the HIV virus?
Although most researchers agree that HIV is involved in the development of AIDS, there is some disagreement over the virus's exact role. The basic beliefs are:

- Many scientists believe that HIV, acting by itself, triggers AIDS.

- A growing second group of scientists takes the position that HIV plays a critical role in causing the immune system cells to attack themselves, possibly in combination with other microorganisms such as fungi.

- Peter Duesberg of the University of California at Berkeley leads a third group that feels that HIV has no connection with AIDS, and that AIDS is not even an infectious disease [11,12].

- HIV, with or without other microorganisms, is more likely to develop into AIDS in a person with an immune system which is already suppressed.

French virologist Luc Montagnier has shown that a simple antibiotic prevented the HIV virus from harming infected T cells, supporting his belief that HIV alone cannot explain the immune system destruction characteristic of AIDS [13].

In 1988, a Walter Reed Hospital study looked at 29 women who were exposed to the HIV virus. Seven women had yeast infections, and six (86%) of these developed AIDS. The remaining 22 women did not have yeast infections, and after a comparable period none of them (0% vs. 86%) developed AIDS. This shows that fungus or a similar cofactor is probably necessary in combination with HIV or to open the door for HIV to cause AIDS.

The African liver fluke may have allowed AIDS to gain a foothold in Africa, where some believe the disease originated.

HIV has been shown to be quite fragile, surviving only about 24 hours outside the body unless it is in a temperature controlled culture medium. However, before donated blood was screened for HIV, infected blood which had been frozen to well below zero degrees in liquid nitrogen for up to six months was capable of infecting the person to whom it was given. Can the fragile temperature-sensitive HIV virus be the AIDS causative agent in frozen blood?

These facts are all parts of the puzzle, making the question "Does HIV cause AIDS?" impossible to answer definitively given the knowledge available today. The most likely answer is that HIV, probably working with fungus or other cofactors, is at least involved in development of AIDS.

Does HIV cause AIDS? The answer is not as clear-cut as some may think.

An immune system depressed by primary toxic suppressors is a likely contributor to the development of AIDS in a person who has been exposed to HIV. A person with a healthy immune system can fight off colds if exposed to the cold virus, and it follows that a healthy immune system can keep HIV at bay indefinitely. Although AIDS is well-known to be a suppressor of the immune system, the converse may well be true.

There is considerable evidence that HIV is not the sole or even primary causative agent for AIDS if indeed it is involved at all. Ideally evidence on both sides of the HIV argument should be considered before making any categorical statements about whether HIV does or does not cause AIDS. One well referenced book (nearly 600 scientific / medical references) giving support for the HIV-doesn't-cause-AIDS side is *AIDS* by Peter Duesberg and John Yiamouyiannis [12]. Another book with a similar view and similarly well researched is *The AIDS War* by John Lauritsen [14].

412

This discussion of the HIV-doesn't-cause-AIDS view is advanced to balance the HIV-causes-AIDS viewpoint so prevalent in the media. There are too many contradictions and not enough evidence to be positive about HIV's role - or lack of it - in the development of AIDS.

Peter Duesberg, leading opponent of the HIV-causes-AIDS hypothesis, researched the literature and found 4621 HIV-free AIDS cases, giving support for his position that HIV is not the causative agent for AIDS [15]. There are 13 million people worldwide who are HIV antibody positive who have no clinical symptoms [16].

One of the leading AIDS researchers in Amsterdam was quoted in *Lancet* as saying, "AIDS does not have the characteristics of an ordinary infectious disease. This view is incontrovertible" [17]. Peter Duesberg says, "...despite enormous efforts, no common active microbe has ever been found in AIDS patients" [18].

Why is HIV antibody tested for in "AIDS tests", rather than HIV itself?
On average 5 million white blood cells must be cultured to isolate enough HIV to show up on tests. Even with these conditions it may take as much as 15 different attempts to get one HIV virus from an HIV carrier. It is unlikely that a virus present in such a tiny amount, as compared with the virus populations in nearly all other viral diseases, could be the sole cause of such a devastating illness [19].

Why is the presence of HIV antibodies unlikely to be a sign of susceptibility to the disease associated with it?
The purpose of antibodies is to protect against a particular disease, and, in fact, the presence of specific antibodies is an indication of immunity to that disease. This is why people who have had measles or mumps and who now have antibodies to these diseases almost never get sick with them again. Yet the argument is put forth that the presence of antibodies to HIV not only doesn't protect against AIDS but is a virtual guarantee that the person *will* get AIDS. There is a certain lack of logic to this position [20-24].

How do mutations of HIV complicate the picture?
The HIV virus, like other retroviruses, lacks a self-correcting mechanism that would prevent genetic errors (mutations) on duplication. The number of genetically distinct strains of the virus increases steadily during the progression towards AIDS [25]. A computer model suggests that full-blown AIDS is not a gradual decrease in immune system response but rather a catastrophic event that occurs when the immune system is suddenly overwhelmed by the large number of different HIV strains [26].

In 1992, 24 to 30 people with AIDS symptoms and high risk factors tested negative for HIV. The causative agent, which these people may or may not have in common, may be either an HIV virus that has mutated into a form undetectable by present tests, or by another rare virus [27].

If HIV were a single virus which caused AIDS, it should be a comparatively simple procedure to develop a vaccine for it. To develop any vaccine, dead or weakened strains of the virus are injected into the body. The immune system is stimulated to form antibodies specific to that virus which will recognize the particular markers of that virus if live virus is introduced into the body. A marker is analogous to the bumps and dips particular to the key which opens your front door.

The fact that no HIV vaccine is even close to being developed points to a virus which mutates, or changes markers, rapidly enough to make a specific vaccine useless. This fact also points to the idea that HIV may not be the primary causative agent of AIDS, since even with mutations a vaccine which worked for a while might still be possible.

How does AIDS disrupt the entire immune system?

T cells that carry what is called the CD4 marker have a regulatory function which is central to the function of the entire immune system. T cells with the CD4 marker are also called T4 cells, or helper T cells. These, as discussed in the chapter on the Immune System in *Thriving In A Toxic World*, turn the immune system on, or notify the various components that their services are needed. The immune system is not actually destroyed, but instead is like a police department with no link to the outside world. The immune system, like the police, are there and ready for action, but with no knowledge of when and where they are needed they are essentially useless.

The HIV virus preferentially infects cells carrying the CD4 marker, thus explaining in part how the virus can disrupt an entire immune system with so many supporting and backup systems. Once infection has occurred, the virus may lie latent for up to twelve years before symptoms develop. During this time, the virus is passed from one CD4-marked cell to another by direct contact, bypassing the antibodies in the blood that might otherwise destroy it at an early stage. Mutations occur as the virus multiplies and spreads.

The disease is characterized by the progressive depletion of T4 lymphocytes. The thymus gland has been found to be eroded in AIDS patients, and swollen lymph nodes signify the involvement of the lymphatic system. There is failure to respond to skin tests which measure cell-mediated immunity [28]. Patients are said to have AIDS when an opportunistic infection and/or overt symptoms (discussed later in this chapter) develop. Once a person is diagnosed with AIDS, that person's chance of surviving more than three years is only about one in ten [1]. AIDS related complex (ARC) is a precursor to full-blown AIDS and this is when symptoms first start to show up.

How is HIV transmitted from one person to another?

HIV is transmitted through transfer of body fluids, especially blood and semen. Consequently, AIDS is most common among intravenous drug users and male homosexuals. Intravenous (IV) drug users often share needles which are contaminated with the infected blood of a person who has himself been infected in the same way.

Anal sex, rather than vaginal sex, accounts for many sexually transmitted cases of AIDS. The disease does not distinguish between a male and a female rectum. The disease is, in fact, epidemic in certain areas of Africa where heterosexual anal sex is used as a method of birth control. Intestinal tissue, including the rectum, is designed to absorb nutrients. In fact, the lower colon is so absorptive that a person getting a colonic in which water is introduced into the colon often needs to urinate afterwards. However, this absorptive design also allows the easy absorption of the HIV virus as well as other infective agents. In addition, rectal tissue, unlike vaginal tissue, was not meant to be stretched, with the result that tiny fissures or tears in the tissue may form and admit the virus to the bloodstream.

Small amounts of the HIV virus have been found in other body fluids such as saliva and tears, but to our knowledge there have been no reported cases from contact with these sources.

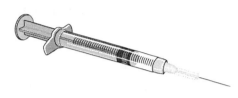

Health-care workers may be at risk, since many of them work around both blood and sharp instruments, and latex surgical gloves are easily pierced. Surgeons get stuck with scalpels and needles 3-5% of the time while operating [29], and infected blood can be transferred either from doctor to patient or vice versa.

AIDS is also acquired prenatally and through breastfeeding by an infected mother. Blood transfusions prior to 1984, when testing of donated blood was instituted, have also been responsible for many cases of AIDS.

Although it has not been proven that this is a method of transmission, it has been shown that HIV stays alive in mosquitoes for 24-48 hours. It is possible that spraying with the insecticide Malathion in California is not for the well-publicized Medfly but rather for mosquitoes which may harbor the virus. If mosquitoes are vectors, or carriers of the virus, it is also possible that fleas are also vectors, as they were of the plague centuries ago.

As far as we know, AIDS is **not** spread by being around a person with AIDS, hugging or touching them, changing diapers of infected babies, or by donating blood. When blood is donated, sterile never-used needles and tubing are used, and blood flows only out from the patient.

Can drugs other than IV drugs contribute to the spread of AIDS?

Non-IV drugs such as marijuana, cocaine, and alcohol do not directly spread the HIV virus. However, most drugs lower immune system function, increasing the chances of becoming infected if exposed to HIV. In addition, most recreational drugs will lower inhibitions and judgment, increasing the dangers of having irresponsible sex. It is likely that the dangers of getting AIDS from using IV drugs comes as much from the immunosuppressive effects of the drugs as from contaminated needles. Both may be required to spread the disease.

There is a very high correlation between drug use and the development of AIDS. Two epidemiological studies done in 1993 showed that every one of several hundred men with AIDS had been using recreational drugs like nitrite inhalants, amphetamines, cocaine, or they were on the drug AZT [30-32].

Consistent use of nitrite inhalants, commonly used as sexual stimulants, provided a 94-100% association with AIDS [33-35].

Cocaine use is correlated with AIDS. In fact, in the early 1900s, heavy cocaine users were reported to have a list of symptoms that looks remarkably like the list of AIDS symptoms [36,37].

What is it about semen that increases the chances of transmitting HIV and other viruses?
It has long been a puzzle to scientists that a woman's immune system does not destroy sperm, a foreign protein, after intercourse. It is fortunate that this does not happen, as conception could then not occur and the human race would have died out long ago. It was theorized that women secreted a local immunosuppressive agent which protected the sperm from immune system attack, but such an agent was never found. It has recently been discovered that the sought-after immunosuppressive agent is in the man's semen.

If a virus, HIV, herpes, fungus, or other infectious agent were in semen along with an immunosuppressive substance, the pathogen could infect the new host without interference from the host's immune system until it was too late.

It is also possible that the local immunosuppressive agents in semen have a relationship to the prevalence of prostate problems in men, especially vasectomized men whose bodies resorb the semen. It has also been found that men who are less or not sexually active have a higher incidence of cancer, and the retention of immunosuppressive semen may partially explain this.

Can semen contribute to problems after infection?
It seems logical that once one is infected with AIDS/HIV, one has nothing to lose by continuing to have sex (other than danger to one's partner). Actually, exposure to more semen, which is both a foreign protein and contains an immunosuppressive agent, will stress the immune system of the recipient. In addition, ejaculation depletes the prostate gland of zinc, a mineral essential to the health of the immune system. It follows that an infected person may live longer by foregoing sex, as well as being safer for potential partners.

How is candida involved?
Records at Walter Reed Hospital show a correlation between candida and the development of AIDS in a group of twenty-nine women, all exposed to AIDS. Seven had fungal infections, and six of those seven developed AIDS. The other 86%, who did not have fungal infections, tested negative for AIDS

Since candida overgrowth has been shown to be linked to the development of AIDS symptoms, it would therefore be wise to limit candida growth by reducing or eliminating refined sugar and simple carbohydrates [38]. Taking lactobacillus bulgaricus, a noncolonizing bacteria with powerful antibiotic and antifungal properties, is also recommended [39].

Why is it sometimes difficult to determine the cause of infection?
The span of years between infection and symptoms or diagnosis often makes it very difficult to determine the cause of the infection.

In addition, there is some difficulty in determining the true cause of infection in many people, as the most common routes of infection, male homosexual contact and intravenous drug use, carry a heavy stigma that would likely motivate people to lie.

Why are some people more susceptible to getting AIDS?

Susceptibility to getting AIDS after exposure to HIV is determined by a number of factors, including:

- Immune system health at the time of infection. Mercury, nickel, other toxins, or allergy can suppress the immune system.

- Age (older people and infants are most susceptible)

- The route of infection

- The quantity of viruses entering the body

- Pre-existing infection such as fungus or bacteria, which is itself more likely if your supply of protective bacteria is low

- Possibly genetics.

While neither men nor women are inherently more susceptible to HIV, women are at far greater risk (17:1) of contracting HIV through intercourse with a man than a man is at risk for getting HIV from a woman. This is due to the immunosuppressive effect of semen, and to the fact that the body fluids are flowing from man to woman.

How can mental outlook affect the lifespan of a HIV infected person?

Bernie Siegel, M.D., in his books *Peace, Love, and Healing* and *Love, Medicine, and Miracles*, and Norman Cousins in his book *Anatomy of an Illness* show how positive mental outlook and hope can increase the quality and quantity of one's life for those who have been diagnosed with an incurable illness. It is therefore quite possible that despair and lack of hope can adversely affect one's lifespan. Since optimism and the will to live have been shown to affect the time of death, and it is quite possible that hearing the news that one has a disease believed to have a 100% fatality rate may itself cause people to give up and die sooner.

Eventual death from AIDS is virtually certain, according to allopathic medicine, but it is infection of various types that overwhelms the marginally functioning immune system that kills the person, rather than any direct effect of HIV.

How can AIDS be prevented?

Prevention of AIDS, or at least minimizing risk, lies in taking the following measures:

- Abstaining from sex, especially intercourse. A lifestyle that promotes sex with multiple partners with a similar history is like playing "HIV Roulette".

- The safest sexual practice other than complete abstinence is mutual lifelong monogamy with an HIV negative partner.

- Abstaining from questionable sexual practices, such as anal sex.

- Do not use intravenous drugs. The sharing of needles among intravenous drug users as been a major route of infection and spread of HIV.

- Do not use any drugs.

A word on monogamy: many people feel that having only one partner at a time is monogamy, even if they change partners every year
or so. If you have sex with six people over ten years, you have had
sex with six people, and it doesn't matter as far as disease spread
whether they were one at a time or all at once. So don't fool yourself into thinking you are safe if
you practice "serial monogamy".

> **When is monogamy
> not really monogamy?**

Do condoms help to prevent infection?

Condoms, when used to prevent pregnancy, have a 5% failure rate even when used correctly, and
a 14% failure rate when errors in use are considered. In other words, sperm will get through
holes or tears in the condom in at least one out of twenty acts of intercourse and impregnate the
woman. Since not every act of unprotected intercourse results in pregnancy, it is likely that
sperm gets through the condom barrier even more than one in twenty times, or one in seven times
if the 14% failure rate figure is used.

The HIV virus is 450 times smaller than a sperm cell. If a sperm cell were blown up to the size
of a volleyball, an HIV virus would be the size of a gnat by comparison. If you had a net which
let one out of twenty volleyballs through, would you trust it to keep out gnats? The same logic
applies to the use of condoms.

Condoms, especially if they contain the spermicide nonoxynol-9, have been shown to reduce the
risk of HIV transmission. This is like saying that having one bullet in the gun's chamber rather
than two will reduce the chances of your being killed in Russian roulette. In either case, are the
odds acceptable? Only you can make that decision for yourself, but it is important to know that
it is definitely possible to contract HIV from an infected partner who is wearing a condom. The
failure rate of condoms in preventing HIV transmission is 38%.

What are the symptoms of AIDS?

Symptoms of AIDS occur from infections which overwhelm the immune system. Not all symptoms occur in all patients, nor do they occur in the same order. Early symptoms are sometimes
called AIDS-related complex (ARC), and include:

- *Fatigue*
- *Fevers*
- *Diarrhea*
- *Yeast infections*
- *Night sweats*
- *Weight loss, sometimes called "the slims"*

- *Shortness of breath*
- *Sores that don't heal*
- *Swollen lymph glands*
- *Bone and joint pains*
- *Tender, bleeding gums*

Later symptoms include:

- Kaposi's sarcoma (KS), a skin cancer characterized by reddish brown raised lesions on the skin, increasing in number as the disease progresses. KS has been identified in men who are free of AIDS, and is believed to be caused by an infectious organism [40]. When KS spreads internally, death results.

- A formerly rare pneumonia caused by pneumocystis carinii. This can be fatal.

- Weight loss progresses to a skeletal stage in most AIDS cases, as absorption of food as well as appetite decline. The illness causes one to be sympathetic-dominant, so the parasympathetic function of digestion and restoration is not fully activated, leading to poor food digestion and absorption.

- Neurological symptoms, including blindness and motor difficulties. Poor absorption of oils can lead to the degeneration of the myelin sheath of the nerve cells, causing neurological problems.

- Almost one third of all AIDS patients develop a brain inflammation called encephalitis. This causes increasing memory loss and dementia as it progresses [41]. AIDS dementia combined with anger and a feeling of victimization can cause a person who is otherwise responsible to go around spreading the virus.

- A nearly unlimited number of viral, bacterial, and fungal infections, alone or in combination, can ravage the body with devastating results. Even a simple cold can be deadly.

What kind of testing is available?
Testing for HIV infection involves testing for antibodies to HIV, rather than for the virus itself. It was believed that antibodies to HIV would develop within six months. This meant that a person who tested negative six months after the most recent possible risk was home free. It is now believed by some that as much as 3 1/2 years may elapse between infection and antibody development [42].

The preliminary test done is the ELISA test (Enzyme Linked Immuno-Sorbent Assay). A negative result means that no HIV antibodies have been found. However, due to the long incubation period this does not necessarily mean that one is free of infection, but only that antibodies have not yet developed. A positive result is not diagnostic for HIV infection alone. Other conditions can also cause one to test positive. A positive result is an indication to perform a more sensitive, discriminating, and expensive test, the Western Blot test. A positive result on this test indicates HIV infection.

What allopathic, or drug, treatments are available for AIDS?
Azidothymidine (AZT) is the best known allopathic drug currently approved for the treatment of AIDS. More recently, DDI is also being used. A number of other drugs are in the lengthy research or clinical testing phases pending approval. Unfortunately, AZT does not cure AIDS but

merely delays the onset of some of the symptoms, and, in fact, may cause other symptoms - including death - to come on faster. In addition, AZT resistant strains of HIV are developing, which is not surprising for a virus which mutates as a matter of course.

AZT was originally a cancer chemotherapeutic agent. It was known in 1961 that, like other chemotherapeutic agents, it actually suppresses the immune system. Also, like other cancer chemotherapeutic agents, it is itself carcinogenic, a particular hazard in someone with a depressed immune system.

Many of the symptoms attributed to AIDS may actually be caused by AZT. The anti-AIDS drug AZT is highly toxic and has been associated with immune suppression and other symptoms usually attributed to AIDS. The *Physician's Desk Reference* (PDR) states that "It was often difficult to distinguish adverse effects possibly associated with Zidovudine [AZT] administration from underlying signs of HIV disease...". AZT is the most toxic drug that has ever been licensed for long-term consumption [43,44].

Other drugs are in the development stage. One such example is Penavir, which acts as an antioxidant and prevents infected cells from reactivating.

Currently, AIDS is considered by the medical establishment to be 100% incurable, i.e. fatal. Cures have been reported and ascribed to everything from faith healing to herbs, but there is little scientific verification with controlled studies at this time. The medical/scientific community does not take non-allopathic methods seriously enough to study them. This does not, however, mean that they don't work. They may at least help to lengthen lifespan, postpone the onset of symptoms, or improve quality of life.

What Can Be Done?

What are some immune-supporting treatments?
Holistic methods exist for the treatment of AIDS. These methods are based on the following principles:

- *Utilization of less toxic virus-killing agents*
- *Detoxification to eliminate metabolic waste*
- *Increasing cellular metabolism to energize the body*
- *Boosting and rebuilding of the immune system via cellular repair*

Holistic protocols, sometimes used alone but usually used in combination, include [40]:

- *Herbs*
- *Colonics*
- *Aloe vera*
- *Nutrients*

- *Lecithin*
- *Ultraviolet therapy*
- *Elimination of parasites, fungus, and bacteria*
- *Treatment of treatable opportunistic infections*
- *Prayer and positive affirmations*

Other supportive treatments include:

- *Oxidants - oxygen kills viruses and other anaerobic microorganisms*
  - *Ozone*
  - *Ozonate, Dioxychlor*
  - *Hydrogen peroxide*

- *Eliminate or reduce suppressors*
  - *Elimination of metals and toxic chemicals*
  - *Metal chelation*
  - *Sauna*
  - *Rife frequencies - the correct ones can kill viruses and other infectious agents*
  - *Hi-Tech Hygiene iodine hand and face wash - stop infection and reinfection*
  - *Copper lysinate - anti-viral*

- *Heat*
  - *Hyperthermia therapy (heating the blood) beyond the viral survival temperature*
  - *Constitutional hydrotherapy - alternate hot and cold*

- *Immune Support*
  - *Transfer factor - improves communication and thus effectiveness of the immune system*
  - *Bee propolis and pollen - feed and support immune system*
  - *Glandulars - thymus, pituitary, adrenal, and others*
  - *PCM-4 (thymus glandular and ginseng)*
  - *Live cell therapy - thymus cells from sharks or other animals regenerate new thymus tissue*
  - *Cyclic AMP to support the energy cycle*

- *Antioxidants / Free radical scavengers*

- *Adaptogens such as ginseng*
- *Vitamin C, bioflavonoids and antioxidants (vitamins A and E)*
- *Kyolic garlic*
- *Coenzyme Q-10 - provides cellular energy by supporting mitochondria*
- *Pycnogenol*

People who are HIV positive and/or have AIDS are most commonly deficient in the following essential nutrients:

- *Vitamin B6 [45]*
- *Vitamin B12 [46,47]*
- *Zinc [49]*
- *Folic acid / folate [46]*
- *Selenium [48]*

It would thus be a good idea to supplement with these especially. Large doses of ascorbate, a salt of vitamin C, can suppress the disease symptoms and have been linked to reduction of diseased lymph glands and the disappearance of Kaposi's sarcoma lesions [50].

A multimodal AIDS treatment program has shown a 95% success rate (measured by normalizing test results and physical and mental well-being). The approach, called Life Science Universal (LSU), combines ozone therapy, nutrient supplementation, herbs, a primarily vegetarian diet, and counseling and goal-setting exercises [51].

Ultraviolet blood irradiation has been used for the treatment of HIV and other bloodborne viruses [52,53].

Hyperthermia, or the induction of a fever for an extended period of time, has been linked to inactivation of the HIV virus, immune system stimulation similar to that caused by a natural fever, release of toxins, a reduction in night sweats, a decrease in secondary infections and a greater sense of well-being. Although high-tech methods of fever induction exist, measures such as sauna, hot baths, hot water bottles, and blankets alone or in combination are often effective. Use these to provoke a heavy sweat for a few hours, then follow with a cool shower. The person undergoing treatment should be monitored for adverse effects such as liver and kidney stress from release of toxins or symptoms such as dizziness [54-56].

Oxygen therapy, in the form of hydrogen peroxide or ozone, helps to provide an inhospitable environment for HIV and other viruses, bacteria and many opportunistic microorganisms. Ozone in water, which is essentially the same as hydrogen peroxide, is either injected intravenously or some blood is removed, treated and reinjected. After treatment it is recommended that antioxidants be taken to protect against free radical damage from the ozone [57-59].

What are some herbal treatments used in AIDS?

- Garlic is used in treatment because of its antibacterial and antiviral qualities [60-62].

- Ginseng increases the ability to withstand stress and has a tonic effect on the thymus gland, which is part of the immune system [63,64].

- St. John's Wort has blocking actions against retroviruses [65].

- Chinese bitter melon, monolaurin and lentinan from shiitake mushrooms also have anti-HIV effects [66-68].

Acupuncture is often used with Chinese herbs to improve immune function and alleviate symptoms such as night sweats and fatigue associated with AIDS. There are even claims that it has converted several patients from HIV positive to HIV negative [69].

Acupuncture alone is also useful in AIDS treatment. Improvement in symptoms [70], increased T-cell counts [71,72] and a reduction in side effects from medicinal AIDS treatment [73] were noted.

29 patients who took IV minerals and followed a protocol to control fungus had an improved T4/T8 ratio and an increase in energy. One 30 year old man, a former weight lifter, came in without enough energy to even talk. After one month of IV and other support he felt much better and had more energy.

What are some suggestions for avoiding developing AIDS if you are HIV positive?

- *Improve your diet - see Nutrition section in* **Thriving In A Toxic World**.
- *Avoid toxic chemicals.*
- *Keep a positive mental attitude.*
- *Exercise regularly to boost your immune system and oxygenate your body.*
- *Get enough sleep [12].*
- *Avoid anal sex and drugs.*

What else can be done?
Many people seem to believe that more money, more research into the cause, and more government involvement are the keys to ending this epidemic. Rather, the government should get out of the way of people building up their immune systems and undergoing treatments that work with the body's systems rather than overriding them.

References and Resources

General

- Brighthope, Ian, *The AIDS Fighters*, Keats Publishing, New, Canaan CT, 1987.

- Chaitow, Leon and S. Martin, *A World Without AIDS*, Thorsons, London, 1989.

- Check, William A. and Ann G. Fettner, *The Truth About AIDS - Evolution of an Epidemic*, Holt, Rinehart and Winston, NY, 1985.

- Fee, E. and DM Fox (eds.), *AIDS: The Making of a Chronic Disease*, University of California Press, Berkeley CA, 1992.

- Gregory, Scott J. and Bianca Leonardo, *They Conquered AIDS!*, True Life Publications, 1989.

Controversies - Does HIV cause AIDS, The use of AZT

- Adams, Jad, *AIDS: The HIV Myth*, St. Martin's Press, New York, 1989. *Explores the hypothesis that HIV is not the causative agent of AIDS.*

- Duesberg, Peter and John Yiamouyiannis, *AIDS*, Health Action Press, Delaware OH, 1995. *Examines the causes of AIDS and concludes that HIV doesn't cause it, but recreational drugs and medications such as AZT do. This book has nearly 600 scientific references backing up their position.*

- Fry, TC, *The Great AIDS Hoax*, Life Science Institute, Austin TX, 1989.

- Fumento, M., *The Myth of Heterosexual AIDS*, Regnery Gateway, Washington DC, 1993.

- Lauritsen, John, *The AIDS War: Propaganda, Profiteering and Genocide From the Medical-Industrial Complex*, Pagan Press, NY, 1993. *The debate about whether HIV causes AIDS, the dangers of the AIDS treatment AZT, and more.*

- Nussbaum, B., *Good Intentions: How Big Business, Politics and Medicine are Corrupting the Fight Against AIDS*, Atlantic Monthly Press, NY, 1990.

- Root-Bernstein, Robert, *Rethinking AIDS*, The Free Press, New York, 1993. *Explores the hypothesis that HIV is not the causative agent of AIDS.*

AZT and Drugs

- Lauritson, John, *Poison By Prescription: The AZT Story*, Asklepios, New York, 1990. *The politics and dangers involved in the use of AZT.*

- Lauritsen, John and H. Wilson, *Death Rush, Poppers and AIDS*, Pagan Press, NY, 1986.

- Loimer, N., R. Schmid and A. Springer (eds.), *Drug Addiction and AIDS*, Springer-Verlag, NY, 1991.

424

- Turner, CF, HG Miller and LE Moses, AIDS, *Sexual Behavior and Intravenous Drug Use*, National Academy Press, Washington DC, 1989.

Natural Healing Methods

- Badgley, Lawrence, *Healing AIDS Naturally*, Healing Energy Press, Foster City CA, 1987.

- The Burton Goldberg Group, *Alternative Medicine: The Definitive Guide*, "AIDS", pp. 494-509, Future Medicine Publishing, Puyallup WA, 1994.

- Callen, Michael, *Surviving AIDS*, Harper Collins, New York, 1990. *The author is one of the longest survivors of AIDS, and he credits natural healing methods and outlines his approach to health.*

- Chaitow, Leon and Simon Martin, *A World Without AIDS*, Thorsons Publishing Group, London England, 1988. *Discusses why conventional medicine doesn't work, and how AIDS can be treated using naturopathic medicine.*

- Gregory, Scott J., *A Holistic Protocol for the Immune System*, Tree of Life Publications, Palm Springs CA, 1989.

- Siegel, Bernie, *Peace, Love and Healing*, Harper and Row, NY, 1989.

- *This book and its companion volume Love, Medicine and Miracles discuss the mind/body connection and the importance of having a positive attitude and its effect on healing.*

Organizations

- **AIDS Alternative Health Project**, 3223 N. Sheffield Avenue, Chicago IL 60657, phone (312) 327-6437. *Offers various comprehensive therapies to HIV+ people for a nominal fee, or free if hardship.*

- **Cure Now**, P.O. Box 29386, Los Angeles CA, 90029, phone (213) 660-7563. *Education on healing alternatives.*

- **HEAL**, 16 East 16th Street, New York NY, 10003, phone (212) 647-HOPE. *Informatiion on alternative healing methods; offers referrals to hypnotherapists trained to deal with fears surrounding HIV diagnosis.*

MYCOPLASMAS

Like Crossing A Bacteria With A Virus

Do you have the following symptoms? You may have a mycoplasma infection.

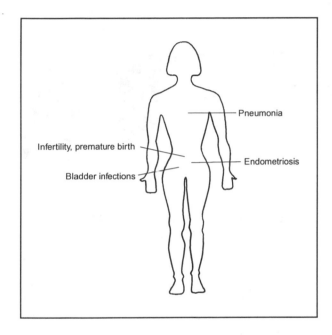

Pneumonia

Infertility, premature birth

Bladder infections

Endometriosis

In this chapter you can learn:

- *What are mycoplasmas, and what types of disease do they cause?*
- *What is the link between mycoplasmas and AIDS?*

What are mycoplasmas?

Mycoplasmas are smaller than bacteria but larger than viruses. Unlike bacteria, they do not have a cell wall. They are gram-negative (do not take a certain type of biological stain) and they do not move on their own. They are considered to be the smallest free-living self-replicating cellular units, with a cell volume about one-fifth that of E. coli bacteria.

What types of disease are caused by mycoplasmas?

Mycoplasmas cause a number of diseases in animals. In humans, the respiratory and genitourinary systems are most affected.

A lung disease known as primary atypical pneumonia is caused by Mycoplasma pneumoniae. It is an acute self-limiting disease, especially affecting children ages 5-15, that begins as an upper respiratory tract infection which then spreads to the lungs. After an incubation period of 2-3 weeks, pneumonia symptoms develop, including paroxysmal cough, headache, and malaise. The attack lasts several weeks and recovery is gradual. Symptoms may be so mild as to go unnoticed. The disease, which is not very contagious, is spread to the upper respiratory tract of the new host via oral or nasal droplets, as in coughing or sneezing.

Genitourinary mycoplasmal infection is spread via sexual activity. The organisms involved are M. hominis, M. genitalium, and ureaplasma urealyticum. These agents cause [1, 2, 3]:

- *Infertility and premature birth*
- *Pelvic inflammatory disease*   *PID*
- *Nongonococcal urethritis*   *inflammation of the urethra*
- *Prostatitis*   *inflammation of the male prostate*
- *Cervicitis*   *inflammation of the female cervix*
- *Cystitis*   *bladder infection*
- *Endometriosis*   *inflammation of the uterine tissue*
  outside the uterus

Pelvic inflammatory disease, which is sometimes caused by mycoplasma, is often also related to exposure to the toxic metal nickel.

How can a doctor tell what organism is causing pneumonia?

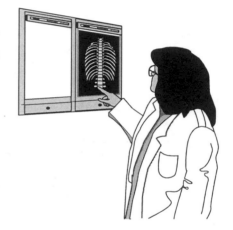

Mycoplasmas can cause pneumonia, but so can bacteria, viruses, and fungi. Different patterns that show up on x-ray can distinguish between these:

- *Bacteria*   *large spots*
- *Mycoplasma*   *small spots*
- *Fungus*   *long wispy lines*

Distinguishing between these is important so the correct treatment can be offered.

What is the link between mycoplasmas and AIDS?

Mycoplasmas are associated with AIDS, according to experiments by Shyh-Ching Lo. Cultured cells, infected with both mycoplasma fermentans and the HIV virus, died more readily than cells infected with HIV alone. The study's implication is that mycoplasmas decrease immune resistance, enhance the pathogenicity of AIDS and/or activate the HIV virus [4]. Mycoplasma incognitus can cause fatal tissue damage in AIDS-infected humans without alerting the immune system [5].

How are mycoplasmas diagnosed and treated?

Diagnosis is made from cell culture, or from observing a rising antibody titer [2]. Since penicillin attacks cell walls, it is ineffective against mycoplasmas. Doxycycline, however, destroys the mycoplasma, and may be of use in treating AIDS patients [6].

References and Resources

Smith, Alice Lorraine, *Principles of Microbiology*, C.V. Mosby Co., St. Louis MO, 9th ed., 1981.

Do you have the following symptoms? You may have a fungus infection.

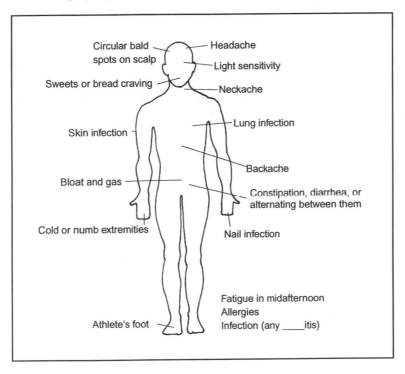

Circular bald spots on scalp — Headache — Light sensitivity — Sweets or bread craving — Neckache — Lung infection — Skin infection — Backache — Bloat and gas — Constipation, diarrhea, or alternating between them — Cold or numb extremities — Nail infection — Athlete's foot — Fatigue in midafternoon / Allergies / Infection (any _____itis)

Things in this chapter that can change your health:

- *A fungus infection is usually a sign of an imbalance in the body that must be dealt with to successfully eradicate the fungus.*

- *If you have a fungus infection that seems to be local, such as skin fungus or a vaginal yeast infection, chances are that the rest of the body is affected.*

- *If you have diabetes or a blood sugar problem, you may be especially susceptible to fungus infection.*

- *Fungal and parasitic infections often go together. You may not be able to get rid of the fungus until you get rid of the parasites.*

What are fungi?
Fungi (singular: fungus) are organisms in the plant kingdom that are characterized by:

- *Having a nucleus*
- *Reproducing both sexually and asexually (without two genders) via spores*
- *Having no chlorophyll, the green matter in most plants*

Fungi vary in size but are larger than bacteria, ranging from single-celled organisms to mushrooms and toadstools. The fungi that are most important medically are single celled or at least microscopic.

What types of fungi are there?
Fungi are loosely divided into two groups:

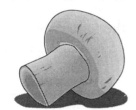

- *One-celled forms, designated as yeasts*
- *Multicellular forms, designated as molds*

Most disease-producing fungi are dimorphic, meaning that they exist in both a yeast and a mold phase.

What are some indications of a fungus infection?
Some fungus infections have specific symptoms as discussed later in this chapter. A general indication of fungus infection is allergy to:

- *Dust*
- *Mildew*
- *Grass*
- *Other sources of mold spores*
- *Cigarette smoke*

What are the basic types of fungus diseases?
Fungus diseases (mycoses) in humans are of three types characterized by both amount of penetration and by seriousness:

- *Superficial*   *on the surface*
- *Subcutaneous*   *under the skin*
- *Systemic*   *throughout the body*

> **If you have an infection on the outside, there's a pretty good chance it's on the inside too.**

Vaginal fungus infections such as candida (discussed in the next chapter) appear to be a different category. However, if you have a vaginal infection chances are that the infection is systemic. Skin fungi may spread throughout the body, causing general symptoms such as fatigue even though the infection looks superficial. If you have the infection on the outside, there's a pretty good chance it's on the inside too.

Is ringworm really caused by a worm?
Superficial fungus infections of the skin, hair, and nails are called tinea or ringworm. The name "ringworm" can cause confusion; it is named for the appearance of the infection on the skin, although worms are not involved. The fungi involved colonize in the keratin, the hard protein that

is the primary constituent of hair, nails, and to a certain extent skin. The disease (tinea or ringworm) is communicable by contact. Damp or dirty conditions favor infection, and secondary bacterial infection can occur. Some common tinea infections include:

- *Scalp ringworm*   *Circular bald spots on scalp*
- *Jock itch*   *Red, scaling, itchy areas in groin*
- *Athlete's foot*   *Itching, scaling lesions between toes*
- *Body ringworm*   *Circular patches with central scaling*
- *Onychomycosis*   *Thickened, crumbly, whitish nails*

Although on the surface, superficial fungus infections may indicate an imbalance within the body that allowed the infection to take hold. These infections may also indicate an internal fungus condition, or can be a result and symptom of immune suppression.

What are some subcutaneous fungus infections?
Fungus infections that get below the skin include sporotrichosis and mycetoma. Sporotrichosis is contracted from contaminated plants and enters the body through open wounds or by inhalation or ingestion. Symptoms are ulcers and nodular masses (lumps) that penetrate the skin but do not travel beyond the local site except in people with compromised immune defenses such as AIDS patients. Mycetoma affects the feet and toenails, causing necrosis (cell death) and swelling.

What are some of the most serious fungus diseases?
Systemic mycoses, the most serious type of fungus infection, include

- *Aspergillosis*   • *Blastomycosis*
- *Rotella*   • *Cryptococcosis*
- *Histoplasmosis*   • *Mucormycosis*
- *Candidiasis*   • *Coccidioidomycosis*

Candidiasis, better known as yeast infection, is probably the most prevalent and the best known. Most of these infections are discussed in the following pages. Candidiasis is discussed in the next chapter.

Aspergillosis is caused by aspergillus mold, which grows on feed, nuts and grain. Aspergillosis usually takes the form of an external ear infection or lung infection. Aflatoxin is a very potent toxin produced by aspergillus mold on peanuts and grains, and on potato skins. As little as 50 ppb (parts per billion) can 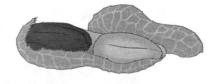 cause liver cancer in animals, and the FDA has set the safe allowable level of aflatoxins in peanuts and peanut butter at 20 ppb. The presence of mold on peanuts and pistachios is one of the major reasons they should not be eaten.

In **blastomycosis,** multiple abscesses form in and under the skin and/or internal organs. The lesions are often mistaken for cancer or tuberculosis. It is most common in the central and south-eastern United States. Cutaneous (skin) blastomycosis enters the body via wound infections, while the internal type of infection enters the body through the lungs.

Coccidioidomycosis is one of the most infectious of the fungus diseases. In the primary, self limiting form, lesions are confined to the lungs, resulting in pulmonary symptoms of varying severity. In a small percentage of cases, the fungus process spreads from the lungs to produce the progressive form, in which the disease spreads to and under the skin, bones, meninges, and internal organs. This form, also known as coccidioidal granuloma, can be fatal. It is most commonly found in the dry, dusty areas of California and the Southwestern United States, and is usually contracted by inhaling spore-bearing dust.

Cryptococcosis, also called torulosis, is caused by a yeastlike organism that infects the lungs and central nervous system. The fungus lives in animal and bird droppings, and humans are infected through the skin, mouth, nose, and throat. Cryptococcal meningitis is most common in cities due to large pigeon populations.

The primary form of **Histoplasmosis** involves the lungs, and is usually benign and self-limiting. In the often fatal progressive form, which rarely affects any but the immunocompromised or AIDS patient, ulcerating lesions are found in the nose and mouth, and there is enlargement of the spleen, liver, and lymph nodes. Humans contract the disease by inhalation of spores from fungi growing in the soil and in caves. The soil is infected by the excreta of birds and bats.

Mucormycosis can be an acute and fatal infection. The fungus, normally harmless, is found in soil and decaying organic matter, and is almost universally found in hospital environments. The most important forerunner of the disease is the ketoacidotic condition found in untreated and out-of-control diabetes.

What can worsen fungus?
Fungi prefer an alkaline environment, and fungi and bacteria set up an alkaline condition in a vicious cycle. Carbonated beverages alkalinize the gut, promoting fungal growth. Sugars and simple carbohydrates such as white flour products provide food for the fungus, causing it to proliferate.

Diabetes or a blood sugar problem can contribute to fungus growth, as there would be more sugar, their food, in the blood. Conversely, fungus can contribute to hypoglycemia, or low blood sugar, by taking sugar that is needed by your cells.

What Can Be Done?

How can you be tested for fungus?
Testing for fungus includes making use of the antibody/antigen relationship to see whether your body had mounted a defense against fungus. IgA testing shows whether you are reacting at the mucosal level. Stool testing can reveal the presence of some fungi directly.

What treatments are available for fungus infections?
Dietary and treatment protocols for candida, one of the most common types of fungus, are discussed in the next chapter. These treatments are also applicable to other types of fungus.

Summary

The type of fungus infection is less important than the fact that one exists. The existence of a fungal infection is an indication of an imbalance in the body that must be cleared up.

References and Resources

- The Burton Goldberg Group, *Alternative Medicine: The Definitive Guide*, Future Medicine Publishing, Puyallup WA, 1994. *The following chapters are relevant to Fungal Infections:*
        "Fungal Infection", p. 922
        "Ringworm", pp. 969-70

- Smith, Alice Lorraine, *Principles of Microbiology*, C.V. Mosby Co., St. Louis MO, 9th ed., 1981.

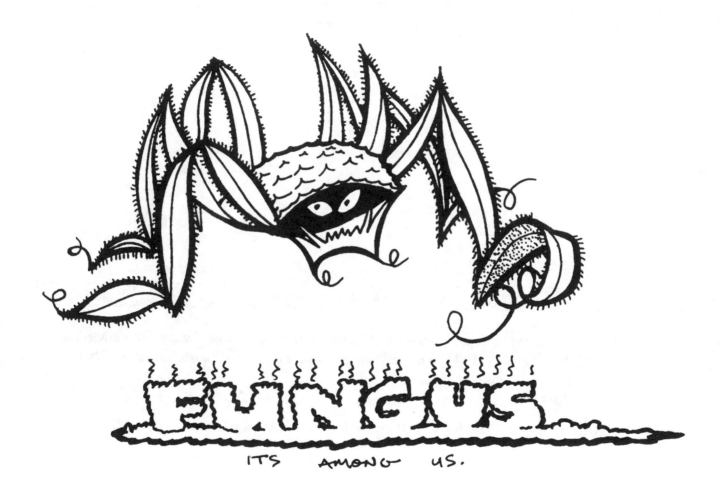

YEAST INFECTIONS

Candida's Not Just A Country North of the U.S.

Do you have the following symptoms? You may have a yeast infection or overgrowth.

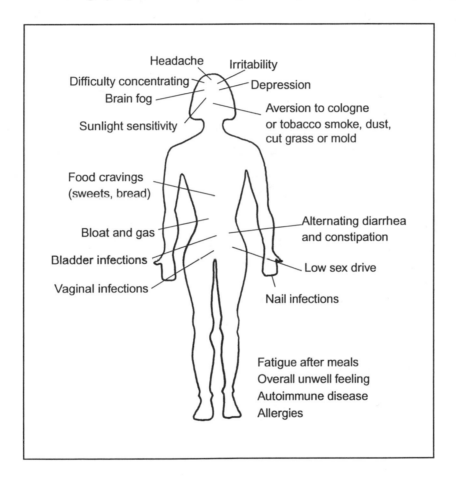

Thirteen things in this chapter that can change your health:

1-9. If you have any of the following, they may be due to yeast overgrowth:

Chronic fatigue	Brain fog	Irritability
Hyperactivity	Low libido	Bladder infections
Food cravings	Allergies	Autoimmune disorders

10. Vaginal yeast infections are a sign of systemic yeast overgrowth, although such overgrowth can be present and detrimental to your health without a visible vaginal infection.

11. Allergies or aversion to perfume or cigarette smoke can be signs of yeast infection.

12. If you have candida, sugar is your worst enemy.

13. Taking acidophilus two hours after each dose of antibiotic can reduce yeast overgrowth.

What is candida?

Candida albicans, also known as monilia, is a yeastlike organism that is found on the skin and mucous membranes of nearly everyone worldwide. It is especially found in the mouth, intestinal tract, and vagina. Candidiasis, which refers to a wide variety of symptoms caused by the overgrowth of candida, can be local or systemic. These symptoms can range from mild to debilitating. Candidiasis can also be called a yeast infection.

Where do such organisms like to live?

Candida and other fungi prefer a place that is moist, dark, and warm; in short, the human body. They prefer an environment with no protective bacteria to get in the way of their multiplying, so one of your first lines of defense is to keep your level of protective bacteria up (no antibiotics or mercury fillings, replenish acidophilus bacteria, etc.).

What's in a name?

Fungi prefer an environment that has plenty of their favorite food, sugar. It may be a coincidence, but it is interesting the first five letters of candida spell "candi".

What are some types of candida infection?

Local manifestations of candidiasis include:

- Vaginal infections in women - these infections cause a cheeselike vaginal discharge and intense itching and burning.

- Thrush is visible as whitish patches in the mouths of newborn and young babies. Thrush can be acquired from the mother during birth, or can be transmitted by contaminated fingers or rubber nipples.

- Skin infections affect mainly the moist warm parts of the body where skin contacts skin with little ventilation. Areas primarily affected are the axilla (armpits), groin, and neck folds in babies, and under the breasts in women with heavy breasts that rest on the underlying skin. Affected areas are reddish and shiny, sometimes with slight slimy or whitish discharge and/or skin soreness.

- Nail infections, in which the nail thickens and raises from its bed.

- Candida may cause disease in lungs, kidneys, and other organs where there is a predisposing condition.

If the candida fungi circulate in the bloodstream, they secrete toxins that create a variety of effects. Systemic infection can follow an untreated local infection, although systemic infection can exist without visible local symptoms.

If a woman has a long history of vaginitis and yeast, chances are good that her husband will have prostate problems later in life.

How common are candida problems?
There is some dispute regarding the prevalence of systemic yeast infections. Some researchers believe that systemic infections are rare and are limited to those with severe immune deficiencies. Others believe that a wide variety of symptoms and conditions, including Chronic Fatigue Syndrome, are attributable to yeast. A culture from, say, a vaginal infection can show whether candida is present in such quantities that it is likely to be the causal organism. However, a blood culture for candida or antibodies to it is nearly useless since nearly everyone would test positive regardless of the presence or absence of symptoms.

How, then, can it be determined whether an overgrowth of yeast is causing your problems?
If certain conditions which favor the overgrowth of yeast are present, then it is more likely that yeast is your problem, or one of them. If measures known to reduce the yeast population are employed, and your symptoms are reduced, this is again diagnostic of a yeast problem.

Yeast overgrowth is actually a symptom, not a root cause of problems. The presence of yeast is usually an indication of other parasites or a primary toxicity.

What are some systemic symptoms of candida overgrowth?
Symptoms that can be caused by yeast (but may also have other causes) are [1]:

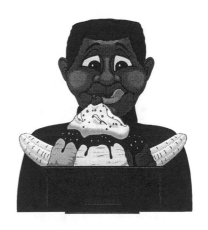

- Chronic fatigue, or fatigue in mid-afternoon or after meals
- Food cravings, especially for sweets (including fruit), cheese, bread, vinegar, alcoholic and carbonated beverages, pickles, or mushrooms
- Depression, brain fog, poor concentration, irritability
- Hyperactivity and learning disabilities in children
- Loss of sexual desire, dry vaginal area
- A reaction or aversion to perfumes, dust, cut grass, tobacco smoke
- Allergies or hypersensitivity to foods, chemicals, molds, pollen, perfume, tobacco smoke
- Immune impairment, autoimmune disorders
- Headaches, stiff neck and back, joint pains

- Alternating constipation and diarrhea, or either one

- Bladder infections, vaginitis

- Sunlight sensitivity, light hurts eyes

- An overall feeling of not being well

- Bloat and gas. Yeast produces gas and thus bloat, like the gas bubbles that cause the rising of bread.

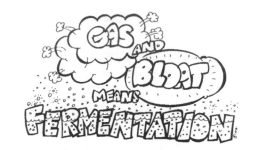

What conditions predispose a person to get candidiasis?

A number of conditions predispose a person to get candidiasis:

- Antibiotics - Friendly bacteria normally coexist with yeast in the gut in a mutually beneficial balance. When antibiotics wipe out the good bacteria (99% of total) along with the bad (1% of total), yeasts can multiply unchecked. Many women on antibiotics can expect a vaginal yeast infection at about the time the antibiotic is used up.

- Birth control pills - Progesterone in birth control pills changes the vaginal lining to make it more hospitable to yeasts. Progesterone also causes the release of yeast-feeding sugar into the bloodstream.

- Cortisone, Prednisone, and other steroid drugs suppress the immune system, thus letting yeast overgrow.

- Suppressed immune system function, whether caused by the presence of allergies, toxins, or other stressors, AIDS, or immunosuppressive drugs.

- Living in a damp, moldy environment.

- Diabetes or a diet high in sugar, including fruit and juices - both conditions raise the blood sugar level, and yeast feeds on sugar.

- Poor diet - yeast-feeding foods are listed later in this chapter.

- Mercury in metal tooth fillings acts as an antibiotic, killing the good bacteria which keep the fungi under control. Every time you eat you may be releasing so much mercury that it is like taking tetracycline at every meal.

How can you tell whether you have a fermentation problem?

Test your urine pH using commercially available pH test paper. The pH should be tested toward the end of your first morning (daytime) urination. The optimal pH is 6.0, and a pH of 7.0 or higher generally means fermentation, which in turn points to yeast and bacteria. (A pH of less than 5.5 can mean metals or chemicals). If you don't solve the underlying problem until your urine pH is 6 on a regular basis, you may end up on a sweets restricted diet for the rest of your life just to feel good.

A person with severe candidiasis may ferment sugar into alcohol to such an extent that there may be detectable amounts of alcohol in body even when none has been consumed. This is called auto-brewery syndrome. Such a person may feel chronically intoxicated, if not hung over [4,5].

How fast can yeast multiply?
A single bacterium can multiply to 16,777 bacteria within 24 hours, and yeast can multiply almost as fast. To see how fast yeast multiply, make a loaf of yeast bread dough. Set it to rise at its preferred temperature, which is about 98 degrees, or about body temperature. Within an hour or so, the size of the loaf has doubled or tripled due to the growth of yeast. The can multiply in your body just about as fast.

When bacteria is cooked, it dies, as in the pasteurization of milk. When yeast is cooked, it forms heat resistant spores. It stops growing, and if in bread the bread stops rising. When bread is eaten the yeast spores are now in your body, where they sense their favorite growing conditions and multiply about as fast as they did in the loaf of bread.

What You Can Do

What can be done if a systemic overgrowth of yeast is known or suspected?
There are a number of options, both allopathic and natural.

- Certain medications, such as Nystatin, Diflucan, and Nizoral, act as fungicides in the body and can be useful for severe infections. Diflucan, Amphotericin B, and Sporinex are cidals, meaning that they kill yeast. Other remedies are statics, meaning that they keep the infection from getting worse. The yeast will probably come back when statics are used unless the primary problem is dealt with, and the protective bacteria reestablished.

- Natural remedies include using acidophilus capsules or plain unsweetened yogurt to repopulate the good bacteria in the gut. A threefold decrease in candidal vaginitis was seen with oral ingestion of active yogurt [2]. Acidophilus or yogurt is recommended while taking antibiotics and for two weeks afterward as a preventive measure. It is best to take acidophilus two hours after each dose of antibiotic. Acidophilus can also be taken vaginally, rectally, or as a gargle. To use vaginally, add two tablespoons of acidophilus to yogurt, wait 30 minutes, then use a plunger tube to inject the mixture into the vagina before bed.

- Garlic (Kyolic brand, for example), whole or in capsules, to create an inhospitable environment for yeast.

- Mycopryl 680 (caprylic acid) is useful [3], although it works by temporarily changing the environment to one less friendly to fungus and thus is only effective while it is being used.

- Aloe vera gel or powder is also useful for controlling yeast in the mouth and intestinal tract.

- Dioxychlor, hydrogen peroxide, or ozone oxygenate the blood, making it in-hospitable for fungi and yeast.

- The herbs myrrh, black walnut, taheebo, pau de arco, melaleuca (tea tree oil)

- Grapefruit seed extract, Citricidal

- Aqua Flora is a homeopathic liquid preparation to treat yeast infections. There is a Phase I and a Phase II of treatment.

- Boric acid powder suppositories (not boric acid crystals) and tea tree oil suppositories have been successful in treating yeast infections.

- Any measures to build up the immune system as discussed elsewhere in this book and *Thriving In A Toxic World* can be of benefit.

What supplements can help?

Recommended nutritional supplements for the direct treatment of candida through the building of immune function includes B vitamins, vitamin A, C and E, antioxidants such as selenium, calcium and zinc, and essential fatty acids [9]. Berberine fights yeast and bacterial overgrowth and normalizes intestinal flora, and can be taken as a tea [10]. Other antifungal herbs include aloe vera, ginger, German chamomile, rosemary, cinnamon, licorice, tea tree oil (melaleuca) [11]. Also useful are myrrh, caprylic, oleic acids, garlic, and Citricidal.

What type of diet is best for controlling or preventing candida?

Diet is important in the control of candida, and to prevent yeast-related problems in the first place. A good diet which includes vegetables, whole grains, quality protein (chicken, turkey, fish, and eggs), and essential fatty acids will help the immune system in general. For yeast in particular, certain types of foods should be avoided [4]:

- **Sugars** - A recipe for yeast bread always includes some kind of sugar, as sugar is the best food for yeast. Since yeast growth and proliferation, desirable in bread, is detrimental to the body, ingested simple sugars should be kept to a minimum. This means eliminating candy, cookies, sodas and other sweets, and fruits and fruit juices. Other sugars - read the package label - are corn syrup, honey, fructose and any ingredient ending in -ose, among others. Fruits and especially their juices are high in sugar. Sweet vegetables such as corn, peas, carrots, and tomatoes should be eliminated in people who are especially sensitive. Intermediate starches such as noodles and crackers break down easily into sugar in the body.

- **Dairy products**, as these contain lactose, a simple sugar.

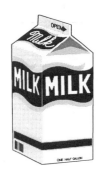

- **Fermented foods** contain fungus spores as part of the fermentation process. These foods include vinegar, by itself and in pickled products, ketchup, and mayonnaise; fermented soy products such as soy sauce, miso, and tempeh; cheeses. Vinegar is a byproduct of fermentation and doesn't contain fungus, although if you have yeast you may be allergic to both the byproduct of the yeast life cycle and to fermentation byproducts such as vinegar.

- **Fungus-containing foods**, such as mushrooms (a type of large fungus), peanut butter and nuts that seem to have a film of mold. Some herb teas contain mold as well.

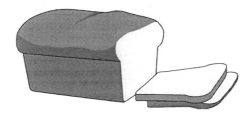

- Foods that directly contain **yeast**, such as breads and Brewer's (nutritional) yeast. Read labels - some unlikely products have torula yeast or other yeasts listed as ingredients. While food yeast and candida are not the same thing, there is likely to be cross-reactivity to yeast in foods.

- All **alcoholic beverages**, which stimulate yeast or decrease yeast resistance. Other beverages in this category are caffeinated beverages (tea, coffee, diet cola) and malted beverages. Alcohol is made from yeast and sugar, and alcohol will eventually turn to vinegar, also a yeast-feeding food.

- **Carbonated beverages,** which make the gut more alkaline and therefore more favorable for yeast growth.

- **Smoked or processed meats**.

Summary

Yeast infections can cause a wide variety of symptoms, not just the vaginal discomfort that many women recognize as a yeast infection. Diet plays an important role in the control of candida, and there are a number of natural remedies.

References and Resources

- The Burton Goldberg Group, *Alternative Medicine: The Definitive Guide*, Future Medicine Publishing, Puyallup WA, 1994. *The following chapters are relevant to Candida:*
  "Candidiasis", pp. 587-594
  "Sexually Transmitted Diseases - Yeast Infections", p. 833

- Crook, William G., *The Yeast Connection*, Vintage Books, NY, 1986.

- Crook, William G., *Chronic Fatigue Syndrome and the Yeast Connection*, Professional Books, Jackson TN, 1992.

- Hunt, Douglas, *No More Cravings*, Warner Books, New York, 1987.

- Kellas, W.R., *Toxic Immune Syndrome Cookbook*, Comprehensive Health Centers, Encinitas CA, 1995. *This book provides recipes which keep yeast-feeding foods to a minimum.*

- Trowbridge, J. and Morton Walker, *The Yeast Syndrome*, Bantam Books, New York.

- Truss, C. Orian, *The Missing Diagnosis*, Missing Diagnosis Inc., Birmingham AL, 1985.

Summary

-

Finding Closure

FINDING CLOSURE

SURVIVING THE TOXIC CRISIS

WHY ARE YOU HAVING PROBLEMS NOW?

You may have been traveling the road to bad health up until the present. Granted, there may have been many positive things that you have done for yourself in that time, but many things mentioned are still exerting a negative effect.

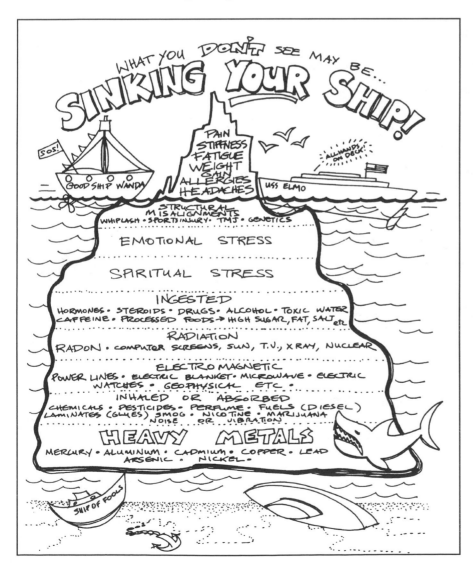

In addition to past influences, there is plenty going on in your present life to cause trouble. You may feel that your fatigue, pain, stiffness, clogged sinuses, or stomachaches are your main problems, but these are just the tip of the iceberg -- the early warning signs. The real underlying problems which are causing these symptoms, and may be seriously endangering your health, are the rest of the iceberg -- the root causes. Lying just below the surface are all of the toxic burdens which are overwhelming your body's defenses.

These toxic burdens and biochemical deficiencies which have been covered in detail in this book and *Thriving In A Toxic World* are briefly summarized here.

TOXIC IMMUNE SYNDROME

A - Primary Toxic Suppressors	B - Biochemical Deficiencies

STRESS
- Spiritual
- Emotional

INHALED OR ABSORBED
Heavy metals, Chemicals, Pesticides, Perfume, Fuels (Diesel), Laminants (glues), Solvents, Paints, Smog, Nicotine, Marijuana

ELECTROMAGNETIC RADIATION
Geophysical, Electric Blanket, Power lines, Electric watches, Computer Screens, TV, Sun, Radon, X-ray, Nuclear

OTHER - Noise, Vibration

INGESTED
Hormones, Steroids, Drugs, Alcohol, Caffeine, Chlorinated/Toxic water, Processed foods, High sugar/fat/salt

STRUCTURAL MISALIGNMENTS
Whiplash, Sports injury, Congenital weakness, TMJ

NUTRIENTS
- Vitamins
  - Fat soluble: E, A, D, K
  - Water Soluble: Bs, C
- Protein, Amino Acids
- Minerals
- Fats and Oils
- Carbohydrates

OTHER REQUIREMENTS
- Pure water
- Clean air / oxygen
- Sleep
- Exercise

DIGESTION
- Hydrochloric Acid
- Enzymes
  - Protein
  - Carbohydrates
  - Insulin / sugars
  - Bile / fats
- Bacteria

SUPPRESSED IMMUNE SYSTEM
C - Secondary Opportunistic Microorganisms
(Transmission by mouth or sex)

PARASITES   FUNGUS   BACTERIA   VIRUSES

The road to disease can begin with either A - Primary Toxic Suppressors or B - Biochemical Deficiencies. Suppression or Deficiency cause the immune system to function incorrectly which allows the C - secondary Opportunistic Microorganisms to take over. The the D - Genetic Predisposed Weaknesses become a factor. (See "Stages of Toxic Immune Syndrome" chart)

Of the many things that could be contributing to your present problems - and there are still others not mentioned due to space limitations - most of them are in the past or are otherwise beyond your control.

Can anything be done?

The picture is not as bleak as it seems. The body and especially the immune system do a pretty good job of repair work even under some fairly adverse conditions. If you tip the balance in your favor, the repair work will proceed even faster and more efficiently and your health will certainly improve. If you do not treat problems in the early stages, they can progress to a more serious and less easily treatable form. They can become chronic.

STAGES OF TOXIC IMMUNE SYNDROME			
D - Genetic Predisposed Weakness			
Affected Body System	**Stage I** Acute stage - Toxicity Body is stressed We see a warning light	**Stage II** Chronic Stage - Inflammatory Body bends We ignore the warning light, then experience steam from under the hood	**Stage III** Degeneration/disease\death Body breaks We reach a point where our engine (body) seizes up and the "vehicle" fails
Immune System	Susceptibility to infections, decrease in immunity protectors, low white cell count, low gamma globulin, colds, allergy	Progressive susceptibility to disease process, any -itis or lupus, multiple sclerosis	Immune system collapse and death, Kaposi's sarcoma, cancer, pneumonia, atrophy, Alzheimer's
Lymphatic System	Poor healing, swollen glands	Edema	Lymphoma
Nervous System - Central and Peripheral	Confusion, irritation, tingling, depression, chills, anxiety, headaches, twitching, loss of balance, dizziness, tremors, forgetfulness	Neuralgias, neuritis, memory loss, loss of consciousness, hallucinations, seizures, multiple sclerosis, Parkinson's disease	Paralysis, stroke, aphasia, convulsions
Musculoskeletal System	Aches, pains, cramps, weakness, subluxation, twitching, tenderness	Arthritis, tendinitis, bursitis, spondylitis, muscles wasting, fibromyalgia	Muscles atrophying, frequent fractures, scoliosis, kyphosis, osteoporosis
Circulatory System (Cardiovascular)	Palpitations, rapid heartbeat, turning blue, cold extremities	Elevated triglycerides, chest pain, arm pain, numbness of extremities	Arteriosclerosis, heart attack, chest pain, heart failure, cardiac arrest, gangrene, amputation
Digestive System	Weight loss or gain, loss of appetite, nausea, vomiting, diarrhea, constipation, gas, bloating	Stool color changes, gastritis, ulcers, colitis, loss of bowel control, diverticulitis, Crohn's disease	GI cancers
Respiratory System	Shortness of breath, coughing, wheezing, choking sensation	Mucus production, sputum color changes, water on lungs, pleurisy	Pneumonia, respiratory failure, collapsed lung, opportunistic infections, emphysema
Reproductive System	Urinary incontinence, bloody urine, dysuria	Urinary infection, vaginitis, prostatitis, endometriosis, painful sex, impotence, herpes	Inability to conceive, reproductive system cancer
Endocrine system	Excessive or insufficient production of hormones (steroids, thyroid hormones), fatigue	Hyperfunction or hypofunction of glands (goiter, nodules hot and cold), chronic fatigue, cold extremities	Organ failure, cancers, exhaustion, feeling of freezing
Skin	Redness, sores, dandruff, itching, dryness, flabbiness, premature greying, acne, blackheads, changes in integrity of skin, oiliness, pimples, sunburn easily	Rashes, carbuncles, hives, abscesses, other lesions, dermatitis, eczema, boils, ulcers, blisters, easy bruising, skin tags, psoriasis	Skin cancer, pemphigus, scleroderma, depigmentation, pigmentation, wrinkling, poor healing
Head, Eyes, Ears	Headaches, poor vision, dry eyes, light sensitivity, tearing, eye discharge, floaters, ear wax	Blurred vision, tearing, ears ringing, earaches, migraines, ear discharge, Sjogren's syndrome	Loss of vision or hearing, cataracts, glaucoma, detached retina
Nose	Runny, itching, sneezing, nosebleeds	Encrusting, sinusitis, stuffiness, rhinitis, mouth breathing	Nasal polyps, spider veins, loss of smell
Mouth	Dry mouth, tongue (sore, furred, coated, red), halitosis	Swelling, geographic tongue, canker sores	Loss of taste, black tongue, oral cancer, tooth loss
Mucous Membranes	Lack of or excessive production of mucus	Infections and inflammations pertaining to organs with mucous lining, polyps, IgA excess	Chronic stages of infections, Cancers (nose, lung, mouth, gastrointestinal)

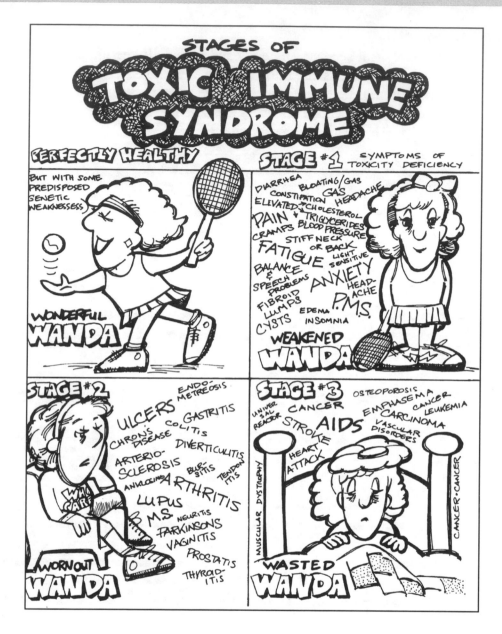

Each of the steps on the Road to Bad Health which were outlined in *Thriving In A Toxic World*, can be compensated for specifically up to a point. For example:

- *Tonsils out*   *- keep lymph system clear in other ways*
- *Gallbladder out* *- take beneficial oils and lecithin, build up liver*
- *No breastfeeding* *- take beneficial bacteria bifidus and acidophilus*
- *Surgical scars*   *- neural-fascial therapy*

How can you tip the balance in your favor?
Tipping the balance in your favor is a process that can be broken down into two basic steps:

1. *Eliminate the negative (suppressors)*
2. *Accentuate the positive (supporters)*

Changing Your Health Results

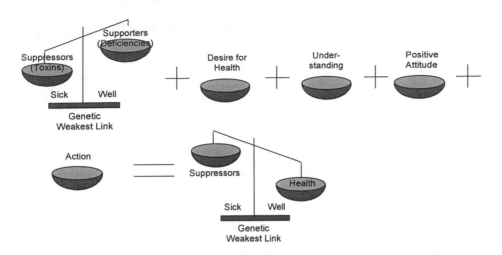

Eliminating the negative refers to removing or minimizing the physical and mental toxic burdens that are slowing you down. If you don't do that first, it is like training for running a race with a heavy knapsack on your back. If you want to really get somewhere, first remove the knapsack, and then you can concentrate on improving your running. And you're more likely to come in a winner.

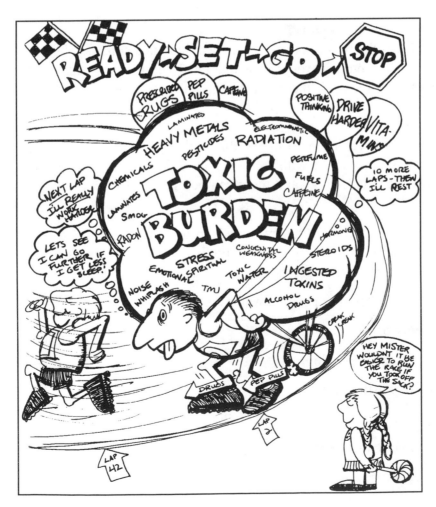

More specifically, eliminating the negative, or toxic suppressors, can include the following:

- Eliminate alcohol and other "recreational" drugs, cigarettes, and caffeine

- Reduce or eliminate sugar, refined carbohydrates, table salt, saturated fats, and processed foods

- Remove chemicals from the home that you might be sensitive to, if it is practical to do so, such as insect sprays and perfumes

- Stop using, or keep your distance from, electrical appliances such as the electric blanket, microwave oven, and television

- Replace heavy metal sources, such as tooth fillings, crowns and root canals, and household plumbing, with a safer substitute

- Reduce sources of stress wherever possible - job, relationship, financial

- Reduce noise levels at home and work if possible; earplugs may be a good idea

There are many other ways to eliminate the negative that are specific to your particular problems, as discussed throughout these books. However, the above suggestions will benefit just about anybody.

How can you accentuate the positive?

Now that the load is off the runner's back, or at least lightened considerably, it is time to work on improving performance. In other words, now that many of the things that are dragging you down have been eliminated or reduced, the good things that you do for yourself will be all the more beneficial.

Accentuating the positive refers to all of the things that you can do to benefit your body, your immune system, or your spirit. As with the items listed for Eliminating the Negative, the following suggestions can benefit anyone, and there can be many more tailored to your specific situation:

- Eat a balanced diet of healthy, minimally processed foods - 30% protein, 40% carbohydrate, and 30% fat (by calories, not weight) as well as sufficient vitamins, minerals, enzymes, and cofactors

- Drink plenty of filtered or purified water

- Breathe plenty of clean air

- Exercise - just don't overdo it

- Repeat positive affirmations

- Develop your spiritual side, pray, meditate

- Get a chiropractic or osteopathic checkup and alignment done

Eliminating the negative and accentuating the positive are the two ways you can start out right. Since you can't change the past, <u>today is your start date</u>. Remember - **you've got to start out right to end up right!**

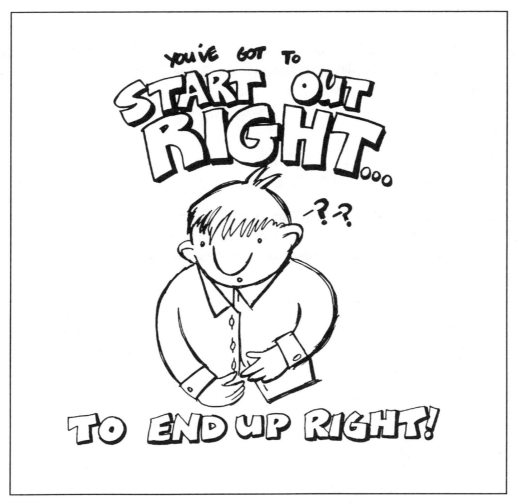

How do you reach your health goals?
In order to reach your health goals, there are several stages to pass through.

Make the decision - Are you sick and tired of feeling sick and tired? Are you fed up enough to do something about it? Are you willing to change your lifestyle to get relief? How much of a change are you really willing to make? Do you just want to get well or do you refuse to stay sick?

If you truly want to get well, your first step is to make a firm decision that you are going to do what it takes to get well, and accepting God's will (if such is your belief), realizing that there is a time frame of healing involved. At this stage the action may consist of learning all you can - seeing doctors, getting tested, reading books. Or you may already know at least some of what is wrong and what to do about it, such as giving up smoking or making dietary changes.

If there are some changes that you are not willing to make, some things you are not willing to give up yet, be honest with yourself about it. There is nothing wrong with respecting your boundaries. Just do so from a position of knowledge, not just amplified ignorance; of looking at what you have to gain or lose by different courses of action or inaction. Be willing to pay the price yourself and not blame anyone else.

It is very possible that you have been to doctors, read books, and tried treatments, without very favorable results. Today is a new day and there are still decisions to be made that can start turning things around for you.

So, now it's decision time:

- From this day on I will _____
- From this day on I will no longer _____

Chances are greater that you will stick to a firm, clear decision than to a vague wishy-washy one. For example, you may decide to go on a detoxification diet to reduce yeast and sweet cravings (described in the Supporters section of ***Thriving In A Toxic World***) to reduce yeast and sweets cravings.

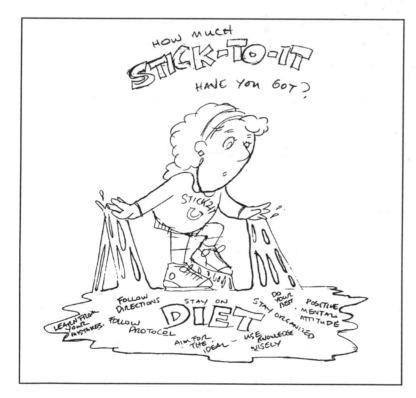

Plan for the long haul - Get organized. It helps to have a plan. Find out what doctor to see, what books to read. Keep a journal. Alternatively, make a list of your symptoms, every one you can think of. Review the list periodically to see which ones are no longer a problem so you can realize that you are actually making progress. Otherwise you may focus only on the symptoms you still have and feel frustrated, even after achieving success in other areas.

Understanding is your key to health - Get external information. External information is obtained from doctors, clinics, blood tests and other tests, and books and magazine articles. People who have gone through what you are going through are one of the best sources if they can spark a "can-do attitude" in you, which you'll need as you look at where you want to be and how you're going to get there. It's true what they say, knowledge is power.

Get internal information - Your own body is the best source of information; tune into what it is saying. Granted, your pain, fatigue, muscle weakness, sleeplessness, and other symptoms are certainly undesirable, but they can be used in a positive manner. They are a signal, like the "idiot lights" on your car, that something is wrong. Symptoms may be your only warning.

Using medication or allopathic treatments to suppress the symptoms is like disconnecting the "idiot light" on the car dashboard. This approach works about as well for your body as it does for you car.

Yes, you already know something is wrong, or you probably wouldn't be reading this book. Your body and its various malfunctions can tell you much more than just the fact that a problem exists.

Any symptom can have a variety of causes. And it's finding the cause that is important so you or your doctor can determine the treatment for the underlying problem.

For example, low back pain can be caused by any of the following, alone or in combination:

- *Spinal disk collapse*
- *Kidney problems such as stones*
- *Mercury, nickel, or copper*
- *Pelvic or tooth inflammation*
- *Muscle strain*
- *Low potassium or other minerals*
- *Allergy*
- *Whiplash*

The picture is complicated considerably since you probably have a variety of symptoms with a number of causes that are affecting each other. In order to narrow down the possible causes, it is good to be aware of all of the symptoms in detail and what affects them. For example:

- The symptoms - be as specific as possible. Saying "I feel generally lousy" doesn't give the doctor much information to go on. Do you feel pain, what kind, and when? Do you have muscle weakness? Do you have a desire to sleep often, and at what time of day?

- Location - where exactly is the pain? What muscles feel weak?

- Quality - is the pain sharp, dull, intermittent?

- Timing - when do you feel these symptoms? A certain time of day, before your or after eating? Continuously or intermittently?

- Correlation - what else is going on before or just after these symptoms occur? Do they come after eating certain foods, or at work, or after exercise? Does one symptom follow another, such as tiredness after a headache?

- Improvement - under what circumstances do you feel better?

Keep a journal of all of this information, even if you aren't sure what is important. In some cases it will enable you to figure out your problem yourself. For example, if your nose clogs up and you have to clear your throat a lot, and the pattern of journal entries shows that this happens after eating or drinking milk products, it doesn't take a medical degree to figure out that you probably have a milk allergy. Sometimes you won't see a pattern, but a knowledgeable doctor will.

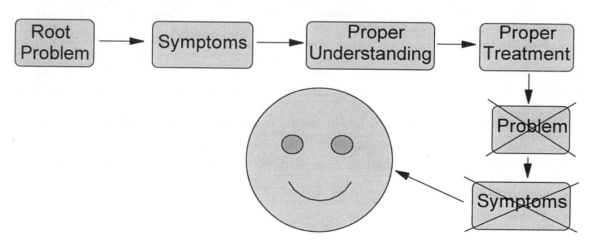

Diagnosis - You may or may not need to be evaluated by a doctor at this point. If you go to a doctor, health practitioner, or clinic, chances are you will be given some tests, starting with a complete blood workup.

At some point, you or the doctor will arrive at a diagnosis, at least a tentative one. Treatment will be prescribed. This may include taking medication, taking supplements, changing your diet, or avoiding certain chemicals or allergens.

Honest follow through - The above steps are necessary, but useless without follow through. Follow through is up to YOU! You are the one who must watch your diet, give up smoking, take your vitamins, and report back to your doctor.

Follow Through is up to YOU!

Why is a positive attitude essential?
It is important to have a positive attitude for several reasons.

Achieving expectations: the mind/body connection - The mind and the body are closely linked, and mental suggestions will affect the outcome for the body. Have you ever heard of the placebo effect? A placebo is a pill that contains no actual medication, but is made to look as if it does. For instance, if a person takes a placebo, thinking that it is a real aspirin tablet, the person's headache may very well go away because of the expectation that it will; this is called the placebo effect.

Similarly, if you expect to be able to stick to your diet, or if you expect the new bottle of supplements to give you more energy, then your expectations will make it more likely that the desired result will occur.

Expectations alone won't get you well. Your problems and symptoms are probably not all in your mind; neither is the cure. However, therapy along with a positive attitude is likely to be more effective than therapy alone.

Lawrence LeShan, a pioneer in mind/body medicine, found and documented that people who took charge of their lives after a cancer diagnosis had markedly better outcomes than those who passively accepted their diagnosis [1]. Taking action also decreases the fear and depression that often accompany life-threatening illnesses, and restores a sense of control [2]. A variation on the placebo effect is that those who have a more positive outlook, i.e. feel they will get better, often have better outcomes than people with similar illnesses who go home and write their wills (figuratively speaking) after diagnosis [3].

Compliance - There are lifestyle changes you have to make in order to get well - pills to take, old habits to break, allergens and toxins to avoid. How likely are you to follow through if you are thinking "This probably won't work"? Your resolve to do what you need to do will likely not last long if you don't think there will be any improvement to show for it. Conversely, you probably will stick with it if you expect a reward at the end. It takes about 21 days to form a new habit.

It takes about 21 days to form a new habit.

Feeling - A cheerful, optimistic outlook certainly *feels* better than a gloomy, pessimistic one. Right? This one is simple, but not easy.

Realistically, it might be hard to stay upbeat, even if you know it's in your best interest to be optimistic. You feel lousy physically. Doctors, tests, and vitamins aren't cheap. Tofu and sprouts are replacing coffee and donuts. And the last five treatments you tried didn't have the outcome you hoped for. So what's to be cheerful about? It helps to look for the lessons in everything you are going through. Your positive outlook and efforts will bolster your immune system which is fighting for you. Why throw in negative, toxic attitudes which unbalance the scales on the side of negative biochemical reactions.

How can you stay on track?
Here are a few more ideas to keep you on track emotionally:

> **Good can come from bad circumstances if you look for it!**

Side benefits - Look at other advantages of the course you are taking, in addition to the hoped-for health benefits. Quitting smoking? Think of the money you'll save, and of the fact that you will no longer smell like a dirty ashtray. Eliminating paints and products in spray cans? Think of the environmental benefits. Getting rid of or reducing use of your microwave oven or waterbed heater? Think of your lowered electric bill. Eliminating sugar? Fewer cavities. Good can come from bad circumstances if you look for it.

Focus of recovery - You will be spending a good bit of time in a state where there is some symptomatic improvement, but optimal health is still some distance away. There is a poem, attributed to Dorothy Parker, that goes:

> "Twixt optimist and pessimist
> The difference is droll;
> The optimist sees the doughnut,
> The pessimist sees the hole."

As it pertains to health, you can choose to focus on what has been accomplished (the doughnut) or on what hasn't been fixed yet (the hole). You can rejoice in the ten pounds you lost or be depressed over the twenty left to go. You can feel good about the fact that you finally slept through the night or you can complain about the headaches you still have. To keep your spirits up, focus on the ways in which you are now feeling better than you did before.

Success stories - It helps to see, hear, or read about people who have overcome or been helped with a problem like yours. Books and magazine articles often contain before-and-after stories and pictures, or maybe someone who has been going to your clinic for a while has some good news. Journal and write your own success story as it unfolds. Set as a goal helping others with similar problems once your own have been successfully dealt with.

Positive affirmations - It helps to repeat positive affirmations to yourself as reminders to keep your good attitude in place. These are things you can say to yourself in the mirror, or write down and tape to the walls, or think about in a spare moment. Remind yourself of these positive affirmations:

- *Others have been successful*
- *Success is a journey, not a destination*
- *There has been improvement already*
- *I'm healthier and stronger and feeling better every day*

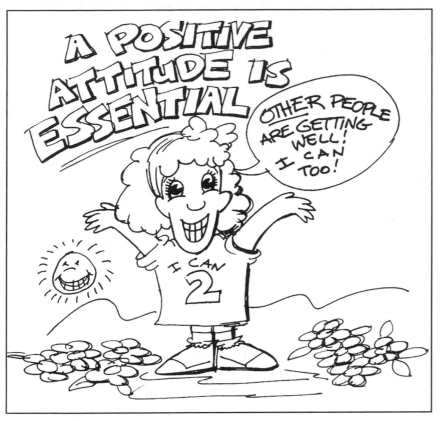

- *I'm overcoming the problem, not just talking about it*
- *I'm in charge of what I contribute to my health*
- *So far I've accomplished _____, _____, and _____*
- *I can do it!*

Acceptance - Accept the Creator's will and timing in your healing. As you continue to go forward positively, your faith will be rewarded.

TAKING STEPS TO YOUR HEALING

Are you sick?

You may have a recognized chronic disease such as chronic fatigue syndrome (CFS), environmental illness (EI), arthritis, or arteriosclerosis. You may simply feel unwell or in less than optimal health without having a specific name for your condition. You may be concerned about future health problems.

Whatever the case, you desire to improve your health. Although specifics will vary depending on your condition, there are certain basic steps on the road back to health. But certain things must be done first to prepare the way, as described in the following analogy.

The Seven Steps Back to Health

7. Rebuild / Restore
6. Eliminate microorganisms
5. Align, balance body structures
4. Biochemical, nutritional support
3. Desensitize allergens, unblock pathways
2. Detoxify and cleanse your body
1. Stop bombing your body with toxins and allergens

A bombed-out city

If you lived in a city that was bombed during wartime, such as Dresden, Germany, and you wanted to rebuild, steps must be taken in a certain order:

1. First the bombing must stop. It is futile to try to rebuild while the onslaught continues.

2. Next, the rubble must be cleared away to provide a clean foundation for rebuilding. Only at this point can meaningful rebuilding start.

3. Now walls are built, water and electrical supply lines are reconnected, appliances are installed.

4. Finally, the houses are functional. Fine-tuning makes the houses into homes: pictures are hung, windows are cleaned, dishes are stored in cabinets. Comfortable living begins.

A bombed-out body? - Prioritizing repair
Rebuilding your health after chronic illness has taken hold is a process similar to that of rebuilding a bombed-out city. The first steps must be completed before later steps can have meaningful results. Eating nutritious food while your teeth are full of mercury fillings, for example, is like repainting the kitchen while bomber planes are still flying overhead.

What are the steps to healing?
As is the case with the bombed-out city, first the bombing (toxic onslaught) must stop. Then the rubble (toxins in the body) must be cleared away before rebuilding can begin.

1. First **stop bombing your body with toxins**. Remove your mercury fillings (mercury leaches out of them and enters the body), stop spraying pesticides, unplug your electric blanket, quit smoking, and take many other steps as described throughout this book. Start with the most offensive toxins first. The chapters in this book have outlined what is toxic, why it is toxic, how to avoid the toxin, and what to substitute where applicable.

2. **Detoxify and cleanse your body.** Clear away the rubble. Even though you have reduced the entry of new toxins into your body to a bare minimum, old toxins are still in your bloodstream, lymph nodes, and organs. Cleansing your body takes many forms:

- *Chelation to remove metals (Metal Detoxification chapter)*
- *Sauna to remove chemicals (Chemical Toxicity chapter)*
- *Gallbladder flush to clear your liver and gallbladder*
- *Constitutional hydrotherapy to cleanse the lymph system*
- *Lymph cleansing exercise and massage*
- *Colonics to cleanse the digestive tract*
- *Counseling to resolve emotional or spiritual issues*
- *Emotional release work*
- *Detoxification diet to remove allergens and yeast-supporting conditions*

Some of these cleansing methods have been described in the Chemical Toxicity and Metal Detoxification chapters. Specific "What You Can Do" suggestions have been given in many of the chapters in this book, discussing what can be done after exposure to the toxin.

Although your body, unlike a city, has many self-cleansing mechanisms, they are probably impaired. Supporting the body's own cleansing processes speeds up this phase of healing.

3. **Desensitize to allergens, unblock pathways** - There are a number of treatments to reduce sensitivity to allergens, including NAET (Nambudripad's Allergy Elimination Treatment, discussed in the Toxic Immune Syndrome chapter in *Thriving In A Toxic World*), low-dose immunotherapy and others.

Unblocking pathways includes the following, which were discussed in the Structural chapters:

- *Nerves*   *- chiropractic*
- *Blood and fluid*   *- osteopathic*
- *Galvanic*   *- acupressure and acupuncture*

4. **Nutritional and biochemical support** - Now that the cleansing has been done, it is time to support the body's natural restoration and defense. This restoration stage can be done concurrently with the other steps. Nutritional and biochemical support includes vitamins, minerals, amino acids, fatty acids, carbohydrates, enzymes, oxygen, water, and herbs. Nutritional support is also important during the cleansing steps. *Thriving In A Toxic World* discusses this support in detail.

5. **Align and balance body structures** - Structural problems, including whiplash injuries, misalignments, foot balancing and dental bite problems, are discussed in detail in the Structural chapters.

6. **Eliminate microorganisms** - Once the primary suppressors and toxins are removed from your environment and your body, it is time to go after the secondary suppressors, or opportunistic microorganisms (parasites, yeast, bacteria, viruses). Eliminating them before the primary suppressors have been dealt with and the body has been supported would likely lead to reinfection and reinfestation, just as squatters evicted from an abandoned decaying building would simply move back in after the police have gone. These are discussed in the Microorganisms section.

7. **Rebuild and restore** - This includes:

- Supporting and balancing the immune system - homeopathics, gamma globulin, herbs, allergy antigens, transfer factor, c-AMP, live cell therapy, glandulars

- Supporting the mind in helping the body through spiritual and emotional counseling and processes

At this point your disease is gone or under control. You are functional and you are feeling pretty good. All of the above suggestions as well as the many other methods described in these books can be used to fine-tune your health as you complete the journey from feeling okay to being optimally healthy. This stage is akin to hanging the pictures, polishing the candlesticks, and arranging the flowers in vases to make your home - or your body - a place you want to live in for the rest of your life.

What kind of healing progress can be expected?

Chances are you have a multitude of symptoms caused by a number of underlying problems which may be interlinked. These problems have likely been building up for years or decades, even if symptoms have only recently begun to show up.

No health care or medicine, whether allopathic or comprehensive, can heal. No doctor can "heal" you, but can guide and assist you in making the choices that will assist your body in the healing process. Only your body, with God's help, can bring about real healing.

Comprehensive integrated health care removes the obstacles to your body's natural healing processes. Remember, it took a long time to reach your present state of ill health and it will usually take month or even years to get your health back as completely as possible. Healing usually occurs as a series of baby steps versus giant strides forward.

With faith and a positive attitude you can tip the scales on the side of healing processes which encourage positive biochemical reactions, versus negative ones which may encourage negative biochemical reactions in your body at a time when your body needs all the support it can get.

A recent television news program featured the story of a young boy diagnosed with a terminal brain tumor. It was his wish to go down in the **Guinness Book of World Records** as receiving the most get well cards. Cards came in by the thousands. Amazingly, his tumor began to shrink, until today he is pronounced totally healed. The tumor is no more. Speculation has it that all those positive wishes and prayers on his behalf, as manifested by the thousands of cards and letters he received, made the difference and tipped the scales on the side of healing.

So it is a good idea, in whatever way you can, to put your spirits in a positive frame and know that every step you take to regain your health is taking you closer to success and you are not alone in resolving this crisis -- and believe that you can once more be filled with vibrant health.

Occasionally, dramatic healing does occur. For example, seizures have been known to cease as soon as root-canaled teeth were extracted. However, this is the exception. The usual course of healing is slow compared to the rapid relief that can come from suppressing symptoms. Treatments which don't provide noticeable relief of symptoms may still be benefiting you in the immediate, and contributing to the eventual long-term success of future treatment.

One patient's course of recovery is typical. She had severe fatigue and multiple chemical sensitivities, which worsened over the years until she hit bottom in early 1993. Over the next year she underwent sauna therapy, had the mercury in her teeth removed, had root-canaled teeth extracted, underwent several types of detoxification procedures, gave up sugar and ate more nutritious food, took nutritional supplements, and did emotional release work.

Although there were a few plateaus and even setbacks along the way, she has gone from being too disabled to stay out of bed for more than a few hours to being a vibrant, optimistic, fully functioning person. Her journey from sickness to health has taken a year and a half and is not yet over. But she's nearing the finish line as she runs her own race. She is now confident she will truly overcome. And you can too.

Your own progress depends on:

- *The number, type, and severity of your problems*

- *The understanding on the part of both you and your health care practitioner of the way the human body and healing work*

- *How closely you follow your health care protocol*

- *Your own body's response, which varies between individuals.*

- *God or circumstances beyond human control.*

As you go forward with a positive attitude you have cleared away perhaps the greatest obstacle standing in your way -- and you must constantly reaffirm and reinforce your determination as you persevere through all the steps you must take, knowing that although it may not happen overnight. it will happen.

WHAT'S THE NEXT STEP

By now you are aware that with all chronic conditions related to Toxic Immune Syndrome, it is important to identify the root cause(s) of the symptoms and treat them. The identification and treatment of these causes have been the focus of this book. Review the <u>Seven Steps to Health</u> and check for, eliminate and treat the primary and secondary toxic suppressors as discussed in this book:

- *Chemicals, including organics, pesticides, cologne, drugs, and food additives*
- *Metals, especially dental mercury and nickel.*
- *Electromagnetic radiation*
- *Structural problems such as whiplash and an unbalanced bite.*
- *Emotional stresses*
- *Microorganisms*

Follow these steps and the sunshine of optimum health will be shinning down on you.

Remember an old Chinese proverb which says, "A journey of a thousand miles begins with one step." And so it is, as you begin your journey back to optimum health.

And why settle for less?

The next step is up to you . . . .

References and Resources

- The Burton Goldberg Group, ***Alternative Medicine: The Definitive Guide***, Future Medicine Publishing Inc., Puyallup WA, 1994.

  *This excellent guide to alternative / progressive medicine is highly recommended for further understanding of the issues in this book. In addition, books, journals, and organizations pertinent to each chapter are found at the end of each chapter. Specific sections of **Alternative Medicine** will be referenced where applicable at the end of chapters in this book.*

- ***Townsend Letter for Doctors*** *is a monthly journal with many articles pertaining to issues raised in this book. Although the journal is geared towards progressive doctors and practitioners, much of the information would be understandable to the layperson.*

- Airola, Paavo, ***How To Get Well***, Health Plus Publishers, Phoenix AZ, 1974.

- **American College of Advancement in Medicine**, P.O. Box 3427, Laguna Hills CA 92654. Phone 714-583-7666. *Provides worldwide listing of practitioners trained in nutritional and preventive medicine.*

- Austin, P., ***Natural Remedies: A Manual***, Yuchi Pines Institute, Seale AL, 1983.

- Beasley, Joseph, ***The Betrayal of Health***, Times Books, NY, 1991. *The effect of lifestyle and nutrition choices on health.*

- ***Better Health Through Natural Healing: How To Get Well Without Drugs or Surgery***, McGraw-Hill, NY, 1985.

- Chopra, Deepak, ***Quantum Healing: Exploring the Frontiers of Mind/Body Medicine***, Bantam Books, NY, 1989.

- Dirchfeld, Friedhelm and Wade Boyle, ***Nature Doctors: Pioneers in Naturopathic Medicine***, Medicina Biologica, Portland OR, 1994.

- Goodheart, RS and MD Shils, ***Health and Disease***, Lea and Febinger, Philadelphia PA, 1980.

- Heimlich, J., ***What Your Doctors Won't Tell You***, Harper Perennial, NY, 1990.

- Hirschberg, Caryle and Marc Ian Barasch, ***Remarkable Recovery***, G.P.Putman's Sons, NY, 1995. *Looks at survivors of cancer and other illnesses who were given a death sentence by their doctors. Discusses the many types of treatment, primarily "alternative", that the survivors credited with their recovery.*

- Moyers, Bill, ***Healing and the Mind***, Doubleday, NY, 1993.

- Page, Melvin, ***Degeneration and Regeneration***, St. Petersburg Beach, FL, 1949.

- Payer, Lynn, ***Medicine and Culture: Varieties of Treatments in the United States, England, West Germany and France***, Henry Holt and Co., NY, 1988.

- Pizzorno, Joseph E. and Michael T. Murray, *A Textbook of Natural Medicine*, John Bastyr College Publications, Seattle WA, 1989.

- Pizzorno, Joseph E. and Michael T. Murray, *Encyclopedia of Natural Medicine*, Prima Publishing, Rocklin CA, 1991.

- Shannon, Sara, *Good Health In A Toxic World: The Complete Guide to Fighting Free Radicals*, Warner Books Inc., NY, 1994. *Fighting free radical damage. Has over 150 pages of resources and references.*

- Shreeve, Caroline M., *The Alternative Dictionary of Symptoms and Cures*, Century Hutchinson Publishing, London England, 1986.

- Simonton, O. Carl and S. Matthews, *Getting Well Again*, Jeremy P. Tarcher, Los Angeles CA, 1978.

- Sinclair, Brett Jason, *Alternative Health Care Resources*, Parker Publishing Co., West Nyack NY, 1992. *A directory of self-help groups, professional care providers, scientific journals, lay magazines and newsletters, and institutes / foundations. These are listed by subject heading.*

- Thomas, John, *Young Again!*, Plexus Press, Kelso WA, 1995. *Techniques and information to maintain youthfulness, including detoxification procedures, colon cleansing and nutrition.*

- Weil, Andrew, *Natural Health, Natural Medicine: A Comprehensive Manual for Wellness and Self-Care*, Houghton Mifflin, Boston MA, 1990.

- Wigmore, Ann, *Be Your Own Doctor: A Positive Guide to Natural Living*, Avery Publishing Co., Garden City Park NY, 1983.

Reference

Abbreviations Used in This Book

AA	Alcoholics Anonymous
AAs	Amino acids, protein building blocks
AC	Alternating Current (electrical)
ADA	American Dental Association
ADD	Attention Deficit Disorder
AIDS	Acquired Immune Deficiency Syndrome
ALS	Amyotrophic Lateral Sclerosis, also called Lou Gehrig's disease
APC	Aspirin-Phenacetin-Caffeine, a pain killing medication combination
ARC	AIDS Related Complex
ASDS	American Society of Dental Surgeons
ASI	Adrenal Stress Index, a test of adrenal function
ATM	Awareness Through Movement, a Feldenkrais structural technique
ATP	Adenosine triphosphate, a cellular form of energy
AZT	Azidothymidine, an allopathic AIDS medication
BHA	Butylated Hydroxyanisole, a food preservative
BHT	Butylated Hydroxytoluene, a food preservative
bid	Twice a day (medicine dosage)
c-AMP	Cyclic Adenosine Monophosphate, an immune system booster
Ca	Calcium
CAT	Computerized Axial Tomography, an x-ray imaging technique, also called CT scan
CB	Citizen's Band radio
Cd	Cadmium
CDC	Centers for Disease Control
CEBV	Chronic Epstein-Barr Virus syndrome, old name for Chronic Fatigue Syndrome
CFIDS	Chronic Fatigue Immune Deficiency Syndrome, same as CFS
cfm	Cubic Feet per Minute, a measure of the ventilation rate of air in a building
CFS	Chronic Fatigue Syndrome
Cl	Chlorine
CMV	Cytomegalovirus
CNS	Central Nervous System
CO	Carbon monoxide
CO$_2$	Carbon dioxide
CSF	Cerebrospinal Fluid
DC	Direct Current (electrical)
DC	Doctor of Chiropractic
DDS	Doctor of Dental Surgery, a dental degree

DDT	A pesticide
DEET	Insect repellent ingredient
DES	Diethylstilbestrol, a synthetic hormone
DHEA	Hormone for adrenal support
DMPS	A chelating agent
DMSA	Dimercaptosuccinic acid, a chelating agent
DMT	Dimethyltriptamine, a hallucinogenic drug
DNA	Deoxyribonucleic acid, a genetic component
DO	Doctor of Osteopathy
DTs	Delirium Tremens, alcohol withdrawal symptom
EBV	Epstein-Barr Virus, which causes mononucleosis
EDB	Ethylene dibromide, a toxin found in pesticides
EDTA	Ethylenediaminetetraacetic acid, a chelating agent
EEG	Electroencephalogram, a measure of the brain's electrical activity
EH	Entamoeba Histolytica
EI	Environmental Illness
EKG	Electrocardiogram, a measure of the heart's electrical activity
ELF	Extra (or Extremely) Low Frequency of electromagnetic radiation
ELISA	Enzyme Linked Immunosorbent Assay, a test for HIV
EM	Electromagnetic
EMR	Electromagnetic Radiation
EMS	Eosinophilia Myalgia Syndrome, caused by a contaminated batch of tryptophan
EPA	Environmental Protection Agency
ER	Emergency Room of the hospital
et al	And others, a Latin abbreviation in journal references
FD & C	Food, Drug, and Cosmetic
FDA	Food and Drug Administration
Fe	Iron
FTFD	Foundation for Toxic Free Dentistry
GABA	Gamma-Aminobenzoic Acid, an amino acid and neurotransmitter
GLA	Gamma-linolenic Acid, an essential fatty acid
GSH	Glutathione, a metal chelator
H_2O	Water
HCl	Hydrochloric acid
Hct	Hematocrit, a measure of red blood cells
HDL	High Density Lipoprotein, "good" cholesterol
Hg	Mercury
Hgb	Hemoglobin, a measure of the oxygen carrying capacity of red blood cells
HIV	Human Immunodeficiency Virus
HTLV	Human T-cell Leukemia Virus

Hz	Hertz, meaning cycles per second (electrical term)
Ig	Immunoglobulin, immune system components IgA, IgE, IgM, IgG, and IgD
IM	Intramuscular
IND	Investigational New Drug
IR	Infrared
IU	International Units, a measure of potency for oil soluble vitamins A, D, E, and K
IUD	Intrauterine Device for birth control
IV	Intravenous
IVF	Intervertebral Foramen, which holds the spinal cord
K	Potassium
KS	Kaposi's Sarcoma, a type of cancer common in AIDS patients
LD50	Lethal Dose for 50% of test animals, a measure of poison potency
LDH	Lactose dehydrogenase, a liver enzyme
LDL	Low Density Lipoprotein, "bad" cholesterol
LSD	Lysergic Acid Diethylamide, a hallucinogenic drug
mcg	Microgram, 1/1,000,000 of a gram (1 gram = 1/28 ounce)
mcg/dl	Micrograms per Deciliter, a measure of concentration
MCS	Multiple Chemical Sensitivity
MD	Medical Doctor
mG	MilliGauss, a measure of electromagnetic radiation
mg	Milligram, 1/1000 of a gram (1 gram = 1/28 ounce)
mg/kg	Milligrams per kilogram, a measure of dosage per unit of body weight
ml	Milliliter, a measure of volume (about 1/1000 of a quart)
MRI	Magnetic Resonance Imaging, a diagnostic technique
MS	Multiple Sclerosis
Na	Sodium
NET	Neuro-Emotional Therapy
NSAIDs	Nonsteroidal Anti-Inflammatory Drugs
OD	Overdose of drugs
OSHA	Occupational Safety and Health Agency
OTC	Over The Counter drugs
PAH	Polycyclic Aromatic Hydrocarbons, toxic chemicals
PCBs	Polychlorinated Biphenyls, a toxin from plastic
PCP	Phencyclidine, a hallucinogenic drug
PDR	Physician's Desk Reference, a book of drug effects
PET	Positron Emission Tomography, an imaging testing technique
PGE1,2,3	Prostaglandins, hormones which cause or inhibit inflammation
pH	Measure of acidity or alkalinity of a solution
PMS	Premenstrual Syndrome
ppb	Parts Per Billion

ppm	Parts Per Million
PVC	Polyvinyl Chloride, a toxin
PVCs	Premature Ventricular Contractions, irregular heartbeat
PZI	Zinc and insulin mixture used to rinse tooth extraction site
qid	Four times a day (medicine dosage)
RBC	Red Blood Cells
RF	Radio Frequency electromagnetic radiation
RFV	Resultant Force Vector analysis, a structural technique
RNA	Ribonucleic acid, a genetic component
SLE	Systemic Lupus Erythematosus, also called lupus, an autoimmune disease
T3	Triiodothyronine, a thyroid hormone
T4	Thyroid hormone; also an unrelated type of immune system cell
TCE	Trichloroethylene, a chemical toxin
TENS	Transcutaneous Electronic Nerve Stimulator for pain relief
THC	Tetrahydrocannabinol, active ingredient in marijuana
tid	Three times a day (medicine dosage)
TIS	Toxic Immune Syndrome
TMD	Temporomandibular joint Dysfunction
TMJ	Temporomandibular joint in the jaw; also used to refer to problems with this joint
TSH	Thyroid Stimulating Hormone
TV	Television
U.S.	United States
UV	Ultraviolet
WBC	White Blood Cells
Zn	Zinc

Glossary

This glossary contains medical and non-lay terms used throughout the book. *Italicized* words within a definition are themselves defined in this glossary. More detailed definitions, or definitions of words not found here, can be located by using the Index at the end of this book.

AC - Alternating current

Acetaldehyde - A toxic metabolic byproduct of ethanol, or beverage alcohol; also called acetyl aldehyde. Can also be produced by fungus

Acidophilus - Protective (beneficial) bacteria, which is produced in the body and can also be taken as a supplement

Acquired Immune Deficiency Syndrome (AIDS) - System-wide immune suppression caused by the incapacitation of *T cells*

Acute - Referring to illness lasting less than 120 days, or that which has a comparatively sudden onset

ADA - American Dental Association

Adrenaline - The fight-or-flight hormone released by the adrenal glands which is responsible for the fight-or-flight reaction to stress and for a feeling of energy or anxiety. Also called epinephrine

Aerobic - Oxygen-using

Aflatoxin - A potent *carcinogen* from the mold that grows on peanuts and potatoes

Agoraphobia - Fear of leaving the house, driving, or shopping

AIDS - *Acquired Immune Deficiency Syndrome*

Alimentary - Referring to the digestive tract

Allergen - Substance which can cause an allergic reaction

Allergy - An excessive immune system response to something which is relatively harmless to most people

Allopathic - The type of medicine most common in the U.S. Also called Western, symptom-suppressing, or drug-oriented medicine.

ALS - Amyotrophic lateral sclerosis, also called Lou. Gehrig's disease; a progressive illness involving the nerves and muscles and loss of muscle control

Alzheimer's disease - A brain disease, sometimes called senility, in which the memory becomes progressively worse

Amalgam - Combination; refers in this context to dental fillings made of mercury, silver, and other metals

Amebiasis - The most deadly parasitic disease

Amino acid - Basic building block of protein; protein is broken down through digestion into amino acids which are used by the body

Amoeba - A type of *parasite*

Amylase - *Enzyme* which digests starches

Anabolic - Building up

Anaerobic - Refers to organisms which thrive best without oxygen or in conditions of low oxygen

Analgesic- Pain relieving

Anaphylaxis - Allergy-induced shock which can be fatal

Anesthetic - Substance which deadens pain or produces unconsciousness

Angiography - X-ray study of blood vessels

Ankylosing spondylitis - An *autoimmune disease* which causes pain and stiffness of the spine

Anorexia - Loss of appetite

Anosmia - Loss of ability to smell

Anoxia - Lack of oxygen

Anthropogenic - Human-made

Antibodies - Immune system components which attack *antigens* and signal other immune system components to attack

Antigens - Foreign protein which stimulates the immune system, including *allergens* and *microbes*

Antihistamines - Medications which suppress the action of *histamines*, reducing uncomfortable symptoms but reducing immune system function

Antioxidant - Substance which counteracts the damaging effects of oxygen and *free radicals*

Arachidonic acid - Substance found in meat and dairy products which stimulates the production of *prostaglandin* E2, which produces inflammation

Arrhythmia - Irregular heartbeat

Arteries - Blood vessels which carry oxygenated blood to organs and tissues

Arteriosclerosis - Hardening of the arteries

Arthritis - Painful inflammation of the joints

Asbestos - Fibrous material used in insulation; the sharp fibers can damage cells

Ascaris - Roundworm

Asphyxia - Lack of oxygen

Asthma - An allergic reaction which causes difficulty in breathing

Atlas - Top vertebra

Atom - A single unit of an *element*

Autoimmune disease - A disease in which the immune system appears to attack the body, causing symptoms

Autonomic - Part of the nervous system not under conscious control, such as that which controls heartbeat and digestion

AZT - Azidothymidine, a drug used to treat *AIDS* patients

B cells - These make *antibodies*

BHT - A food preservative containing the toxic solvent toluene

Bifidus - Protective (beneficial) bacteria, which are produced in the body and colonize in the colon. They can also be taken as a supplement. Bifidus has a role in the production of B vitamins, especially biotin, and helps with digestion and keeping fungus under control.

Bile - Substance produced by the liver to aid in digestion of fats. It also digests fat, stores *enzymes*, and carries certain toxic wastes out of the body

Bioavailable - Usable by the body

Biopsy - Removal of a small amount of body tissue for diagnostic purposes

Brain fog - Inability to concentrate, impairment of short-term memory, confusion, spaciness, difficulty in thinking

Bruxism - Grinding the teeth

Cadmium - A toxic metal, found in cigarettes as well as other sources

Candidiasis - Yeast infection

Capillaries - Tiny blood vessels

Carcinogenic - Cancer-causing

Cardiac - Pertaining to the heart

Cardiovascular - Referring to the *circulatory system*

Carpal tunnel syndrome - Pain in the wrist

Casein - Milk protein, a common *allergen*

CAT scan - Computerized axial tomography, an x-ray diagnostic technique

Caustic - Chemical causing destruction of cells and tissue

Cells - The microscopic building blocks of all living things, including ourselves

Cervical - Referring to the neck bones

Cesarean - Type of birth in which the baby is surgically removed through the abdomen

Chelation - A technique for removing metals from the blood and tissues

Chelator - Substance which latches onto metals and eliminates them from the body

Chiropractic - A medical specialty in which the focus is on adjusting spinal *misalignment*s

Chlamydia - Most widespread sexually transmitted disease, caused by bacteria

Cholesterol - A fatty component of the blood which helps to build and repair cell membranes and make *hormones*

Choline - B vitamin needed for building *neurotransmitters*

Chromosomes - *Cell* component which contains genetic material

Chronic - Long-term, referring to illness usually defined as lasting over 120 days

Circulatory system - Heart and blood vessels

Cirrhosis - Hardening and scarring of the liver

Cis - A chemical configuration, referring to oils which are beneficial

CNS - Central Nervous System, which consists of the brain and spinal cord

Coccyx - Tailbone

Colitis - Inflammation of the *colon*, causing diarrhea and malabsorption of food

Collagen - Major structural component of skin and cartilage

Colon - Lower part of the digestive tract

Colonic - Mechanical cleansing of the digestive tract

Colostrum - A component of breast milk which contains *antibodies* to help the baby's immune system

Compound - A new chemical entity formed when two or more *molecules* or *elements* combine (react)

Comprehensive health care - Healing based on finding and treating the root causes of disease. Also called holistic or alternative medicine.

Concussion - A head injury

Condyloma - Genital warts

Congener - Grain or carbohydrate from which a particular type of beverage alcohol is made. Congeners are often *allergens*.

Conjunctivitis - An eye infection, sometimes called pinkeye

Coronary - Referring to the heart

Cortisol - An anti-inflammatory substance naturally produced by the adrenal glands

Creosote - *Carcinogenic* wood preservative

Crohn's disease - An *autoimmune disease* which affects the intestines, causing chronic diarrhea

Cross-linking - Hardening of *collagen*

Cyst - Egg or inactive form of *protozoa* or worms

Cystitis - Urinary tract infection

Cytochrome P450 - One of the body's detoxification systems

Cytoplasm - The jellylike material in the *cell*

Cytotoxicity - Poisoning of cells

Decongestants - Drugs which dry up the nasal passages and mucous membranes

Degenerative diseases - Diseases such as cancer and high blood pressure which take a long time to develop (are *chronic*) and tend to worsen without treatment

Denatured - Chemically changed, usually referring to protein

Dentin - Part of tooth

Dermatitis - Skin inflammation and rashes, often caused by allergy

Dermatology - Study of skin diseases

Detergent - Capable of dissolving oils

DNA - Deoxyribonucleic acid, which contains information needed for a *cell* to replicate itself

DTs - Delirium tremens, mental symptoms of alcohol withdrawal

Dysentery - *Amoebic* disease characterized by diarrhea and vomiting

Eczema - An itchy, unsightly skin rash, usually allergic in origin

Edema - Fluid collecting in the body, usually to try to dilute poisons; swelling due to water retention

Eicosanoids - *Hormones* which regulate and balance many body systems. Also called prostaglandins

Electricity - The flow of *electrons* outside a wire or through a conductive medium

Electrolyte - A mineral in *ion*ic form necessary to the body

Electromagnetic radiation - Harmful radiation given off by electrical appliances

Electrons - Negatively charged particles around the outside of an *atom*; the number of electrons determines the types of chemical reactions in which the *element* participates.

Element - A chemical entity defined by the number of *protons* in its *nucleus*, and which has specific properties

Endocrine - Referring to glands which secrete *hormones*. Endocrine means ductless, and these hormones are secreted directly into the body

Endodontist - Dental specialist who does root canals

Endogenous - Naturally occurring within the body

Entamoeba histolytica - The *protozoon* responsible for *amebiasis*

Environmental Illness (EI) - Sensitivity to many chemicals and artificial substances. Sometimes called Multiple Chemical Sensitivity (MCS)

Enzymes -   Biological substances which help to speed up biochemical reactions in the body or enable them to occur

Eosinophil -   A type of white blood cell

EPA -   Environmental Protection Agency, which monitors environmental hazards

Epidermis -   Outer layer of skin

Epinephrine - Another name for *adrenaline*

Epithelium -   Top intestinal layer

Erythrocytes - Red blood cells

Ethanol -   Beverage alcohol, a poison

Exogenous -   Introduced from outside the body

Fatty acids -   Components of fats; fats are broken down through digestion into fatty acids which are used by the body

FD&C -   Food, Drug, and Cosmetic

FDA -   Food and Drug Administration, which monitors drugs and food additives

Fermentative - Refers to cells such as yeast and cancer cells which are more primitive and prefer an *anaerobic* environment

Fermented -   Changed to alcohol or vinegar

Fibromyalgia - Pain throughout the body due to inflamed tissue

Fluoride -   Harmful chemical compound used in toothpaste and added to water, supposedly for the prevention of dental cavities

Fluoroscope - Imaging technique using x-rays to see moving parts of the body

Free radicals - *Atoms* with unpaired *electrons* which are extremely reactive and damaging in the body

Galvanic -   Referring to the electrical pathways of the body, the *meridians*

Gastrointestinal - Pertaining to the stomach and digestive tract

Giardia -   Common parasite

Glutathione - Sulfur-containing *amino acid* which detoxifies metals and chemicals

Goiter -   A form of *hypothyroidism* due to iodine deficiency, characterized by fatigue and swollen neck

Halogens -   Also called halides; these are the elements chlorine, fluorine, iodine, and bromine

Hematocrit - Measure of the number of red blood cells

Hemoglobin - The oxygen-carrying component of blood

Hepatic - Pertaining to the liver

Hepatitis - Liver infection which can be fatal

Herniate - Squeeze out of proper location

Histamines - Immune system components which attack invaders and whose presence causes typical cold or allergy symptoms

HIV - Human immunodeficiency virus, believed by many to cause *AIDS*

Hormone - A substance which helps regulate a cell's activity

Humectants - Food additives which keep food moist

Hydrogenation - A process by which beneficial liquid oils are changed to harmful solid or semi-solid fats

Hypercholesterolemia - High blood *cholesterol*

Hypertension - High blood pressure

Hypoglycemia - Low blood sugar

Hypothyroidism - Underactivity of the thyroid gland, which can cause fatigue

Hysterectomy - Surgical removal of the uterus

Iatrogenic - Caused by doctors or the medical system

Idiopathic - Of unknown cause

Ileocecal valve - Valve in the small intestine

Immunoglobulins - Types of *antibodies*, called IgA, IgG, IgM, IgE, and IgD

Impingement - Pinching of a nerve

Inert - Not chemically active

Insulin - Hormone which regulates glucose (sugar) metabolism

Ion - Form of an *element* which has an electrical charge due to changes in the number of *electrons*

Ionizing - Electromagnetic frequencies above the frequencies of light, which are usually more powerful and damaging than nonionizing radiation (lower frequencies)

Ischemic - Diseased, usually referring to body tissue

Isolate - Single part of an herb or natural substance

Itis - Suffix meaning infection or inflammation

Jaundice - Skin yellowing caused by a liver problem

Kaposi's sarcoma - A type of cancer which often afflicts *AIDS* patients

Keratin - Calcium-containing material which forms hair and nails

Kinesiology - Refers to muscle testing

Laminants - Toxic chemicals used to glue together sawdust and wood chips to make plywood and particle board

Latent - Resting phase

LD50 - Lethal dose for 50% of test animals, a measure of *acute* chemical toxicity

Leaky gut - Condition in which food is not digested, or broken down into small enough component parts, leading to allergy

Leukemia - A type of cancer affecting the bone marrow's production of white blood cells

Libido - Sex drive

Lipid - Fat

Lipophilic - Oil soluble

Lupus erythematosus - An autoimmune disease affecting the kidneys, skin, and other parts of the body. Usually just called lupus.

Lymph nodes - Collection points in the lymph system, which collect toxins

Lymphocyte - A type of white blood cell and immune system component

Lymphoma - Cancer of the lymph system

Macronutrients - Proteins, carbohydrates, and fatty acids

Macrophages - Immune system components which attack invaders and clean up after a battle with these invaders

Malaise - Fatigue and weakness, flu-like feelings

Malignant - Referring to a cancer that can spread to other parts of the body, with the potential for fatal results

Mammography - X-ray examination of the breast

Mastectomy - Breast removal for cancer

Mcg - Microgram, a unit of weight which is one millionth of a gram, or one-thirty-millionth of an ounce

Melatonin - Hormone which regulates sleep cycles and fights cancer

Meningeal system, or meninges - Outer covering of the brain and spinal cord which acts as shock absorber

Meningeal - Referring to the meninges

Mercury - A toxic metal, most commonly found in amalgam tooth fillings

Meridian - Electrical pathway in the body, usually just under the skin

Metabolite - Breakdown product of a chemical formed in the body

Metallothionein - A sulfur containing *chelator* which clears metals from the body

Metastasis - The spreading of cancer cells to other parts of the body

Microbes - Parasites; literally small living things

Microbiology - The study of small (micro) living things such as *parasites*; the existence of these parasites in your body

Micronutrients - Vitamins and minerals

MilliGauss - The measure of electromagnetic field strength; abbreviated mG

Mineral - A chemical element, usually in charged (ionic) form, which is necessary for bodily function

Misalignment - A condition in which the *vertebrae* of the spine do not line up properly

Mitochondria - The power plants of the *cell*

Mixture - A combination of two or more chemical entities which do not react and whose essential nature does not change

Molecule - A chemical entity which is electrically neutral that can stand alone without immediately reacting

Mononucleosis - An acute infectious viral disease

MRI - Magnetic resonance imaging, a diagnostic technique

Multiple sclerosis (MS) - An *autoimmune disease* in which the *myelin sheath* of the nerves is partially dissolved, leading to loss of control of the muscles served by those nerves

Mutation - Genetic change

Myalgia - Muscle aches

Mycoplasmas - Parasites which are smaller than bacteria

Mycoses - Fungus diseases

Myelin sheath - The fatty covering around the nerve cell

Myocardial infarction - Heart attack

Necrosis - Cell or tissue death

Neurons - Nerve cells

Neurotoxic - Poisonous to nerves

Neurotransmitters - Biochemicals which transmit nerve impulses across the *synapse*

Nickel - Toxic metal, found in root canal posts and dental braces

Noradrenaline - Also called norepinephrine; hormone which allows you to stay asleep and constricts blood vessels in response to shock

Nosocomial - Referring to infections contracted in the hospital

Nucleus - Center, as of a cell or an *atom*

Occiput - Back of head

Olfactory - Referring to the nose

Oncologist - Doctor who focuses on treating cancer

Oncology - The medical specialty that studies and treats cancer

Ophthalmic - Relating to the eye

Organic - a.) A chemical compound which contains carbon

b.) Food which is grown without pesticides or artificial fertilizers

Organophosphate - Toxic pesticide which blocks nerve activity in pests

OSHA - Occupational Safety and Health Agency, which monitors workplace health hazards

Osteoporosis - A condition in which bones become porous and brittle, leading to height loss and fractures

Ozone - Component of smog which can cause *free radical* damage

Pancreas - Organ which produces both digestive enzymes and insulin to regulate blood sugar

Parasite - A living organism that stays alive through dependence on a host such as ourselves. These include bacteria, viruses, and worms

Parasympathetic - The part of the *autonomic* nervous system which is responsible for digestion and for repairing and restoring body function; the opposite of sympathetic

Particulates - Tiny particles of solids and liquids in air pollution

Pathogen - Harmful disease-causing microorganism

Pathogenic - Disease-causing, usually referring to bacteria

Penetrants - Chemicals used in pesticides and cologne which penetrate the skin for both staying power and greater toxicity

Periodic Table - A chemical table which is a simplified model of chemical relationships

Peritonitis - Intestinal infection

Pesticide - Generic term for poisons made to kill bugs, rodents, or weeds

Petrochemicals - Toxic chemicals which are byproducts of the oil industry

pH - Measure of the acidity or alkalinity of a solution

Pituitary gland - Small gland in the base of the brain which regulates activity of the other *endocrine* glands

Placebo - An *inert* substance which physically resembles a drug and is used as a control in studies to evaluate drugs. It can have a positive effect due to the mind's effect on the body

480

Plaque - Calcium-containing substance which forms on artery walls

Plasma - The liquid part of the blood

Platelets - Blood components responsible for clotting

Pleomorphism - Having different forms during different parts of the life cycle

PMS - Premenstrual syndrome, characterized by depression, irritability, breast soreness, cramps, and/or headache

Prostaglandins - *Hormones* which regulate and balance many body systems. Also called eicosanoids

Proton - A part of the *nucleus* of an *atom* which has a positive charge; the number of protons determines an *element*'s identity

Protozoa - A type of *parasite*; a single-celled organism. Singular: protozoon

Psoriasis - An itchy, unsightly skin rash, usually allergic in origin

Psychotropic - Affecting the mind; the term usually refers to certain types of drugs

Pulmonary - Pertaining to the lungs

Putrefaction - Rotting

Putrefied - Rotten, usually referring to proteins in the digestive tract

PVC - Polyvinyl chloride, a toxic component of some plastics

PVCs - Premature ventricular contractions, or irregular heartbeat

Radon - Naturally produced radioactive gas; a radioactive byproduct of uranium decay

Radura - Symbol identifying irradiated food

Rebound effect - Tendency of most drugs to cause the symptom they were designed to treat after continued use

Redox - Type of chemical reaction combining oxidation and reduction

Referred pain - Pain that is perceived by the brain as coming from a site other than its true origin

Renal - Pertaining to kidneys

Respiratory - Referring to breathing; also referring to oxygen-using cells

RF - Radio frequency

Rhinorrhea - Nasal discharge

Salmonella - Bacteria which can cause food poisoning

Salt - A *compound* formed from a metal and a nonmetal

Saturated - Refers to a fat which contains all the hydrogen it can hold. Saturated fats are usually solid at room temperature. They are toxic to the body.

Sciatica - Nerve pain in the upper part of the leg

Scoliosis - Sideways curvature of the spine

Secondary toxic suppressor - A *suppressor*, usually a parasite, which gains a foothold in the body once the immune system is compromised by a primary toxic suppressor

Serotonin - *Neurotransmitter* which promotes feeling of well-being and restful sleep

Specialist - Doctor who focuses on one disease or system of the body, such as a heart specialist or *oncologist* (cancer doctor)

Spleen - Makes antibodies and gets rid of old red blood cells

Steroids - Anti-inflammatory drugs which depress the immune system

Subcutaneous - Under the skin

Subluxation - A *misalignment* of the spinal *vertebrae*

Suppressor - Something which decreases the efficiency of the immune system or body systems in general

Sutures - Divide the bony plates of the skull

Symbionts - Organisms which interact with another for mutual benefit

Sympathetic dominance - A condition in which the adrenal glands are stimulated to release *adrenaline*

Sympathetic - The part of the *autonomic* nervous system which is responsible for fight-or-flight responses to stress

Symptoms - Early warning signs of a problem; examples of symptoms are headaches and rashes

Synapse - Gap between nerve cells

Syndrome - Collection of *symptoms* which usually occur together to form a recognizable entity, such as Chronic Fatigue Syndrome

Synthetic - Human-made, not natural

Thermography - Diagnostic technique using heat sensing

Thimerosal - A mercury-containing preservative

Thymus - Gland behind the breastbone which is part of the immune system and manufactures *lymphocytes*

Tinea - Fungus infection of the skin

Tinnitus - Ringing in the ears

TMJ - Temporomandibular joint, where the upper and lower jaws meet

Topical - On or through the skin

Toxic Immune Syndrome - A collection of symptoms caused by interference with the function of the immune system

Toxic - Poisonous

Toxoplasmosis - *Protozoal* disease transmitted by cats, especially dangerous to a developing fetus

Trans - A chemical configuration, referring to oils which are made harmful by heating or *hydrogenation*

Trapezius - Muscles between the shoulder blades

Trichomonas - Gynecological infection caused by a *protozoal parasite*

Triglycerides - Fats in the blood

Trophozoites - Active form of protozoa

Tryptophan - An amino acid which converts to *serotonin*

Tumor - An abnormal growth of cells which forms a mass; some but not all tumors are cancerous

Ultrasound - The part of the electromagnetic spectrum just above sound; can be used for diagnostic testing

Urticaria - Hives, which are an allergic skin swelling

Valence - Electrical charge of an *ion*

Vascular - Referring to the blood vessels

Veins - Blood vessels which carry deoxygenated blood back to the heart

Verapamil - A drug which regulates the heartbeat by blocking calcium and increasing magnesium uptake

Vermifuge - Medicine which kills worms

Vertebrae - Bony segments of the spine. Singular form is vertebra

Villi - Fingerlike projections in the *cell* and in the digestive tract which increase surface area

Virulence - Ability to cause disease

Vitiligo - Lightening of skin, usually in blotches

Whiplash - An injury, most common in automobile accidents, in which the neck is snapped back and then forward

Zinc - A necessary *mineral*, a deficiency of which can cause loss of smell and taste among other symptoms.

Sources for Products Named in This Book

The following are the sources for some of the nutritional and supportive products named in this book. Years of clinical experience have shown these particular brands to be among the best of their type. Most if not all products named can be ordered directly through:

Comprehensive Health Centers
4403 Manchester Avenue, Suite 107
Encinitas CA 92024
Phone 619-632-9042 Fax 619-632-0574

Product	Brand Name	Company
Cellular support	Mitochondrial Resuscitate	Metagenics
Phosphatidyl choline	Maxicholine	Phillips Nutritionals
Liver cleanse	Lipotropic Plus	Ethical Nutrients
Liver cleanse	Lipogen	Metagenics
Liver cleanse	LiverTox	Enzymatic Therapy
Liver cleanse, digestion	Boldo	Rainforest Bio-Energetics
Liver cleansing homeopathic	LGB-414	
Garlic extract	Kyolic	Wakunaga
Chlorophyll	Sun Chlorella	Sun Wellness / Integris
Flax oil	Flax Oil	Barleans
GLA oils	GLA Softgels	Carlson / Phillips Nutritionals
Salmon oil	Salmon Oil Softgels	Carlson
Acidophilus	Megadophilus / UltraDophilus	Metagenics / Ethical Nutrients
Acidophilus	Kyodophilus	Wakunaga
Bifidus	Ultra Bifidus / Megabifidus	Metagenics / Ethical Nutrients
Bacteria	Latero-Flora	Metagenics / Ethical Nutrients
Control microorganisms	Replenz	Integris
Digestive enzymes	Bio-Zyme	Enzymatic
Vitamins A, C, E, selenium	ACES	Carlson
Bioflavonoids	Inflavonoids	Metagenics / Ethical Nutrients
Vitamin A	NutriSorb A	Interplexus
Vitamin E	E-Gems	Carlson
Multinutrient preparation, women	Perfect Equation for Women	Professional Preference
Multinutrient preparation, men	Perfect Equation for Men	Professional Preference
Multinutrient preparation, low blood pressure or underweight	Lo-Balance	Professional Preference
Multinutrient preparation, high blood pressure or overweight	Hi-Balance	Professional Preference
CoQ10	CoQ10	Metabolic Maintenance
Glutathione complex	Glutathione complex	Professional Preference
Minerals	Kona Gold	Integris
Calcium supplement	Osteo-Citrate	Metagenics
Calcium / magnesium supplement	Cal-Mag 2:1	Enzymatic Therapy

Iodine	Dulse	Carlsons
Rice protein	Life Solubles / Life Wafer	Integris
Protein powder	Ultra Clear Plus	Metagenics
Glutamine	L-Glutamine	Metabolic Maintenance
Detoxification	Lymph Clear	Enzymatic Therapy
Detoxification, especially metals	Toxi-Cleanse	Metagenics
Metal detoxification - DMSA	Chemet	McNeil
DHEA	Colloidal DHEA	Royal Scandinavian
Oxygenation	Dioxychlor	
Pycnogenol	Pycnogenol	Phillips Nutritionals
Bee propolis	Propolis Extract	Dragon River Herbals
Milk thistle	Super Thistle X	Enzymatic
Air purifier	Alpine Air	Environmental Health Systems
Cookbook	Toxic Immune Syndrome Cookbook - Kellas	Comprehensive Health Centers
For worms	Paragone I	Integris
For amoebas	Paragone II	Integris
Candida homeopathic	Aqua Flora I and II	Aqua Flora / East West
Antiparasitic	AP Mag	InterPlexus
Aloe vera powder for yeast	OriFresh	Amni
Aloe vera	Aloe Vera	Innovative Natural Products
Worm medication (mebendazole)	Vermox*	Janssen Pharmaceuticals
For worms	Wormwood Combination	Kroeger Herb Products
Antifungal (caprylic acid)	Mycopril 680	T.E. Neesby
Antifungal (caprylic acid)	Caprol oil	Attogram Corp.
Antiparasitic	Citricidal / Nutricidal	BioChem Research
Antiparasitic	Artemisia annua	
Antiparasitic	Black walnut tincture	Holistic Labs Inc.
Anti-amoebic (metronidazole)	Flagyl*	Searle
Anti-amoebic (tinidazole)	Fasigyn**	Pfizer
Virus fighter	Livit I	Interplexus
Virus fighter	Colloidal silver	Royal Scandinavian
Virus fighter, immune booster	SSKI	Scientific Botanicals Inc.
Virus fighter, immune booster	L-Lysine	Carlson
Immune booster	Immuplex lozenges	Tyler
Prevent reinfection	Hi-Tech Hygiene	Hi-Tech Hygiene
Prevent release of stomach acid	Zantac*	Glaxo
Prevent release of stomach acid	Prilosec*	Astra Merck
Coat stomach	Bismogel	Clark's Pharmacy
Anti-yeast	Nystatin*	Squibb
Anti-yeast	Diflucan*	Roerig

*   Available by prescription only

**   Available outside of U.S. (e.g. Mexico or Canada)

References

Basic Chemical Concepts

1. Kervran, C. Louis, *Biological Transmutations*, Happiness Press, Magalia CA, 1966.

Chemical Toxicity

1. Schnare, DW et al, "Body Burden Reductions of PCBs, PBBs and Chlorinated Pesticides in Human Subjects", *Ambio: A Journal of the Human Environment*, Vol. 13, No. 5-6, 1984, pp. 378-380.

2. Langer, Stephen, "Keeping Environmental Toxins at Bay", *Better Nutrition for Today's Living*, July 1993, pp. 28-32.

3. Sherman, Janette D., *Chemical Exposure and Disease*, Princeton Scientific Publishing Co., Princeton NJ.

4. Rogers, Sherry A., *Tired or Toxic?*, Prestige Publishing, Syracuse NY, 1990.

5. Dager, S.R. et al, "Panic Disorder Precipitated By Exposure to Organic Solvents in the Workplace", *American Journal of Psychiatry*, Vol. 144, No. 8, August 1987, pp. 1056-8.

6. Rea, William J., *Chemical Sensitivity*, Volume 1, Lewis Publishers, Boca Raton FL, 1992.

7. Langer, Stephen, "Keeping Environmental Toxins at Bay", *Better Nutrition for Today's Living*, July 1993, pp. 28-32.

8. Bodin, F., and C.F. Chernisse, *Poisons*, McGraw-Hill Book Co., New York, 1970.

9. *Los Angeles Times*, August 18, 1992, page H3.

10. Heuser, G., Mena, I. and F. Alamos, "NeuroSPECT Findings in Patients Exposed to Neurotoxic Chemicals", *Toxicol. Ind. Health*, Vol. 10, No. 4-5, July-Oct. 1994, pp. 561-71.

11. Dienhart, Charlotte M., *Basic Human Anatomy and Physiology*, W.B. Saunders Co. Philadelphia PA, 1973, 2nd ed.

12. Casaret and Doull, *Toxicology*, Macmillan Publishing Co., New York, 1986, 3rd ed.

13. Schnare, DW et al, "Evaluation of a Detoxification Regimen for Fat Stored Xenobiotics", *Medical Hypotheses*, Vol. 9, no. 3, 1982, pp. 265-282.

14. Gard, Zane and Erma Brown, "Literature Review and Comparison Studies of Sauna/Hyperthermia in Detoxification", *Townsend Letter For Doctors*, No. 107, June 1991, pp. 470-8.

15. The Burton Goldberg Group, *Alternative Medicine: The Definitive Guide*, "Hydrotherapy", pp. 281-298, Future Medicine Publishing, Puyallup WA, 1994.

16. Nambudripad, Devi, *Say Goodbye To Illness*, Delta Publishing Company, Buena Park CA, 1993.

17. Nambudripad, Devi, *The NAET Guidebook*, Delta Publishing Company, Buena Park CA, 1994.

18. *McGraw-Hill Encyclopedia of Science and Technology*, McGraw-Hill Book Co., 1992, 7th ed.

19. Arena, Jay M., *Poisoning: Toxicology, Symptoms, Treatments*, Charles C. Thomas (publisher), 1974, 3rd ed.

20. Vojdani, Aristo, *New Immunobiologic Markers for Diagnosis of Toxic Chemical Exposure*, Immunosciences Lab Inc., Los Angeles CA.

Organic Chemicals and Solvents

1. Bodin, F., and C.F. Chernisse, *Poisons*, McGraw-Hill Book Co., New York, 1970.

2. Pacific Toxicology Labs, Volume 1, Issue 3.

3. Ward, A.M. et al, "Immunological Mechanisms in the Pathogenesis of Vinyl Chloride Disease", *British Medical Journal*, Vol. 1, 1976, pp. 936-8.

4. Graestrom, R.C. and A.J Fornore et al, "Formaldehyde Damage to DNA and Inhibition of DNA Repair in Human Bronchial Cells", *Science*, Vol. 220, April 8, 1983, pp. 216-8.

5. Abedin, Z. et al, "Cardiac Toxicity of Perchloroethylene", *S. Med. Journal*, Vol. 73, pp. 1081-3.

6. Mago, L., "The Effects of Industrial Chemicals on the Heart", *Cardiac Toxicology*, T. Balazo (ed.), CRC Press, Boca Raton FL, 1981.

7. King, G.S., "Sudden Death in Adolescents Resulting From the Inhalation of Typewriter Correction Fluid", *Journal of the American Medical Association*, Vol. 253, 1985, pp. 1604-6.

8. Zimmerman, S.W. et al, "Hydrocarbon Exposure and Chronic Glomerulonephritis", *The Lancet*, August 2, 1975, pp. pp. 199-201.

9. Raunskov, G. et al, "Glomerulonephritis in Exposure to Organic Solvents", *Acta. Medi. Scand.*, Vol. 205, 1979, pp. 575-9.

10. Dager, S.R. et al, "Panic Disorder Precipitated by Exposure to Organic Solvents in the Workplace, *American Journal of Psychiatry*, Vol. 144, No. 8, August 1987, pp. 1056-8.

11. Feldman, *American Journal of Industrial Medicine*, 1980.

12. Klotter, Jule, "Toluene", *Townsend Letter for Doctors*, No. 118, May 1993, p. 518.

13. Rogers, Sherry A., *The E.I. Syndrome*, Prestige Publishing, Syracuse NY, 1986.

14. Meyer, Beat, *Indoor Air Quality*, Addison-Wesley Publishing Co., Reading MA, 1983.

15. Dadd, Debra Lynn, *Nontoxic and Natural*, Jeremy P. Tarcher Inc., Los Angeles CA, 1984.

16. Kaura, S.R., *Understanding and Preventing Cancer*, Health Press, Santa Fe NM, 1991.

17. Rogers, Sherry A., *Tired or Toxic?*, Prestige Publishing, Syracuse NY, 1990.

18. Vaughn, TL, DS Strader, S. Davis and JR Daling, "Formaldehyde and Cancers of the Pharynx, Sinus and Nasal Cavity, II. Residential Exposures", *International Journal of Cancer*, Vol. 38, 1986, p. 685.

19. Kane, L.E. and T. Alaria, "Sensory Irritation to Formaldehyde and Acrolein During Single and Repeated Exposures in Mice", *American Industrial Hyg. Assoc. Journal*, Vol. 38, 19177, p. 509.

20. Main, D.M. and T.J. Hogan, "Health Effect of Low-Level Exposure to Formaldehyde", *Journal of Occupational Medicine*, Vol. 25, 1983, pp. 896-900.

21. Cox, J.E., "OSHA Reconsidering Formaldehyde", *ASHRAE Journal*, Sept. 1985, p. 10.

Pesticides

1. Zenz, C., "Occupational Health Aspects of Pesticides", Chapter 46, *Occupational Medicine*, Yearbook Medical Publishers Inc., Chicago IL, 1988.

2. Rogers, Sherry A., *Tired or Toxic?*, Prestige Publishers, Syracuse NY, 1990.

3. Hodgson et al, "Organophosphate Poisoning in Office Workers", *Journal of Occupational Medicine*, Vol. 28, 1986.

4. Mott, Lawrie, and Karen Snyder, *Pesticide Alert*, Sierra Club Books, San Francisco CA, 1987.

5. Brown, Ellen, "Crystal Power", *Townsend Letter for Doctors*, No. 124, Nov. 1993, p. 1107.

6. Millichap, J. Gordon, *Environmental Poisons In Our Food*, PNB Publishers, Chicago IL, 1993.

7. Jaffe, Russell, "16 Million Americans Sensitive to Pesticides", *Townsend Letter for Doctors*, Dec. 1990, pp. 869-872.

8. Regenstein, Lewis, *America the Poisoned*, Acropolis, 1982.

9. Langer, Stephen, "Keeping Environmental Toxins at Bay", *Better Nutrition for Today's Living*, July 1993, pp. 28-32.

10. Bland, Jeffrey S. "Managing Endo- and Exotoxicity", *Townsend Letter for Doctors*, No. 108, July 1992, pp. 590-3.

11. Costa, I.G. et al, "Interaction Between Acetaminophen and Organophosphates in Mice", *Research Communications in Clinical Pathology and Pharmacology*, Vol. 44, No. 3, June 1984, pp. 389-400.

12. Lipscomb, J.W., J.E. Kramer and J.B.Leikin, "Seizure Following Brief Exposure to the Insect Repellent N,N-diethyl-m-toluamide", *Annals of Emergency Medicine*, Vol. 21, No. 3, March 1992, pp. 3115-7.

13. Metcalf and Holmes, *Annals of the New York Academy of Science*, Vol. 160.

14. Forasteire F., A Quercia et al, "Cancer Among Farmers In Central Italy", *Scand. Journal of Work and Environmental Health*, Vol. 19, No. 6, Dec. 1993, pp. 382-9.

15. Aesoph, Lauri, "The Poisonous Legacy of Pesticides", *Delicious*, April 1994, pp. 32-4.

16. McDuffie, H.H., "Women at Work: Agriculture and Pesticides", *Journal of Occupational Medicine*, Vol. 36, No. 11, Nov. 1994, pp. 1240-6.

17. Fleming, L., J.B. Mann et al, "Parkinson's Disease and Brain Levels of Organochlorine Pesticides", *Annals of Neurology*, Vol. 36, No. 1, July 1994, pp. 100-3.

18. Butterfield, P.G., B.G. Valanis et al, "Environmental Antecedents of Young-Onset Parkinson's Disease", *Neurology*, Vol. 43, No. 6, June 1993, pp. 1150-8.

19. Cellini, A. and A. Offidani, "An Epidemiological Study on Cutaneous Diseases of Workers Authorized to Use Pesticides", *Dermatology*, Vol. 189, No. 2, 1994, pp. 129-32.

20. "Acute Pancreatitis Following Continuous Exposure to Organophosphate Insecticide, *Internal Medicine World Report*, March 1-14, 1989.

21. Allazov, S., "The Characteristics of Acute Infectious-Inflammatory Kidney Diseases in Pesticide Exposure", *Urol. Nefrol. Mosk.* (Russian), No. 2, March-April 1994, pp. 14-6.

22. Colborn, Theo and Coralie Clement (editors), *Chemically Induced Alterations in Sexual and Functional Development*, Princeton Scientific Publishing Co., Princeton NJ, 1992.

23. Petty, C.S., "Organic Phosphate Insecticide Poisoning", *American Journal of Medicine*, Vol. 24, 1958, pp. 467-470.

24. Raloff, Janet, "That Feminine Touch", *Science News*, Vol. 145, Jan. 22, 1994, pp. 56-8.

25. Ortiz-Martinez, A and E. Martinez-Conde, "The Neurotoxic Effects of Lindane at Acute and Subacute Dosages", *Ecotoxicology and Environmental Safety*, Vol. 30, No. 2, March 1995, pp. 101-5.

26. Klotter, Jule, "Toxins in Pesticides", *Townsend Letter for Doctors*, No. 118, May 1993, p. 518.

27. Dadd, Debra Lynn, *Nontoxic and Natural*, Jeremy P. Tarcher Inc., Los Angeles CA, 1984.

28. Hallenbeck, W.H., and K.M. Cunningham-Burns, *Pesticides and Human Health*, Springer-Verlag, New York, 1985.

Personal Care Products

1. Ashford, Nicholas A. and Claudia S. Miller, *Chemical Exposures: Low Levels, High Stakes*, 1991.

2. *Neurotoxins: At Home and the Workplace*, Report by the Committee on Science and Technology, U.S. House of Representatives, Sept. 16, 1986, Report 99-827.

3. "Making Sense of Scents", *Townsend Letter for Doctors*, No. 132, July 1994, pp. 765-7.

4. Manning, Betsy Russell (editor), *Candida, Silver Mercury Fillings and the Immune System*, Greensward Press, San Francisco CA, 1985, p. 136.

5. Cooper, S.D., J.H. Raymer, E.D. Pellizzari and K.W. Thomas, "The Identification of Polar Organic Compounds Found in Consumer Products and Their Toxicological Properties", *Journal of Expo. Environ. Epidemiology*, Vol. 5, No. 1, Jan-Mar. 1995, pp. 57-75.

6. Klotter, Jule, "Toluene", *Townsend Letter for Doctors*, No. 118, May 1993, p. 518.

7. Shim, Chang and M. Henry Williams, *American Journal of Medicine*, Vol. 80, Jan. 1986.

8. *Ugeskr. Laeer.* (Danish journal), Vol. 153, Issue 13, 1991, pp. 939-940.

9. Dadd, Debra Lynn, *Nontoxic and Natural*, Jeremy P. Tarcher Inc., Los Angeles CA, 1984.

10. Arnold, Kathryn, "Is Your Hair Dye Safe?", *Delicious*, July/Aug. 1993, pp. 50+.

11. The Burton Goldberg Group, *Alternative Medicine: The Definitive Guide*, "Body Odor", pp. 890-1, Future Medicine Publishing, Puyallup WA, 1994.

Air Pollution

1. Dadd, Debra Lynn, *Nontoxic and Natural*, Jeremy P. Tarcher Inc., Los Angeles CA, 1984.

2. Brenner, I., "Cadmium Toxicity", *World Review of Nutrition and Diet*, Vol. 32, pp. 165-197.

3. Meyer, Beat, *Indoor Air Quality*, Addison-Wesley Publishing Co., Reading MA, 1983.

4. "When Your Office Makes You Sick", *Lear's*, Jan. 1993.

5. *McGraw-Hill Encyclopedia of Science and Technology*, McGraw-Hill Book Co., 1992, 7th ed.

6. Environmental Protection Agency, "EPA Data Show Steady Progress in Cleaning Nation's Air", *Environmental News*, Oct. 1992.

7. Lee, Douglas H.K., *Environmental Factors in Respiratory Disease*, Academic Press, New York, 1972.

Water Pollution, Fluoride and Chlorine

1. Environmental Protection Agency, "130 Cities Exceed Lead Levels for Drinking Water", *Environmental News*, Oct. 1992.

2. Schnare, DW, *The Unpolluting of Men*, Foundation Essay Series, Foundation for Advancements in Science and Education, Los Angeles CA.

3. Environmental Protection Agency, "819 Cities Exceed Lead Level for Drinking Water", *EPA Environmental News* Publication No. A-107, May 11, 1993, p. R110.

4. Steinman, David, *Diet For A Poisoned Planet*, Ballantine Books, NY, 1990.

5. "Tap Water as Bad as We've Suspected - Possibly Worse", *Townsend Letter for Doctors and Patients*, No. 151/152, Feb./Mar. 1996, p. 41.

6. McCleary, Kathleen, "Trouble From the Tap", *Health*, May 1990, pp. 32+.

7. Dunnick, J.K and R.L. Melnick, "Assessment of the Carcinogenic Potential of Chlorinated Water: Experimental Studies of Chlorine, Chloramine and Trihalomethanes", *Journal of the National Cancer Institute*, Vol. 85, No. 10, May 19, 1993, pp. 817-22.

8. Whitfield, GM, "Acute and Chronic Fluoride Toxicity", *Journal of Dental Research*, Vol. 71, No. 5, May 1992, pp. 1249-54.

9. Casarett and Doull, *Toxicology*, Macmillan Publishing Company, New York, 1986, 3rd edition.

10. Maugh, TH, "Experts Downplay Cancer Risk of Chlorinated Water", *Los Angeles Times*, July 2, 1992.

11. Yiamouyiannis, John, *Fluoride: The Aging Factor*, Health Action Press, Delaware OH, 1986.

12. Williams and Wilkins, *Clinical Toxicology of Commercial Products*, 1984, pp. II-4, 112, 129, 138.

13. "The Village Where People Are Old Before Their Time", *Stern*, Vol. 30, 19178, pp. 107-112.

14. Foulkes, Richard G., "Fluoridation of Community Water Supplies - 1992 Update", *Townsend Letter for Doctors*, No. 107, June 1992, pp. 450-6.

15. Yiamouyiannis, John, *Fluoride: The Aging Factor*, Health Action Press, Delaware, OH, 3rd ed., 1993.

16. Stannard, JG et al, "Fluoride Levels and Fluoride Contamination of Fruit Juices, *J. Clin. Pediatr. Dent.*, Vol. 16, 1991, pp. 38-40.

17. Saunders, Milton A., "Fluoride Toothpastes: A Cause of Acne-Like Eruptions", *Archives of Dermatology*, Vol. 111, 1975, p. 793.

18. Mellette, J. Ramsey et al, "Fluoride Toothpaste: A Cause of Perioral Dermatitis", *Archives of Dermatology*, Vol. 112, 1976, pp. 730-1.

19. Dadd, Debra Lynn, *Nontoxic and Natural*, Jeremy P. Tarcher Inc., Los Angeles CA, 1984.

20. Roberts, H.J., "Toxicology of Fluoride", *Townsend Letter for Doctors*, No. 108, July 1992, pp. 623-4.

21. "Fluoridation Death", *Townsend Letter for Doctors*, No. 112, Nov. 1992, p. 988.

22. Drozdz, Marian et al, "Studies on the Influence of Fluoride Compounds Upon Connective Tissue Metabolism in Growing Rats", *Toxiligical European Research*, Vol. 3, No. 5, 1981, pp. 237-241.

23. Susheela, AK and Mohan Jha "Effects of Fluoride on Cortical and Cancellous Bone Composition", *IRCS Medical Sciences: Library Compendium*, Vol. 9, No. 11, 1981, pp. 1021-2.

24. Sharma, YD, "Effect of Sodium Fluoride on Collagen Cross-Link Precursors, *Toxicological Letters*, Vol. 10, 1982, pp. 97-100.

25. Sharma, YD, "Variations in the Metabolism and Maturation of Collagen After Fluoride Ingestion, *Biochemica et Biophysica Acta*, Vol. 715, 1982, pp. 137-141.

26. Farley, John R. et al, "Fluoride Directly Stimulates Proliferation and Alkaline Phosphatase Activity of Bone Forming Cells", *Science*, Vol. 222, 1983, pp. 330-2.

27. Smid, JR et al, "Effect of Long-Term Administration of Fluoride on the Levels of EDTA-Soluble Protein and Gamma Carboxyglutamic Acid in Rat Incisor Teeth", *Journal of Dental Research*, Vol. 63, 1984, pp. 1061-3.

28. Bowes, JH and MM Murray, "A Chemical Study of 'Mottled Teeth' from Maldon, Essex", *British Dental Journal*, Vol. 60, 1936, pp. 556-562.

29. Abishev, Kh. A. et al, "Molecular Composition of Bones During Chronic Fluoride Poisoning", *Zdravookr. Kaz*, Vol. 30, No. 5, 1971, pp. 28-30.

30. Bhussry, BR, "Chemical and Physical Studies of Enamel From Human Teeth", *Journal of Dental Research*, Vol. 38, 1959, pp. 369-373.

31. Singh, Amarjit and SS Jolly, "Chronic Toxic Health Effects on the Skeletal System", *Fluorides and Human Health*, World Health Organization, Geneva Switzerland, 1970, pp. 238-249.

32. Singh, Amarjit et al, "Skeletal Changes in Endemic Fluorosis", *Journal of Bone and Joint Surgery*, Vol. 44B, No. 4, 1962, pp. 806-815.

33. Waldbott, George et al, *Fluoridation: The Great Dilemma*, Coronado Press, Lawrence KS, 1978.

34. Jacobson, Steven et al, "Regional Variation in the Incidence of Hip Fracture", *Journal of the American Medical Association*, Vol. 264, 1990, pp. 500-502.

35. Cooper, Cyrus et al, "Water Fluoridation and Hip Fracture", *Journal of the American Medical Association*, Vol. 266, July 1991, pp. 513-514.

36. Danielson, C. et al, "Hip Fractures and Fluoridation in Utah's Elderly Population, *Journal of the American Medical Association*, Vol. 268, 1992, pp. 746-8.

37. , MF et al, "A Prospective Study of Bone Mineral Content and Fracture in Communities with Differential Fluoride Exposure", *American Journal of Epidemiology*, Vol. 133, 1991, pp. 649-660.

38. Riggs, B. Lawrence, "Effect of Fluoride Treatment on the Fracture Rate in Postmenopausal Women With Osteoporosis", *New England Journal of Medicine*, Vol. 322, 1990, pp. 802-9.

39. Hedlund, LR and JC Gallagher, "Increased Hip Fractures in Osteoporotic Women Treated With Sodium Fluoride", *Journal of Bone and Mineral Research*, Vol. 4, 1989, pp. 223-5.

40. Zong-Chen, Lian and Wu En-Huei, "Osteoporosis - An Early Radiographic Sign of Endemic Fluorosis, *Skeletal Radiology*, Vol. 15, 1986, pp. 350-3.

41. Marks, Stephen, "Restraint and Use of High-Dose Fluorides to Treat Skeletal Disorders", *Journal of the American Medical Association*, Vol. 240, No. 15, 1978, pp. 1630-1.

42. Robin, JC et al, "Studies on Osteoporosis III. Effect of Estrogens and Fluoride", *Journal of Medicine*, Vol. 11, 1980, pp. 1-14.

43. Robin, JC and JL Ambrus, "Studies on Osteoporosis IX, Effect of Fluoride on Steroid Induced Osteoporosis", *Research Communications in Chemical Pathology and Pharmacology*, Vol. 37, No. 3, 1982, pp. 453-461.

44. Schnitzler, CM et al, "Histomorphometric Analysis of a Calcaneal Stress Fracture: A Possible Complication of Fluoride Therapy for Osteoporosis", *Bone*, Vol. 7, 1986, pp. 193-198.

45. Dumbacher, MA et al, "Long-Term Fluoride Therapy of Postmenopausal Osteoporosis", *Bone*, Vol. 7, 1986, pp. 199-205.

46. Schnitzler, CM et al, "Bone Fragility of the Peripheral Skeleton During Fluoride Therapy for Osteoporosis", *Clin. Orthop.*, Vol. 261, 1990, pp. 268-275.

47. Marcelli, C. et al, "Bone Complications During The Treatment of Osteoporosis with Fluoride", *Rev. Med. Interne*, Vol. 10, 1989, pp. 118-126.

48. Segrettom, Vincent A. et al, "A Current Study of Mottled Enamel in Texas", *Journal of the American Dental Association*, Vol. 108, 1984, pp. 56-59.

49. Brown, JP, "Fluoride Supplements and Fluorosis of Enamel", *Journal of Dental Research*, Vol. 64, 1985, p. 225.

50. DePaola, PF, "History of Fluoride Ingestion Among Children Diagnosed With And Without Fluorosis", *Journal of Dental Research*, Vol. 64, 1985, p. 226.

51. Woltgens, JH, et al, "Prevalence of Mottled Enamel in Permanent Dentition of Children Participation in a Fluoride Programme at the Amsterdam Dental School", *J. Biol. Buccale*, Vol. 17, 1989, pp. 15-20.

52. Little, John, "Relationship Between DNA Repair Capacity and Cellular Aging, *Gerontology*, Vol. 22, 1976, pp. 28-55.

53. Voroshilin, SI et al, "Cytogenetic Effect of Inorganic Fluorine Compounds on Human and Animal Cells in Vivo and in Vitro, *Genetika*, Vol. 9, No. 4, 1973, pp. 115-120.

54. Jagiello, Georgianna and Ja-Shein Lin, "Sodium Fluoride as Potential Mutagen in Mammalian Eggs", *Archives of Environmental Health*, Vol. 29, 1974, pp. 230-5.

55. Mohamed, Aly and ME Chandler, "Cytological Effects of Sodium Fluoride on Mice", *Fluoride*, Vol. 15, No. 3, 1983, pp. 110-8.

56. Tsutsui, Takeki et al, "Cytotoxicity, Chromosome Aberrations and Unscheduled DNA Synthesis in Cultured Human Diploid Fibroblasts Induced by Sodium Fluoride", *Mutation Research*, Vol. 139, 1984, pp. 193-8.

57. Thompson, EJ et al, "The Effect of Fluoride on Chromosome Aberration and Sister-Chromatid Exchange Frequencies in Cultured Human Lymphocytes", *Mutation Research*, Vol. 144, pp. 89-92.

58. Mukherjee, RN and FH Sobels, "The Effect of Sodium Fluoride and Iodoacetamide on Mutation Induction by W-Irradiation in Mature Spermatazoa of Drosophila", *Mutation Research*, Vol. 6, No. 2, 1968, pp. 217-225.

59. "Re: Fluoridation", *Townsend Letter for Doctors*, No. 115/116, Feb./Mar. 1993, p. 206.

60. Taylor, Alfred and Nell Carmichael Taylor, "Effect of Sodium Fluoride on Tumor Growth", *Proceedings of the Society for Experimental Biology and Medicine*, Vol. 119, 1965, pp. 252-5.

61. *Merck Index*, Merck and Co. Inc, Rahway NJ, 1968, p. 959.

Carcinogens

1. "Pesticides and Groundwater: A Health Concern for the Midwest", Proceedings of the Freshwater Foundation Conference, Navarre MN, Oct. 16-17, 1986.

2. Vaughn, TL, DS Strader, S. Davis and JR Daling, "Formaldehyde and Cancers of the Pharynx, Sinus and Nasal Cavity, II. Residential Exposures", *International Journal of Cancer*, Vol. 38, 1986, p. 685.

3. Levitt, Paul M. and Elissa S. Guralnick, *The Cancer Reference Book*, Facts on File Inc., New York, 1983, 2nd ed.

4. Kaura, S.R., *Understanding and Preventing Cancer*, Health Press, Santa Fe NM, 1991.

Drugs

1. *Webster's II New Riverside University Dictionary*, Houghton Mifflin Co., Boston MA, 1994, p. 880.

2. Roe, D.A., "Nutrient and Drug Interactions", *Nutrition Reviews*, Vol. 42, No. 4, April 1984, pp. 141-154.

3. Carson, Robe B., "Pharmaceutical Nemesis: Medical Drugs are Ersatz Biochemicals That Shorten Life", *Townsend Letter for Doctors*, Vol. 123, Oct. 1993, pp. 948-952.

4. Whitaker, Julian, "Act Now To Protect Your Health", *Health and Healing*, Sept. 1993.

5. *Physician's Desk Reference*, Medical Economics Co., Oradell NJ, 1993.

6. Cooley, Leland and Lee Morrison Cooley, *Pre-Medicated Murder?*, Chilton Book Co., Radnor PA, 1974.

7. Crook, William G., *Chronic Fatigue Syndrome and The Yeast Connection*, Professional Books, Jackson TN, 1984, 1992.

8. "Survey Shows Link Between Antibiotics and Developmental Delays in Children", *Townsend Letter for Doctors and Patients*, No. 147, Oct. 1995, p. 9.

9. Newman, NM and RSM Ling, "Acetabular Bone Destruction Related to Nonsteroidal Anti-Inflammatory Drugs", *Lancet*, Nov. 13, 1985.

10. Brandt, KD, "Effects of Nonsteroidal Anti-Inflammatory Drugs on Chondrocyte Metabolism In Vitro and In Vivo", *American Journal of Medicine*, Vol. 83, 1987, pp. 29-34.

11. Gaby, Alan R., "Do Non-Steroidal Anti-Inflammatory Drugs Damage Cells?", *Townsend Letter for Doctors*, Vol. 126, Jan. 1994, p. 13.

12. Copeland, P.M., "Renal Failure Associated With Laxative Abuse", *Psychother.Psychosom.*, Vol. 62, No. 3-4, 1994, pp. 200-2.

13. Wen, AH and SY Cheung, "How Acupuncture Can Help Addicts", *Drugs and Society*, 1973, pp. 18-20.

14. Malone, Joan, "Marijuana Makes a Comeback", *Mademoiselle*, Vol. 96, Oct. 1990, pp. 184-7.

15. Beardsley, Tim, "Cannabis Comprehended", *Scientific American*, Vol. 263, Oct. 1990, p. 38.

16. Schwartz, R.H. and R.A. Beveridge, "Marijuana as an Antiemetic Drug: How Useful is it Today? Opinions From Clinical Oncologists", *Journal of Addict. Dis.*, Vol. 13, No. 1, 1994, pp. 53-65.

17. Bandow, Doug, "Sometimes Marijuana is the Best Medicine, *Townsend Letter for Doctors*, Vol. 123, Oct. 1993, p. 1022.

18. Solowij, N., P.T Michie and A.M. Fox, "Differential Impairments of Selective Attention Due To Frequency and Duration of Cannabis Use", *Biol. Psychiatry*, Vol. 37, No. 10, May 15, 1995, pp. 731-9.

19. Solowiz, N., "Do Cognitive Impairments Recover Following Cessation of Cannabis Use?", *Life Science*, Vol. 56, 1995, pp. 2119-26.

20. Solowij, N., "Do Cognitive Impairments Recover Following Cessation of Cannabis Use?", *Life Science*, Vol. 56, No. 23-24, May 5, 1995, pp. 2119-26.

21. Oliwenstein, Lori, "The Perils of Pot", *Discover*, Vol. 9, June 1988, p. 18.

22. Sherman, M.P., Aeberhard E.E. et al, "Effects of Smoking Marijuana, Tobacco or Cocaine Alone or in Combination on DNA Damage in Human Alveolar Macrophages", *Life Science*, Vol. 56, No. 23-24, May 5, 1995, pp. 2201-7.

23. Nahas, G. and C. Latour, "The Human Toxicity of Marijuana", *Med. Journal Aust.*, Vol. 156, No. 7, April 6, 1992, pp. 495-7.

24. Barnes, B. and SG Bradley, *Planning for a Healthy Baby*, Ebury Press, London, 1990.

25. Stenchever, MA, TJ Kunysz and MA Allen, "Chromosome Breakage in Users of Marijuana", *American Journal of Obstetrics and Gynecology*, Vol. 118, No. 1, Jan. 1974, pp. 106-113.

26. Siegel, B.Z., Lindley Garnier, and S.M. Siegel, "Mercury in Marijuana", *BioScience*, Vol. 38, Oct. 1988, pp. 619-23.

27. Levy, Stephen J., *Managing the Drugs in Your Life*, McGraw-Hill Publishing Co., New York, 1983.

28. Pearson, Durk, and Sandy Shaw, *Life Extension*, Warner Books, New York, 1982.

29. Enwonwu, C.O. and V.I. Meeks, "Bionutrition and Oral Cancer in Humans", *Crit. Review Oral Bio. Medicine*, Vol. 6, No. 1, 1995, pp. 5-17.

30. Dominguez-Rojas, V. et al, "Spontaneous Abortion in a Hospital Population: Are Tobacco and Coffee Intake Risk Factors?", *European Journal of Epidemiology*, Vol. 10, No. 6, Dec. 1994, pp. 665-8.

31. Hudson, Tori, "Women and Substance Abuse", *Townsend Letter for Doctors and Patients*, No. 151/152, Feb./Mar. 1996, p.158.

32. Behnegar, Atoosa, "The Cigarette Plague", *American Health*, March 1993, pp.11-12.

33. Turk, Michele, "Cutting Heart Attack Risk", *American Health*, March 1993, pp. 12-14.

34. Krogh, David, *Smoking: The Artificial Passion*, W.H. Freeman and Co., New York, 1991.

35. Etzel, RA et al, "Passive Smoking and Middle Ear Effusion Among Children in Day Care", *Pediatrics*, Vol. 90, 1992, pp. 228-232.

36. Abramson, R., "EPA Officially Links Passive Smoke, Cancer", *Los Angeles Times*, Vol. 112, June 8, 1993, p. A27.

37. Janerich, D.T. et al, "Lung Cancer and Exposure to Tobacco Smoke in the Household", *New England Journal of Medicine*, Vol. 323, 1990, pp. 632-6.

38. Hampton, NB, "Smokeless is Not Saltless", *New England Journal of Medicine*, Vol. 312, No. 14, April 11985, pp. 919-920.

39. Roberts, Marjory, "Mouth Cancer from a Morning Gargle?" *U.S. News and World Report*, Vol. 111, July 1, 1991, p. 63.

40. Gloeckner, Carolyn, "From Drinking to Disease", *Current Health*, Vol. 17, Oct. 1990, pp. 23-5.

41. Longnecker, M.P., P.A. Newcomb et al, "Risk of Breast Cancer in Relation to Lifetime Alcohol Consumption", *Journal of the National Cancer Institute*, Vol. 87, No. 12, June 21, 1995, pp. 923-9.

42. Buglass, E., "Links between Alcohol Misuse and Cancers of the Head and Neck", *Professional Nurse*, Vol. 10, No. 12, Sept. 1995, pp. 789-90.

43. Chermack, S.T. and S.P. Taylor, "Alcohol and Human Physical Aggression: Pharmacological Versus Expectancy Effects", *J. Stud. Alcohol*, Vol. 56, No. 4, July 1995, pp. 449-56.

44. Tivis, R., W.W. Beatty, S.J. Nixon and O.A. Parsons, "Patterns of Cognitive Impairment Among Alcoholics: Are There Subtypes?", *Alcohol Clin. Exp. Res.*, Vol. 19, No. 2, April 1995, pp. 496-500.

45. Anderson, RA Jr. et al, "Male Reproductive Tract Sensitivity to Ethanol: A Critical Overview", *Pharmacol. Biochem. Behav.*, Vol. 18, 1983, pp. 305-310.

46. Werbach, Melvin R., "Male Infertility", *Townsend Letter for Doctors and Patients*, No. 147, Oct. 1995, p. 20.

47. Anderson RA Js. et al, "Spontaneous Recovery from Ethanol-Induced Male Infertility", *Alcohol*, Vol. 2, No. 3, 1985, pp. 479-84.

48. Rico, H., "Alcohol and Bone Disease", *Alcohol and Alcoholism*, Vol. 25, No. 4, 1990, pp. 345-352.

49. Lalor, BC, MW France, D. Powell, PH Adams and TB Counihan, "Bone and Mineral Metabolism and Chronic Alcohol Abuse", *Quarterly Journal of Medicine*, Vol. 59, No. 229, May 1986, pp. 497-511.

50. Casagrande, G. and F. Michot, "A Randomized Bone Marrow Study in Alcohol-Dependent Individuals", *Blut.*, Vol. 59, No. 3, Sept. 1989, pp. 231-6.

51. Sandler, RS, "Diet and Cancer: Food Additives, Coffee and Alcohol", *Nutrition and Cancer*, Vol. 4, No. 4, 1983, pp. 273-8.

52. "Beer Drinking and the Risk of Rectal Cancer", *Nutrition Reviews*, Vol. 42, No. 7, July 1984, pp. 244-7.

53. Potter, JD and AJ McMichael, "Alcohol, Beer and Lung Cancer: A Meaningful Relationship?", *International Journal of Epidemiology*, Vol. 13, No. 2, June 1984, pp. 240-2.

54. Savage, D. and J. Lindenbaum, "Anemia in Alcoholics", *Medicine*, Vol. 65, No. 5, Sept. 1986, pp. 322-338.

55. Fortmann, SP et al, "The Association of Blood Pressure and Dietary Alcohol: Differences by Age, Sex and Estrogen Use", *American Journal of Epidemiology*, Vol. 118, No. 4, Oct. 1983, pp. 497-507.

56. Gruchow, HW, KA Sobocinski and JJ Barboriak, "Alcohol, Nutrient Intake, and Hypertension in U.S. Adults", *Journal of the American Medical Association*, Vol. 253, No. 11, March 1985, pp. 1567-70.

57. Gaby, Alan, "Is a Little Alcohol Good for You?", *Townsend Letter for Doctors*, No. 100, Nov. 1991, p. 898.

58. Dadd, Debra Lynn, *Nontoxic and Natural*, Jeremy P. Tarcher Inc., Los Angeles CA, 1984.

59. Thompson, W.G., "Coffee: Brew or Bane?", *American Journal of Medical Science*, Vol. 3308, No. 1, July 1994, pp. 49-57.

60. Shirlow, MJ and CD Mathers, "A Study of Caffeine Consumption and Symptoms: Indigestion, Palpitations, Tremor, Headache and Insomnia", *Int. Journal of Epidemiology*, Vol. 14, No. 2, 1985, pp. 239-248.

61. Greden, JF et al, "Caffeine Withdrawal Headache: A Clinical Profile", *Psychosomatics*, Vol. 21, 1980, pp. 411-8.

62. Silverman, K., SM Evans, EC Strain and RR Griffiths, "Withdrawal Syndrome After the Double-Blind Cessation of Caffeine Consumption", *New England Journal of Medicine*, Vol. 327, 1992, pp. 1109-14.

63. Lang, T. et al, "Relation Between Coffee Drinking and Blood Pressure: Analysis of 6321 Subjects in the Paris Region", *American Journal of Cardiology*, Vol. 52, No. 10, Dec. 1983, pp. 1238-42.

64. Sahl, W.J., S. Glore, P. Garrison, K. Oakleaf and S.D. Johnson, "Basal Cell Carcinoma and Lifestyle Characteristics", *Int. Journal of Dermatology*, Vol. 34, No. 6, June 1995, pp. 398-402.

65. Simon, D., S. Yen and P. Cole, "Coffee Drinking and Cancer of the Lower Urinary Tract", *Journal of the National Cancer Institute*, Vol. 54, No. 3, March 1975, pp. 587-591.

66. Mulvehill, JJ, "Caffeine as Teratogen and Mutagen", *Teratology*, Vol. 8, No. 1, Aug. 1973, pp. 69-72.

67. Weinstein, D., I. Maurer and HM Solomon, "The Effects of Caffeine on Chromosomes of Human Lymphocytes: In Vivo and In Vitro Studies", *Mutation Research*, Vol. 16, No. 4, Dec. 1972, pp. 391-9.

68. Harris, S.S. and B. Dawson-Hughes, "Caffeine and Bone Loss in Healthy Postmenopausal Women", *American Journal of Clinical Nutrition*, Vol. 60, No. 4, Oct. 1994, pp. 573-8.

69. Kiel, DP et al, "Caffeine and the Risks of Hip Fracture: The Framingham Study", *American Journal of Epidemiology*, vol. 132, No. 4, Oct. 1990, pp. 675-684.

70. Palmer, J.R., L. Rosenberg, R.S. Rao and S. Shapiro, "Coffee Consumption and Myocardial Infarction in Women", *American Journal of Epidemiology*, Vol. 141, No. 8, April 15, 1995, pp. 724-31.

71. Wilcox, A., C. Weinberg and D. Baird, "Caffeinated Beverages and Decreased Fertility", *Lancet*, Vol. 2, Nos. 8626-7, Dec. 1988, pp. 1453-6.

Additives

1. Herbert, Victor, and Genell J. Subak-Sharpe (editors), *The Mount Sinai School of Medicine Complete Book of Nutrition*, St. Martin's Press, New York, 1990.

2. Schnare, DW, *The Unpolluting of Men*, Foundation Essay Series, Foundation for Advancements in Science and Education, Los Angeles CA.

3. Saifer, P. and M. Zellerbach, *Detox*, Jeremy P. Tarcher Inc., Los Angeles CA, 1984.

4. Langer, Stephen, "Keeping Environmental Toxins at Bay", *Better Nutrition for Today's Living*, July 1993, pp. 28-32.

5. Allan, Jane E., "Allergic Eaters Warned About Hidden Flavorings", *Health and Science*, March 9, 1994.

6. Null, Gary and Steve, *The New Vegetarian*, William Morrow and Co., New York, 1978.

7. Graham, JR, "Headache Related to a Variety of Medical Disorders", in Appenzeller, O. (ed.), *Pathogenesis and Treatment of Headache*, Spectrum Publications, NY, 1976.

8. "Color Johnny Hyperactive", *Townsend Letter for Doctors*, No. 119, June 1993, pp. 642-4.

9. Roberts, H.J., "Re: Article in Wall Street Journal", *Townsend Letter for Doctors*, No. 112, Nov. 1992, pp. 977-8.

10. Roberts, H.J., "Joint Pain Associated with Aspartame Use", *Townsend Letter for Doctors*, No. 94, May 1991, pp. 375-6.

11. Van den Eeden, S.K., T.D. Koepsell et al, "Aspartame Ingestion and Headaches: A Randomized Crossover Trial", *Neurology*, Vol. 44, No. 10, Oct. 1994, pp. 1787-93.

12. Walton, R.G., R. Hudak and R.J. Greene-Waite, "Adverse Reactions to Aspartame: Double- Blind Challenge in Patients From a Vulnerable Population", *Biol. Psychiatry*, Vol. 34, No. 1-2, July 1-15, 1993, pp. 13-17.

13. "MSG", *Townsend Letter for Doctors*, No. 124, Nov. 1993.

14. Samuels, Adrienne, "Trial Begins on MSG Near-Death", *Townsend Letter for Doctors and Patients*, No. 150, Jan. 1996, p. 17.

15. Bland, Jeffrey, *Your Health Under Siege*, The Stephen Greene Press, Brattleboro VT, 1981.

Mercury

1. Veron et al, "Amalgam Dentaires et Allergies", *J. Biol. Buccale*, Vol. 14, 1986, pp. 83-100.

2. Gordon, "Pregnancy in Female Dentists - A Mercury Hazard", Proceedings of International Conference on Mercury Hazards in Dental Practice, Glasgow Scotland, 1981.

3. Butler, J., Proceedings of the First International Conference on Biocompatibility, 1988.

4. Mandel, Irwin, "Amalgam Hazards - An Assessment of Research", *Journal of the American Dental Association*, Vol. 122, August 1991.

5. Ziff, Sam, *Silver Dental Fillings - The Toxic Time Bomb*, Aurora Press, Santa Fe NM, 1984.

6. Langan, Fan, Hoos, "The Use of Mercury in Dentistry: A Critical Review of the Literature", *Journal of the American Dental Association*, Vol. 115, Dec. 1987, p. 867.

7. W.H.O., "Environmental Health Criteria 118: Inorganic Mercury", World Health Organization, Geneva Switzerland, 1991.

8. Begley, Sharon, and Patricia King, "Drilling for Danger", *Newsweek*, Oct. 15, 1990.

9. Huggins, Hal, and Sharon Huggins, *It's All in Your Head*, Life Sciences Press, Colorado Springs CO, 1986.

10. Heintz, Edwardson, Derand and Birkhed, "Methylation of Mercury From Dental Amalgam and Mercuric Chloride by Oral Streptococci", *Scandinavian Journal of Dental Research*, Vol. 91, 1983, pp. 150-2.

11. Taylor, Joyal, *The Complete Guide to Mercury Toxicity from Dental Fillings*, Scripps Publishing, San Diego CA, 1988.

12. Patterson, J.E., B.G. Weisberg and J.P. Dennison, "Mercury in Human Breath From Dental Amalgam", *Bull. Environ. Contam. Toxicol.*, Vol. 34, 1985, pp. 459-468.

13. Nielsen-Kudsk, F., "Absorption of Mercury Vapor From the Respiratory Tract in Man", *Acta Pharmacol. Toxicol.*, Vol. 23, 1965, pp. 250-62.

14. Till, T. and K. Maaly, "Mercury in Tooth Roots and in Jaw Bones", *ZRW*, Vol. 87, Issue 6, 1978, pp. 288-90.

15. Hanson, Mats, "Why is Mercury Toxic: Basic Chemical and Biochemical Properties of Mercury Amalgam in Relation to Biological Effects", ICBM Conference, Colorado, 1988.

16. Till et al., *Zahnarztl. Welt/Reform*, Vol. 87, 1978, pp. 1130-4.

17. Lorscheider, Fritz L., "Whole-Body Imaging of the Distribution of Mercury Released From Dental Fillings Into Monkey Tissues", *FASEB Journal*, Vol. 4, Nov. 1990, pp. 3256-60.

18. Rowland, I.R., P. Grasso and M.J. Davies, "The Methylation of Mercuric Chloride By Human Intestinal Bacteria", *Experientia*, Vol. 31, 1975, pp. 1064-5.

19. Hanson, Mats, "Amalgam Hazards in Your Teeth", *Journal of Orthomolecular Psychiatry*, Vol. 3, No. 3, Sept. 1983.

20. Stortebecker, Patrick, "Mercury Poisoning from Dental Amalgam - A Hazard to the Human Brain", Karolinska Institute, Stockholm, Sweden.

21. Huggins, Hal, "Observations From the Metabolic Fringe", ICBM Conference, Colorado, 1988.

22. Goyer, R.A., "Toxic Effects of Metals", *Cassarett and Doull's Toxicology - The Basic Science of Poisons*, Macmillan Publishing Co., New York, 1986, pp. 582-609.

23. Nylander et al, Fourth International Symposium Epidemiology in Occupational Health, Como Italy, Sept. 1985.

24. Schaumberger, H.H. and P.S. Spencer, "Clinical and Experimental Studies of Distal Axonopathy - A Frequent Form of Brain and Nerve Damage Produced by Environmental Chemical Hazards", *Annals of New York Academy of Science*, Vol. 329, 1979, pp. 14-29.

25. Nilner, K., S. Akerman and B. Klinge, "Effect of Dental Amalgam Restorations on the Mercury Content of Nerve Tissues", *Acta Odont. Scand.*, Vol. 43, 1985, pp. 303-7.

26. Arvidson, B., "Retrograde Axonal Transport of Mercury in Primary Sensory Neurons Innervating the Tooth Pulp in the Rat", *Acta Neurol. Scan.*, Vol. 82, No. 4, Oct. 1990, pp. 234-7.

27. Schiele, R. et al, "Studies on the Mercury Content in Brain and Kidney Related to Number and Condition of Amalgam Fillings", presented at the "Amalgam - Viewpoints from Medicine and Dental Medicine Symposium", March 12, 1984, Cologne, West Germany.

28. Massler, M. and T.K. Barber, "Action of Amalgam on Dentin", *Journal of the American Dental Association*, Vol. 47, Oct. 1953, pp. 415-22.

29. Halse, A., "Metals in Dentinal Tubules Beneath Amalgam Fillings in Human Teeth", *Arch. Oral Biol.*, Vol. 20, 1975, pp. 87-88.

30. Frykholm, K.O. and E. Odeblad, "Studies on the Penetration of Mercury Through the Dental Hard Tissues Using Hg203 in Silver Amalgam Fillings", Acta Odont. Scand., Vol. 13, 1955, pp. 157-65.

31. Jones, D.W., E.J. Sutton and E.L. Milner, "Survey of Mercury Vapor In Dental Offices in Atlantic Canada", *Canadian Dental Association Journal*, Vol. 4906, 1983, pp. 378-395.

32. Vimy, M.J., Y. Takahashi and F.L. Lorscheider, "Maternal-Fetal Distribution of Mercury Released From Dental Amalgam Fillings", *FASEB Journal*, 1990.

33. Lorscheider and Vimy, *The Lancet*, Vol. 337, May 4, 1991.

34. Denton, Sandra, Proceedings of the First International Conference on Biocompatibility, 1988.

35. Chandler, H.H., N.W. Rupp and G.C. Paffenbarger, "Poor Mercury Hygiene From Ultrasonic Amalgam Condensation", *Journal of the American Dental Association*, Vol. 82, 1971, pp. 553-7.

36. Nixon, G.S. and T.C. Rowbotham, "Mercury Hazards Associated with High Speed Mechanical Amalgamators", *British Dental Journal*, Vol. 131, 1971, pp. 308-11.

37. Soremark, R., O. Ingels, H. Plett and K. Samsahl, "Influence of Some Dental Restorations on the Concentrations of Inorganic Constituents of the Teeth", *Acta Odont. Scand.*, Vol. 20, 1962, pp. 215-224.

38. Svare, C.W., C.W. Frank and K.C. Chan, "Qualitative Measure of Mercury Vapor Emission From Setting Dental Amalgam", *Journal of Dental Research*, Vol. 52, No. 4, 1973, pp. 740-3.

39. Soremark, R., K. Wing, K. Olsson and J. Goldin, "Penetration of Metallic Ions from Restorations Into Teeth, *Journal of Prosthetic Dentistry*, Vol. 20, 1968, pp. 531-540.

40. Reinhardt, J.W., D.B. Boyer et al, "Mercury Vapor Expired After Restorative Treatment: Preliminary Study", *Journal of Dental Research*, Vol. 58, No. 10, 1979, p. 2005.

41. Nicholson, R.J., M.M. Stark and K.B. Soelberg, "Dissemination of Mercury During Preparation and Trituration of Amalgam", *Journal of Prosthetic Dentistry*, Vol. 20, 1968, pp. 248-254.

42. Capdebosq, C.B. and W.N. von der Lehr, "Mercury Leakage During Trituration: An Evaluation of Capsules", *Oper. Dent.*, Vol. 4, 1979, pp. 39-42.

43. Barkmeier, W.W. and R.L. Cooley, "Mercury Leakage During Amalgam Trituration: Evaluation of Reusable Capsules", *Journal of the Indiana Dental Association*, Vol. 60, 1981, pp. 8-11.

44. Brune, D., A. Hensten-Pettersen and H. Beltesbrekke, "Exposure to Mercury and Silver During Removal of Amalgam Restorations", *Scandinavian Journal of Dental Research*, Vol. 88, No. 5, 1980, pp. 460-3.

45. "Mercury Vapor Released During the Removal of Old Amalgam Restorations".

46. Reinhardt, J.W., K.C. Chan and T.M. Schulein, "Mercury Vaporization During Amalgam Removal", *Journal of Prosthetic Dentistry*, Vol. 50, 1983, pp. 62-64.

47. Fisher, A., *Contact Dermatitis*, Lea and Febinger, Philadelphia PA, 1973.

48. Cutright, D.E., R.A. Miller, G.C. Battistone and L.J. Millikan, "Systemic Mercury Levels Caused by Inhaling Mist During High-Speed Amalgam Grinding", *Journal of Oral Medicine*, Vol. 28, 1973, pp. 100-4.

49. Cooley, R.L. and W.W. Barkmeier, "Mercury Vapor Emitted During Ultraspeed Cutting of Amalgam", *Journal of the Indiana Dental Association*, Vol. 57, 1978, pp. 28-31.

50. Gay, D.D., R.D. Cox and J.W. Reinhardt, "Chewing Releases Mercury From Fillings", *Lancet*, Vol. 1, No. 8123, 1979, pp. 985-6.

51. Svare, C.W., L.C. Peterson et al, "The Effect of Dental Amalgams on Mercury Levels in Expired Air", *Journal of Dental Research*, Vol. 60, 1981, pp. 1668-71.

52. Vimy, M.J. and F.L. Lorscheider, "Intra-Oral Air Mercury Released from Dental Amalgam", *Journal of Dental Research*, Vol. 64, No. 8, 1985, pp. 1069-71.

53. Vimy, M.J., A.J. Luft and F.L.Lorscheider, "Estimation of Mercury Body Burden from Dental Amalgam Computer Simulation of a Metabolic Compartment Model", *Journal of Dental Research*, Vol. 65, No. 12, Dec. 1986, pp. 1415-9.

54. Svare, C.W., L.C. Peterson et al, "Dental Amalgam: A Potential Source of Mercury Vapor Exposure", *Journal of Dental Research*, Vol. 59, 1980, p. 341.

55. Emler, B.F. and M. Cardone, "An Assessment of Mercury in Mouth Air", *Journal of Dental Research*, Vol. 64, March 1985, p. 247.

56. Sheppard, A.R. and M. Eisenbud, "Biological Effects of Electric and Magnetic Fields of Extremely Low Frequency", *New York University Press*, 1977.

57. Ott, K. et al., "Mercury Burden Due to Amalgam Fillings", *Dtsch. Zahnarztl. Z.*, Vol. 39, No. 9, 1984, pp. 199-205.

58. Brune, D. "Corrosion of Amalgams", *Scandinavian Journal of Dental Research*, Vol. 89, 1981, pp. 506-514.

59. Skare, I. and A. Engqvist, "Amalgam Restorations - An Important Source of Human Exposure to Mercury and Silver", *Lakartidningen*, Vol. 15, 1992, pp. 1299-1301.

60. Stofen, D., "Dental Amalgam - A Poison in Our Mouth?", *Toxicology*, Vol. 2, No. 4, 1974, pp. 355-8.

61. Sarkar, N.K, G.W. Marshall, J.B.Moser and E.H. Greener, "In Vivo and In Vitro Corrosion Products of Dental Amalgam", *Journal of Dental Research*, Vol. 54, 1975, pp. 1031-8.

62. Marek, M., R.F. Hochman and T. Okabe, "In Vitro Corrosion of Dental Amalgam Phases", *Journal of Biomed. Mater. Research*, Vol. 10, 1976, pp. 789-804.

63. Guthrow, C.E., L.B. Johnson and K.R. Lawless, "Corrosion of Dental Amalgam and Its Component Phases, *Journal of Dental Research*, Vol. 46, 1967, pp. 1372-81.

64. Godfrey, Michael, "Chronic Illness in Association with Dental Amalgam: Report of Two Cases", *Journal of Advancement in Medicine*, Vol. 3, No. 4, Winter 1990.

65. Clarkson, TW, "Biochemical Aspects of Mercury Poisoning", *Journal of Occupational Medicine*, Vol. 10, July 1968, pp. 351-5.

66. Clarkson, TW, "Mercury Poisoning, Clinical Chemistry and Chemical Toxicology of Metals", Amsterdam, Elsevier Science Publishers, 1977, pp. 189-200.

67. Dahhan, SS and H. Orfaly, "Electrocardiographic Changes in Mercury Poisoning", *American Journal of Cardiology*, Vol. 14, 1964, pp. 178-183.

68. Ellis, RW and SC Fang, "Elimination, Tissue Accumulation and Cellular Incorporation of Mecury in Rats Receiving an Oral Dose of 203Hg-Labeled Phenylmercuric Acetate and Mercuric Acetate", *Toxicology and Applied Pharmacology*, Vol. 11, 1967, pp. 104-113.

69. Amin Zaki, L and Clarkson TW et al, "Prenatal Methylmercury Poisoning", *American Journal of Disabled Children*, Vol. 133, 1979, pp. 172-7.

70. Ziff, Michael, "The Missing Link? A Persuasive New Look at Heart Disease as it Relates to Mercury", BioProbe Inc., 1991.

71. Siblerud, Robert, "Evidence That Mercury From Silver Dental Fillings May be an Etiological Factor in Multiple Sclerosis", *The Science of the Total Environment*, Vol. 142, 1994, pp. 191-205.

72. Abraham, J., C. Svare and C. Frank, "The Effects of Dental Amalgam Restorations on Blood Mercury Levels", *Journal of Dental Research*, Vol. 63, No. 1, 1984, pp. 71-73.

73. Gallagher, PJ and RL Lee, "The Role of Biotransformation in Organic Mercury Neurotoxicity", *Toxicology*, Vol. 15, 1980, pp. 129-134.

74. Hanson, Mats (translator), "Amalgam Removal Improves Overall Health and Reduces Health Care Costs", Swedish Health Insurance Bureau, Stockholm, Sweden.

75. Cassano GB, Viola PL, Ghetti B, Amaducci L, "Distribution of Inhaled Mercury (Hg203) Vapor in the Brain of Rats and Mice", *Journal of Neuropathol. Exp. Neurol.*, Vol. 28, pp. 308-20.

76. Fukuda, K, "Metallic Mercury Induced Tremor in Rabbits and Mercury Content of the Central Nervous System", *Br. Journal Ind. Medicine*, Bol. 28, 1971, pp. 308-311.

77. Miller, JM, DB Chaffin and RG Smith, "Subclinical Psychomotor and Neuromuscular Changes in Workers Exposed to Inorganic Mercury", *A. Indus. Hyg. Association Journal*, Vol. 36, 1975, pp. 725-733.

78. Chaffin, DB, BD Dinman, JM Miller, RG Smith and DH Zontine, "An Evaluation of the Effects of Chronic Mercury Exposures on EMG and Psychomotor Functions", National Institute for Occupational Safety and Health, Contract No. HSM-099-71-62, Jan. 1973.

79. Ganote, CE, KA Reimer and RB Jennings, "Acute Mercuric Chloride Nephrotoxicity. An Electron Microscopic and Metabolic Study", *Lab Invest.*, Vol. 31, 1974, pp. 633-47.

80. Shoemaker, HA, "The Pharmacology of Mercury and Its Compounds", *Annals of the New York Academy of Science*, Vol. 65, 1957, pp. 504-510.

81. Cook, TA and PO Cook, "Fatal Mercury Intoxication in Dental Surgery Assistant", *British Dental Journal*, Vol. 127, 1969, pp. 553-5.

82. "Mercury Induced Glomerulonephritis", *Archives of Toxicology*, Vol. 50, 1982, p. 187.

83. Verschoor, MA, RFM Herbert and RL Zielhuis, "Urinary Mercury Levels and Early Changes in Kidney Function in Dentists and Dental Assistants", *Community Dentistry and Oral Epidemiology*, Vol. 16, No. 3, June 1988.

84. Weeden, RP, "Lead, Mercury and Cadmium Nephropathy", Neurotoxicology, Vol. 4, No. 3, 1983, pp. 134-146.

85. Ziff, Sam and Michael Ziff, *Infertility and Birth Defects*, BioProbe Inc., Orlando FL, 1987.

86. Khera et al., "Teratogenic and Genetic Effects of Mercury Toxicity: The Biochemistry of Mercury in the Environment", Nriagu, J.O. (editor), *Amsterdam Elsevier*, 1979, pp. 503-518.

87. Babich et al., "The Mediation of Mutagenicity and Clastogenicity of Heavy Metals by Physiochemical Factors", *Environmental Research*, Vol. 37, 1985, pp. 253-286.

88. "EPA Mercury Health Effects Update Health Issue Assessment", Office of Health and Environmental Assessment, Washington DC.

89. Lee, L.P. and Dixon, "Effects of Mercury on Spermatogenesis", *Journal of Pharmacol. Exp. Thera.*, Vol. 194, No. 1, 1975, pp. 171-181.

90. Kuhnert, P., B.R.R. Kuhnert and P. Erkard, "Comparison of Mercury Levels in Maternal Blood, Fetal Cord Blood and Placental Tissue", *American Journal of Obstetrics and Gynecology*, Vol. 1139, 1981, pp. 209-212.

91. Brodsky, J.B., "Occupational Exposure to Mercury in Dentistry and Pregnancy Outcome", *Journal of the American Dental Association*, Vol. 111, No. 11, 1985, pp. 779-780.

92. Mohamed et al., "Laser Light Scattering Study of the Toxic Effects of Methylmercury on Sperm Motility", *Journal of Androl.*, Vo9l. 7, No. 1, 1986, pp. 11-15.

93. Inouye, M., K. Murao and Y. Kajiwara, "Behavioral and Neuropathological Effects of Prenatal Methylmercury Exposure in Mice", *Neurobehav. Toxicol. Teratol.*, Vol. 7, 1985, pp. 227-232.

94. Koos, BJ and LD Lango, "Mercury Toxicity in Pregnant Women, Fetus and Newborn Infant - A Review", *American Journal of Obstetrics and Gynecology*, Vol. 126, No. 3, 1976, pp. 390-409.

95. Kennedy DC, "Toxics in Dentistry", International Academy or Oral Medicine and Toxicology Scientific Symposium, Atlanta, GA, Sept. 14-15,1990.

96. Synder RD, "Congenital Mercury Poisoning", *New England Journal of Medicine*, Vol. 18, 1971, pp. 1014-16.

97. Rowland et al, "Reduced Fertility Among Dental Assistants with Occupational Exposure to Mercury", *The Toxicologist*, Vol. 12, No. 1, Feb. 1992, p. A246.

98. Panova, Z and G. Dimitrov, "Ovarian Function in Women Having Professional Contact with Metallic Mercury", *Akusherstvoi Ginekologiya*, Vol. 13, No. 1, 1974, pp. 29-34.

99. Mikhailova LM et al, "The Influence of Occupational Factors on Disease of the Female Reproductive Organs", *Pediatriya Akusherstvoi Ginekologiya*, Vol. 33, No. 6, 1971, pp. 56-58.

100. Goncharuk, GA, "Problems Relating to Occupational Hygiene of Women in Production of Mercury", *Gigiena Truda i Professional nye Zabolevaniya*, Vol. 5, 1977, pp. 17-20.

101. Gerhard, B., "Toxic Materials and Infertility: Heavy Metals and Minerals", *Obstetrics and Gynecology*, Vol. 52, 1992, pp. 383-396.

102. Gelbier, S. and J. Ingram, "Possible Fetotoxic Effects of Mercury Vapor: A Case Report", *Public Health*, Vol. 103, No. 1, Jan. 1989, pp. 35-40.

103. Berlin, M., "Prenatal Exposure to Mercury Vapor: Effects on Brain Development", *Fundamentals of Applied Toxicology*, Vol. 19, 1992, pp. 319-329.

104. Wannag, Axel and Julie Skjaersen, "Mercury Accumulation in Placenta and Foetal membranes: A Study of Dental Workers and Their Babies", *Environmental Physiol. Biochem.*, Vol. 5, 1975, pp. 348-352.

105. Fujita, M. and E.T. Takabatake, "Mercury Levels in Human Maternal and Neonate Blood, Hair and Milk", *Bull. Environ. Contam. Toxicol.*, Vol. 18, 1977, pp. 205-9.

106. Vimy, M., L.J. Hahn, R. Klober, Y. Takahashi and F.L. Lorscheider, "Mercury Uptake in Sheep Fetus From Dental Fillings", 32nd annual meeting of the Canadian Federation of Biological Societies, June 14-17, 1989.

107. Soremark, R., D. Misbah and K. Arvidson, "Autoradiographic Study of Distribution Patterns of Metals Which Occur as Corrosion Products From Dental Restorations", *Scandinavian Journal of Dental Research*, Vol. 87, 1979, pp. 450-8.

108. Holt, D., "Comparisons of the Biochemical Effect of Teratogenic Doses of Mercury and Cadmium in the Pregnant Rat", *Arch.Toxicol.*, Vol. 58, 1986, p. 243.

109. Kuntz, WD, RM Pitkin, AW Bostrom and MS Hughes, "Maternal and Cord Blood Background Mercury Levels: A Longitudinal Surveillance", *American Journal of Obstetrics and Gynecology*, Vol. 143, No. 4, 1982, pp. 440-3.

110. Clarkson, TW, L. Magos and MR Greenwood, "The Transport of Elemental Mercury Into Fetal Tissues", *Biol. Neonate*, Vol. 21, 1972, pp. 239-44.

111. Sundberg, Johanna, Agneta Oskarsson and Kerstin Bergman, "Milk Transfer of Inorganic Mercury to Suckling Rats: Interaction With Selenite", *Biological Trace Element Research*, Vol. 28, 1991.

112. Hansen, K. et al., "A Survey of Metal Induced Mutagenicity In Vitro and In Vivo", *Journal of the American Coll. Toxicology*, Vol. 3, 1984, pp. 381-430.

113. Verchaeve, L. et al, "Comparative In Vitro Cytogenetic Studies in Mercury Exposed Human Lymphocytes", *Mutation Research*, Vol. 157, 1985, pp. 221-6.

114. Pelletier, L. et al, "In Vivo Self Reactivity of Mononuclear Cells to T Cells and Macrophages Exposed to $HgCl_2$", *European Journal of Immunology*, 1985, pp. 460-5.

115. Stortebecker, Patrick, *Mercury Poisoning From Dental Amalgam - A hazard to the Human Brain*, Bioprobe Publications, Orlando FL, 1985.

116. Dzeracy, E. and M. Semerdzieva, "A Proposal of Allergization to Silver Amalgam Mercury", *Stomatologiia*, Vol. 55, 1973, 391-4.

117. Djerassi, E. and N. Berova, "The Possibilities of Allergic Reactions from Silver Amalgam Restorations" *Int. Dent. Journal,* Vol. 19, 1969, pp. 481-8.

118. White, RR and RL Brandt, "Development of Mercury Hypersensitivity Among Dental Students", *Journal of the American Dental Association*, Vol. 9, No. 2, pp. 1204-7, 1976.

119. Miller EG, Perry WL, Wagner MJ: "Prevalence of Mercury Hypersensitivity in Dental Students", *Journal of Dental Research*, Vol. 64, March 1985, p. 338.

120. Burrows, D, "Hypersensitivity to Mercury, Nickel and Chromium in Relation to Dental Materials", *Int. Dental Journal*, Vol. 36, 1986, p. 30-4.

121. Simon, E., Buchner A., Bubis JJ, "Asteroid Bodies in Foreign-Body Reaction to Amalgam", *Oral Surgery*, Vol. 33, 1972, pp. 772-4.

122. Nakayama H., Niki F., Shono M, Hada S, "Mercury Exanthem", *Contact Dermatitis,* Vol. 9, No.5, 1983, pp. 411-7.

123. Koller, LD, "Immunotoxicology of Heavy Metals", *Int. Journal of Immunopharmacology*, Vol. 2, 1980, pp. 269-279.

124. Koller, LD, "Immunosuppression Produced by Lead, Cadmium, Mercury", *American Journal of Vet. Research*, Vol. 34, 1973, pp. 1457-8.

125. Fiskesjo, G, "The Effect of Two Organic Mercury Compounds on Human Leukocytes inVitro", *Hereditas*, Vol. 64, 1970, pp. 142-6.

126. Eggleston, DW, "Effect of Dental Amalgam and Nickel Alloys on T-Lymphocytes: Preliminary Report", *Journal of Prosthetic Dentistry*, Vol. 51, 1984, pp. 617-23.

127. Druet, P, F. Hirsch, C. Sapin, E. Druet and B. Bellon, "Immune Dysregulation and Auto- Immunity Induced by Toxic Agents", *Transplantation Proceedings*, Vol. 14, Sept. 1982, pp. 482-4.

128. "Mercury Induced Autoimmunity", *Journal of Immunology*, 1986, pp. 137+.

129. Djerassi, E and N. Berova, "The Possibilities of Allergic Reactions from Silver Amalgam Restorations", *Int. Dental Journal*, vol. 19, 1969, pp. 481-8.

130. Nebenfuhrer, L, S. Korossy, E. Vincze and M. Gozony, "Mercury Allergy in Budapest", *Contact Dermatitis*, Vol. 10, No. 2, 1984, pp. 121-2.

131. Witek, E., "A Case of Hypersensitivity to mercury Released from Amalgam Fillings", *Czas. Stomat.*, Vol. 22, pp. 311-5.

132. Manning, Betsy Russell (editor), *Candida: Silver (Mercury) Fillings and the Immune System*, Greensward Press, San Francisco CA, 1985.

133. James, J, MM Ferguson and A. Forsyth, "Mercury Allergy as a Cause of Burning Mouth", *British Dental Journal*, Vol. 159, 1985, p. 392.

134. Summers, AO, MJ Vimy and F. Lorscheider, "'Silver' Dental Fillings Provoke an Increase in Mercury and Antibiotic Resistant Bacteria in the Mouth and Intestines of Primates", *The Alliance for Prudent Use of Antibiotics*, Vol. 9, No. 3, Fall 1991.

135. Summers, AO, J Wireman, MJ Vimy et al, "Mercury Released from Dental 'Silver' Fillings Provokes an Increase in Mercury and Antibiotic Resistant Bacteria in Primates' Oral and Intestinal Flora", *Antimicrobial Agents and Chemotherapy*, Vol. 37, 1993, pp. pp. 825-834.

136. Huggins, Hal A., *Position Papers: The Amalgam Issue, Root Canals, Cavitations*, Huggins Diagnostic Center, Colorado Springs CO, 1991.

137. Null, Gary, "Mercury Dental Amalgams - Analyzing the Debate", *Townsend Letter for Doctors*, No. 109/110, Aug./Sept. 1992, pp. 760-9.

138. Malmstroum, C. M. Hansson and M. Nylander, Conference on Trace Elements in Health and Disease, Stockholm Sweden, May 25, 1992.

139. Chang, LW and HA Hartman, "Blood-Brain Barrier Dysfunction in Experimental Mercury Intoxication", *Acta Neuropathology*, Vol. 21, 1972, pp. 179-184.

140. Shapiro, IM, AJ Sumner et al, "Neurophysiological and Neuropsychological Function in Mercury-Exposed Dentists", *Lancet*, Vol. 8282, 1982, pp. 1147-50.

141. Chang, LW, "Neurotoxic Effects of Mercury - A Review", *Environmental Research*, Vol. 14, 1977, pp. 329-373.

142. Vroom, FQ and M. Greer, "Mercury Vapor Intoxication", *Brain*, Vol. 95, 1972, pp. 305- 318.

143. Ross, WD, AS Grechman, MC Sholiton et al, "Need for Alertness to Neuropsychiatric Manifestations of Inorganic Mercury Poisoning", *Compr. Psychiatry*, Vol. 18, 1977, pp. 595-8.

144. Siblerud, Robert, "The Relationship Between Mercury From Dental Amalgam and Mental Health", *American Journal of Psychiatry*, Vol. 43, No. 4, Oct. 1989.

145. Siblerud, Robert, "Psychometric Evidence That Mercury from Silver Dental Fillings May Be an Etiological Factor in Depression, Excessive Anger and Anxiety", *Psychological Reports*, Vol. 74, 1994, pp. 67-80.

146. "Multiple Sclerosis", *American Journal of Forensic Path.*, Vol. 4, 1983, p. 55.

147. "MS", *Journal of Epidemol. Comm. Health*, Vol. 32, 1978, p. 155.

148. Ahlrot-Westerlund, *Nutr. Research*, Suppl. 1, 1985, p. 403; Second Nordic Symposium on Trace Elements in Human Health and Disease, Odense Denmark, Aug. 1987.

149. Mayhazati, H., "Psychiatric Aspects of Methyl Mercury Poisoning", *Journal of Neurol. Neurosurg. Psychiatry*, Vol. 37, 1974, pp. 954-8.

150. Kantarjiam, AD, "A Syndrome Clinically Resembling Amyotrophic Lateral Sclerosis Following Chronic Mercurialism", *Neurology*, Vol. 11, 1961, pp. 639-641.

151. "Amyotrophic Lateral Sclerosis", *American Journal of Medicine*, Vol. 53, 1972, p. 219.

152. Barber, TE, "Inorganic Mercury Intoxication Reminiscent of Amyotrophic Lateral Sclerosis", *Journal of Occupational Medicine*, Vol. 20, 1978, pp. 667-9.

153. "Amyotrophic Lateral Sclerosis", *Journal of Occupational Medicine*, Vol. 20, 1978, p. 667.

154. Thompson, CM, WR Markesbery, WD Ehmann, Y-X Mao and DE Vance, "Regional Brain Trace-Element Studies in Alzheimer's Disease", *Neurotoxicology*, Vol. 9, No. 1, 1988, pp. 1-8.

155. Markesbery, WR, WD Ehmann, M Alauddin and T.I.M. Hossain, "Brain Trace Element Concentrations in Aging", *Neurobiology of Aging*, Vol. 5, 1984, pp. 19-28.

156. Ehmann, WD, WR Markesbery, M Alauddin, T.I.M. Hossain and EH Brubaker, "Brain Trace Elements in Alzheimer's Disease", *Neurotoxicology*, Vol. 7, No. 1, 1986, pp. 196-206.

157. Ehmann, WD et al, "Application of Neutron Activation Analysis to the Study of Age Related Neurological Diseases", *Biological Trace Element Research*, Vol. 13, 1987, pp. 19-33.

158. Duhr, E., C. Pendergrass, E. Kasarskis, J. Slevin and B. Haley, "Hg 2+ Induces GTP-Tuberculin Interactions in Rat Brain Similar to Those Observed in Alzheimer's Disease", *FASEB* meeting, Atlanta GA, April 21-25, 1991, Abstract 493.

159. Bjorklung, G., "Mercury as a Potential Source for the Etiology of Alzheimer's Disease", *Trace Element Medicine*, Vol. 8, No. 4, 1991, p. 208.

160. Wenstrup, D., Ehmann, WD and WR Markesbery, "Trace Element Imbalances in Isolated Subcellular Fractions of Alzheimer's Disease Brains", *Brain Research*, Vol. 533, 1990, pp. 125-131.

161. Smith, DL, "Mental Effects of Mercury Poisoning", *South. Medical Journal*, Vol. 71, 1978, pp. 904-5.

162. "Mercury in Fish", *Bulletin of W.H.O.*, Vol. 64, No. 5, 1986, p. 634.

162a. "Board Investigates Mercury-Free Dentistry", *FDA Hotline*, Oct. 1995.

163. "Dental Group Agrees With FDA and EPA on Issue of Toxic Mercury", *Townsend Letter for Doctors*, No. 88, Nov. 1990, p. 720.

164. "Amalgam Moratorium Called For", *Townsend Letter for Doctors*, No. 109/110, Aug./Sept. 1992, pp. 734-6.

165. Siblerud, Robert L., "The Relationship Between Mercury from Dental Amalgam and Oral Cavity Health", *Townsend Letter for Doctors*, No. 100, Nov. 1991, pp. 901-2.

166. Gerhard, P., H. Waldberenner et al, "Diagnosis of Heavy Metal Loading by the Oral DMPS and Chewing-Gum Tests", *Clinical Lab*, Vol. 38, 1992, pp. 404-411.

167. Campbell, J.R., Clarkeson, T.W. and M.D. Omar, "The Therapeutic Use of 2,3-Dimercaptopropane-1-Sulfonate in Two Cases of Inorganic Mercury Poisoning", *Journal of the American Medical Association*, Vol. 256, 1986, pp. 3127-30.

168. Aposhian, H.V. et al, "Urinary Mercury After Administration of 2,3-Dimercaptopropane-1- Sulfonic Acid: Correlation With Dental Amalgam Score", *FASEB Journal*, Vol. 6, No. 6, 1992, pp. 2472-6.

169. Friedheim, E. et al, "Meso-Dimercaptosuccinic Acid: A Chelating Agent for the Treatment of Mercury and Lead Poisoning", *Journal of Pharm. Pharmac.*, Vol. 28, 1976, pp. 711-2.

170. Fournier, L., "2,3-Dimercaptosuccinic Acid Treatment of Heavy Metal Poisoning in Humans", Medical Toxicology, Vol. 3, pp. 499-504.

171. Graziano, J.H., "Role of 2,3-Dimercaptosuccinic Acid in the Treatment of Heavy Metal Poisoning", *Medical Toxicology*, Vol. 1, 1986, pp. 155-162.

172. Hahn et al, *The FASEB Journal*, Vol. 3, Dec. 1989, pp. 2643+.

173. Danscher, G., P. Horsted-Bindslev and J. Rungby, "Traces of Mercury in Organs from Primates with Amalgam Fillings", *Exp. Mol. Pathol.*, Vol. 52, 1990, pp. 2911-9.

174. Friberg, L., L. Kullman, B. Lind and M. Nylander, "Mercury in the Central Nervous System in Relation to Dental Amalgam", Lakartidningen, Vol. 83, 1986, pp. 519-22.

175. Nylander, M. et al, "Mercury Concentration in the Human Brain and Kidneys in Relation to Exposure From Dental Amalgam Fillings", *Swedish Dental Journal*, Vol. 11, 1987, pp. 179-187.

176. Nylander, M., "Mercury in Pituitary Glands of Dentists", *Lancet*, Vol. 442, Feb. 22, 1986.

177. Eggleston, D.W., M. Nylander et al, "Correlation of Dental Amalgam with Mercury in Brain Tissue", *Journal of Prosthetic Dentistry*, Vol. 58, 1987, pp. 704-7.

178. Joselow, M.M., L.J. Goldwater, A. Alvarez and J. Herndon, "Absorption and Excretion of Mercury in Man - Occupational Exposure Among Dentists", *Archives of Environmental Health*, Vol. 17, 1968, pp. 39-43.

179. Stock, A. and F. Cucuel, "The Mercury Content of Human Excretions and Human Blood", *Zeitschr. Angew. Chem.*, Vol. 47, 1934, pp. 641-7.

180. Joselow, M.M., L.J. Goldwater, A. Alvarez and J. Herndon, "Absorption and Excretion of Mercury in Man - Salivary Excretion of Mercury and Its Relationship to Blood and Urine Mercury", *Archives of Environmental Health*, Vol. 17, 1968, pp. 35-38.

181. Hursh, JB, TW Clarkson and MG Cherian et al, "Clearance of Mercury (Hg-197, Hg-203) Vapor Inhaled by Human Subjects", *Archives of Environmental Health*, Vol. 31, 1976, pp. 302-9.

182. Goldwater, LJ, AC Ladd and MB Jacobs, "Absorption and Excretion of Mercury in Man: Significance of Mercury in Blood", *Archives of Environmental Health*, Vol. 9, 1964, pp. 835+.

183. Molin, Margareta, "Mercury Released From Dental Amalgam in Man", *Swedish Dental Journal Suppl.*, Vol. 71, 1990.

184. Hoover, AW. and LJ Goldwater, "Absorption and Excretion of Mercury in Man - Dental Amalgams as a Source of Urinary Mercury", *Archives of Environmental Health*, Vol. 12, 1966, pp. 506-8.

185. Siedlicki, JT, "Long-Term Exposure of Dentist to Mercury", *Journal of Oral Medicine*, Vol. 25, 1971, p. 93.

186. Weening, JJ et al, "Mercury Induced Immune Complex Glomerulopathy: An Experimental Study", *VanDendergen*, 1980, pp. 36-66.

187. Wong, S., "Effectiveness of Special Garlic Preparation on Dental Patients With Mercury Restorations", *Health Consciousness*, 1982.

188. Pallotti, G, B. Bencivenga and T. Simonetti, "Total Mercury Levels in Whole Blood, Hair and Fingernails for a Population Group from Rome and its Surroundings", *Sci. Total Environ.*, Vol. 11, 1979, pp. 69-72.

189. Reinhardt, JW, DB Boyer et al, "Exhaled Mercury Following Removal and Insertion of Amalgam Restorations", *Journal of Prosthetic Dentistry*, Vol. 49, 1983, pp. 652-6.

190. Berlin, MH, GF Nordberg and F. Serenius, "On The Site and Mechanism of Mercury Vapor Resorption in the Lung", *Archives of Environmental Health*, Vol. 18, 1969, pp. 42-50.

191. Ziff, Sam, Michael Ziff and Mats Hansen, *Mercury Detoxification*, BioProbe Inc., Orlando FL, 1990.

192. Dickey, LD, *Clinical Ecology*, Charles C. Thomas, Springfield IL, 1976, pp. 294-5.

193. U.S.E.P.A. Mercury Effects Update, Final Report, 1984, EPA-600/8-84-019F.

194. Socialstyrelsen Report, May 20, 1987 as reported in Svenska Dagbladet Bioprobe 4, June 1987, Issue 3.

195. Simonsen, RJ and NA Landy, "Preventive Resin Restorations: Fracture Resistance and Seven Year Clinical Results", *Journal of Dental Research*, Vol. 63, Abstract #39, March 1984.

196. Loe, Harold, "Research in Progress: Voices from NIDR", *Dentistry Today*, Sept. 1993.

197. Leverett, DH, CM Brenner, SL Hendelman and HP Iker, "Use of Sealants in the Prevention and Treatment of Early Carious Lesions: Cost Analysis", *Journal of the American Dental Association*, Vol. 106, 1983, pp. 39-42.

198. Cataldo, E. and H. Santis, "Response of the Oral Tissue to Exogenous Foreign Materials", *Journal of Periodontology*, Vol. 45, 1974, pp. 93-106.

199. Nasjleti, CE, WA Castelli and RG Caffesse, "Effects of Amalgam Restorations on The Periodontal Membrane in Monkeys", *Journal of Dental Research*, Vol. 56, 1977, pp. 1127-31.

200. Larsen, TO, WM Douglas and RE Geistfield, "Effect of Prepared Cavities on the Strength of Teeth", *Operative Dentistry*, Vol. 6, 1981, pp. 2-5.

201. Kanca, J., "The Single Visit Heat Processed Indirect Composite Resin Inlay", *Journal of Esthetic Dentistry*, Oct. 1988, pp. 31-34.

202. Hornbrook, DSM "Direct Composite Resin Inlay Technique and Materials", *Esthetic Dentistry Update*, Vol. 1, No. 1, April 1990.

203. Wendt, S., "The Effect of Heat Used as a Secondary Cure Upon the Physical Properties of Three Composite Resins", *Quint. Int.*, Vol. 18, pp. 265-271.

204. Foundation for Toxic Free Dentistry, *Dental and Health Facts*, Vol. 6, No. 1, January 1993, pp. 1-2.

Nickel and Root Canals

1. Manning, Betsy Russell (editor), "Benefits of Electroacupuncture by Voll", *Candida, Silver Mercury Fillings, and the Immune System*, Greensward Press, San Francisco CA, 1985, pp. 69-71.

2. Medical Immunotoxicology / Immunologic Consequences of Poisoning.

3. "Nickel May Pose Health Hazard", *Dentistry Today*, April 1985, p. 8.

4. Casarett and Doull, *Toxicology*, Macmillan Publishing Company, New York, 3rd edition, 1986.

5. Balch, James F. and Phyllis A. Balch, *Prescription for Nutritional Healing*, Avery Publishing Group, Garden City Park, NY, 1990.

6. Huggins, Hal, *Position Papers: Amalgam Issue, Root Canals, Cavitations*, Huggins Diagnostic Inc., Colorado Springs CO, 1991.

7. Huggins, Hal, "The Hazards of Root Canal", *Townsend Letter for Doctors*, No. 87, Oct. 1990, pp. 659-60.

Other Metals

1. Shroeder, Henry A., *The Poisons Around Us*, Indiana University Press, Bloomington IN, 1974.

2. Shroeder, Henry A., *The Trace Elements and Man*, The Devin-Adair Co., Old Greenwich CT, 1973.

3. Klotter, Jule, "Lead Poisoning", *Townsend Letter for Doctors*, No. 107, June 1992, p. 533.

4. Campbell, Joseph D., "Hair Tissue Mineral Analysis: A Review", *Townsend Letter for Doctors*, No. 118, May 1993, pp. 436-44.

5. Pirkle, JL et al, "The Relationship Between Blood Lead Levels and Its Cardiovascular Risk Implications", *American Journal of Epidemiology*, Vol. 121, No. 2, Feb. 1985, pp. 246-258.

6. Glauser, SC, CT Bello and EM Gauser, "Blood Cadmium Levels in Normotensive and Untreated Hypertensive Humans", *Lancet*, Vol. 1, April 1976, pp. 717-8.

7. "Acid Rain, Aluminum, and Alzheimer's Disease", *The Futurist*, Vol. 21, Jan/Feb. 1987, p. 36.

8. Campbell, Joseph D., "Aluminum and Alzheimer's Disease", *Townsend Letter for Doctors*, No. 108, July 1992, pp. 624-5.

9. Neri, LC and D. Hewitt, "Aluminum, Alzheimer's Disease and Drinking Water", *Lancet*, Vol. 338, 1991, p. 390.

10. Martyn, CN et al, "Geographical Relation between Alzheimer's Disease and Aluminum in Drinking Water", *Lancet*, Vol. 1, 1989, pp. 59-62.

11. Zatta, P. et al, "Alzheimer Dementia and the Aluminum Hypothesis", *Medical Hypotheses*, Vol. 26, 1988, pp. 139-142.

12. McLachlan, DRC et al, "Intramuscular Desferrioxamine in Patients with Alzheimer's Disease", *Lancet*, Vol. 337, 1991, pp. 1304-8.

13. Ward, NI and JA Mason, "Neutron Activation Analysis Techniques for Identifying Elemental Status in Alzheimer's Disease", *Journal of Radioanalytical Nuclear Chemistry*, Vol. 113, No. 2, 1987, pp. 515-526.

14. Wenk, GL and KL Stemmer, "Suboptimal Dietary Zinc Intake Increases Aluminum Accumulation Into the Rat Brain", *Brain Research*, Vol. 288, 1983, pp. 393-5.

15. Balch, James F. and Phyllis A. Balch, *Prescription for Nutritional Healing*, Avery Publishing Group, Garden City Park, NY, 1990.

16. Jackson, J.A., H.D. Riordan, and C.M. Poling, "Aluminum From A Coffee Pot", *Lancet*, Vol. 1, 1989, pp. 781-2.

17. Millichap, J. Gordon, *Environmental Poisons In Our Food*, PNB Publishers, Chicago IL, 1993.

18. Harrison, DP, "Copper as a Factor in the Dietary Precipitation of Migraine", *Headache*, Vol. 26, No. 5, 1986, pp. 248-250.

19. Nieper, Hans A., "Catalytic Converters and Chronic Fatigue Syndrome", *Townsend Letter for Doctors*, No. 96, July 1991, pp. 546-7.

Metal Detoxification

1. Clarkson, Thomas W., "Some Naturally Occurring Detoxification Systems", *Mercury Free News*, Vol. 5, No. 2, May 1992, p. 12.

2. "N-Acetylcysteine: More Than a Mucolytic", *Capsulations*, No. 19, Nov. 1990.

3. Hruby, K., and A. Donner, "2,3-Dimercapto-1-Propanesulfate in Heavy Metal Poisoning", Poison Information Center, University of Vienna, Austria, 1987, pp. 317-323.

4. Cutler, Paul, "Desferoxamine Therapy in High-Ferritin Diabetes", *Diabetes*, Vol. 38, Oct. 1989, pp. 1207-1210.

5. *BioProbe Newsletter*, Nov. 1989, p. 6.

6. Olszewer, E., and Carter, J.P., "EDTA Therapy in Chronic Degenerative Disease", *Medical Hypotheses*, Vol. 27, No. 1, Sept. 1988, pp. 41-49.

7. The Burton Goldberg Group, "Chelation Therapy", pp. 126-133, *Alternative Medicine: The Definitive Guide*, Future Medicine Publishing, Inc., Puyallup WA, 1994, pp. 126-133.

8. Farr, CH, R. White and M. Schacter, "Chronological History of EDTA Chelation Therapy". Presented to the American College of Advancement in Medicine, Houston TX, May 1993.

9. Olszewer, E. and JP Carter, "EDTA Chelation Therapy: A Retrospective Study of 2,870 Patients", in *A Textbook on EDTA Chelation Therapy*, Elmer M. Cranton (ed.), *Journal of Advancement in Medicine*, Vol. 2, NOs. 1-2, Human Sciences Press, NY, 1989, pp. 197-211.

10. Alsleben, HR and WE Shute, *How To Survive The New Health Catastrophes*, Survival Publications Inc., Anaheim CA, 1973.

11. Casdorph, HR, "EDTA Chelation Therapy: Efficacy in Brain Disorders", in *A Textbook on EDTA Chelation Therapy*, Elmer M. Cranton (ed.), *Journal of Advancement in Medicine*, Vol. 2, Nos. 1-2, Human Sciences Press, NY, 1989, pp. 131-153.

12. McDonagh, E., C. Rudolph and E. Cheraskin, "An Oculocerebrovasculometric Analysis of the Improvement in Arterial Stenosis Following EDTA Chelation Therapy", in *A Textbook on EDTA Chelation Therapy*, Elmer M. Cranton (ed.), *Journal of Advancement in Medicine*, Vol. 2, Nos. 1-2, Human Sciences Press, NY, 1989, p. 155.

13. The Burton Goldberg Group, *Alternative Medicine: The Definitive Guide*, "Cadmium Toxicity", pp. 896-7, Future Medicine Publishing, Puyallup WA, 1994.

Battery Effect

1. The Burton Goldberg Group, *Alternative Medicine: The Definitive Guide*, "Biological Dentistry", Future Medicine Publishing, Puyallup WA, 1994, pp. 88-9.

2. Ziff, Sam, *Silver Dental Fillings - The Toxic Time Bomb*, Aurora Press, Santa Fe NM, 1986. Chapter 5, "Do We Really Have Electricity In Our Mouths?", pp. 65-70.

3. Schoonover, IC and W. Souder, "Corrosion of Dental Alloys", *Journal of the American Dental Association*, Vol. 28, Aug. 1941.

4. Chase, H.S., "Some Observations and Experiments Connected With Oral Electricity", *American Journal of Dental Science*, Vol. 12, 1878, pp. 18-23.

5. Palmer, SB, "Dental Decay and Filling Materials Considered in Their Electrical Relations", *American Journal of Dental Science*, Vol. 12, 1878, pp. 105-111.

6. Lippman, *Deutsche Med. Wchnschr.*, 1930.

7. Ullman, *Wein. Klin. Wchnschr.*, 1932.

8. Freidlander, *Monat. F. Zahnheilk*, 1932.

9. Hyams, BL, *International Journal of Orthodontia*, 1933.

10. Macdonald, *New England Journal of Medicine*, 1934.

11. Rattner, *Arch. Derm. and Syph.*, 1935.

12. Lain, ES and GS Caughron, "Electrogalvanic Phenomena of the Oral Cavity Caused By Dissimilar Metallic Restorations", *Journal of the American Dental Association*, Vol. 23, Sept. 1936.

13. Lain, ES, W. Schriever and GS Caughron, "Problems of Electrogalvanism in the Oral Cavity Caused By Dissimilar Dental Metals", *Journal of the American Dental Association*, Vol. 27, Nov. 1940.

14. Solomon, HA, MC Reinhard and HI Goodale, "The Possibility of Precancerous Oral Lesions from Electrical Causes", *Dental Digest*, Vol. 39, April 1933, pp. 142-4.

15. Hyams, BL and HC Ballon, "Dissimilar Metals in the Mouth as a Possible Cause of Otherwise Unexplainable Symptoms", *Canadian Medical Association Journal*, Vol. 29, Nov. 1993, pp. 488-491.

16. Huggins, Hal A., "Proposed Role of Dental Amalgam Toxicity in Leukemia and Hematopoietic Dyscrasias", *International Journal of Biosocial and Medical Research*, Vol. 11, No. 1, 1989, pp. 84-93.

17. Huggins, Hal, and Sharon Huggins, *It's All in Your Head*, Life Sciences Press, Colorado Springs CO, 1986.

18. Taylor, Joyal, *The Complete Guide to Mercury Toxicity from Dental Fillings*, Scripps Publishing, San Diego CA, 1988.

Radiation - Basic Concepts

1. Becker, Robert O., *Cross Currents*, Jeremy P. Tarcher Inc., Los Angeles CA, 1990.

2. Schechter, Steven R., *Fighting Radiation with Foods, Herbs, and Vitamins*, East West Health Books, Brookline MA, 1988.

3. Handler, Sheldon Saul, *The Oxygen Breakthrough*, William Morris and Co., NY, 1989.

4. Lee, Lita, *Radiation Protection Manual*, Grassroots Network, Redwood City CA, 1990, 3rd ed.

5. Wadsworth, Chloe, "Electromagnetic Radiation and What You Can Do To Neutralize Its Harmful Effects", *Townsend Letter for Doctors*, No. 114, Jan. 1993, pp. 14-15.

Radiation - Electricity

1. Maugh, Thomas H., "Studies Stir Fears Over Cancer Risk for Children", *Los Angeles Times*, Nov. 8, 1992, p. A3.

2. Brodeur, Paul, *The Great Power-Line Cover-Up*, Little, Brown, and Co., New York, 1993.

Radiation - Other Frequencies

1. *McGraw-Hill Encyclopedia of Science and Technology*, McGraw-Hill Book Co., 7th ed., 1992.

2. Ott, John Nash, *Light, Radiation, and You*, The Devin-Adair Co., Old Greenwich CT, 1982.

3. "New Study Shows Driving and Dialing As Dangerous as Driving and Drinking", *Townsend Letter for Doctors and Patients*, No. 151/152, Feb./Mar. 1996, p. 41.

4. Freeman, Ira M., *Light and Radiation*, Random House, NY, 1968.

5. Gofman, John W., *Preventing Breast Cancer: The Story of a Major, Proven, Preventable Cause of the Disease*, Committee for Nuclear Responsibility, San Francisco CA, 1995.

6. Sharn, Lori, "Fliers Face Increased Risk from Radiation", *USA Today*.

7. Jule Klotter, "Food Irradiation", *Townsend Letter for Doctors*, No. 121/122, Aug./Sept. 1993, p. 816.

8. Millichap, J. Gordon, *Environmental Poisons In Our Food*, PNB Publishers, Chicago IL, 1993.

9. Schechter, Steven R., *Fighting Radiation with Foods, Herbs, and Vitamins*, East West Health Books, Brookline MA, 1988.

Structural

1. The Burton Goldberg Group, *Alternative Medicine: The Definitive Guide*, "Carpal Tunnel Syndrome", pp. 898-900, Future Medicine Publishing, Puyallup WA, 1994.

2. Dworkin, Barry et al, "Behavioral Method for the Treatment of Idiopathic Scoliosis", *Proceedings of the National Academy of Science*, April 1985, pp. 2493-7.

3. Altman, Nathaniel, *Everybody's Guide to Chiropractic Health Care*, Jeremy P. Tarcher Inc., Los Angeles CA, 1990.

4. Langone, John, *Chiropractors: A Consumer's Guide*, Addison-Wesley Publishing Co., Reading MA, 1982.

5. Tousley, Dick, *The Chiropractic Handbook for Patients*, White Dove Publishing Co., Kansas City MO, 1983.

6. Feitis, R., *Ida Rolf Talks About Rolfing and Physical Reality*, Rolf Institute, Boulder CO, 1978.

7. Rolf, Ida P., *Rolfing: The Integration of Human Structures*, Harper and Row Publishers, NY, 1977.

8. Rolf, Ida P., *Structural Integration: Gravity, An Unexplored Factor in a More Human Use of Human Beings*, Rolf Institute, Boulder CO, 1962.

9. Juhan, Deane, "The Trager Approach", *The Trager Journal*, Vol. 2, Fall 1987, pp. 1-3.

10. Barlow, Wilfred, *The Alexander Technique*, Alfred A. Knopf, NY, 1973.

11. Jones, Frank Pierce, "Body Awareness in Action" in Murphy, M., *The Future of the Body*, Jeremy P. Tarcher Inc., Los Angeles CA, 1992.

Structural / Cranial / Dental

1. Upledger, John, *Your Inner Physician and You: Craniosacral Therapy SomatoEmotional Release*, North Atlantic Books, Berkeley CA, 1992.

2. Biser, Sam, and Dean Howell, "Cranial Therapy: The Most Neglected Treatment in Natural Healing", *The Last Chance Health Report*, Vol. 4, No. 3, 1994, pp. 1-7.

3. Manning, Betsy Russell (editor), *Candida, Silver Mercury Fillings, and the Immune System*, Greensward Press, San Francisco CA, 1985, pp. 163-5.

4. Price, Weston A., *Nutrition and Physical Degeneration*, The Price-Pottinger Nutrition Foundation Inc., La Mesa CA, 1945, 1970.

5. Wang, K., "A Report of 22 Cases of Temporomandibular Joint Dysfunction Syndrome Treated With Acupuncture and Laser Radiation", *Journal of Traditional Chinese Medicine*, Vol. 12, No. 2, June 1992, pp. 116-8.

6. Gole, Daniel R., "The Resultant Force Vector Technique (RFV)", West Michigan Pain Seminars, Hastings MI, 1993.

7. Porterfield, Kay Marie, "Jaws", *Current Health*, Vol. 16, Jan. 1990, pp. 12-13.

8. Kaplan, Andrew S. and Gary Williams, "Self-Help for TMJ", *Prevention*, Vol. 40, Nov. 1988, pp. 46-54.

9. "TMJ - When Your Joint is Out of Joint", *Prevention*, Vol. 38, March 1986, pp. 46-7.

Microorganisms

1. *McGraw-Hill Encyclopedia of Science and Technology*, McGraw-Hill Book Co., 1992, 7th ed.

2. Bland, Jeffrey, "New Perspectives in Nutritional Therapies", Seminar held Feb. 4, 1996, Los Angeles CA.

3. Pacific Research Distributors, Inc. (information sheets), 1990, 1991.

4. Sapolsky, Robert M. , "Why You Feel Crummy When You're Sick", *Discover*, July 1990, pp. 66-70.

5. Todd, SC et al, "Cryptosporidium and Giardia in Surface Water In and Around Manhattan, Kansas", *Transactions of the Kansas Academy of Science*, Vol. 94, Nos. 3-4, 1991, pp. 101-6.

6. Graham, Barbara, "A New Bug in Town", *Health*, Oct. 1990, pp. 38-40.

7. Shepherd, R.W. and P.F.L. Boreham, "Recent Advances in the Diagnosis and Management of Giardiasis", *Scand. J. Gastroenterology*, 1989, Vol. 24, pp. 60-64.

8. The Burton Goldberg Group, *Alternative Medicine: The Definitive Guide*, "Parasitic Infections", pp. 782-9, Future Medicine Publishing, Puyallup WA, 1994.

Amoebas and Protozoa

1. Juranek, Dennis, "Giardiasis", Centers for Disease Control, Division of Parasitic Infection, Atlanta GA.

2. Keystone, JS et al, "Intestinal Parasites in Metropolitan Toronto Day Care Centers", *Canadian Medical Association Journal*, Vol. 131, No. 7, 1984, pp. 733-5.

3. Spencer, MJ et al, "Parasitic Infections in a Pediatric Population", *Pediatric Infectious Diseases*, Vol. 2, No. 2, March/April 1983, pp. 110-3.

4. Schmidt, Gerald D, and Larry S. Roberts, *Foundations of Parasitology*, Times Mirror/Mosby College Publishing, St. Louis MO, 3rd ed., 1985.

5. Galland, Leo, "Intestinal Protozoan Infection is a Common Unsuspected Cause of Chronic Illness", *Journal of Advancement in Medicine*, Vol. 2, No. 4, Winter 1989, pp. 539-552.

6. Weller, Peter F., "Amebiasis and Giardiasis are Indigenous - and Spreading", *Consultant*, April 1983, pp. 115+.

7. "Giardiasis and You", County of San Diego, California Dept. of Health Services, Sept. 1987 (pamphlet).

8. Parrish, Louis, "The Protozoal Syndrome", *The Nutrition and Dietary Consultant*, March 1991, pp. 5+.

9. Galland, Leo, Marty Lee, Hermann Bueno, and Colette Heimowitz, "Giardia Lamblia Infection as a Cause of Chronic Fatigue", *Journal of Nutritional Medicine*, Vol. 1, 1990, pp. 27-31.

10. Troiano, Linda, "Stomach Distress from a Gut-Gripping Bug", *Redbook*, August 1990, pp. 32-34.

11. Beaver, Paul Chester, *Animal Agents and Vectors of Human Disease*, Lea and Febinger, Philadelphia PA, 5th ed. 1985.

12. Pacific Research Distributors, Inc. (info. sheets), 1990, 1991.

13. Shepherd, R.W. and P.F.L. Boreham, "Recent Advances in the Diagnosis and Management of Giardiasis", *Scand. J. Gastroenterology*, 1989, Vol. 24, pp. 60-64.

14. The Burton Goldberg Group, *Alternative Medicine: The Definitive Guide*, "Sexually Transmitted Diseases", pp. 827-837, Future Medicine Publishing, Puyallup WA, 1994.

15. Willmott, F. et al, "Zinc and Recalcitrant Trichomoniasis", *Lancet*, Vol. 1, No. 8332, May 1983, p. 1053.

16. Russo, A.R., S.L. Stone, M.E. Taplin, H.J. Snapper, and G.V. Doern, "Presumptive Evidence for Blastocystis Hominis as a Cause of Colitis", *Archives of Internal Medicine*, May 1988, Vol. 148, No. 5, p. 1064.

17. Guirges, S.Y., N.S. Al-Waili, "Blastocystis Hominis: Evidence for Human Pathogenicity and Effectiveness of Metronidazole Therapy", *Clinical Exp. Pharmacol. Physiol.*, April 1987, Vol. 14, No. 4, pp. 333-5.

18. Diaczok, B.J., J. Rival, "Diarrhea Due to Blastocystis Hominis: An Old Organism Revisited", *Southern Medical Journal*, July 1987, Vol. 80, No. 7, pp. 931-2.

19. Rosenbaum, Michael and Murray R. Susser, *Solving the Puzzle of Chronic Fatigue Syndrome*, Life Sciences Press, Tacoma WA, 1992.

20. Turner, J.A., *Parasitic Disease Newsletter*, Fall 1984.

Worms

1. Seaton, Kenneth, "Allergies", High Technology Hygiene Inc., Costa Mesa CA, May 1990 (info. sheet).

2. Leventhal, R. and R.F. Cheadle, *Medical Parasitology: A Self-Instructional Text*, F.A. Davis Company, Philadelphia PA, 3rd ed., 1989.

3. Schmidt, Gerald D, and Larry S. Roberts, *Foundations of Parasitology*, Times Mirror / Mosby College Publishing, St. Louis MO, 3rd ed., 1985.

4. Beaver, Paul Chester, *Animal Agents and Vectors of Human Disease*, Lea and Febinger, Philadelphia PA, 5th ed. 1985.

5. Pacific Research Distributors, Inc. (info. sheets), 1990, 1991.

6. *McGraw-Hill Encyclopedia of Science and Technology*, McGraw-Hill Book Co., 1992, 7th ed.

7. Smith, Alice Lorraine, *Principles of Microbiology*, C.V. Mosby Co., St. Louis MO, 9th ed., 1981.

Bacteria

1. Smith, Alice Lorraine, *Principles of Microbiology*, C.V. Mosby Co., St. Louis MO, 9th ed., 1981.

2. *Fact Acts*, Food Animal Concerns Trust, Chicago IL (newsletter).

3. Rodolsky, Doug M., "Kill the Bug and You Kill the Ulcer". *U.S. News and World Report*, Vol. 110, May 13, 1991, p. 94.

4. McAuliffe, Kathleen, "In the Belly of the Bug", *Omni*, Vol. 12, Aug. 1990, pp. 20+.

5. Foley, Denise, "Ulcers: On the Brink of a Cure", *Prevention*, Vol. 39, May 1987, pp. 49-52.

6. Cerda, James J., Mae F. Go and Tadataka Yamada, "Peptic Ulcer Disease: Now You Can Cure", *Patient Care*, Dec. 15, 1995, pp. 101+.

7. Wallach, Joel, "Dead Doctors Don't Lie" (tape).

8. Purvis, Andrew, "Cancer from Germs", *Time*, Vol. 138, Oct. 28, 1991, p. 88.

9. "Allergies Linked to Same Germ That Can Cause Peptic Ulcers", *Health and Science*, March 9, 1994.

10. Bland, Jeffrey, "New Perspectives in Nutritional Therapies", Seminar held Feb. 4, 1996, Los Angeles CA.

11. Laino, C., "H. Pylori Implicated In Allergies", *Medical Tribune*, March 24, 1994, p. 1.

12. Gaby, Alan R., "Does Helicobacter Pylori Cause Allergies?", *Townsend Letter for Doctors*, No. 132, July 1994, p. 713.

13. Thrasher, Jack and Alan Broughton, *The Poisoning Of Our Homes and Workplaces*, Seadora, Inc., 1989.

14. Fraser, DW, Tsai TF, Orenstein W. et al, "Legionnaire's Disease: Description of an Epidemic", *New England Journal of Medicine*, Vol. 297, 1977, p. 1189.

15. Bennett, Dawn D., "Pelvic Inflammatory Disease: Pill Risk", *Science News*, Vol. 127, April 27, 1985, p. 263.

16. Gibbons, Wendy, "Clueing in on Chlamydia", *Science News*, Vol. 139, April 20, 1991, pp. 150-2.

17. Boyd, Elizabeth, "What is Chlamydia?", *Ms.*, Vol. 14, Feb. 1986, pp. 64-6.

18. Rapp, Ellen, "Chlamydia: The Sexual Disease Your Body Keeps Secret", *Mademoiselle*, Vol. 92, Feb. 1986, p. 80.

19. "Comprehensive Digestive Stool Analysis", Great Smokies Diagnostic Laboratory, Asheville NC, 1994.

20. Ebringer, A., S. Khalafpour et al, *Rheumatology Int.*, Vol. 9, 1989, pp. 223-8.

21. Ebringer, A., N. Cox et al, *British Journal of Rheumatology*, Vol. 27, 1988, pp. 72-85.

22. Begley, Sharon, "The End of Antibiotics", *Newsweek*, March 28, 1994, pp. 46-52.

23. Lappe, Marc, *When Antibiotics Fail*, North Atlantic Books, Berkeley CA, 1986.

24. Neu, HC, "The Crisis in Antibiotic Resistance", Science, Vol. 257, 1992, pp. 1064-73.

25. Cohen, SR and JW Thompson, "Otitic Candidiasis in Children: An Evaluation of the Problem and Effectiveness of Ketoconazole in 10 Patients", *Annals of Otology, Rhinology, and Laryngology*, Vol. 99, 1990, pp. 427-431.

Viruses

1. Fettner, Ann Giudici, *Viruses: Agents of Change*, McGraw-Hill Publishing Co., New York, 1990.

2. Smith, Alice Lorraine, *Principles of Microbiology*, C.V. Mosby Co., St. Louis MO, 9th ed., 1981.

3. *McGraw-Hill Encyclopedia of Science and Technology*, McGraw-Hill Book Co., 1992, 7th ed.

4. Pizzorno, Joseph E. and Michael T. Murray, *A Textbook of Natural Medicine*, John Bastyr College Publications, Seattle WA, 1989.

5. Neiman, DC et al, "The Effects of Moderate Exercise Training on Natural Killer Cells and Acute Upper Respiratory Tract Infections", *International Journal of Sports Medicine*, Vol. 11, No. 6, 1990.

6. Cohen, S., DA Tyrell and AP Smith, "Psychological Stress and Susceptibility to the Common Cold", *New England Journal of Medicine*, Vol. 325, Aug. 1991, pp. 606-612.

7. *Harvard Mental Health Letter*, Vol. 8, No. 7, Jan. 1992.

8. Pennebaker, JW, *Opening Up: The Healing Power of Confiding in Others*, Avon, NY, 1991.

9. Tutelian, Louise, "Herpes Update", *New York*, Vol. 24, June 3, 1991, pp. 55-6.

10. Brown, Zane A., "Mom's Symptomless Herpes Threatens Baby", *Science News*, Vol. 139, June 22, 1991, p. 398.

11. SerVaas, Cory, "Baylor College Lysine-Herpes Study", *The Saturday Evening Post*, Vol. 258, Dec. 1986, pp. 108-9.

12. Pompei, R. et al, "Glycyrrhizic Acid Inhibits Virus Growth and Inactivates Virus Particles", *Nature*, Vol. 281, No. 5733, Oct. 1979, p. 690.

13. The Burton Goldberg Group, *Alternative Medicine: The Definitive Guide*, "Cold Sores", pp. 905-7, Future Medicine Publishing, Puyallup WA, 1994.

14. Valnet, Jean, *The Practice of Aromatherapy*, Healing Arts Press, Rochester VT, 1980.

15. Derman, RJ, "Counseling the Herpes Genitalis Patient", *Journal of Reproductive Medicine*, Vol. 31, Suppl. 5, May 1986, pp. 439-444.

16. Fackelmann, Kathy, "Herpes, HIV and the High Risk of Sex", *Science News*, Vol. 141, Feb. 1, 1992, p. 68.

17. Cowen, Ron, "Herpes May Disarm Immune System", *Science News*, Vol. 137, May 26, 1990, p. 326.

18. Berton, Paul, "A New Theory on Herpes", *Maclean's*, Vol. 99, Dec. 15, 1986, p. 61.

19. Dix, Richard, "Killer Herpes", *USA Today*, Vol. 1114, Oct. 1985, p. 3.

20. Kaura, S.R., *Understanding and Preventing Cancer*, HealthPress, Santa Fe NM, 1991.

21. Silberner, Joanne, "AIDS: A Role for CMV?", *Science News*, Vol. 130, Oct. 11, 1986, p. 238.

22. Melnick, Joseph L., "CMV and Heart Disease", *Science News*, Vol. 137, May 5, 1990, p. 277.

23. Ellison, James Whitfield, "A Separate Peace", *American Health*, Vol. 9, May 1990, pp. 64-8.

24. Fackelmann, Kathy, "Survival Bonus for People with AIDS", *Science News*, Vol. 140, Oct. 26, 1991, p. 260.

25. Jones, James F., "Chronic Fatigue Syndrome", *The Human Ecologist*, No. 38, pp. 16-19.

26. Stoff, Jesse A. and Charles R. Pellegrino, *Chronic Fatigue Syndrome: The Hidden Epidemic*, Random House, New York, 1988.

27. Pacific Research Distributors, Inc. (information sheets), 1990, 1991.

28. "Chronic Epstein-Barr Virus Infections and Persistent Illness", *Research Perspectives in Allergy and Immunology*.

29. Holland, Lee, "The ABCs of Hepatitis", *Good Housekeeping*, Vol. 212, April 1991, p. 239.

30. Tanne, Janice Hopkins, "The Other Plague (Hepatitis B)", *New York*, Vol. 21, July 11, 1988, pp. 34-40.

31. Whitman, Sylvia, "Hepatitis", *Current Health*, Vol. 18, Sept. 1991, pp. 12-13.

32. Thyagarajan, S.P. et al, "Effect of Phyllanthus Amarus on Chronic Carriers of the Hepatitis B Virus", *The Lancet*, Oct. 1, 1988, p. 764.

33. Findlay, Steven, "Herpes, AIDS, and Now a Cancer Virus", *U.S. News and World Report*, Vol. 105, Oct. 24, 1988, p. 80.

34. Eisenberg, Steve, "From One Lover to Another: The Infection That Can Lead to Cancer", *Health*, Vol. 20, Sept. 1988, pp. 62-64+.

35. Webb, Lillian Frier, "Venereal Warts", *Essence*, Vol. 19, March 1989, p. 12.

36. Fackelmann, Kathy, "The Cervical Dilemma", *Science News*, Vol. 139, June 8,1991, pp. 362-3.

37. The Burton Goldberg Group, *Alternative Medicine: The Definitive Guide*, "Sexually Transmitted Diseases", pp. 827-837, Future Medicine Publishing, Puyallup WA, 1994.

HIV and AIDS

1. Adler, Jerry, "Living with the Virus: When and How HIV Turns Into AIDS", *Newsweek*, Vol. 118, Nov. 18, 1991, pp. 63-4.

2. Alexander, Susan, and Jennifer Rapaport, "The Real AIDS Numbers", *Mademoiselle*, Vol. 98, March 1992, p. 104.

3. Duesberg, Peter H., "AIDS Acquired by Drug Consumption and Other Noncontagious Risk Factors", *Pharm. and Therap.*, Vol. 55, 1992, pp. 210-277.

4. Duesberg, Peter H., "Infectious AIDS - Stretching the Germ Theory Beyond Its Limits", *Int. Arch. Allergy Immunol.*, Vol. 103, 1994, pp. 131-142.

5. Greene, Warner C., "AIDS and the Immune System", *Scientific American*, Vol. 269, No. 3, Sept. 1993, pp. 99-105.

6. Montagna, Richard, "HTLV-1: A New AIDS-like Threat?" *The Saturday Evening Post*, Vol. 261, July/Aug. 1989, pp. 82+.

7. Fettner, Ann Giudici, *Viruses: Agents of Change*, McGraw-Hill Publishing Co., New York, 1990.

8. Beardsley, Tim, "Multiple Choice", *Scientific American*, Vol. 260, April 1989, pp. 34-5.

9. Iwakura, Yoichiro, Mariko Tosu, and Emi Yoshida, "Induction of Inflammatory Arthropathy Resembling Rheumatoid Arthritis in Mice Transgenic for HTLV-1", *Science*, Vol. 253, Aug. 30, 1991, pp. 1026-8.

10. Clark, Matt, "AIDS's Cancerous Cousin", *Newsweek*, Vol. 109, June 8, 1987, p. 73.

11. Fennell, Tom, "What Causes AIDS", *Maclean's*, Vol. 105, June 1, 1992, pp. 32-3.

12. Duesberg, Peter and John Yiamouyiannis, *AIDS*, Health Action Press, Delaware OH, 1995.

13. Brady, Diane, "New AIDS Doubts", *Maclean's*, Vol. 103, Nov. 12, 1990, p. 68.

14. Lauritsen, John, *The AIDS War: Propaganda, Profiteering and Genocide From the Medical-Industrial Complex*, Pagan Press, NY, 1993.

15. Duesberg, Peter H., "The HIV Gap in National AIDS Statistics", *Biotechnology*, Vol. 11, 1993, pp. 955-6.

16. Merson, MH, "Slowing the Spread of HIV: Agenda for the 1990s", *Science*, Vol. 260, 1993, pp. 1266-8.

17. Goudsmit, Jaap, "Alternative View on AIDS", *Lancet*, Vol. 339, 1992, pp. 1289-90.

18. Duesberg, Peter and John Yiamouyiannis, *AIDS*, Health Action Press, Delaware OH, 1995.

19. Weiss, SH, JJ Goedert, S. Gartner et al, "Risk of Human Immunodeficiency Virus (HIV) Infection Among Laboratory Workers", *Science*, Vol. 239, 1988, pp. 68-71.

20. Duesberg, Peter H., "Does HIV Cause AIDS?", *Journal of AIDS*, Vol. 2, 1989, pp. 514-5.

21. Duesberg, Peter H., "Human Immunodeficiency Virus and Acquired Immunodeficiency Syndrome: Correlation But Not Causation", *Proc. Natl. Academy of Science*, Vol. 86, 1989, pp. 755-764.

22. Duesberg, Peter H., "AIDS Epidemiology: Inconsistencies With Human Immunodeficiency Virus and With Infectious Disease", *Proc. Natl. Academy of Science*, Vol. 88, 1991, pp. 1575-9.

23. Evans, AS, "Does HIV Cause AIDS? An Historical Perspective", *Journal of AIDS*, Vol. 2, 1989, pp. 107-113.

24. Duesberg, Peter H., *Cancer Research*, March 1, 1987.

25. Nowak, Martin A., Roy M. Anderson, and Angela R. McLean, "Antigenic Diversity Thresholds and the Development of AIDS, *Science*, Vol. 254, Nov. 15, 1991, pp. 963-9.

26. Nowak, Rachel, "Diversity Equals Death", *Discover*, Vol. 13, May 1992, p. 16.

27. Findlay, Steven, "The Shock of the New", *U.S.News and World Report*, Vol. 113, Aug. 3, 1992, p. 14.

28. Redfield, Robert R. and Donald S. Burke, "HIV Infection: The Clinical Picture", *Scientific American*, Vol. 259, Oct. 1988, pp. 90-8.

29. Day, Lorraine, "AIDS Plague", Oct. 14, 1991 [tape].

30. Ascher, MS, HW Sheppard, et al, "Does Drug Use Cause AIDS?", *Nature* (London), Vol. 362, 1993, pp. 103-4.

31. Duesberg, Peter H., "Can Epidemiology Determine Whether Drugs or HIV Cause AIDS?", *AIDS Forschung*, Vol. 12, 1993, pp. 627-635.

32. Schechter, MT, KJ Kraib, et al, "HIV-1 and the Etiology of AIDS", *Lancet*, Vol. 341, 1993, pp. 658-9.

33. Marmor, M.., Friedman-Kien, AE et al, "Risk Factors for Kaposi's Sarcoma in Homosexual Men", *Lancet*, 1982, pp. 1083-7.

34. Jaffe, HW, K. Choi et al, "National Case-Control Study of Kaposi's Sarcoma and Pneumocystis Carinii Pneumonia in Homosexual Men", *Annals of Internal Medicine*, Vol. 99, 1983, pp. 145-151.

35. Newell, GR, P. Mansell et al, "Risk Factor Analysis Among Men Referred for Possible Acquired Immune Deficiency Syndrome", *Preventive Medicine*, Vol. 14, 1985, pp. 81-91.

36. Duesberg, Peter and John Yiamouyiannis, *AIDS*, Health Action Press, Delaware OH, 1995.

37. Terry, CE and M. Pellens, The Opium Problem, Bureau of Social Hygiene of New York, 1928.

38. Crook, William, *The Yeast Connection*, Professional Books, Jackson TN, 1984.

39. Chaitow, Leon and N. Trenev, *Probiotics*, HarperCollins, NY, 1990.

40. Silberner, Joanne, "Chipping Away at AIDS", *U.S. News and World Report*, Vol. 108, April 9, 1990, p. 47.

41. Walker, Tim, "AIDS Dementia: Neurons Nixed by Virus, *Science News*, Vol. 139, May 18, 1991, p. 311.

42. Gregory, Scott J., *A Holistic Protocol for the Immune System*, Tree of Life Publications, Palm Springs CA, 1989.

43. Kolata, G., "Imminent Marketing of AZT Raises Problems; Marrow Suppression Hampers AZT Use in AIDS Victims", *Science*, Vol. 235, 1987, pp. 1462-3.

44. Kolata, G., "After Five Years of Use, Doubt Still Clouds Leading AIDS Drug", *The New York Times*, June 2, 1992.

45. Mantera-Tienza, E. et al, "Low Vitamin B6 in HIV Infections", *Fifth International Conference on AIDS*, June 1989, p. 468.

508

46. Herbert, Victor, "Vitamin B12, Folate and Lithium in AIDS".

47. Harriman, G. et al, "Vitamin B12 Malabsorption in AIDS", *Archives of Internal Medicine*, Vol. 149, No. 9, 1989, pp. 2039-41.

48. Dworkin, Barry et al, "Selenium Deficiency in AIDS", *Journal of Parenteral and Enteral Nutrition*, Vol. 10, No. 4, 1986, pp. 405-7.

49. Fabris, N. et al, "AIDS, Zinc Deficiency andThymic Hormone Failure", *Journal of the American Medical Association*, Vol. 259, 1988, pp. 839-840.

50. Cathcart, Robert, "Vitamin C in the Treatment of AIDS", *Medical Hypotheses*, Vool. 14, 1984, pp. 432-4.

51. "AIDS 1982-1992. Hope and Challenge of 10 Years of LSU AIDS Therapy with Ozone and a Multimodal Treatment Program", *Townsend Letter for Doctors*, Aug./Sept. 1995, pp. 52-61.

52. Schleicher, "Application of Ultraviolet Blood Irradiation for Treatment of HIV and Other Bloodborne Viruses", *Townsend Letter for Doctors and Patients*, No. 147, Oct. 1995, pp. 66-72.

53. Bisaccia, E., C. Berger and A. Klainer, "Extracorporeal Photopheresis in the Treatment of AIDS-Related Complex"", *Annals of Internal Medicine*, Vol. 113, pp. 270-5.

54. Spire, B. et al, "Inactivation of Lymphadenopathy-Associated Virus by Heat, Gamma Rays, and Ultraviolet Light", *Lancet*, Vol. 1, No. 8422, Jan. 1985, pp. 188-9.

55. Weatherburn, H., "Hyperthermia and AIDS Treatment", *British Journal of Radiology*, Vol. 61, No. 729, Sept. 1988, p. 862.

56. Standish, Leanna, et al, "One Year Open Trial of Naturopathic Treatment of HIV Infection Class IV-A in Men", *Journal of Naturopathic Medicine*, Vol. 3, No. 1, 1992, pp. 42-64.

57. Nault, K., "AIDS, Cancer - An Answer (Ozone Therapy)", report in *Crosswinds*, Santa Fe NM, Dec. 1988.

58. Well, K. et al, "Inactivation of Human Immunodeficiency Virus Type I by Ozone in Vitro", *Blood*, Vol. 78, 1991, pp. 1882-90.

59. Vallancien, Bertrand and Jean-Marie Winkler, "Immunomodulating Effect of Ozone Among Patients With AIDS", *Conference Report*, NY, 1989.

60. Adetumbi, M. et al, "Allium Sativum: A Natural Antibiotic", *Medical Hypotheses*, Vol. 12, 1983, pp. 227-237.

61. Vahora, S et al, "Medicinal Use of Indian Vegatables", *Planta Medica*, Vol. 23, 1973, pp. 381-393.

62. "Garlic in Cryptoccal Meningitis", *Chinese Medical Journal*, Vol. 93, 1980, pp. 123-6.

63. Brekhmann, E., *Man and Biologically Active Substances*, Pergamon Press, London England, 1980.

64. Takada, A. et al, "Restoration of Radiation Injury by Ginseng", *Journal of Radiation*, Vol. 22, 1981, pp. 323-5.

65. Meruelo, D. et al, "Therapeutic Agents with Dramatic Retroviral Activity", *Proceedings of the National Academy of Sciences*, Vol. 85, 1988, pp. 5230-4.

66. Zhang, QC, "Preliminary Report on the Use of Momordica Charantia Extract by HIV Patients", *Journal of Naturopathic Medicine*, Vol. 3, No. 1, 1992, pp. 65-69.

67. Hierholzer, J. et al, "In Vitro Effects of Monolaurin Compounds on Enveloped RNA and DNA Viruses", *Journal of Food Safety*, Vol. 4, No. 1, 1982.

68. Aoki, T. et al, "Antibodies to HTLV-1 and HTZLV-3 in Sera From Two Japanese Patients", *Lancet*, Vol. 20, Oct. 1984, pp. 936-7.

69. NADA Newsletter Committee, *National Acupuncture Detoxification Association Newsletter*, Dec. 1992, pp. 1-6.

70. Orman, D. and D. Margetis, "Effectiveness of Acupuncture and Chinese Phytomedicals in the Treatment of HIV and AIDS", *Journal of Naturopathic Medicine*, Vol. 3, No. 1992, pp. 80-82.

71. Smith, Michael and N. Rabinowitz, "Acupuncture Treatment of AIDS", Lincoln Hospital Acupuncture Clinic, NY, March 1985.

72. Smith, Michael, "Research in Use of Acupuncture With AIDS", *American Journal of Acupuncture*, Vol. 16, No. 2, April-June 1988.

73. Chaitow, Leon and S. Martin, *A World Without AIDS*, Thorsons, London, 1989, p. 131.

Mycoplasmas

1. *McGraw-Hill Encyclopedia of Science and Technology*, McGraw-Hill Book Co., 1992, 7th ed.

2. Smith, Alice Lorraine, *Principles of Microbiology*, C.V. Mosby Co., St. Louis MO, 9th ed., 1981.

3. Taylor-Robinson, David, and Joseph G. Tully, "Sexual Mycoplasmas", *Science News*, Vol. 131, Sept. 20, 1986, p. 184.

4. Ezzell, Carol, "New Evidence Supports a Cofactor in AIDS", *Science News*, Vol. 139, March 2, 1991, p. 133.

5. McKenzie, Aline, "An AIDS-Associated Microbe Unmasked", *Science News*, Vol. 136, Dec. 2, 1989, p. 356.

6. Silberner, Joanne, "Chipping Away at AIDS", *U.S. News and World Report*, Vol. 108, April 9, 1990, p. 47.

Fungi

1. Smith, Alice Lorraine, *Principles of Microbiology*, C.V. Mosby Co., St. Louis MO, 9th ed., 1981.

Yeast Infections

1. Buttram, Harold E., "Overuse of Antibiotics and the Need for Alternatives", *Townsend Letter for Doctors*, No. 100, Nov. 1991, pp. 867-72.

2. Hilton, E., "Ingestion of Yogurt as Prophylaxis for Candidal Vaginitis", *Annals of Internal Medicine*, Vol. 116, 1992, pp. 353-7.

3. Crook, William G., *Chronic Fatigue Syndrome and the Yeast Connection*, Professional Books, Jackson TN, 1992.

4. Hunt, Douglas, *No More Cravings*, Warner Books, New York, 1987.

Closure

1. LeShan, Lawrence, *Cancer as a Turning Point: A Handbook for People with Cancer, Their Families and Health Professionals*, Plume, NY, 1990.

2. Seligman, ME, *Learned Optimism*, Alfred A. Knopf, NY, 1991.

3. Achterberg, J., *Imagery in Healing: Shamanism and Modern Medicine*, Shambala, Boston MA, 1985.

Index

Mouth sores, 130
Mouthwash, 74, 78, 84, 108, 109, 119, 149
Mucous membranes, 84, 95, 106, 185, 214, 231, 368, 377, 395, 436
Mucus, 215, 216, 356, 362, 363, 366, 382
Multiple Chemical Sensitivity, 57, 366
Multiple sclerosis (MS), 5, 52-54,75, 191, 208, 209, 231, 242, 266, 326, 341, 342, 385, 411
Muscle, 16, 17, 39, 42, 43, 53, 91, 111, 133, 136, 138, 164, 187, 193, 202, 217, 248-250, 257, 261, 262, 267, 288, 302-307, 309, 311-318, 321, 324-327, 329, 332, 335-337, 339-341, 353, 363, 366, 376, 453, 454
Muscle cramps, 187, 193, 267
Muscle spindle bundle fiber, 325
Muscle testing, 321357
Muscle weakness, 43, 63, 67, 78, 187, 193, 217, 228, 261, 282, 286, 340, 453, 454
Muscular dystrophy, 5, 326
Musculoskeletal, 302, 316
Mushrooms, 27, 42, 423, 430, 437, 441
Musk, 75
Mutation, 388, 411
Myalgia, 363
Mycoplasmas, 351, 392, 427, 428
Mycoses, 430, 431
Myelin sheath, 42, 53, 75, 419
Myrrh, 440

-N-

N-acetylcysteine, 240
NAET allergy treatment, 49, 322, 459
Nail products, 82
Nailbiting, 348, 352, 371, 377
Nails, 82, 352, 356, 359, 361, 372, 374, 430, 431
Narcotics, 126
Nasal polyps, 194, 248
Nasal specific therapy, 330, 332, 342, 343
Nausea, 38, 54, 56, 66, 70, 91, 110, 111, 120, 128, 130, 140, 144, 149, 156, 169, 170, 217, 228, 234, 242, 337, 362, 365, 369, 373, 405
Near field, 271, 283
Neck, 302-304, 306, 308-313, 315-317, 319-321, 326, 327, 331, 334, 336, 341, 352, 436
Neckaches, 215, 307
Necrosis, 43, 44, 67, 366431
Nerve, 3, 28, 29, 35, 41, 42, 52, 53, 57, 62, 65, 67, 75, 136, 167, 185, 186, 219, 231, 232, 248, 250, 257, 294, 303, 305, 306, 308, 311-315, 317-320, 322-324, 326, 331, 335, 341, 394, 395, 399, 401, 419, 459
Nervous system, 4, 6, 27, 28, 31, 36, 37, 41, 42, 52, 54, 60, 66-68, 74, 78, 167, 187, 190, 204, 226, 246, 248, 261, 267, 287, 306, 327, 368, 432
Neuro-Emotional Therapy (NET), 322, 326
Neurological effects, 110, 111, 191, 382, 419
Neurons, 13, 14
Neurotransmitter, 42, 43, 135, 144, 167, 191, 192
Niacin, 48
Nickel, 4, 20, 47, 53, 77, 118, 121, 144, 148, 176, 178, 185, 193, 194, 204, 205, 207, 213-224, 229, 232, 247, 266, 335, 336, 341, 342, 417, 428, 453, 461
Nickel carbonyl, 216
Nicotine, 142-144, 147
Night sweats, 422, 423
NIOSH, 196
Nitrates, 101, 165, 166
Nitrogen, 20, 27, 36, 40, 69, 70, 88, 89, 93, 95, 96, 166, 191, 412

Nitrogen oxides, 89, 93
Noise, 30, 272, 279, 354, 450
Nonionizing radiation, 260
Noradrenaline, 42
Norepinephrine, 42
Nose, 56, 89, 91, 132, 185, 194, 232, 248, 332, 333, 342, 359, 361, 368, 432
Nose fatigue, 77
Nose picking, 352
Nosocomial infection, 388
NSAIDs, 127, 134
Nuclear medicine, 293
Nuclear radiation, 255
Nucleus, 13, 21, 216, 393, 430
Numbness, 187, 209, 222, 305, 333
Nutrients, 4, 5, 7, 20, 43, 48, 124-126, 135, 151, 164, 170, 219, 279, 294, 295, 317, 369, 420, 422
Nutrisweet (see Aspartame)
Nutrition, 9, 10, 170, 205, 406, 462, 463
Nuts, 400, 431, 441
Nystatin, 127, 439

-O-

Occiput, 312316
Oil, 4, 31, 35, 44, 48, 52, 60, 64, 65, 69, 70, 74-76, 80-83, 91, 93, 106, 118, 134, 136, 137, 148, 151, 152, 161, 166, 168, 193, 218, 297, 318, 338, 361, 362, 400, 419, 440, 448
Oleic acid, 440
Olfactory, 76, 232
Omega-3 oils, 148
Optimism, 208, 417
Oral contraceptives, 387
Organic, 11, 20, 51, 100, 102, 103, 160, 163, 165, 171, 177, 183, 184, 216, 233, 316, 432
Organic chemicals, 26, 51-58, 62, 105
Organic compounds, 43, 75, 89, 103, 105, 183
Organic produce, 61, 163
Organophosphate pesticides, 62, 65
Orthodontia, 321, 331, 336, 341
OSHA, 57, 95, 195, 196
Osteoarthritis (also see Arthritis), 134, 369
Osteopathy, 3, 302, 306, 316, 320, 322-324, 328, 329, 331, 336, 338, 450, 459
Osteoporosis, 5, 46, 112, 133, 151, 156, 239
Ott, John Nash, 282, 286, 298
Outlook, 190, 417, 455, 456
Overweight, 4, 39, 60, 70, 137, 151
Oxidant, 18, 94
Oxygen, 17, 20, 21, 26, 32, 34, 36, 37, 40, 41, 48, 51, 56, 65, 66, 69, 82, 88, 92, 93, 95, 100, 104-106, 120, 121, 136, 144, 149, 177, 187, 191-193, 197, 201, 216, 381, 421, 459
Ozone, 40, 88, 89, 94, 95, 104, 106, 397, 421, 422, 440

-P-

PABA, 137
Pacemaker, 246-248, 282
PAH, 47
Pain, 3, 5, 39, 42, 45, 53, 56, 61, 66, 111, 126, 130-132, 134, 136, 140, 155, 156, 170, 187, 194, 205, 209, 217, 219, 221, 222, 228, 230, 233, 242, 248, 250, 303, 305-308, 310, 312-314, 316, 317, 319-321, 324-326, 332-334, 337, 339, 340, 352, 354, 363, 369, 376, 382, 384, 385, 399, 445, 453, 454
Pain relievers, 132, 338
Paint, 26, 27, 29, 30, 32, 38, 40, 45, 52, 54, 63, 69, 80, 91, 96, 177, 178, 197, 226, 227, 229, 232, 233, 285, 286, 288, 456

Sun Chlorella, 49, 98, 243, 297
Sunburn, 95, 120, 288, 367, 383
Sunglasses, 30, 278, 285-289
Sunlight, 78, 88, 93, 286-288
Sunlight sensitivity, 78, 319, 337, 438
Sunscreen, 80
Supplements, 15, 22, 53, 58, 70, 112, 124, 136, 227, 230, 234, 241, 397, 440, 454, 455, 460
Surgery, 35, 104, 241, 244, 288, 323, 324, 342, 360, 363, 371, 373, 382, 406
Sweat, 48, 62, 82, 203, 209, 235, 243, 418, 422
Sweat glands, 82
Sweetener, 166, 168, 169, 209
Swelling, 5, 133, 385, 405, 431
Swollen glands, 187, 368, 399
Sympathetic nervous system, 4, 5, 31, 78, 279, 306, 308, 353, 419
Symptom-suppressing drugs, 131, 132, 135
Synapse, 42
Synthetic vitamins, 170
Syphilis, 129, 388

-T-

T cells, 411, 412, 414, 423
T4, 307, 393, 414, 423
Tablets, 108, 110, 112, 132, 155, 203
Tagamet, 65
Tai Chi, 98, 322, 325
Talc, 85, 119
Tampons, 74, 83, 84, 294
Tapeworm, 372, 375
Tar, 119, 141, 144
Tartrazine, 167, 318
Tea, 218, 243, 440, 441
Tea tree oil (melaleuca), 83, 440
Teeth, 4, 46, 84, 85, 100, 109-112, 115, 152, 184, 185, 194, 198, 201-209, 215, 217, 219-222, 238, 241, 247, 248, 250, 289, 302, 312, 321, 331-340, 342, 363, 458, 460
Teflon, 109, 232
Television (TV), 261, 270, 273, 275, 278, 280-282, 296, 450
Temperature, 113, 182, 186, 187, 190, 206, 230, 235, 283, 284, 353, 412, 421, 439
Temporomandibular joint *(see TMJ/TMD)*
Tendons, 111, 326
Testosterone, 127, 144, 188, 230
Tetracycline, 45, 127, 132, 367, 382, 383, 387, 389, 438
Tetrahydrocannabinol (THC), 141
Thalidomide, 132
Theobromine, 154
Theophylline, 127, 154
Thermography, 284
Thermometer, 182, 184, 185
Thimerosal, 47
Thriving In A Toxic World, 35, 46, 49, 93, 98, 111, 122, 126, 130, 132, 136, 137, 152, 154, 169, 171, 205, 208, 210, 294, 296, 320, 395, 403, 414, 423, 440, 446, 448, 452, 459
Throat, 56, 89, 128, 144, 145, 147, 215, 216, 306, 342, 362, 396, 399, 432, 454
Thrush, 436
Thymus, 285, 400, 414, 421, 423
Thyroid gland, 21, 104, 113, 127, 137, 187, 189, 190, 228, 230, 234, 284, 285, 289, 293, 296, 306, 319, 352, 387
Thyroxin, 190
Timidity, 190, 191
Tin, 43, 47
Tinea, 430
Tingling, 187, 209, 245, 246, 249

Tinnitus, 132
TMJ/TMD, 217, 249, 302, 309, 312, 316, 319, 323, 331, 334-338, 341-343
Tobacco, 69, 84, 96, 97, 118, 123, 124, 138, 141-150, 157, 195, 218, 258, 437
Toluene, 28, 46, 54, 75, 119, 404
Tonsillitis, 399
Tonsils, 448
Tooth decay, 100, 114
Toothpaste, 74, 80, 84, 100, 108-110, 115, 119, 226, 232
"Tourist trots", 379, 385
Toxic attitudes, 456
Toxic Immune Syndrome, 5, 34, 49, 442, 459, 461
Toxic Immune Syndrome Cookbook, 442
Toxoplasmosis, 355, 368
Trager work, 326, 330
Transfer factor, 397, 402, 421, 459
Transformer, 260, 261, 266, 269-272, 287
Transformer effect, 287
Trapezius muscles, 307, 316, 319, 326
Tremors, 54, 75, 153, 187, 217, 228
Trichinosis, 355, 372, 375, 376
Trichomonas, 83, 368, 369
Trigeminal neuralgia, 209
Triglycerides, 137
Trophozoite, 360, 361, 366
Tropical diseases, 350
Tryptophan, 136, 197
Tuberculosis, 90, 129, 388, 389
Tumor, 113, 122, 130, 216, 283, 284, 290, 291, 460
TV *(see Television)*
Tylenol *(see Acetaminophen)*
Tyrosine, 137

-U-

Ulcers, 64, 65, 125, 134, 135, 187, 216, 217, 249, 307, 324, 363, 379, 382, 431
Ultrasound, 202, 279-281, 323, 325
Ultraviolet (UV), 94, 95, 256, 285, 288, 289, 421, 422
Uric acid, 398
Urinary tract infection, 385, 386
Urination, 45, 156, 187, 242, 307, 386, 438
Urine, 19, 44, 45, 67, 70, 120, 167, 198, 200, 236, 238, 240, 377, 380, 405, 438
Urine tests, 198, 236, 238
Urticaria *(see Hives)*
Uterus, 262, 305, 308, 386, 428

-V-

Vaccination, 395, 397
Vaccine, 396, 397, 404, 413, 414
Vacuum, 201, 269, 272
Vagina, 355, 368, 399, 405, 436, 439
Vaginal deodorants, 83
Vaginal discharge, 368, 386, 436
Vaginal odor, 83
Vaginitis, 437-439
Valence, 15, 17, 18, 94, 102, 176, 183, 209
Valium, 125, 126
Valve, 317
Vanadium, 97
Varicose veins, 307
Vegetables, 61, 63, 137, 161, 163, 168, 294, 355, 356, 440
Vegetarian diet, 21, 422
Veins, 36, 204, 205, 238, 283, 291, 292, 305, 324

-W-

-X-

-Y-

-Z-